# HEPATOCELLULAR CARCINOMA – BASIC RESEARCH

Edited by **Wan-Yee Lau**

**Hepatocellular Carcinoma – Basic Research**
Edited by Wan-Yee Lau

**Published by InTech**
Janeza Trdine 9, 51000 Rijeka, Croatia



**Publishing Process Manager** Vedran Greblo

**Technical Editor** Teodora Smiljanic

**Cover Designer** InTech Design Team

Additional hard copies can be obtained from orders@intechopen.com

Hepatocellular Carcinoma – Basic Research, Edited by Wan-Yee Lau
p. cm.
ISBN 978-953-51-0023-2

For EU product safety concerns:
IN TECH d.o.o., Prolaz Marije Krucifikse Kozulić 3, 51000 Rijeka, Croatia,
info@intechopen.com or visit our website at intechopen.com.

# Meet the editor

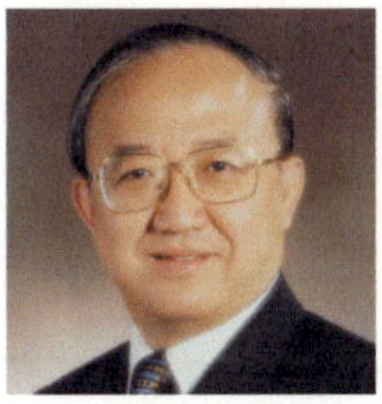

Professor Lau is currently Professor of Surgery, Faculty of Medicine and Master of Lee Woo Sing College at The Chinese University of Hong Kong. He is active both at the international and local surgical scene and holds a number of key positions in government and professional organizations. He is an editorial board member of 29 national and international journals, reviewer of 19 international journals. He is President of the International Hepato-Pancreato-Biliary Association for 2002-2004 and President of Asian-Pacific Hepato-Pancreato-Biliary Association for 2009-2011. He was elected as an academician of the Chinese Academy of Sciences, and was awarded Honorary FRACS in 2003. He has won many scholarships and awards. He is honorary/visiting professor to 29 universities/hospitals in countries around the world. He has published over 380 peer-reviewed papers in international journals, 55 papers in Chinese journals, 90 books/chapters, 3 monographs, 50 reviews/editorials/letters to editor and over 270 abstracts. He has been invited to deliver over 200 lectures to national/international societies.

# Contents

**Preface XI**

**Part 1 Biomarker / Therapeutic Target 1**

Chapter 1 **LAPTM4B: A Novel Diagnostic Biomarker and Therapeutic Target for Hepatocellular Carcinoma 3**
Rou Li Zhou

Chapter 2 **Novel Therapeutic Targets for Hepatocellular Carcinoma Treatment 35**
Yangchao Chen and Chi Han Li

Chapter 3 **Clinical Significance of Serum Ornithine Carbamoyltransferase in Liver Diseases – Is the Ratio of OCT/ALT a New Tumor Marker? 61**
Katsutoshi Tokushige, Etsuko Hashimoto, Noriko Matsushita, Nobuyuki Torii, Makiko Taniai, Keiko Shiratori and Hiroshi Maruyama

Chapter 4 **New Molecular Biomarkers Candidates for the Development of Multiparametric Platforms for Hepatocellular Carcinoma Diagnosis, Prognosis and Personalised Therapy 73**
Annalucia Serafino and Pasquale Pierimarchi

**Part 2 Carcinogenesis / Invasion / Metastasis 101**

Chapter 5 **Modulation of Cell Proliferation Pathways by the Hepatitis B Virus X Protein: A Potential Contributor to the Development of Hepatocellular Carcinoma 103**
Jessica C. Casciano, Sumedha Bagga, Bei Yang and Michael J. Bouchard

Chapter 6 **Vascular Adhesion Protein-1 and Hepatocellular Cancer 153**
Ozgur Kemik, Ahu Sarbay Kemik and A. Cumhur Dulger

Chapter 7 **Tissue Factor Pathway Inhibitor-2 Inhibits the Growth and Invasion of Hepatocellular Carcinoma Cells and is Inactivated in Human Hepatocellular Carcinoma 161**
Yong Xu, Xiaolin Qin, Jinjing Zhou, Zhiguang Tu, Xiao Bi, Wuxian Li, Xiaoqing Fan and Yi Zhang

Chapter 8 **Proteoglycans in Chronic Liver Disease and Hepatocellular Carcinoma: An Update 171**
Péter Tátrai and Ilona Kovalszky

Chapter 9 **Chemically Induced Hepatocellular Carcinoma and Stages of Development with Biochemical and Genetic Modulation: A Special Reference to Insulin-Like-Growth Factor II and Raf Gene Signaling 201**
Biswajit Mukherjee, Miltu Kumar Ghosh and Chowdhury Mobaswar Hossain

Chapter 10 **Hepatocellular Carcinoma: Insights from the Centrosome Abnormalities 219**
Ying Chen and Qingzhong Kong

Chapter 11 **Cytoplasmic Connexin32 and Self-Renewal of Cancer Stem Cells: Implication in Metastasis 235**
Yasufumi Omori, Yohei Kawasaki, Qingchang Li, Toshiaki Yoshioka, Yohei Yamamoto and Katsuhiko Enomoto

Chapter 12 **The Involvement of the ERK-Hypoxia-Angiogenesis Signaling Axis and HIF-1 in Hepatocellular Carcinoma 253**
Ilias Mylonis and George Simos

Chapter 13 **Gap Junction Intercellular Communication and Connexin Expression Profile in Normal Liver Cells and Hepatocarcinoma 275**
Glaucia M. Machado-Santelli and Marisa Ionta

Chapter 14 **Mechanisms of HBx Mediated Liver Cancer: Multiple Pathways and Opportunities 287**
Mark A. Feitelson, Alla Arzumanyan, Tiffany Friedman, N. Lale Tufan, Zhaorui Lian, Marcia M. Clayton, Joyce Kang, Helena M. G. P. V. Reis, Jingbo Pan, Jie Liu, Patrick Arbuthnot and Michael Kew

Chapter 15 **Molecular Mechanism of DNA Damage Response Pathway During Hepatic Carcinogenesis 313**
Yasunobu Matsuda and Toshifumi Wakai

**Part 3 Detection / Prevention / Prevalence 325**

Chapter 16 **Hepatocellular Carcinoma: Methods of Circulating Tumor Cells (CTC) Measurements 327**
Natalia Olaya and Franck Chiappini

Chapter 17 **Use of a Human–Derived Liver Cell Line for the Detection of Protective Effect of Dietary Antioxidants Against Food Mutagens 357**
Paloma Morales and A.I. Haza

Chapter 18 **Reviews on the Epidemiology, Quality of Life, and Management of Chronic Hepatitis B (CHB) 373**
Elegance T.P. Lam and Cindy L.K. Lam

# Preface

Hepatocellular Carcinoma represents a leading cause of cancer death and a major health problem in developing countries. It has also become increasingly important with the increase in hepatitis C infection in developed countries.

Knowledge of hepatocellular carcinoma has progressed rapidly. This book is a compendium of papers written by experts to present the most up-to-date knowledge of hepatocellular carcinoma. We have decided to divide this book on Hepatocellular Carcinoma into two books because of the overwhelming number of excellent book chapters we received from scientists and clinicians from all parts of the world:- Hepatocellular Carcinoma – Basic Research, and Hepatocellular Carcinoma – Clinical Research.

Hepatocellular Carcinoma – Basic Research is divided into three sections: (I) Biomarkers / Therapeutic Target; (II) Carcinogenesis / Invasion / Metastasis; and (III) Detection / Prevention / Prevalence. There are 18 chapters in this book.

This book is an important contribution to the field of hepatocellular carcinoma with an emphasis on basic research. The intended readers of this book are scientists and clinicians who are interested in research on hepatocellular carcinoma. Epidemiologists, pathologists, hospital administrators and drug manufacturers will also find this book useful.

**Dr. Wan-Yee Lau**
Department of Surgery, The Chinese University of Hong Kong,
Prince of Wales Hospital, Hong Kong SAR,
China

# Part 1

## Biomarker / Therapeutic Target

# LAPTM4B: A Novel Diagnostic Biomarker and Therapeutic Target for Hepatocellular Carcinoma

Rou Li Zhou
*School of Basic Medical Sciences, Peking University*
*China*

## 1. Introduction

The carcinogenesis and progression of hepatocellular carcinoma (HCC) are complicated processes which evolve through distinct stages associated with cumulative genomic alterations, which result in deregulation of proliferation, metastasis and recurrence, leading to poor prognosis. Despite the fact many new therapeutic and diagnostic strategies for cancer have been developed in recent years, the cure rate for HCC has not satisfactorily improved and biomarkers currently used for HCC diagnosis are not satisfactory in either their specificity or sensitivity.

More than one thousand cancer-associated genes and proteins have been identified, but the pathogenesis of hepatocellular carcinoma is still incompletely understood. Identifying the as yet unknown pivotal genes and proteins will be critical for early diagnosis, effective monitoring and novel therapies for this highly aggressive cancer. In previous work we cloned and identified a novel HCC-associated gene (lysosomal protein transmembrane 4 beta, *LAPTM4B*). Its complementary mRNA is highly expressed in the vast majority of HCC samples as compared with paired noncancerous liver from the same patient (PNL), fetal liver, and normal liver (Shao et al., 2003). Over our past decade studies have demonstrated that the *LAPTM4B* gene and the LAPTM4B-35 protein which it encodes would be pivotal diagnostic biomarkers and therapeutic targets for hepatocellular carcinoma.

## 2. *LAPTM4B*: A novel gene associated with hepatocellular carcinoma

### 2.1 Identification and cloning of the *LAPTM4B* gene

To search for genes involved in deregulation of proliferation and aberrant differentiation for hepatocellular carcinoma, fluorescent-differential display was performed using human liver tissues, including adult liver, fetal liver, HCC and its paired samples of noncancerous liver from the same patient (paired noncancerous liver). A cDNA fragment, which was not a part of any known gene, was found from 110 differential display fragments obtained. This cDNA fragment was highly expressed in HCC, significantly expressed in fetal liver and the paired noncancerous liver, but showed very low expression in normal adult liver (JJ. Liu et al., 2000). Cloning the full length cDNA (NM_018407, ID=55353, Figure 1) harboring this fragment was performed by Expressed Sequence Tag (EST) splicing, 5′ rapid amplification of cDNA ends (FACE) and reverse transcription-polymerase chain reaction (RT–PCR). Based on the lysosome-targeting signal (YXXΦ) found on the encoded protein this gene was originally designated by the HUGO Gene Nomenclature Committee as "lysosomal-associated protein transmembrane 4 beta" (*LAPTM4B)* and this designation was then revised as "lysosomal protein transmembrane 4 beta" (*LAPTM4B)*. Importantly, it should be emphasized that reverse-transcription from total RNA to synthesize this cDNA must be conducted at 65° C using the ThermoScript RT-PCR Systems (Gibco-BRL) as there is very high content of GC at the 5′ terminus (Shao et al., 2003), otherwise full length LAPTM4B cDNA cannot be obtained. BLAST program analysis shows that the *LAPTM4B* gene maps to chromosome 8q22.1, spanning at least 50 kb composed of seven exons separated by six introns, and contains a 951bp open reading frame (ORF). LAPTM4B mRNA is approximately 2.16 kb in length and which is consistent with the size of the mRNA observed in Northern blots. Two polyadenylation signal sites, AATAAA and AATTAAA are present at the 3′ UTR (Figure 1). The former polyadenylation site (AATAAA) may result in another 1.42 kb mRNA variant (Shao et al., 2003).

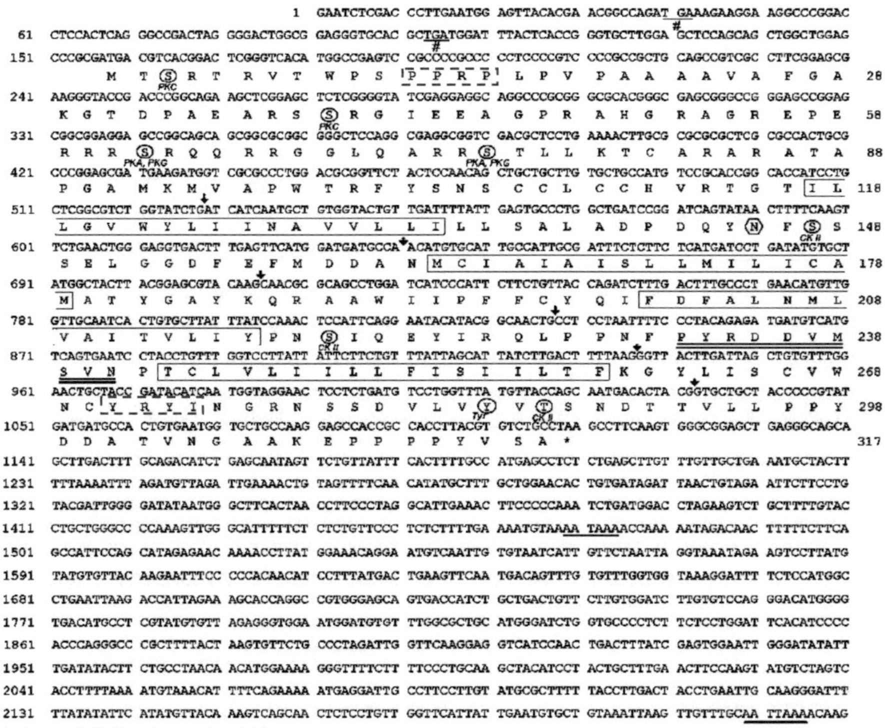

Fig. 1. The nucleotide sequence of LAPTM4B cDNA and the deduced amino-acid sequence. The sequence numbers of the first nucleotide (left) and the final amino acid (right) in each row is indicated, respectively. Exon divisions are indicated by ▼. The polyadenylation consensus sequences (AATAAA, AATTAAA) are underlined. Transmembrane regions are boxed. The putative N-glycosylation site is marked with a ring of hexagon; potential phosphorylation sites are circled, with the corresponding kinases indicated in italic characters. Stop codon or inframe stop codons are indicated as # or *. The PPRP and YXXΦ motifs are boxed with red line of dashes. (Shao et al., 2003)

### 2.2 Bioinformatics analysis of LAPTM4B proteins

Bioinformatics shows that the full-length cDNA sequence of LAPTM4B contains two translational initiation codons (ATG) separated by an interval of 273 bp and therefore, encodes two protein isoforms with apparent molecular weights of 35 kDa containing 317 amino acid residues and 24 kDa containing 226 amino acid residues, which are designated LAPTM4B-35 and LAPTM4B-24. LAPTM4B-35 has a pI at 9.07 due to its high content of arginine residues, while LAPTM4B-24 has a pI at 4.65 resulting from a high content of acidic amino acid residues. Computer analysis shows that LAPTM4B is an integral membrane glycoprotein (Figure 2), with four transmembrane regions, two extracellular domains (EC1 and EC2), one small intracellular loop, together with one N-terminal and one C-terminal tail which reside in the cytoplasm. One potential N-glycosylation site is present in the EC1 domain and several O-glycosylation sites may also be present. LAPTM4B-35 contains six putative intracytoplasmic phosphorylation sites, including one tyrosine phosphorylation site at Try 285, and four N-myristylation sites. Compared to LAPTM4B-24, LAPTM4B-35 has an extra 91 amino acid sequence in its N-terminus that harbors a proline-rich domain, which serves as the binding site of the SH3 domain in some signaling molecules. A conserved YXXɸ (Y represents tyrosine, ɸ represents a large hydrophobic amino acid, X represents any amino acid) motif in the C-terminal tail is believed to function as a signal for targeting to lysosomal membranes and sorting.

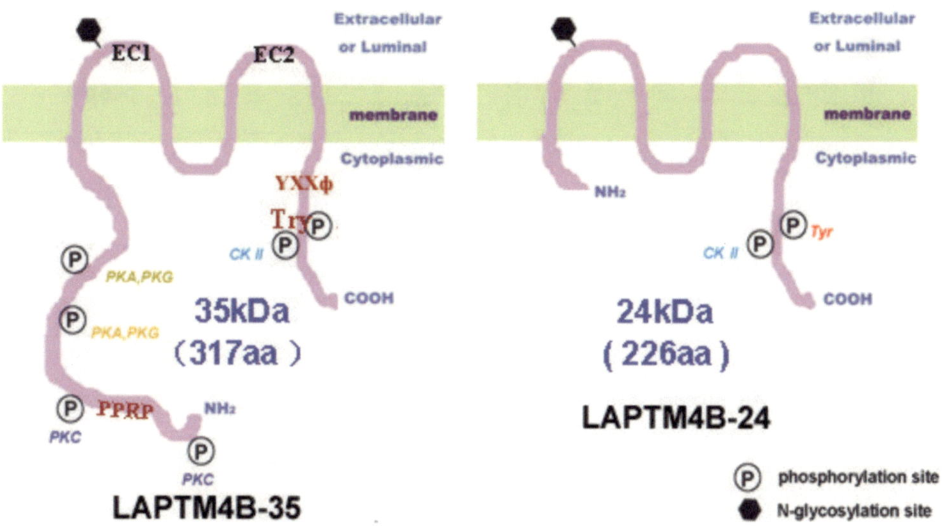


Fig. 2. Topology of LAPTM4B-35 (left) and LAPTM4B-24 (right) proteins

### 2.3 Expression of LAPTM4B mRNA and protein in normal tissues and cancer tissues

Expression of LAPTM4B mRNA has been evaluated by Northern blot and RT-PCR, and found to be widely expressed in human tissues. Its expression is highest in the heart, skeletal muscle and uterus, and more high in testis and ovary. Expression is moderate in the kidney and pancreas, and low in the liver, spleen and thymus, but is lowest in the lung and peripheral leukocytes (Figure 3a) (Shao et al., 2003; Kasper et al., 2005). High expression is also seen in fetal heart, kidney and spleen (Figure 3b). Expression of LAPTM4B mRNA in HCC has been confirmed by Northern blot (Figure 4a), RT-PCR and hybridization in situ (Figure 4b). The frequency of LAPTM4B mRNA over-expression as demonstrated by Northern blot is as high as 87.3% (Shao et al., 2003); Expression of LAPTM4B-35 and LAPTM4B-24 proteins in tissues have been demonstrated by Western blot and immunohistochemistry (IHC). As shown by Western blot (Figure 5a), LAPTM4B-35 is much more abundant than LAPTM4B-24 in the liver and HCC. In other words, over-expression of LAPTM4B-35 but not LAPTM4B-24 presents in HCC, and the ratio of LAPTM4B-35 to LAPTM4B-24 is thus markedly increased in HCC (X. Liu et al., 2004). The frequency of LAPTM4B-35 up-regulation is also extremely high (Figure 5b), and it has been shown that T/N>1.5 [T=tumor)/N =paired non-cancerous liver] is found in 87.7% (57/65) of HCC, T/N>2 in 76.9% (50/65) of HCC and T/N>4 in 61.5% (40/65) of HCC (Yang et al., 2010a). More importantly, the levels of LAPTM4B-35 in HCC tissues are significantly associated with pathological grades, TNM staging, portal vein invasion and recurrence, but not with age, gender, viral status, tumor size and serum AFP levels (Table 1, Yang et al., 2010a). Moreover, LAPTM4B mRNA and LAPTM4B-35 over-expression also occurs in a wide range of hepatocellular carcinoma- and other cancer-derived cell lines (Shao et al., 2003; XR. Liu et al., 2004).

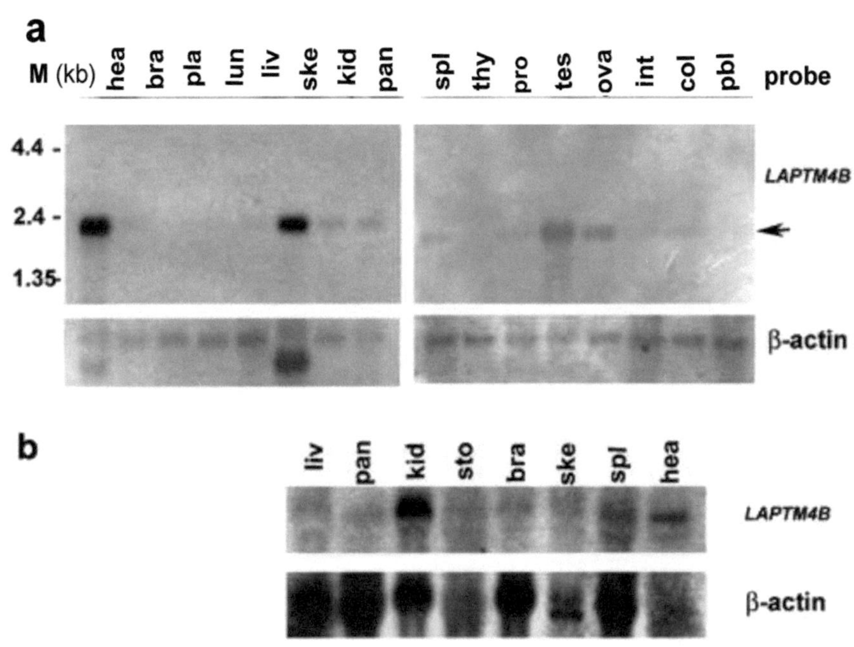


Fig. 3. *LAPTM4B* mRNA expression in normal human tissues analyzed by Northern blot with a *LAPTM4B* prob (corresponding to nt 1876-2171 on NM_018407).
(a) Expression of LAPTM4B mRNA in adult human tissues (b) Expression of LAPTM4B mRNA in fetal human tissues (Shao et al., 2003)

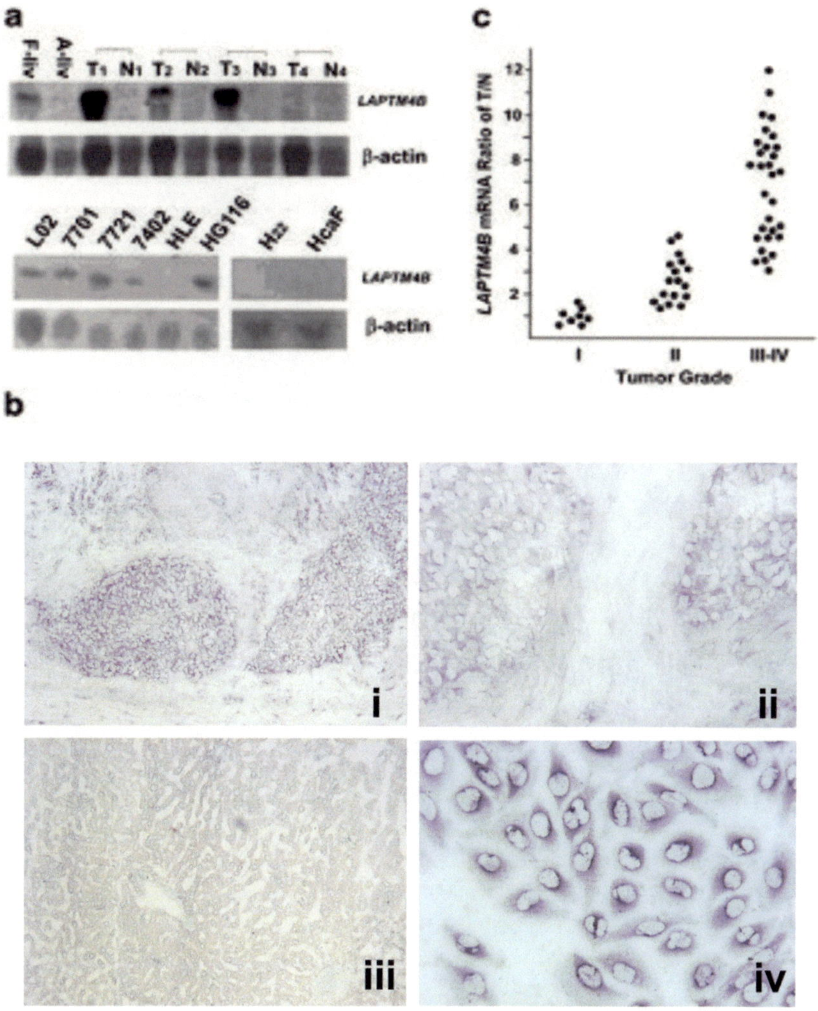


Fig. 4. LAPTM4B mRNA expression in hepatocellular carcinomas (HCCs) tissues and HCC-derived cell lines analyzed by Northern blot with a LAPTM4B prob (corresponding to nt 1876-2171 on NM_018407). (a) Northern blot analysis of LAPTM4B. Upper panel: HCC tissues (T), paired noncancerous liver tissues (N), fetal and adult normal liver tissues (F- & A-liv); Lower panel: The human liver- and HCC-derived cell lines, and mouse HCC-derived cell lines. (b) Hybridization in situ was performed on tissue sections. LAPTM4B mRNA expressions in HCC tissue (i, ii), paired noncancerous tissue (iii), and BEL7402 cells (iv). Positive LAPTM4B mRNA expression was preferentially in hepatic cancerous cells as indicated by blue-purple staining. Original magnification, 40 (i, iii) or 100 (ii, iv). (c) Positive correlation between LAPTM4B mRNA levels and tumor grades. Each spot in the figure represents the ratio of tumor vs. paired noncancerous liver tissue (T/N) of the LAPTM4B mRNA expression evaluated by Northern blot. These spots derived from 55 HCC patients. (Shao et al., 2003)

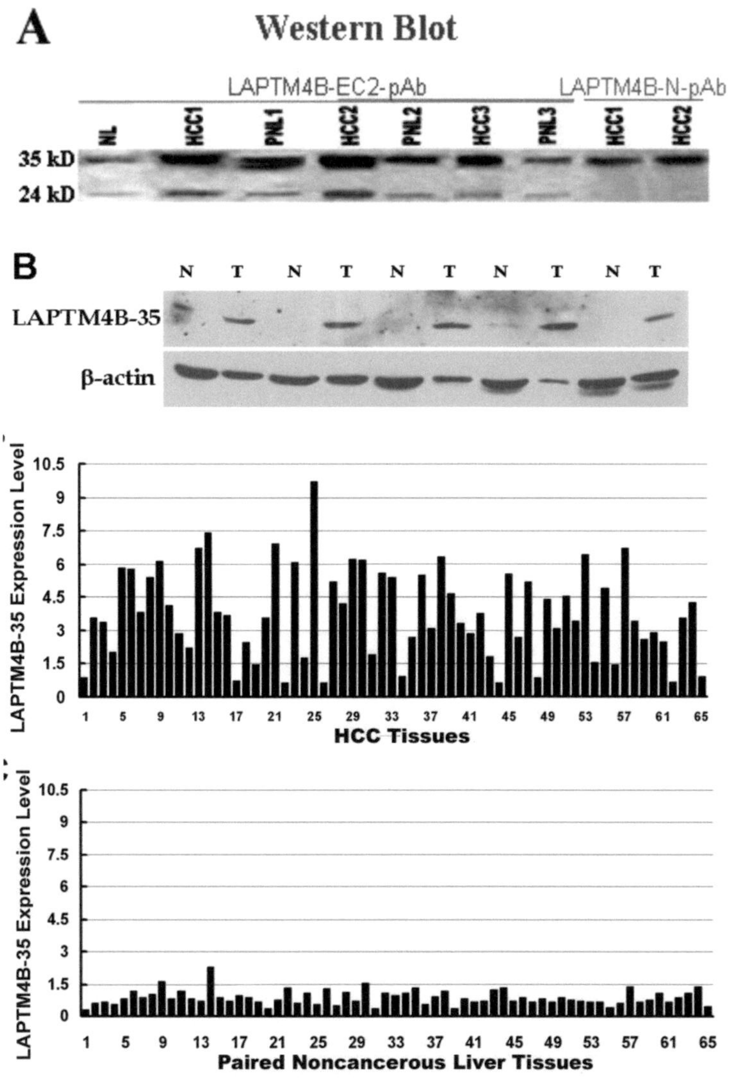


Fig. 5. Expression of LAPTM4B-35 and LAPTM4B-24 protein identified by Western blot in HCCs and paired noncancerous liver tissues (PNL) from the same one patient.
(a) Expression of LAPTM4B-35 and LAPTM4B-24 was evaluated by Western blot with an anti-LAPTM4B-EC2 pAb, which reacts with both LAPTM4B-35 and LAPTM4B-24, and anti-LAPTM4B-N-pAb, which reacts with merely LAPTM4B-35. It is shown that LAPTM4B-35 is much more abundant than LAPTM4B-24 in the normal liver (NL) and HCC. (b) Expression of LAPTM4B-35 detected with Anti-LAPTM4B-N-10 pAb. The upper panel shows the expression of LAPTM4B-35 in HCC (T) and paired noncancerous liver tissues (N) tissues. Densitometry was normalized with β-actin. The middle panel shows the levels of LAPTM4B-35 in HCC tissues derived from 65 patients. The lower panel shows the levels of LAPTM4B-35 in the paired noncancerous liver tissues derived from the same 65 patients. (Yang et al., 2010a).

| Variables | Patients (n) | LAPTM4B-35 expression | | | $P^a$ |
|---|---|---|---|---|---|
| | | Low | Middle | High | |
| All cases | 65 | 15 | 30 | 20 | |
| Gender | | | | | 0.434 |
| Male | 53 | 11 | 24 | 18 | |
| Female | 12 | 4 | 6 | 2 | |
| Age (years) | | | | | 0.544 |
| <60 | 42 | 8 | 21 | 13 | |
| ≥60 | 23 | 7 | 9 | 7 | |
| Cirrhosis | | | | | 0.013 |
| Yes | 44 | 6 | 25 | 13 | |
| No | 21 | 9 | 5 | 7 | |
| Viral status | | | | | 0.766 |
| Hepatitis virus B | 46 | 9 | 23 | 14 | |
| Hepatitis virus C | 12 | 4 | 5 | 3 | |
| Both hepatitis virus B and C | 2 | 0 | 1 | 1 | |
| Non-B, Non-C | 5 | 2 | 1 | 2 | |
| Tumor size | | | | | 0.421 |
| <5 cm | 34 | 10 | 15 | 9 | |
| ≥5 cm | 31 | 5 | 15 | 11 | |
| Invasive tumor | | | | | <0.001 |
| Yes | 17 | 0 | 4 | 13 | |
| No | 48 | 15 | 26 | 7 | |
| Histopathological differentiation | | | | | <0.01[b] |
| Well Differentiation (WD) | 18 | 6 | 8 | 4 | |
| Middle Differentiation (MD) | 24 | 7 | 11 | 6 | |
| Poor Differentiation (PD) | 23 | 2* | 11 | 10* | |
| Serum AFP level | | | | | 0.517 |
| <25 ng/ml | 32 | 6 | 17 | 9 | |
| ≥25 ng/ml | 33 | 9 | 13 | 11 | |
| TNM stage | | | | | <0.001 |
| I | 16 | 11 | 3 | 2 | |
| II | 21 | 2 | 14 | 5 | |
| III−IV | 28 | 2 | 13 | 13 | |

*a*: Chi-square test;
*b*: p<0.01: Low expression vs. High expression for PD group.

Table 1. Relationship between LAPTM4B-35 expression and Clinical-pathological features of HCC (Yang et al., 2010a)

In addition, over-expressions of LAPTM4B mRNA and LAPTM4B-35 protein have also been found in other solid cancers. Kasper et al. (2005) reported that LAPTM4B mRNA tested by Northern Blot is over-expressed in 88% of lung cancer, 50.9% of breast cancers, 67% of colon cancers, 68% of uterus cancers, and 37% of gastric cancers. Peng et al. (2005) reported that LAPTM4B-35 protein as evaluated by immuno-histochemistry (IHC) is highly expressed in lung cancer, stomach cancer, colon cancer and breast cancer. Subsequently, the frequency of over-expression of LAPTM4B-35 in more cases of various cancers was determined, and was found in 76 % of gallbladder cancers (Zhou et al., 2007), 72 % of cholangiocarcinomas (Zhou et al.,. 2008), 63.5% of ovarian cancers (Yang et al., 2008; Yin et al., 2010), 72.57% of cervical cancers (Meng et al., 2010a) and 70.91% of endometrial cancers (Meng, et al., 2010b). However, the mechanism for over-expression of LAPTM4B in HCC and other cancers has not as yet been completely elucidated. Mutation and demethylation of *LAPTM4B* gene has not been found. Nevertheless, it has been reported in a large number of articles that the chromosome 8q region harboring *LAPTM4B* gene is amplified as shown by fluorescence in situ hybridization (FISH) or gained as shown by comparative genomic hybridization (CGH) in both hepatoblastoma and hepatocellular carcinoma (Buendia et al., 2002; Longerichet al., 2011; Marchio et al., 1997). More precisely, it has been recently reported that chromosome 8q 22 where the *LAPTM4B* gene localizes is amplified or gained in breast cancer (Hu et al., 2009; Y. Li. et al., 2010). Therefore, gene amplification may be the cytogenetic basis of LAPTM4B over-expression. However, the genomic DNA copy number alterations of most genes in general do not appear to parallel corresponding transcriptional expression (Huang et al., 2006). It is reasonable to propose that transcriptional up-regulation by transcription factors and/or microRNAs may also contribute to LAPTM4B-35 over-expression in cancers. A more in-depth analysis will be required to clarify these points.

### 2.4 *LAPTM4B* alleles and their significance in susceptibility for hepatocarcinogenesis

Two alleles of the *LAPTM4B* gene have been identified in our laboratory and designated *LAPTM4B *1* and **2*. Allele **2* differs from allele **1* in that it contains an extra tandemly arranged 19-bp (gcttggagctccagcagct) sequence at the 5'UTR in the first exon. A PCR-based method was established for genotyping of this gene using the primers 5' GCCGACTAGGGGACTGGCGGA 3' and 5' CGAGAGCTCCGAGCTTCTGCC 3' to amplify the partial sequence of exon 1, and using genomic DNA as the template. To investigate the relationship between the allelic variants of *LAPTM4B* and the susceptibility to HCC or esophageal squamous cell carcinoma (ESC), patients with HCC or ESC, and two control groups of normal individuals from the corresponding regions were analyzed. Significant differences in the frequency of genotype *LAPTM4B*2/2* were found in patients with HCC (17.4%) as compared with the controls (10.2%) ($p<0.05$), indicating that individuals with the **2/*2* genotype are more susceptible to HCC than **1/*1* and **1/*2* individuals (Table 2). However, no difference was observed in the frequencies of *LAPTM4B* genotypes in patients with ESC as compared with corresponding controls. These results suggest that allele *2 may be associated specifically with susceptibility to HCC. In conclusion, our data suggest that *LAPTM4B*2/*2* is associated with susceptibility to HCC and the *LAPTM4B* genotype provides a new means for screening for people who are susceptible to primary hepatocellular carcinoma. This may be of importance for the assessment and prevention of developing hepatocellular carcinoma in high risk populations, in particular for the patients with liver cirrhosis of small liver nodule from HBV and HCV chronic infection (Shao et al., unpublished data). In addition, allele *2 has been found to be associated with increased risk of lung cancer (Deng et al., 2005), stomach cancer (Liu et al., 2007), cervical carcinoma (Meng et al., 2011) and colon cancer but not of rectal cancer (Cheng et al., 2008). These results indicate that *LAPTM4B* *2 is also a potential risk factor for the development of some solid cancers.

| | N (%) | | *P* value |
|---|---|---|---|
| | Controls (n=206) | HCC (n=184) | |
| LAPTM4B genotype | | | |
| *1/1 | 97 (47.1) | 77(41.8) | |
| *1/2 | 88 (42.7) | 75 (40.8) | |
| *2/2 | 21 (10.2) | 32 (17.4) | 0.038[a] |
| Allele frequency | | | |
| *1 | 0.68 | 0.62 | |
| *2 | 0.32 | 0.38 | |

[a]: when compared with the combined frequency of 1/1 and 1/2;
OR: 1.855, 95%CI: 1.027 - 3.348

Table 2. Distribution of *LAPTM4B* genotypes in HCC and Controls

### 2.5 LAPTM family

In addition to LAPTM4B, LAPTM4A (Hogue et al., 1996) and LAPTM5 (Adra et al., 1996) are also members of lysosome-associated protein transmembrane (LAPTM) family. LAPTM4A (27kDa) shows a 46% homology with LAPTM4B in amino acid sequences. In comparison with LAPTM4B-35 containing 317 amino acid residues, LAPTM4A containing 233 amino acid residues and LAPTM5 containing 262 amino acid residues both are of the N-terminus-truncated molecules of LAPTM family. The three members in the LAPTM family all localize at late endosomes and lysosomes, and play an important role in lysosomal function, including transporting structurally unrelated amphiphilic molecules between cytosol and lysosomes, and are involved in autophagocytosis. Moreover, LAPTM4B, LAPTM4A and LAPTM5 interact and co-localize with mucolipin 1, which is a lysosomal ion channel that belongs to the transient receptor potential (TRP) superfamily and their loss-of-function mutations result in mucolipidosis type IV (MLIV), a lysosomal storage disorder characterized by severe mental and psychomotor retardation (Vergarajauregui et al., 2011). LAPTM4A is involved in the subcellular compartmentalization of diverse hydrophobic small molecules and contributes to the inherent drug sensitivity or resistance of the mammalian cell (Hogue et al., 1999). The *LAPTM5* gene maps to chromosome 1p34 and is expressed mainly in hematopoietic cells and immune cells (Adra et al., 1996). LAPTM5 protein physically interacts with the B cell receptor (BCR) complex and promotes its degradation in the lysosomal compartment in mouse B cells, and thus negatively regulates cell surface BCR levels and B cell activation (Ouchida, 2010). The expression of LAPTM5 gene is usually down-regulated through DNA methylation in a neuroblastoma cell-specific manner, while over-expression of this gene may induce spontaneous regression of neuroblastomas. It is believed that caspase-independent lysosomal cell death due to lysosomal destabilization resulted from LAPTM5 up-regulation is closely associated with the spontaneous regression (Inoue et al., 2009).

Notably, LAPTM family shows similarity in some functional characteristics to "tetraspanin" family, but difference in the structural characteristics, including lacking some conserved amino acid residues and having a smaller EC2 domain. (Maecker et al., 1997; Martin, 2005).

Evolutionarily, *LAPTM* is an ancient and conserved gene family in mammalian species as well as in lower eukaryotic organisms, including zebrafish (Danio rerio) and Drosophila. The phylogenic tree shown in Figure 6 is constructed according to multiple sequence alignment results. It shows that *LAPTM4B* and the other two genes in the *LAPTM* family, *LAPTM4A* and *LAPTM5*, are distributed in clusters. Human *LAPTM4B* shows the closest similarity to Bos Taurus, and also shows some similarity to its zebrafish homolog. In addition, *LAPTM4B* is more related to *LAPTM4A* than *LAPTM5*.

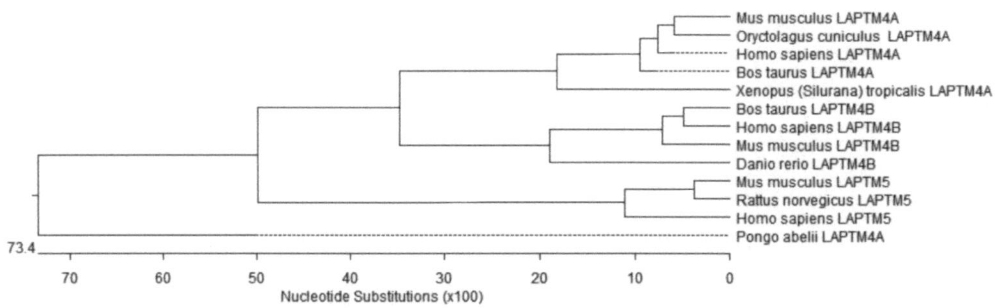


Fig. 6. The evolutionary lineage tree for LAPTM family (This figure was prepared by Shuang Shi)

## 3. Functions of *LAPTM4B*-encoding proteins and the mechanisms thereof

Functional studies of *LAPTM4B*-encoding proteins and the mechanisms thereof have been performed via transgenic and gene knockdown techniques. *LAPTM4B* cDNA is introduced into plasmids with or without a FLAG tag, or into an E1/E3-deleted replication-deficient adenovirus type 5 (Ad5) vector. The LAPTM4B-35 expressing plasmids and cells are all designated in our publications as "AF" if they have a FLAG tag or as "AE" if they do not have a FLAG tag. Similarly, LAPTM4B-24 expressing plasmids and cells are designated as "BF" or "BE". LAPTM4B-35 knockdown is performed by transfection of shRNA-expressing plasmids (Yang et al., 2010c). These functional studies of LAPTM4B-35 and LAPTM4B-24 have determined that these two isoforms of LAPTM4B proteins have antagonistic functions, namely up-regulation of LAPTM4B-35 and LAPTM4B-24 respectively promotes and suppresses hepatocarcinogenesis and metastasis.

### 3.1 Over-expression of LAPTM4B-35 promotes carcinogenesis and metastasis of hepatocellular carcinoma

The effect of LAPTM4B over-expression on carcinogenesis was first explored using mouse NIH3T3 fibroblast cell line (He et al., 2003). Two cell lines stably over-expressing both LAPTM4B mRNA and LAPTM4B-35 were obtained from transfection of *LAPTM4B* cDNA integrated in plasmids. The LAPTM4B-35 over-expressing NIH3T3-AE cells generated a palpable mass by day 7 in all sites of inoculation in NIH3T3 mice, while in the control groups inoculated with NIH3T3-Mock cells or NIH3T3 parent cells, no tumor appeared within an 80 day period following inoculation. Half of the tumor masses generated from LAPTM4B-overexpressing NIH3T3-AE cells showed growth and were histochemically identified as malignant fibrosarcoma; the other half of these masses regressed and were finally identified as liquid lymphoid tissue. Further, the L02 cell line which originated from normal human liver was then used to generate a LAPTM4B-35 over-expressing cell model by infection with replication deficient adenovirus Ad-AE containing LAPTM4B-35 full length cDNA (Lily et al., 2011). Inoculation of LAPTM4B-35 over-expressing L02-AE cells can result in rapidly growing carcinoma xenografts in 100% (6/6) of inoculated sites in the left axilla of nude mice (Figure 7a and 7b) and shorten their live span (Figure 7d) , as

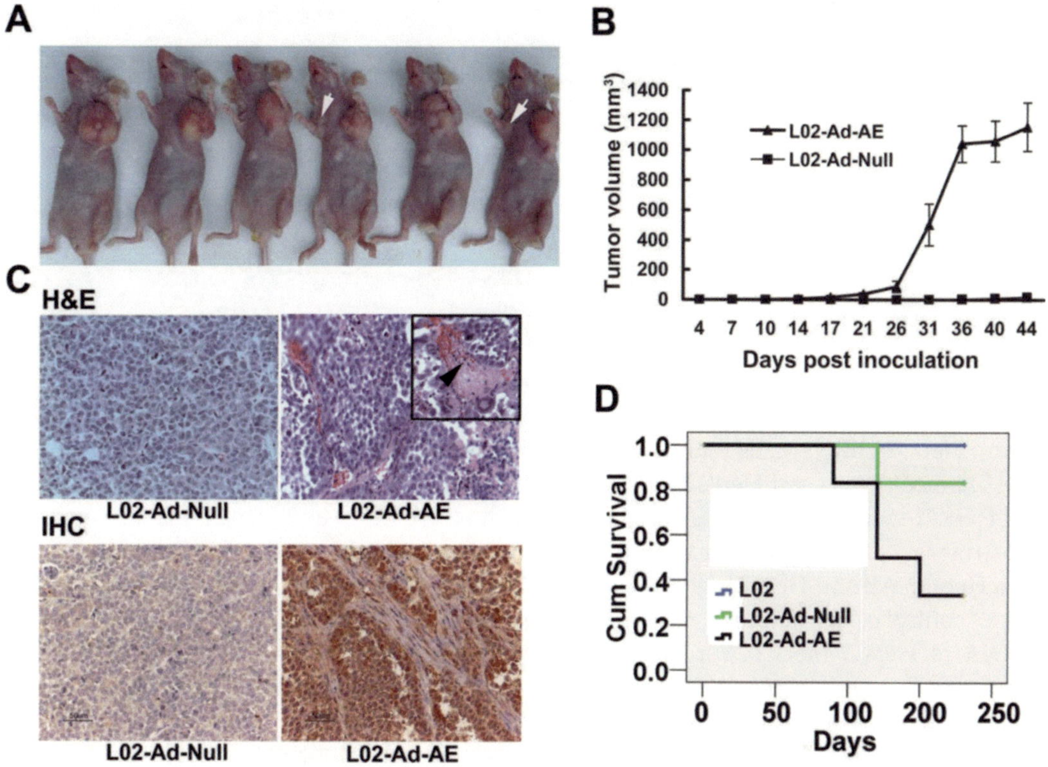


Fig. 7. Upregulation of LAPTM4B-35 promotes tumorigenesis in nude mice. (a) Xenograft tumors formed from L02-Ad-AE cells, in which LAPTM4B-35 is overexpressing, and tumors formed from L02-Ad-Null cells which are indicated by white arrows. (b) Tumor growth curves from L02-Ad-AE cells and L02-Ad-Null cells. (c) Top panel: H&E staining of tumor formed from L02-Ad-Null cells (left) and L02-Ad-AE cells (right). Black arrows indicate the cancer cells in blood vessel. Bottom panel: immunohistochemical evaluation of LAPTM4B-35 expression in xenografts. Tumors derived from L02-Ad-AE cells showed high expression of LAPTM4B-35 (right), but tumors derived from L02-Ad-Null cells showed very low expression of LAPTM4B-35 (left). An anti-LAPTM4B-N10 pAb, which specifically reacts with LAPTM4B-35, was used for IHC (original magnification 200X). (d) Kaplan–Meier survival curves plotted with SPSS 16.0 (n=6). LAPTM4B-35 up-regulation shortened the live span of mice challenged with L02-Ad-AE cells, as compared to the control group infected by Ad-null, the empty Ad vectors. P=0.049 L02-Ad-AE versus L02-Ad-Null. (Lily et al., 2011).

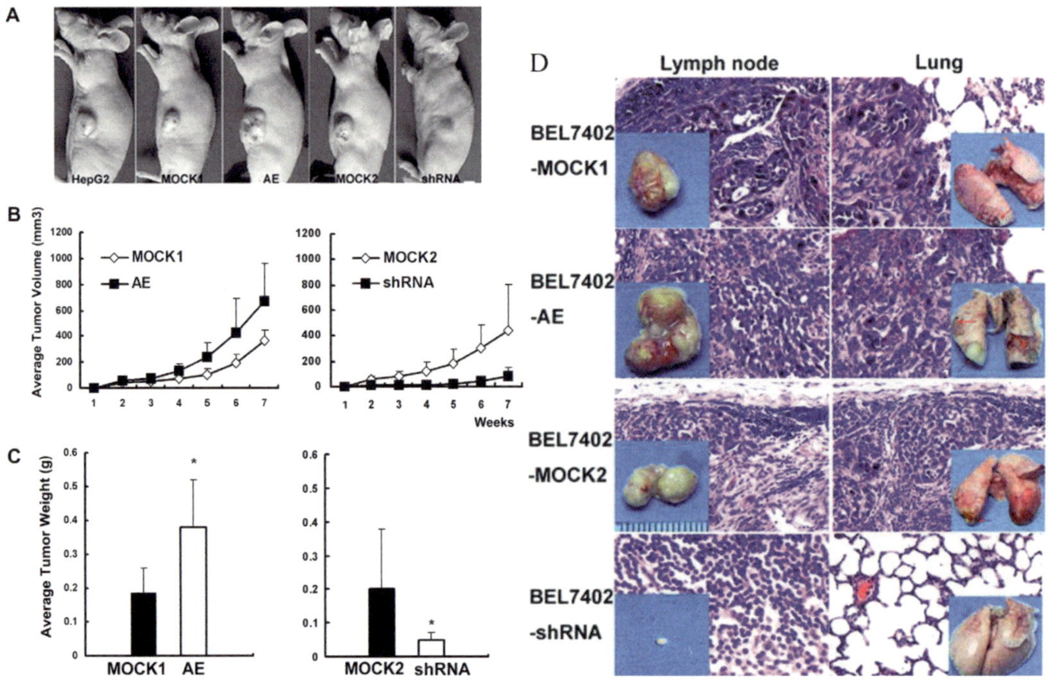


Fig. 8. LAPTM4B-35 promotes tumor growth and metastasis in nude mice. (a) Representative xenograft tumors formed from HepG2-AE cells over-expressing LAPTM4B-35 and HepG2-shRNA cells with LAPTM4B-35 knockdown, and corresponding controls (HepG2-mock1 cells and HepG2-mock2 cells), (b) Tumor growth curves from HepG2-AE and HepG2-mock1 control cells (left), and from HepG2-shRNA and HepG2-mock2 control cells (right). (c) Average tumor weight in nude mice sacrificed 7 weeks after inoculation with HepG2-AE and HepG2-mock1 control cells (left), and with HepG2-shRNA and HepG2-mock2 control cells (right). n = 6. ($P < 0.001$: HepG2-AE vs. HepG2-mock1 and HepG2-shRNA vs. HepG2-mock2). For all data the mean and standard deviation represent the average of three independent experiments. (d) LAPTM4B-35 promotes tumor metastasis in nude mice: Macroscopic photos and microscopic photos shown by H&E staining of tumor metastases in lymph nodes and lungs of mice subcutaneously inoculated with BEL7402-AE cells (upper panels), BEL7402–shRNA cells (lower panels) or corresponding control cells. (Yang et al., 2010c)

compared to the control group infected by Ad-null, in which very small tumors were formed in the right axilla of nude mice (Figure 7a as indicated by the white arrows). The xenografts, which were generated from L02-AE cells, expressed high levels of LAPTM4B-35 as shown by immunohistochemistry (Figure 7c bottom right panel), and these tumors were very well vascularized and tumor blood vessels showed invasion of cancer cells by H&E staining (Figure 7c top right panel). These findings demonstrated that LAPTM4b-35 over-expressing liver cells have potential for hepatocarcinogenesis and metastasis. In addition, the HepG2 cell line which originated from human hepatoblastoma and the BEL7402 cell line which originated from human hepatocellular carcinoma were used for generating up-regulated and down-regulated cell models to study the effects of LAPTM4B-35 on tumor growth and metastasis (Yang et al., 2010c). The xenografts in nude mice originating from HepG2-AE and BEL7402-AE cells, in which LAPTM4B-35 has been up-regulated, grow significantly faster (Figure 8a, 8b and 8c left pannel) and with greater numbers of more widespread metastases in the lymph nodes and lungs than the control group transfected by Mock (empty) plasmids (Figure 8d upper panels). Conversely, the xenografts in nude mice originating from HepG2-RNAi and BEL7402-RNAi cells, in which endogenous LAPTM4B-35 has been knocked down, grow significantly slower (Figure 8a, 8b and 8c right panel). At the same time, metastases in the lymph nodes and lungs in the HepG2-shRNA and BEL7402-shRNA groups were also fewer and smaller than in the corresponding control groups (Figure 8d lower panels). Overall these experiments demonstrate that up-regulation of LAPTM4B-35 promotes HCC growth and metastasis, while down-regulation has an inhibitory effect.

### 3.2 Over-expression of LAPTM4B-35 induces deregulation of proliferation

Promotion and inhibition of proliferation by LAPTM4B-35 up-regulation and down-regulation respectively has been demonstrated conclusively using L02-AE, BEL7402-AE, HepG2-AE and HLE-AE cell lines, together with BEL7402-RNAi and GepG2-RNAi cells (L. Li et al,. 2011; XR. Liu et al., 2009; H.Yang et al., 2010c). Except the L02 cell line was originally derived from normal liver, the BEL7402, HepG2 and HLE cell lines were all originally derived from human HCCs. It is noteworthy that up-regulation of LAPTM4B-35 not only accelerates cell proliferation (Figure 9a, 9b and 9c), but also induces deregulation of proliferation, which is a characteristically neoplastic phenotype. HLE-AE, BEL7402-AE and HepG2-AE cells in which LAPTM4B-35 has been up-regulated, generate colonies which are significantly larger and greater in number; whereas HepG2-RNAi and BEL7402-RNAi cells in which the endogenous LAPTM4B-35 has been down-regulated produce markedly smaller and fewer colonies in soft agar (Figure 9d), respectively demonstrating enhancement and diminution of anchorage-independent growth which is a fundamental criterion for evaluation of proliferative deregulation in malignant transformation (XR.Liu et al., 2009; H.Yang et al., 2010). In addition, growth of HLE-AE cells is less dependent on exogenous growth factors derived from serum supplement as compared with control HLE-MOCK cells, representing auto-secretion of growth factor by LAPTM4B-35 overexpressing cells which is another criterion of proliferative deregulation and malignant transformation (XL.Liu et al., 2009).

Moreover, LAPTM4B-35 over-expression alters not only the proliferation-associated malignant cellular phenotype, but also the proliferation-regulatory proteins encoded by oncogenes and tumor suppressor genes (He et al., 2003; XR. Liu et al., 2009; H. Yang et al., 2010c). We have found that cell cycle-promoting proteins including cyclin D1, cyclin E and p-Rb are up-regulated in LAPTM4B-35 over-expressing HepG2-AE, BEL7402-AE and HLE-AE cells. At the same time, the transcription factors c-Myc, c-Fos and c-Jun that positively regulate expression of cyclins, are also significantly up-regulated. Conversely, the cell cycle-inhibiting proteins of cyclin-dependent kinase inhibitor (CKI) family, including p16, p21 and in particular p27 are markedly down-regulated in these LAPTM4B-35 over-expressing HCC cell lines. At the same time, knockdown of endogenous LAPTM4B-35 gives reverse effects (Figure 10). These studies serve to identify the molecular basis for deregulated malignant proliferation resulting from LAPTM4B-35 over-expression.

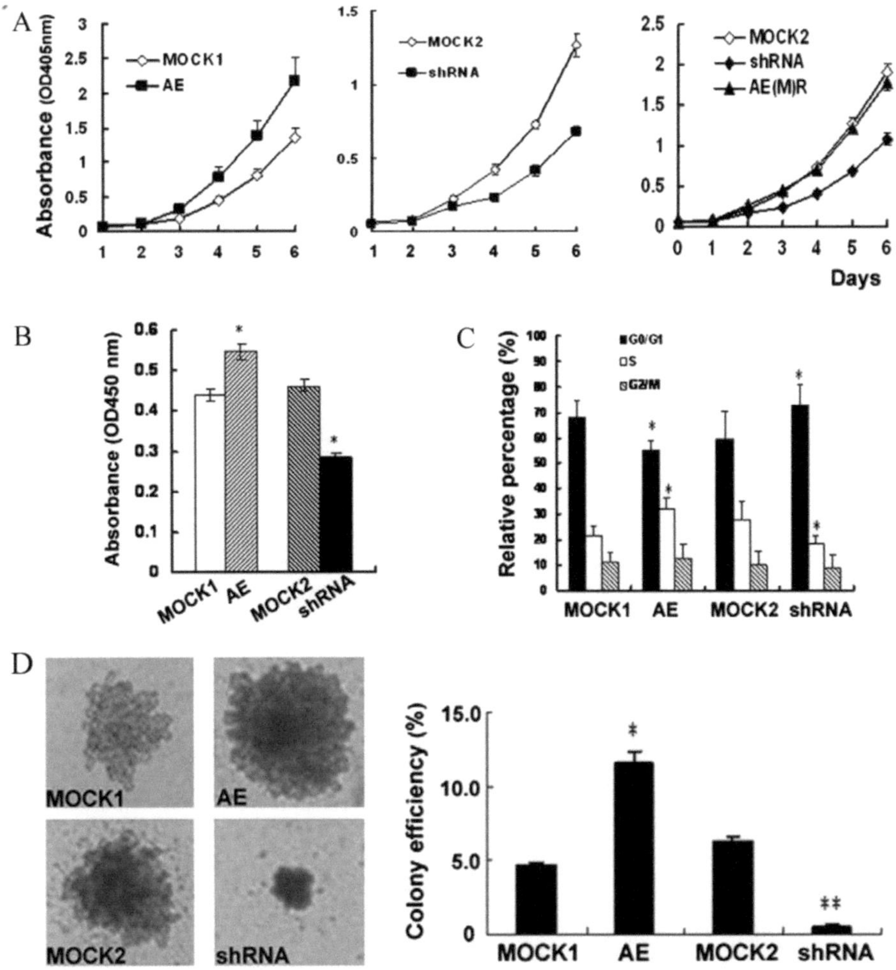


Fig. 9. Over-expression of LAPTM4B-35 promotes cell proliferation and induces deregulation of proliferation. (a) Growth curves determined by MTT assay. Left panel: overexpression of LAPTM4B-35 promotes rapid increase in cell viability/proliferation compared with the control. Middle panel: knockdown of LAPTM4B-35 inhibits increase in cell viability/proliferation as compared with the control. Right panel: restoration of LAPTM4B-35 expression in HepG2(M)R cells, in which the RNAi target was mutated, so that the siRNA produced from shRNA can not bind to the target mRNA, reverses inhibition of cell viability/proliferation resulting from knockdown of LAPTM4B-35. (b) DNA synthesis analyzed by BrdU incorporation assay. $P < 0.05$: HepG2-AE vs. HepG2-mock1, and HepG2-shRNA vs. HepG2-mock2. (c) Cell cycle analyzed by FACS. $P < 0.05$: HepG2-AE vs. HepG2-mock1, and HepG2-shRNA vs. HepG2-Mock2. (d) LAPTM4B-35 promotes colony formation in soft agar. Left panel: overexpression of LAPTM4B-35 promoted colony formation (upper); knockdown of endogenous LAPTM4B-35 inhibited colony formation (down). Right panel: a histogram showing colony numbers larger than 50 μm that were counted 4 weeks after seeding. *$P < 0.05$: HepG2-AE vs. HepG2-mock1; **$P < 0.001$: HepG2-shRNA vs. HepG2-mock2. (H. Yang et al., 2010c)

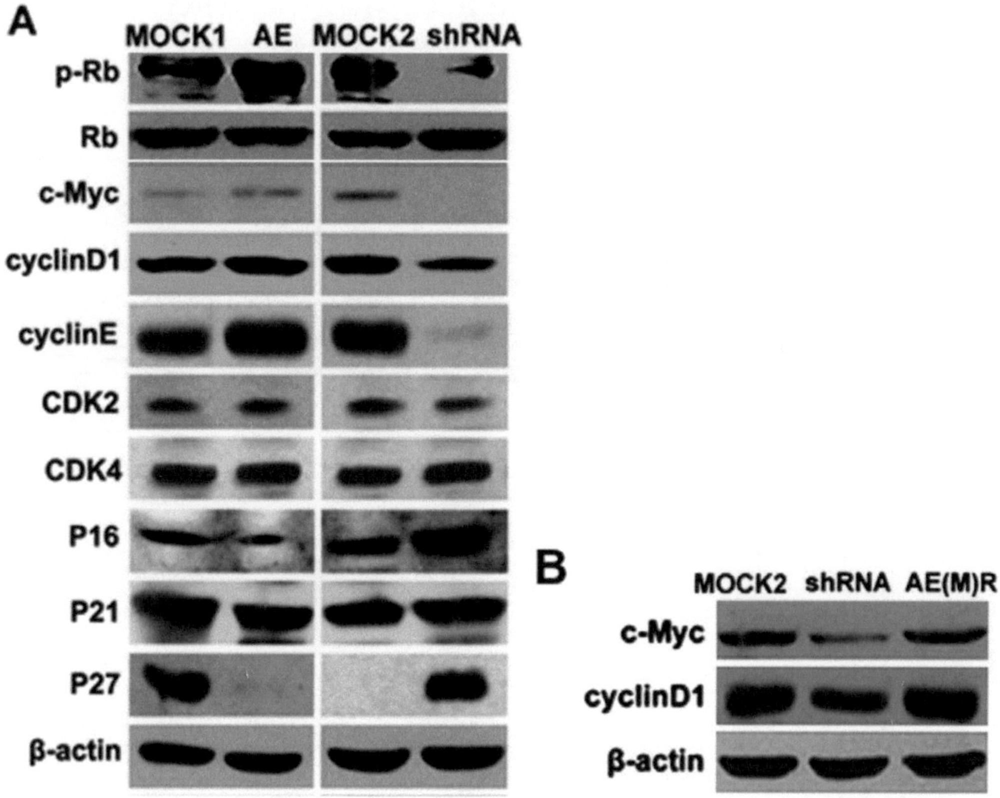


Fig. 10. LAPTM4B-35 alters levels of proliferation-regulating proteins analyzed by Western blot: (a) Level of p-Rb, c-Myc, cyclinD1 and cyclinE protein was significantly increased by over-expression and decreased by knockdown of LAPTM4B-35, respectively. Conversely, level of tumor suppressor gene products, p16 and p27, was significantly decreased by over-expression and increased by knockdown of LAPTM4B-35, respectively. But level of CDK2, CDK4 and p21 was not altered, (b) Restoration of LAPTM4B-35 expression in HepG2-AE(M)R cells reversed the decrease in c-Myc and cyclinD1 proteins resulting from knockdown of endogenous LAPTM4B-35 in HepG2-shRNA cells. (H. Yang et al., 2010c).

### 3.3 Over-expression of LAPTM4B-35 enhances resistance to induced apoptosis

Resistance to apoptosis is one of fundamental characteristics of cancer cells. LAPTM4B-35 over-expressing L02-AE, HepG2-AE and BEL7402-AE cells show marked resistance to drug-induced apoptosis (Figure 11-13). However, down-regulation of endogenous LAPTM4B-35 can restore sensitivity of cancer cells to drug-induced apoptosis (L.Li et al., 2010; H.Yang et al., 2010c). In addition, up-regulation of LAPTM4B-35 inhibits activation of the apoptosis executive caspase 3, up-regulates the anti-apoptotic gene bcl-2, bcl-xL and phosphorylated Bad, and also down-regulates the pro-apoptotic gene Bax and Bid (Figure 12, L.Li et al., 2011; L. Zhou, 2011). Moreover, PI3K/AKT, a fundamental signaling pathway for cell survival is activated by up-regulation of LAPTM4B-35, and is inhibited by down-regulation of endogenous LAPTM4B-35 (L.Li et al., 2010, 2011; H. Yang et al., 2010c). This data serves to establish the cellular and molecular basis of resistance to apoptosis promoted by over-expression of LAPTM4B-35.

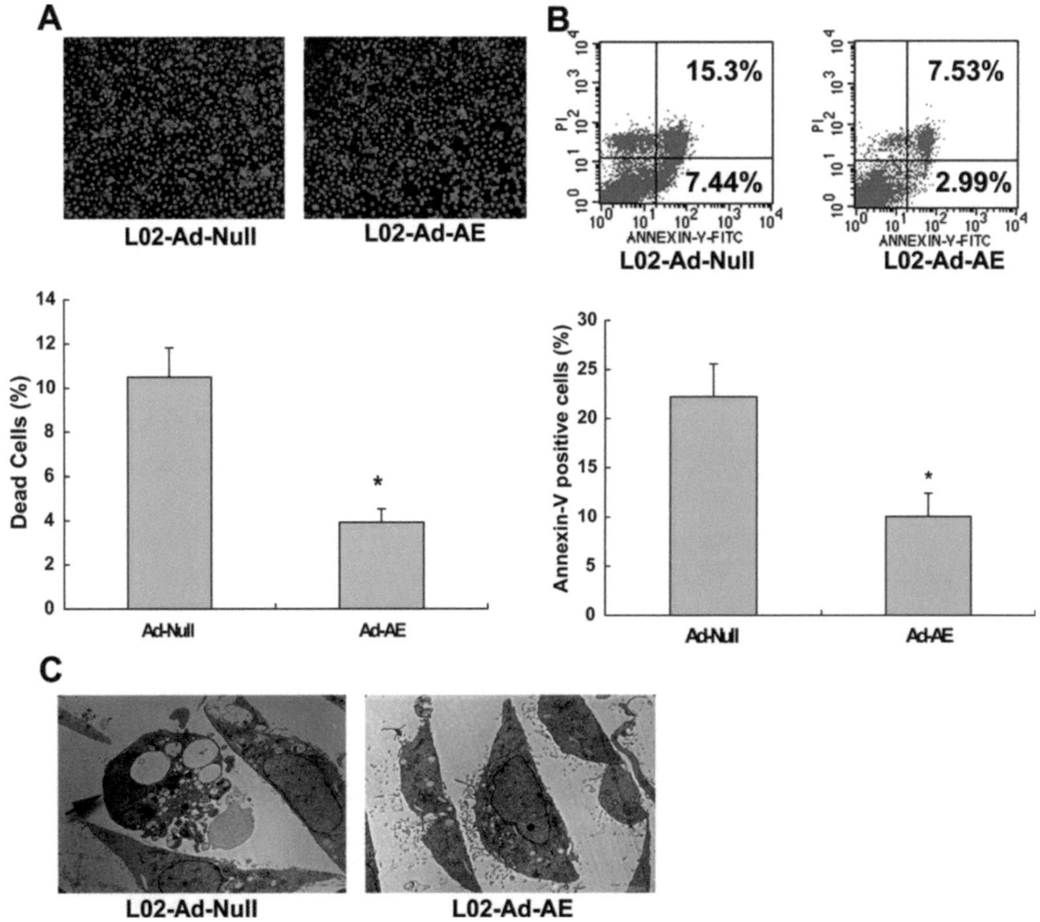


* P<0.05: Ad-Null vs. Ad-AE

Fig. 11. Up-regulation of LAPTM4B-35 protects L02-AE cells from adriamycin induced apoptosis. (a) LIVE/DEAD Viability/Cytotoxicity Kit assay. Green-stained cells are viable cells; cells with red stained nuclear are late apoptotic and dead cells. The LAPTM4B-35 over-expressing L02-Ad-AE cells show less apoptotic cells as compared with L02-Ad-Null control cells. (b) Upper panel: Flow cytometry analysis of apoptosis by Annexin V and PI staining. The number of apoptotic L02-Ad-AE cells appeared in early-, late-phase of apoptosis and dead phase were all less than L02-Ad-Null cells. Lower panel: The histograms showing the cell percentage of dead cells (left) and Annexin V-positive cells in early plus late apoptotic phases (right). (c) Apoptosis shown by transmission electron microscopy. Black arrow indicates the apoptotic L02-Ad-Null control cell induced by adriamycin; this was not seen in L02-Ad-AE cells (L. Li et al., 2011).

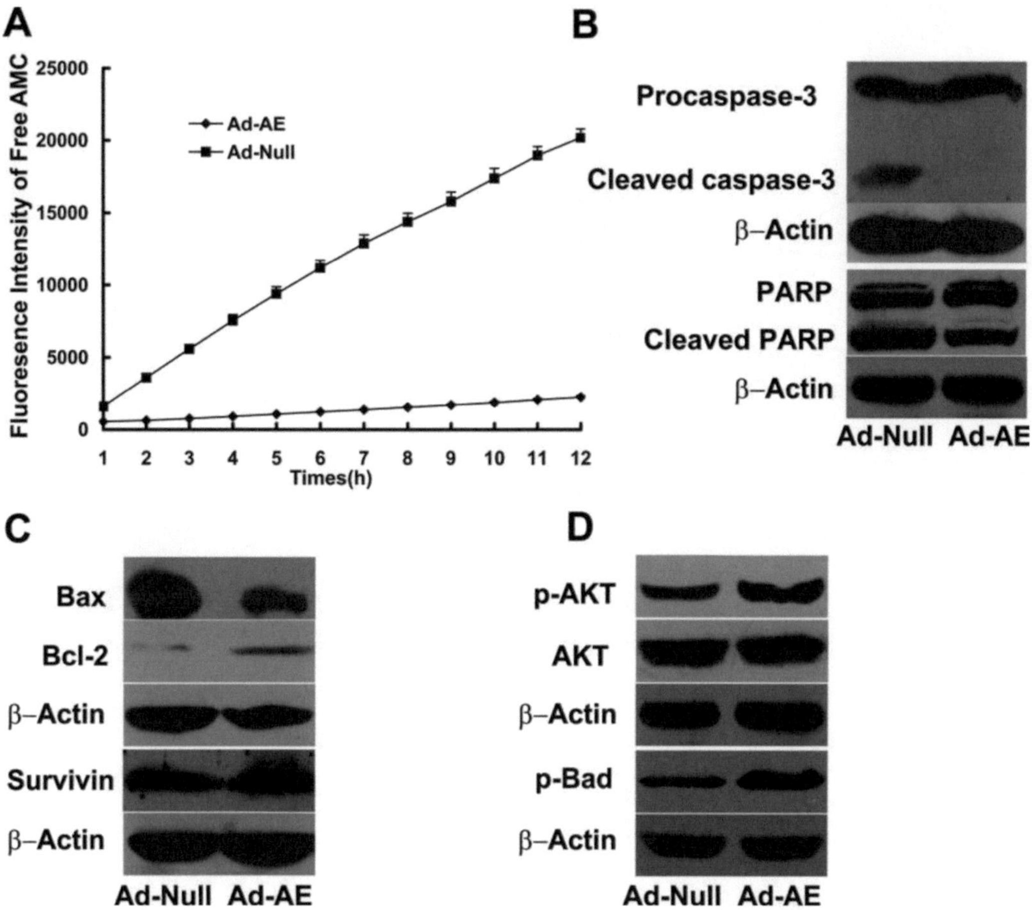


Fig. 12. Up-regulation of LAPTM4B-35 effects activation or expression of apoptosis-associated molecules in L02-AE cells. (a) Inhibition of caspase-3 activation in LAPTM4B-35 over-expressing L02-Ad-AE cells measured by the DEVD cleavage assay. Datum in each point represents the mean SD of three independent experiments. ***P < 0.001: L02-Ad-AE vs. L02-Ad-Null. (b) Cleavage of procaspase-3 and PARP was inhibited by up-regulation of LAPTM4B-35, demonstrating the inhibition of apoptosis. (c) Up-regulation of the anti-apoptotic bcl-2 protein and down-regulation of the pro-apoptotic Bax protein in L02-Ad-AE cells analyzed by Western blot. (d) Increase of phosphorylated AKT and Bad in L02-Ad-AE cells, suggesting the activation of PI3K/AKT signaling and inhibition of apoptosis. (Li et al., 2011).

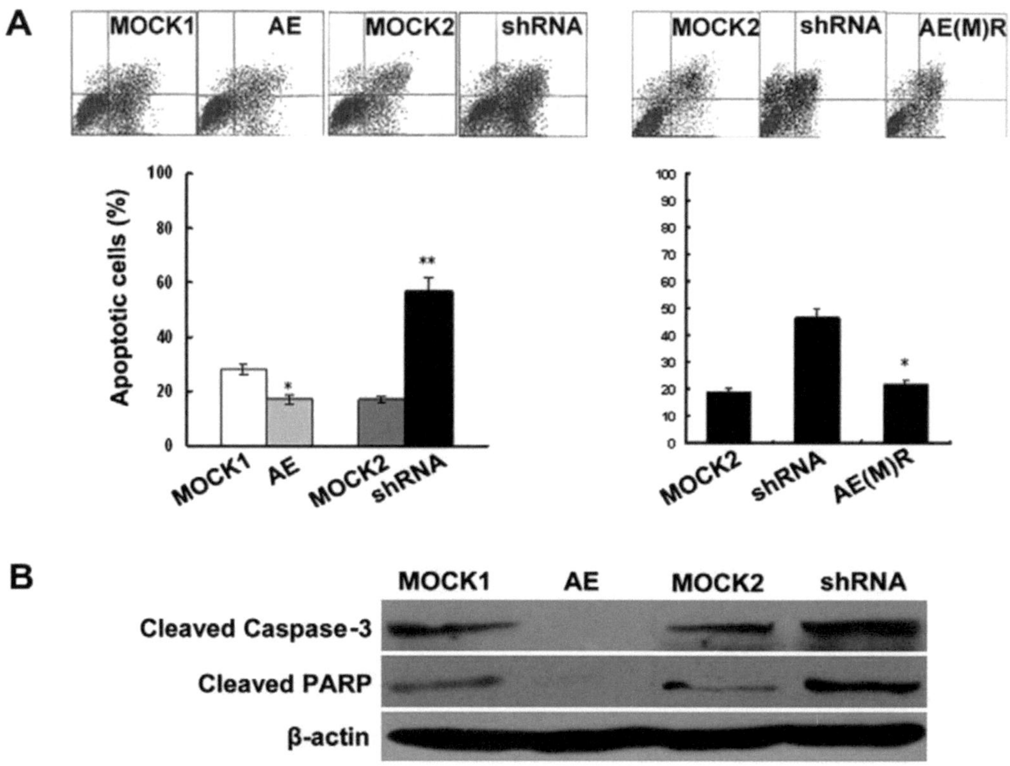


Fig. 13. Up-regulation and down-regulation of LAPTM4B-35 respectively inhibits and promotes HepG2 cells apoptosis induced by adriamycin. (a) Adriamycin (15 μg/ml) induced apoptosis analyzed by FACS in HepG2-AE, HepG2-shRNA, HepG2-AE (M)R cells and corresponding controls. $P < 0.05$: HepG2-AE cells vs. HepG2-mock1, and HepG2-AE (M) R vs. HepG2-shRNA, $P < 0.001$: HepG2-shRNA vs. HepG2-mock2. (b) Analysis of cleaved caspase-3 and PARP by Western blot, demonstrating activation and inhibition of the apoptotic pathway respectively by up-regulation and down-regulation of LAPTM4B-35 in HepG2 cells.

### 3.4 Over-expression of LAPTM4B-35 enhances migration and invasion

Cell migration and invasion are prerequisites for metastasis. Using LAPTM4B-35 over-expressing HCC cells, including HLE-AE, HepG2-AE and BEL7402-AE cells, it has been demonstrated that the cells over-expressing LAPTM4B-35 display enhanced capacity for migration and invasion (XR. Liu et al., 2009; H. Yang et al., 2010c). Conversely down-regulation of endogenous LAPTM4B-35 by RNAi inhibits migration and invasion of HCC cells (Figure 14, H. Yang et al., 2010c). In addition, the matrix metal proteases (MMP2 and MMP9) and urine plasminogen activator (uPA) which are key proteases for cancer cell invasion, are up-regulated and/or activated by over-expression of LAPTM4B-35 (L. Zhou et al., 2010).

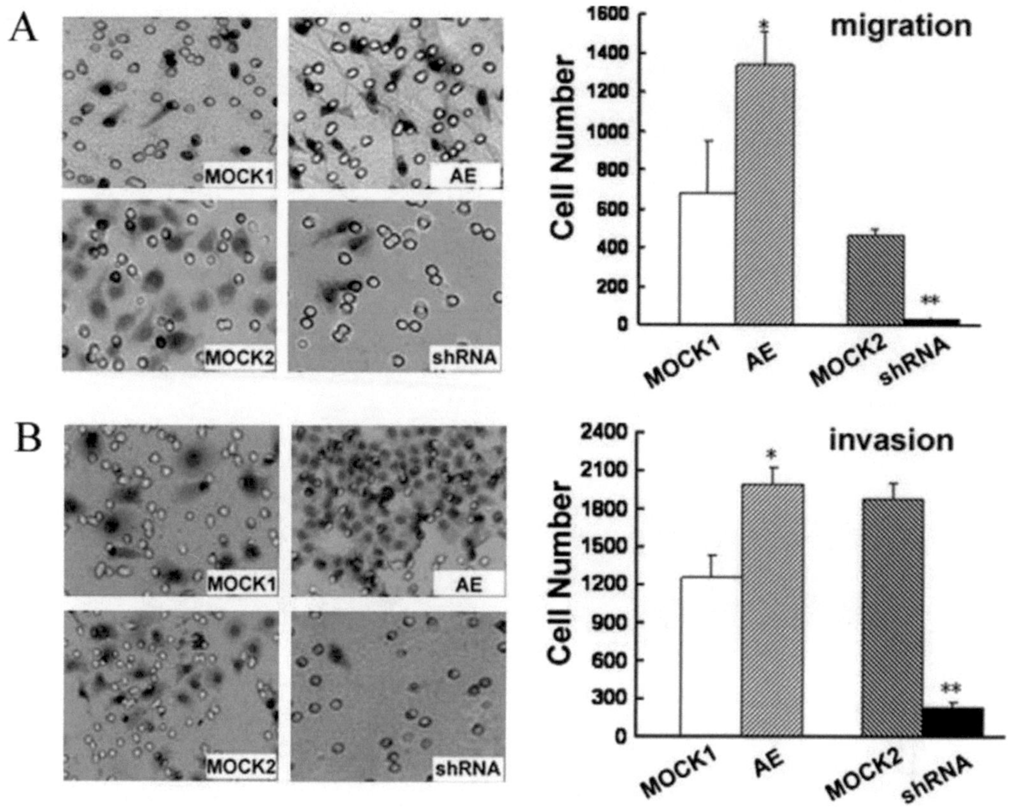


Fig. 14. Over-expression of LAPTM4B-35 promotes migration and invasion. The left panels: (a) Cell migration measured by Boyden chamber assay was promoted and inhibited, respectively, by over-expression (upper panel) and knockdown (lower panel) of LAPTM4B-35 in HepG2 cells. (b) Cell invasion measured by Boyden chamber assay in the presence of Matrigel is promoted and inhibited, respectively, by over-expression (upper panel) and knockdown (lower panel) of LAPTM4B-35 in HepG2 cells. The right panels are the histograms showing number of migratory and invasive cells. *$P < 0.05$: HepG2-AE vs. HepG2-mock1; **$P < 0.001$ HepG2-shRNA vs. HepG2-mock2.

### 3.5 Over-expression of LAPTM4B-35 motivates multi-drug resistance

Multi-drug resistance is a significant obstacle in cancer chemotherapy. We have demonstrated (L Li et al., 2010) that drug efflux and resistance to multiple drugs including doxorubicin, paclitaxel and cisplatin, are enhanced in LAPTM4B-35 over-expressing L02-AE cells that were originally derived from normal liver (Figure 15a), whereas these phenomena are reversed in LAPTM4B-35 down-regulated HeLa-RNAi cells (Figure 15b). In addition, the drug retention in HeLa-RNAi cells was significantly more than in HeLa-Mock control cells (Figure 15c). These findings imply multi-drug resistance is promoted by over-expression of LAPTM4B-35 (L Li et al., 2010). At the same time, LAPTM4B associated multi-drug resistance has also been demonstrated in breast cancer (Hu, 2009; Y.Li., 2010) and ovarian cancer (Yin, 2011a) by other research groups. Y Li et al. (2010) demonstrated that amplification of LAPTM4B and YWHAZ, which was shown by fluorescence in situ

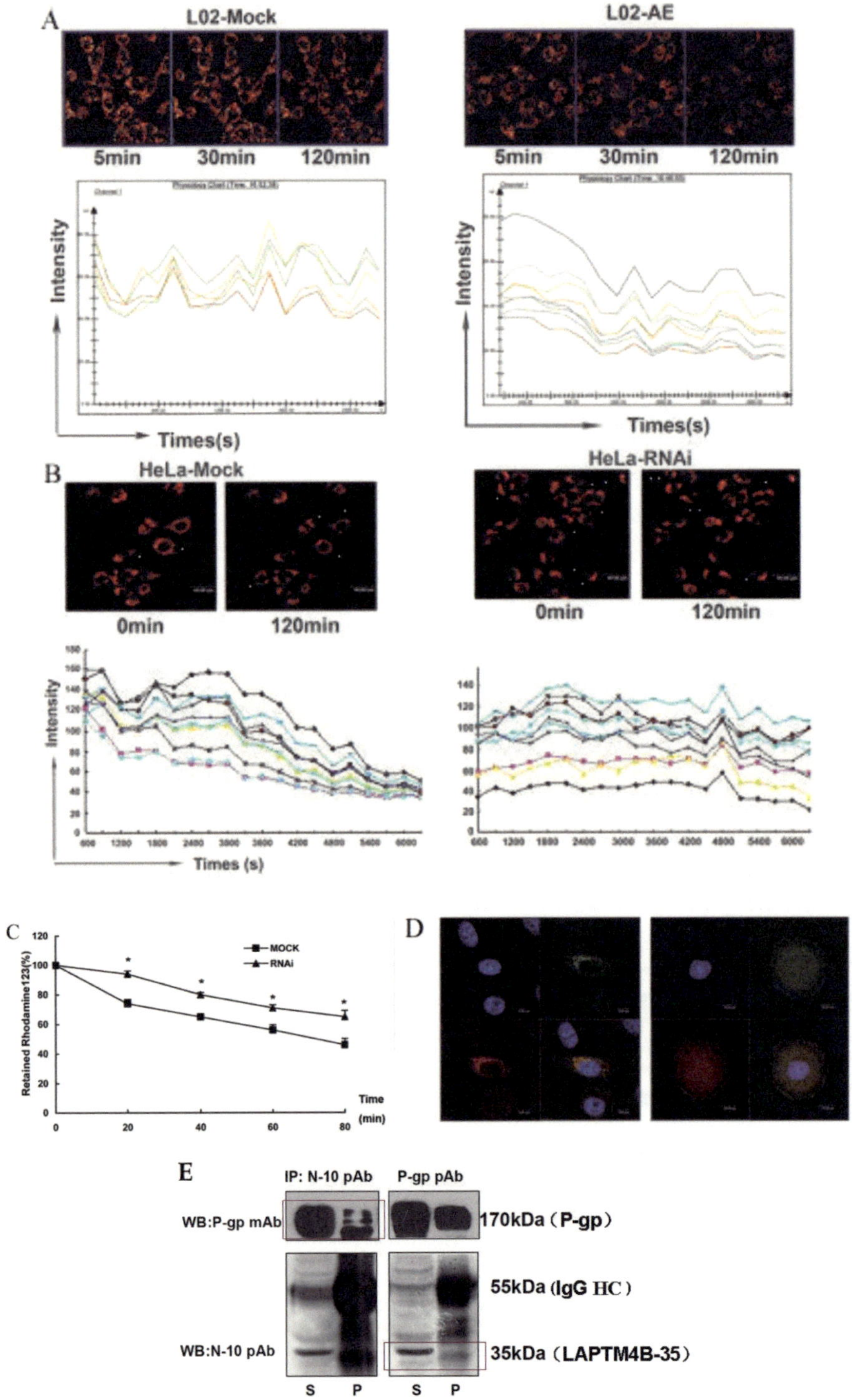


Fig. 15. LAPTM4B-35 motivates multi-drug efflux by interaction with P-gp. (a) Upper panel: The LAPTM4B-35 over-expressing L02-AE cells show faster efflux of Rhodamine-123 as

compaired with L02-Mock control cells. (b) Upper panel: The LAPTM4B-35 knocking down HeLa-RNAi cells show slower drug efflux as compaired with HeLa-Mock cells. The drug efflux was measured by Laser Scanning Confocal Microscopy (LSCM). Lower Panels of (a) and (b): The fluorescence intensity in each cell was monitored and recorded separately as each curve. (c) The Rhodamine-123 retention in HeLa-RNAi cells is significantly greater than that of HeLa Mock control cells (*P<0.05). The time course of Rhodamine-123 retention in LAPTM4B-35 knocking down HeLa-RNAi cells and HeLa-Mock cells was analyzed by a FACS. (d) Left panel: LAPTM4B-35 is co-localized with P-gp (MDR1) mainly at endomembrane organelles in HeLa cells (Bar, 8 mm). Right panel: LAPTM4B-35 is co-localized with P-gp mainly on plasma membrane in PC-3 cells which are spreading onto fibronectin substrate (Bar, 20 mm). Co-localization of LAPTM4B-35 and P-gp was analyzed by Triple-staining immunofluorescence and LSCM. Yellow color is the overlapping of green (P-gp) and red (LAPEM4B-35) signals. (e) Interaction of LAPTM4B-35 with P-gp analyzed by Co-immunoprecipitation (Co-IP). The antibodies used for immuno-precipitation were anti-LAPTM4B-35-N10pAb (left panel) and anti-P-gp pAb (right panel). The antibodies used for immuno-blotting (Western blot) were anti-P-gp mAb (upper panel) and anti-LAPTM4B-35-N10pAb (lower panel). Interaction of LAPTM4B-35 with P-gp is demonstrated by Co-IP analysis of both sets marked with a box with red line. (L Li et al., 2010)

hybridization (FISH), contributes to chemotherapy resistance of breast cancer. Hu et al (2009) reported activation of *MTDH* and *LAPTM4B* (which are localized at the same gene locus) determined by gain of 8q22 via comparative genomic hybridization (CGH) promotes chemoresistance and metastasis of breast cancer. These observations are consistent with our current results. All these studies indicate that LAPTM4B plays an important role in multi-drug resistance. Our study on the mechanism indicates that there is a molecular interaction and co-localization between LAPTM4B-35 and P-gp (MDR1). P-gp is a classic transporter that results in multi-drug resistance by enhancing drug efflux from cancer cells. Interestingly, the co-localization presents at the plasma membrane when cancer cells are spreading onto extracellular matrix component fibronectin, but at intracellular membrane compartments (this may mainly involve endosomes and lysosomes based on the distribution pattern) when cancer cells are not spreading onto extracellular matrix component (Figure 15d). Since P-gp trafficking between lysosomes and plasma membrane plays a critical role in multi-drug resistance (Fu et al., 2004, 2007), our results suggest that LAPTM4B-35 may be a significant factor that is involved in the trafficking of LAPTM4B-35 and P-gp between plasma membrane and intracellular compartments in giving rise to multi-drug resistance. The detailed mechanism for this combined trafficking remains to be further studied. Additionally, increasing numbers of experiments have recently shown that activation of the PI3K/AKT signaling pathway can regulate or enhance multi-drug resistance (Abdul-Ghani et al., 2006; Knuefermann et al., 2003; McCubrey et al., 2006; Tazzari et al., 2007). Our study indicates that PI3K/AKT signaling pathway is remarkably activated by over-expression of LAPTM4B-35 (see section 3.6). Accordingly, PI3K inhibitors can inhibit AKT phosphorylation/activation and increase the sensitivity of cancer cells over-expressing LAPTM4B-35 to doxorubicin, paclitaxel and cisplatin (L Li et al., 2010). Overall, our data provide new insight into the molecular mechanisms of multi-drug resistance and open a novel avenue for overcoming multi-drug resistance in chemotherapy by targeting LAPTM4B-35.

### 3.6 Over-expression of LAPTM4B-35 activates a signaling network associated with carcinogenesis

Over-expression of LAPTM4B-35 in liver and hepatocellular carcinoma cell lines enhances a wide range of malignant cellular and molecular phenotypes. The mechanism for the wide variety of roles played by over-expression of LAPTM4B-35 is therefore of great interest and has provoked scientific attention. We believe the most likely mechanism which may account for the findings and phenotypic changes described above is the involvement of LAPTM4B-35 in a signaling network. Based on the striking similarity of the proline-rich motifs at the N-terminus of LAPTM4B-35 and at the PI3K p85α regulatory subunit, we first explored the effect of LAPTM4b-35 over-expression in HCC cells on activation of the PI3K/AKT signaling pathway. We found that LAPTM4b-35 up-regulation constantly activates PI3K/AKT signaling which has been shown by increased phosphorylation of AKT and its down stream signaling molecules (Figure 16a) in HepG2, BEL7402 HCC cells and HeLa cells (L Li et al., 2010; Yang et al., 2010). Furthermore, interaction between the proline-rich motif of LAPTM4B-35 N-terminal tail and the PI3K p85α regulatory subunit is demonstrated by site-specific mutations, GST-pull down and co-immunoprecipitation (Co-IP) (L Li et al., 2010; XR Liu et al., 2009; and unpublished data). It is believed that binding of the proline-rich motif of LAPTM4B-35 to the SH3 domain of PI3K p85α regulatory subunit may release the inhibitory effect of p85α regulatory subunit of PI3K on kinase activity of the p110 catalytic subunit of PI3K. We then found that the phosphorylation of GSK3β and FOXO4, both of which are downstream signaling molecules of phosphorylated/activated AKT, is promoted by over-expression and attenuated by knockdown of LAPTM4B-35 in HepG2-AE cells (Figure 16a). Since GSK3β (Glycogen synthase kinase 3 beta) is inactivated after phosphorylation by AKT, as a result the phosphorylation of c-Myc and cyclinD1, which are the GSK3β down stream effectors, is thus diminished and increased, respectively, in LAPTM4B-35 over-expressing and knocking down cancer cells (Figure16b). Sequentially, because diminished phophorylation of c-Myc and cyclinD1 can lead to decrease of degradation by proteosomes via ubiqutination (Diehl J et al., 1998), as a result, c-Myc and cyclinD1 become more stable and thus accumulate in LAPTM4B-35 over-expressing cancer cells (Figure 10a and 16c) playing roles in carcinogenesis. On the other hand, FOXO4 is a transcription factor of p27. It is known that phosphorylation of FOXO4 may result in sequestration in the cytoplasm with resultant loss of its function (Medema et al., 2000). This may be the reason that expression of p27 is dramatically diminished by overexpression of LAPTM4B-35, but restored by its knockdown via RNAi (Figure 10a). Based on the fact that p27 is a member of the cyclin-dependent kinase inhibitor (CKI) family, and that restored expression of p27 may inhibit cell proliferation and thus be a favorable prognostic indicator for patients with HCC (M.Fiorentino et al., 2000), it is possible that clinical therapy using LAPTM4B-35 specific RNA interference may improve the prognosis of HCC patients. In addition, the integrin/FAK, RTK/Ras/ERK and Wnt signaling pathways are also activated by LAPTM4B-35 over-expression (unpublished data). It has been demonstrated via GST-pull down, Co-IP and site-specific mutations that LAPTM4B-35 can interact with several signal molecules in cytoplasm and plasma membrane, such as PI3K p85α, FAK, integrins (α5 and α6) and RTKs (for example IGF1R), and so on. Taken together, it is evident that LAPTM4B-35 over-expression activates a signaling network, consisting of at least four signaling pathways which are closely associated with hepatocarcinogenesis, metastasis and multi-drug resistance (Whittaker, 2010). It is proposed that LAPTM4B-35 may act as an organizer or platform of signal molecules which functions at signal network upstream. Further investigation of this point will greatly improve our understanding on hepatocarcinogenesis, metastasis and recurrence of hepatocellular carcinoma, and will thus provide novel strategies for targeted chemotherapy of hepatocellular carcinoma.

Overall our studies demonstrate there is a relationship of LAPTM4B-35 over-expression with up-regulation of proliferation-promoting proteins and down-regulation of proliferation-inhibiting proteins in hepatocellular carcinoma cells. This relationship is mediated by a signaling network.

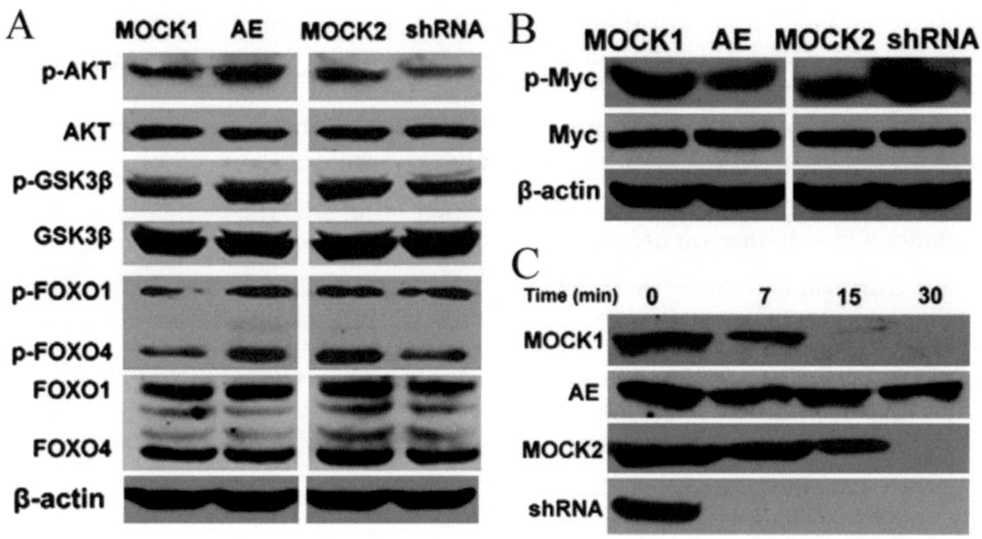


Fig. 16. LAPTM4B-35 over-expression activates a signaling network. (a) Over-expression and knockdown of LAPTM4B-35, respectively, activates and inhibits PI3K/AKT signaling pathway shown by Western blot. AKT activation is generally evaluated by its phosphorylations at S 308 and S473 resulting from PI3K activation through its phosphorylating product PIP3 and two additional kinases. GSK3β and FOXO4 are both down stream effectors of AKT and thus phosphorylated by this activated kinase. (b) Phosphorulated c-Myc (p-Myc) is diminished and increased, respectively, by over-expression and knockdown in HepG2 cells. (c) Degradation of c-Myc is respectively diminished by over-expression of LAPTM4B-35 and enhanced by knowdown of LAPTM4B-35. This experiment was performed via cycloheximide pulse-chase assay, in which stably transfected HepG2 cells were treated with 50 μg/ml of cycloheximide to inhibit biosynthesis of proteins and harvested at 0, 7, 15 and 30 min., then Western blot with anti-Myc Ab was performed to evaluate degradation of c-Myc. The results indicates that up-regulation of LAPTM4B-35 enhances stability of c-Myc, and *vice versa*.

### 3.7 LAPTM4B-24 up-regulation induces apoptosis and autophagocytosis, and abolishes carcinogenicity of hepatocellular carcinoma cells

LAPTM4B-24 is an isoform encoded by the *LAPTM4B* gene. It is a truncated form of LAPTM4B-35 by lacking a 91 amino acid sequence at the N-terminus (Shao et al., 2003). We have demonstrated that up-regulation of LAPTM4B-24 via transfection with plasmids pcDNA-BE or infection with replication-deficient adenovirus Ad-BE induces apoptosis and autophagocytosis of HCC cells, as well as associated cellular and molecular alterations. At the same time LAPTM4B-24 up-regulated HCC cells lose its carcinogenicity (unpublished data). These studies indicate that LAPTM4B-24 plays an antagonistic role in hepatocarcinogenesis.

In summary, the LAPTM4B-35 plays pivotal roles in keeping cell survival, proliferation, migration and invasion, and so on; whereas LAPTM4B-24 plays critical roles in regulating programmed cell death, including apoptosis and autophagocytosis. The expressive equilibrium of LAPTM4B-35 and LAPTM4B-24 maintains physiological homeostasis of cells. Destroy of this equilibrium would lead to diseases. Up-regulation of LAPTM4B-35 leads to oncogenesis, while up-regulation of LAPTM4B-24 may plays a role in cancer regression.

## 4. *LAPTM4B* gene and the encoded LAPTM4B-35 protein are predicted to be novel markers for diagnosis of hepatocellular carcinoma

### 4.1 LAPTM4B-35 is predicted to be a novel marker for diagnosis, pathological grading and progression-monitoring of hepatocellular carcinoma

We have demonstrated via Western blot and immuno-histochemistry that the expression levels of LAPTM4B-35 in HCC tissues show a significant positive correlation with pathological grade (Figure 17a, and Table 1 and 3), intrahepatic and extrahepatic metastasis (figure 17b), TNM stage (Table 1 and 3) and recurrence of HCC (Table 3), and show a negative correlation with overall and disease-free postoperative survival (Figure 17c). Upon multivariate analysis, elevated expression of LAPTM4B-35 was found to be an independent

| Variables | Patients | LAPTM4B-35 expression | | $P^a$ |
|---|---|---|---|---|
| | | Low | High | |
| All cases | 71 | | | |
| Tumor size | | | | |
| <5 cm | 38 | 10 | 28 | 0.710 |
| ≥5 cm | 33 | 10 | 23 | |
| Portal vein invasion | | | | |
| No | 52 | 20 | 32 | 0.001 |
| Yes | 19 | 0 | 19 | |
| Serum AFP level | | | | |
| <25 ng/ml | 35 | 13 | 22 | 0.097 |
| ≥25 ng/ml | 36 | 7 | 29 | |
| TNM stage | | | | |
| I–II | 25 | 14 | 11 | <0.001 |
| III–IV | 46 | 6 | 40 | |
| Recurrence | | | | |
| No | 17 | 13 | 4 | <0.001 |
| Yes | 54 | 7 | 47 | |

Table 3. Expressive level of LAPTM4B-35 in HCC tissues shown by IHC shows significant positive correlation to portal vein invasion, TNM staging and recurrence. (H.Yang et al., 2010b).

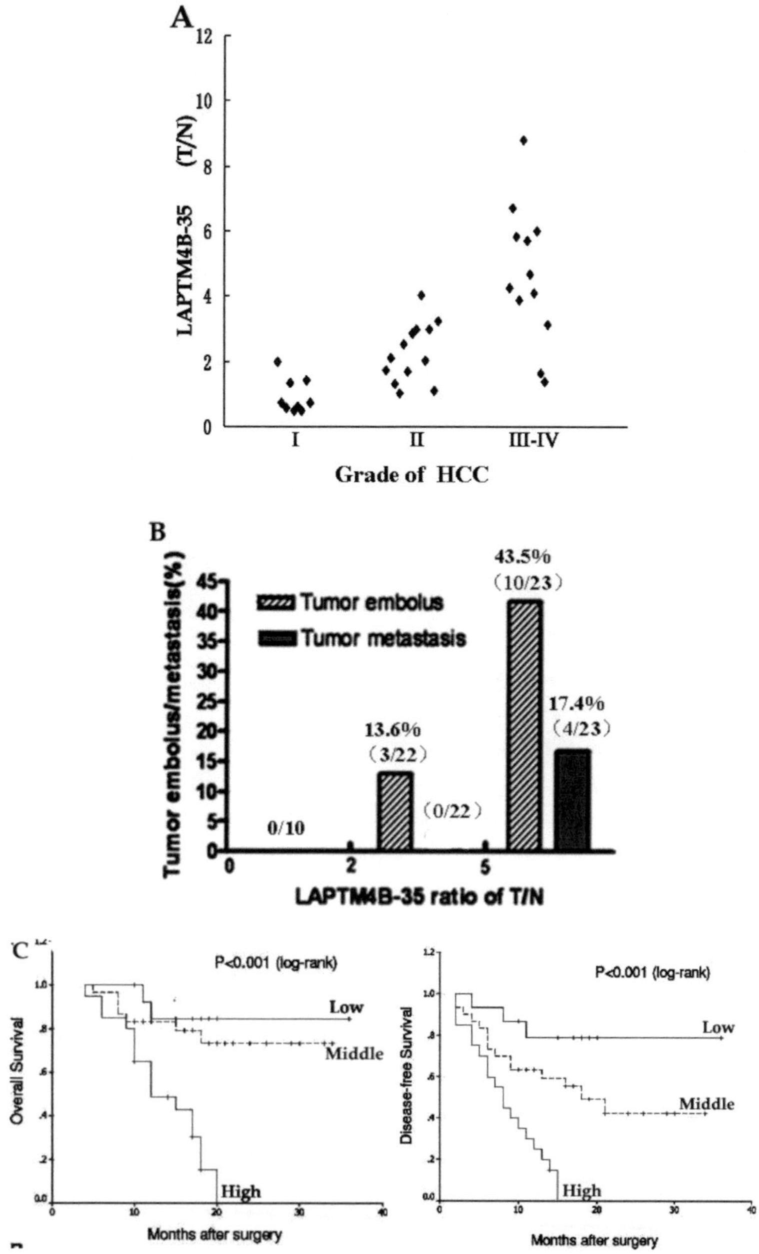


Fig. 17. Correlation of LAPTM4B-35 expression levels in HCC tissues with pathological grading, metastasis and postoperative survival time. (a) Level of LAPTM4B-35 protein in HCCs shows positive correlation with pathological grade. (b) LAPTM4B-35 expressions in HCCs from 65 patients were divided into three groups: "Low," "Mediate," and "High." Level of LAPTM4B-35 in HCC shows significant positive correlation with intrahepatic and extrahepatic metastasis. *P<0.05. (c) Levels of LAPTM4B-35 in HCCs show significantly negative correlation with overall (left) and disease-free (right) postoperative survival of cancer patients. (H.Yang et al., 2010a, 2010b).

prognostic factor for hepatocellular carcinoma (Yang et al., 2010a, 2010b). In our preliminary study we found that about 40% of paired non-cancerous liver tissues in the same HCC patients express elevated LAPTM4B mRNA (JJ. Liu et al., 2000). We believe that the non-cancerous liver tissue of the same one patient with HCC is representing the precancer status to variant extents. We therefore suggest that LAPTM4B-35 may be an important and novel biomarker for early diagnosis, mornitoring of progression, prediction of metastasis and recurrence of HCC, as well as for evaluating prognosis of HCC patients. In addition, we have demonstrated that LAPTM4B-35 protein can be released into the blood in the form of exosomes. The levels of LAPTM4B-35 in serum of HCC patients are significantly higher than those from normal individuals (unpublished data).

Moreover, a number of other cancers also show the similar association of LAPTM4B-35 with clinical and pathological criteria. Cancers which have been evaluated include gallbladder cancer (L. Zhou et al., 2007), cholangiocarcinoma (L. Zhou et al., 2008), ovarian cancer (Y Yang, 2008; Yin et al., 2011a, 2011b), cervical cancer (Meng et al., 2010), and endometrial cancer (Meng et al., 2010). It is likely that LAPTM4B-35 may also find use as a biomarker for other solid cancers.

### 4.2 *LAPTM4B* mRNA expressed in circulating tumor cells can be used for predicting metastasis

It is well known that circulating cancer cells have more highly metastatic potential. We found that the highly metastatic cancer cell lines derived from one cancer mass express higher levels of LAPTM4N-35 than syngenic cancer cell lines of low metastatic potential (XR. Liu et al., 2003). We have determined that the LAPTM4B mRNA expressed by a few circulating HCC cells can be measured by nested RT-PCR and real time RT-PCR. Therefore, testing LAPTM4B mRNA in circulating HCC cells with real time RT- PCR shows promise for application of prediction and evaluation of metastasis occurring at an early stage.

## 5. *LAPTM4B* gene and the encoded LAPTM4B-35 protein as a novel therapeutic targets

### 5.1 Adjusting the expression equilibrium between LAPTM4B-35 and LAPTM4B-24 can be a novel strategy for biotherapy of hepatocellular carcinoma

As described in section 3, the expression equilibrium of LAPTM4B-35 and LAPTM4B-24 plays a pivotal role in maintaining the physiological status of cells. LAPTM4B-35 promotes resistance to apoptosis, deregulation of proliferation, enhancement of migration and invasion, and multi-drug resistance. On the other hand, up-regulation of LAPTM4B-24 increases sensitivity to induction of apoptosis and autophagocytosis. As we have demonstrated in our laboratory knockdown of the high expression of the endogenous cancer-promoting protein LAPTM4B-35 via RNAi, or elevating the relatively low expression of the cancer-inhibiting protein LAPTM4B-24 by transgenic therapy can significantly inhibit cancer growth and metastasis and thus may be applicable in cancer biotherapy. Therefore, we suggest knockdown of LAPTM4B-35 expression via RNAi or microRNA, and/or up-regulation of LAPTM4B-24 expression may provide effective strategies for treatment of HCC and possibly other cancers.

### 5.2 LAPTM4B-35 is a novel therapeutic target for neoadjuvant chemotherapy

Neoadjuvant chemotherapy generally targets one or more molecules in signaling pathways. As discussed in section 3, over-expression of LAPTM4B-35 promotes hepatocarcinogenesis, faster growth of human HCC xenografts and metastasis in mice, and leads to anti-apoptosis, deregulation of proliferation, and enhancement of migration and invasion and multi-drug resistance. In addition, over-expression of LAPTM4B-35 leads to accumulation of a number of cell cycle promoting proteins and survival proteins, and results in down-regulation of a number of cell cycle inhibiting proteins and proapoptotic proteins by activating a signaling network including at least 4 different signaling pathways. Based on our studies in vitro and in vivo, it is clear that LAPTM4B-35 has significant potential as an important novel target for cancer treatment. Recently, we have screened out a few small molecules from various libraries containing nearly 2000 chemically synthetic compounds. These small molecules are able to kill a variety of cancer cells that over-express the *LAPTM4B* gene and LAPTM4B-35 protein in vitro, but do not harm the normal fetal liver cells which do not over-express this gene. One of these small molecules has been demonstrated to inhibit growth and metastasis of human HCC xenografts in nude mice, and results in cellular and molecular alterations opposite to those that result from over-expression of LAPTM4B-35 in HCC cells. Some of these active small molecules have been demonstrated to be inhibitors of tyrosine kinase (unpublished data).

In summary, this gene and the proteins it encodes harbor great potential for application in cancer biotherapy and chemotherapy.

## 6. Conclusion and prospective

*LAPTM4B* gene and its encoding LAPTM4B-35 protein are over-expressed in 87% of HCC and some solid cancers with varying frequencies. The level of LAPTM4B-35 expression in HCC tissues shows significant positive correlation with pathological grade, intrahepatic and extrahepatic metastasis, and recurrence, and negative correlation with overall and disease-free postoperative survival of cancer patients, and is thus an independent prognostic factor for HCC. Over-expression of LAPTM4B-35 promotes malignant transformation of cell lines from normal tissues, including human liver tissue. This result implies that over-expression of the *LAPTM4B* gene and LAPTM4B-35 protein may play pivotal roles in hepatocarcinogenesis and progresion. Up-regulated LAPTM4B-35 promotes faster growth and metastasis of human HCC xenografts in nude mice, and results in resistance to apoptosis, deregulation of proliferation, and enhancement of migration and invasion, as well as multi-drug resistance. In addition, overexpression of LAPTM4B-35 leads to accumulation of a number of oncoproteins encoded by oncogenes and down-regulation of a number of tumor suppressing proteins. In contrast, knockdown of endogenous LAPTM4B-35 via RNA interfering leads to significant inhibition of growth and metastasis of human HCC xenografts in nude mice, and reversion of the cellular and molecular malignant phenotypes. The extensive effects caused by LAPTM4B-35 over-expression result from its function in activation of a signaling network, including at least 4 signaling pathways that are commonly known to be associated with hepatocarcinogenesis (K. Breuhahn, 2010; Takigawa, 2008; XH L 2011). Taken together, our studies suggests that LAPTM4B-35 is a key molecule which functions upstream of a cancer associated signaling network and plays pivotal roles in hepatocarcinogenesis, progression, metastasis, multi-drug resistance and recurrence. Conversely, up-regulation of LAPTM4B-24, an truncated isoform that lacks a 91 amino acid sequence at the N-terminus of LAPTM4B-35, promotes apoptosis and autophagocytosis, and therefore plays an antagonistic role in hepatocarcinogenesis. Overall, these data provide new insight into genes and proteins that are potentially important in the pathogenesis of liver carcinoma. This harbors great potential for future application as novel biomarkers for cancer diagnostics, pathological grading, progression monitoring and prognosis, and as novel molecular targets providing new strategies for biotherapy and chemotherapy of HCC.

Up-regulation of expression of the *LAPTM4B* gene and LAPTM4B-35 protein occur in a broad range of human solid cancers and are often associated with poor prognosis, indicating there is a common key role for this oncogentic gene and protein in cancer development.

Although *LAPTM4B* gene and the encoded LAPTM4B protein have been the subject of more than a decade of study, there are still important issues which remain to be resolved. These include (1) the underlying mechanism(s) responsible for up-regulation of the *LAPTM4B* gene and LAPTM4B-35 protein in neoplastic transformation; (2) the possibility LAPTM4B may be associated with cancer stem cells. Our previous studies indicate that LAPTM4B-35 over-expressing cancer cells possess characteristics typical of cancer stem cells, including apoptosis-resistance, unlimited renewal capacity, metastatic potential and multi-drug resistance. In addition, a study by Lee et al., (2010) suggests that LAPTM4B together with Gp49a, Sox4, and CD34 genes may be "stemness-related" genes in a primitive hematopoietic progenitor cell line EML, and this study demonstrates that these genes are preferentially expressed in hematopoietic stem cells and down-regulated in mature hematopoietic cells. Study of whether LAPTM4B-35 protein is a marker of cancer stem cells is therefore warranted; (3) as it has been shown in our study that LAPTM4B protein localizes at late endosomes, lysosomes, mitochondria, and the plasma membrane (unpublished data), it may be supposed that trafficking of LAPTM4B protein in cells would be very important for execution of its functions, thus it is worthwhile studying when and how LAPTM4B-35 and LAPTM4B-24 trafficking functions in normal cells and in cancer cells; (4) the detailed molecular mechanism for enhancing function of multi-drug resistance of p-gp (MDR1) by LAPTM4B-35 over-expression; (5) the underlying mechanism for metastasis promoted by LAPTM4B-35 over-expression; (6) the detailed molecular mechanism for signaling network activation by LAPTM4B-35 over-expression in HCC; (7) the sensitivity and specificity of LAPTM4B mRNA and LAPTM4B-35 protein as a marker for HCC diagnosis; (8) the underlying molecular mechanism for which targeted chemotherapy of small compounds depends on LAPTM4B-35 over-expression.

## 7. Acknowledgment

I sincerely appreciate all the members of my laboratory who have worked on and are currently working on LAPTM4B for their valuable contributions, and I appreciate the work which has been done by other groups on this topic. These studies of LAPTM4B have been supported by grants from 211 and 985 Foundation of Peking University, National High-tech R&D Program (863 Program) (2006AA02A305), 248 major R&D program of Beijing (H020220020310), NNSFC (90408018) and the Creative Drugs Foundation from Beijing Fangzheng Group.

I would also like to sincerely thank Professor Da Long Ma and his Colleges who have given me great encourage and help, and Dr. Michael A. McNutt who has provided great help in use of the English language.

## 8. References

Abdul-Ghani R., Serra V., Gyo¨ rffy B., Ju¨ rchott K., Solf A., Dietel M.et al. (2006). The PI3K inhibitor LY294002 blocks drug export from resistant colon carcinoma cells overexpressing MRP1. *Oncogene* ,Vol.25, pp.1743–1752.

Adra CN., Zhu S., Ko JL., Guillemot JC., Cuervo AM., Kobayashi H., Horiuchi T., Lelias JM., Rowley JD, Lim B. (1996) LAPTM5: a novel lysosomal-associated multispanning membrane protein preferentially expressed in hematopoietic cells. Genomics. 35(2):328-37.

Breuhahn K. & Schirmacher P. (2010). Signaling networks in human hepatocarcinogenesis--novel aspects and therapeutic options. *Prog Mol Biol Transl Sci.* Vol.97, pp.251-77.

Buendia MA. (2002) Genetic alterations in hepatoblastoma and hepatocellular carcinoma: common and distinctive aspects. *Med Pediatr Oncol.* Vol.39, No.5, pp.530-5.

Longerich T., Mueller MM., Breuhahn K., Schirmacher P., Benner A. & Heiss C. (2011). Oncogenetic tree modeling of human hepatocarcinogenesis. *Int J Cancer.* Mar 11. doi: 10.1002/ijc.26063. [Epub ahead of print]

Cheng XJ., Xu W., Zhang QY. & Zhou RL. (2008). Relationship between *LAPTM4B* gene polymorphism and susceptibility of colorectal and esophageal cancers. *Annals of Oncology* , Vol.19, No.3, pp.527-32

Deng LJ. , Zhang QY., Liu B. & Zhou RL. (2005). Relationship between LAPTM4B gene polymorphism and susceptibility of lung cancer, *J Peking University (health Sciences)* , Vol.37, No.3, pp.302-305

Diehl JA., Cheng M., Roussel MF. & Sherr CJ. (1998). Glycogen synthase kinase-3beta regulates cyclin D1 proteolysis and subcellular localization. *Genes Dev,* Vol.12, pp.499-3511.

Fiorentino M., Altimari A., D'Errico A., Cukor B., Barozzi C., Loda M. & Grigioni WF. (2000). Acquired expression of p27 is a favorable prognostic indicator in patients with hepatocellular carcinoma. *Clin. Cancer Res.* Vol.6, No.10, pp.3966–3972.

Fu D., Bebawy M., Kable EP. and Roufogalis BD. (2004a). Dynamic and intracellular trafficking of P-glycoprotein-EGFP fusion protein: Implications in multidrug resistance in cancer. *Int J Cancer,* Vol.109, pp.174–181

He J., Shao GZ & Zhou RL. (2003), Effects of the novel gene, LAPTM4B, high expression in hepatocellular carcinoma on cell proliferation and tumorigenesis of NIH3T3 cells, *J Peking University (health Sciences),* Vol.35, No.4, (December 2002), pp.348－352, ISSN1671-167X

Hogue DL., Ellison MJ., Young JD. & Cass CE. (1996). Identification of a novel membrane transporter associated with intracellular membranes by phenotypic complementation in the yeast Saccharomyces cerevisiae. *J Biol Chem.,* Vol.271, No.16, pp.9801-8

Hogue DL., Kerby L. & Ling V.A. (1999). Mammalian lysosomal membrane protein confers multidrug resistance upon expression in Saccharomyces cerevisiae. *J Biol Chem,* Vol.274, No.18, pp.12877-82

Hu, GH., Chong, RA., Yang, QF., Wei, Y., Blanco, MA., Li, F., , Reiss, M., Au, JL.-S., Haffty, BG. & Kang, YB. (2009). MTDH Activation by 8q22 Genomic Gain Promotes Chemoresistance and Metastasis of Poor-Prognosis Breast Cancer. *Cancer Cell*, Vol.15, pp.9–20.

Huang J., Sheng HH., Shen T., Hu YJ., Xiao HS., Zhang Q., Zhang QH. & Han ZG. (2006). Correlation between genomic DNA copy number alterations and transcriptional expression in hepatitis B virus-associated hepatocellular carcinoma. *FEBS Lett.* Vol.580, No.15, pp.571-81.

Kasper G., Vogel A., Klaman I, et al. (2005). The human LAPTM4b transcript is upregulated in various types of solid tumours and seems to play a dual functional role during tumour progression. *Cancer Letters*, Vol.224, pp.93–103

Knuefermann C., Lu Y., Liu B., Jin W., Liang K., Wu L. et al. (2003). HER2/PI-3K/Akt activation leads to a multidrug resistance in human breast adenocarcinoma cells. Oncogene 22: 3205–3212.

Lee H M., Zhang H., Schulz V., Tuck DP., & Forget BG. 2010, Downstream targets of HOXB4 in a cell line model of primitive hematopoietic progenitor cells. *Blood*, Vol.116, No.5, pp.720-730

Li, L., Wei, XH., Pan, YP., Shan, Y., Li, HC., Yang, H., Pang, Y., Xiong, FX., Shao, GZ. & Zhou RL. (2010). LAPTM4B：A novel cancer-associated gene motivates multi-drug resistance through efflux and activating PI3K/Akt signaling. *Oncogene*, Vol.29, No.43, pp.5785-95.

Li Y., Zou L., Li Q., Haibe-Kains B., Tian1 R., Li,Y., Desmedt C., Sotiriou C., Szallasi Z., Iglehart JD., Richardson AL. & Wang ZC. (2010). Amplification of LAPTM4B and YWHAZ contributes to chemotherapy resistance and recurrence of breast cancer. *Nature Medicine*; Vol.16, pp. 214-8.

Liu J., Zhang J., Zhang N., Rui J., Jin C. & Zhou R. (2000), Identification of new hepatocellular carcinoma genes by fluorescent differential display. *J Peking University (health Sciences)*, Vol.32, No.5, (October 2000), pp. 411-14, ISSN 1000-1530.

Liu XR., Zhou RL.，Zhang QY.., Zhang Y., Shao GZ., Jin YY., Zhang S., Lin M., Rui JA. & Ye DX. (2003). Identification and characterization of LAPTM4B encoded by a human hepatocellular carcinoma-associated novel gene, *J Peking University (health Sciences)*, Vol.35, No.4, (May 2003), pp.340-347, ISSN1671-167X

Liu XR., Zhou RL., Zhang QY., Zhang Y., Jin YY., Lin M, Rui JA. & Ye DX. (2004). Structure analysis and expressions of a novel tetratransmembrane protein, LAPTM4B, associated with hepatocellular carcinoma. *World J Gestroenterology*, Vol.10, No.11, pp.1555－1559.

Liu XR., Xiong FX., Wei XH., Yang H. & Zhou RL. (2009). LAPTM4B-35, a Novel Tetratransmembrane Protein and its PPRP Motif Play Critical Roles in Proliferation and Metastatic Potential of HCC Cells, *Cancer Sci*, Vol.100, No.12, pp.2335-2340.

Liu Y., Zhang QY., Qian N. & Zhou RL. (2007). Relationship between LAPTM4B gene polymorphism and susceptibility of gastric cancer， *Annals of Oncology*，Vol.18, No.2, pp.311-316

Longerich T., Mueller MM., Breuhahn K., Schirmacher P., Benner A., Heiss C., Marchio A., Meddeb M., Pineau P., Danglot G., Tiollais P., Bernheim A. & Dejean A. (1997). Recurrent chromosomal abnormalities in hepatocellular carcinoma detected by comparative genomic hybridization. *Genes Chromosomes Cancer.* Vol.18, No.1, pp.59-65.

Martin E. H. (2005). Tetraspanin functions and associated microdomains, *Nature Reviews Molecular Cell Biology,* Vol.6, pp. 801-811

McCubrey JA., Steelman LS., Abrams SL., Lee JT., Chang F., Bertrand FE., Navolanic PM., Terrian DM., Franklin RA., D'Assoro AB., Salisbury JL., Mazzarino MC., Stivala F. & Libra M. (2006). Roles of the RAF/MEK/ERK and PI3K/PTEN/AKT pathways in malignant transformation and drug resistance. *Adv Enzyme Regul.* Vol.46, pp.249-79.

Medema RH., Kops GJ., Bos JL., Burgering BM. (2000). AFX-like Forkhead transcription factors mediate cell-cycle regulation by Ras and PKB through p27kip1. *Nature,* Vol.404, No.6779, pp.782-787.

Meng FL., Luo C., Hu YL., Yin MZ., Lin M., Lou G. & Zhou RL. (2010a). Over-expression of LAPTM4B-35 in Cervical Carcinoma. *Int J Gynecol Pathol,* Vol.29, No.6, pp.587-93.

Meng FL., Yin MZ., Hong-tao Song, T Hua Yang, t Ge Lou,* & Zhou RL. (2010b). LAPTM4B-35 Over-expression Is an Independent Prognostic Marker in Endometrial Carcinoma. *Int J Gynecol Cancer,* Vol.20, No.5, pp.745-50.

Meng F., Song H., Luo C., Yin M., Xu Y., Liu H., Zhou R., & Lou G. (2011). Correlation of LAPTM4B polymorphisms with cervical carcinoma. *Cancer*, Vol.117, No.12, pp.2652-8.

Ouchida R., Kurosaki T. & Wang JY. (2010). A role for lysosomal-associated protein transmembrane 5 in the negative regulation of surface B cell receptor levels and B cell activation. *J Immunol.* Vol.185, No.1, pp.294-301.

Peng C., Zhou RL., Shao GZ., Rui JA., Wang SB., Lin M., Zhang S & Gao ZF. (2005). The expressions of LAPTM4B-35, a novel tetratransmembrane protein, in cancers and the correlation with the differentiation status of HCC. *World J Gestroenterology*, Vol.11, No.18, pp.2704-2708. ISSN 1007-9324

Sears R., Nuckolls F., Haura E., Taya Y., Tamai K. & Nevins J R. (2000). Multiple Ras-dependent phosphorylation pathways regulate Myc protein stability. *Genes Dev;*Vol.14, pp.2501-2514.

Seimiya M., O-Wang J., Bahar R., Kawamura K., Wang Y., Saisho H. & Tagawa M. (2003). Stage-specific expression of Clast6/E3/LAPTM5 during B cell differentiation: elevated expression in human B lymphomas. *Int J Oncol.* Vol..22, No.2, pp.301-4.

Shao GZ., Zhou RL., Zhang QY., Zhang Ye., Liu JJ.,. Rui JA., Wei XH. & Ye DX. (2003). Molecular cloning and characterization of LAPTM4B, a novel gene upregulated in hepatocellular carcinoma. *Oncogene,* Vol.22, pp.5060–5069

Takigawa Y. & Brown AM. (2008). Wnt signaling in liver cancer. *Curr Drug Targets.* Vol.9, No.11, pp.1013-24.

Tazzari PL., Cappellini A., Ricci F., Evangelisti C., Papa V., Grafone T.et al. (2007). MRP1 & PI3K/Akt multidrug resistance-associated protein 1 expression is under the control of the phosphoinositide 3 kinase/Akt signal transduction network in human acute myelogenous leukemia blasts. *Leukemia,* Vol.21, pp.427–438.

Vergarajauregui S., Martina JA. & Rosa Puertollano. (2011). LAPTMs regulate lysosomal function and interact with mucolipin 1: new clues for understanding mucolipidosis type IV. *Journal of Cell Science,* Vol.124, pp.459-468

Wang XH., Meng XW., Sun X., Liu BR., Han MZ., DU YJ., Song YY. & Xu W. (2011). Wnt/β-catenin signaling regulates MAPK and Akt1 expression and growth of hepatocellular carcinoma cells. *Neoplasma.* Vol.58, No.3, pp.239-44.

Whittaker S., Marais R. & Zhu AX., 2010, The role of signaling pathways in the development and treatment of hepatocellular carcinoma. *Oncogene,* Vol.29, pp.4989–5005

Yang, H., Xiong, FX., Lin, M., Qi, RZ., Liu, ZW., Rui, JA., Su, J. & Zhou, RL. (2010a). LAPTM4B-35 Is a Novel Diagnostic Marker and a Prognostic Factor of Hepatocellular Carcinoma. *J Surgical Oncology,* Vol.101, pp.363–369.

Yang H, Xiong FX, Lin M, Yang Y, Nie X and Zhou RL. (2010b) LAPTM4B-35 over-expression is a risk factor for tumor recurrence and poor prognosis in hepatocellular carcinoma, *J Cancer Res Clin Oncol.* , Vol.136, pp.275-281.

Yang H., Xiong F., Wei X., Yang Y., McNutt MA. & Zhou RL. (2010c). Over-expression of LAPTM4B-35 promotes growth and metastasis of hepatocellular carcinoma in vitro and in vivo. *Cancer Lett* , Vol.294, pp.236–244.

Yang Y., Yang H. , Mcnutt MA., Xiong FX., Nie X., Li L. & Zhou RL. (2008). LAPTM4B over-expression is an independent prognostic marker in ovarian carcinoma, *Oncology Reports,* Vol.20, No.5, pp.1077-1083.

Yin M., Li C., Li X., Lou G., Miao B., Liu X., Meng F., Zhang H., Chen X., Sun M., Ling Q. & Zhou RL. (2011a). Over-expression of LAPTM4B is associated with poor prognosis and chemotherapy resistance in stages III and IV epithelial ovarian cancer. *J Surg Oncol.* Vol.104, No.1, pp.29-36.

Yin M., Xu Y., Lou G., Hou Y., Meng F., Zhang H., Li C. & Zhou RL. (2011b). LAPTM4B over-expression is a novel predictor of epithelial ovarian carcinoma metastasis. *Int J Cance,* Vol.129, No.3, pp.629-35

Zhou L., He XD., Chen J., Cui QC., Qu Q., Rui JA. & Zhao YP. (2007) Overexpression of LAPTM4B-35 closely correlated with clinicopathological features and post-resectional survival of gallbladder carcinoma. Eur J Cancer. Vol.43, No.4, pp.809-15.

Zhou L., He XD., Cui QC., Zhou WX., Qu Q., Zhou RL., Rui JA. & Yu JC. (2008), Expression of LAPTM4B-35: A novel marker of progression, invasiveness and poor prognosis of extrahepatic cholangiocarcinoma. *Cancer Lett.* Vol.264, No.2, pp.209-217.

Zhou L., He XD., Yu JC., Zhou RL., Yang H., Qu Q. &, Rui JA. (2010a). Over-expression of LAPTM4B promotes growth of gallbladder carcinoma cells in vitro. *Am J Surg* , Vol.199, No.4, pp.515-21.

Zhou L., He XD., Yu JC., Zhou RL., Xiong FX., Qu Q., Rui JA. (2010b). Expression of LAPTM4B in gallbladder carcinoma cells: the role in invasive potential. *Hepatogastroenterology,* Vol. 57, No.98, pp.207-11.

Zhou L., He XD., Yu JC., Zhou RL., Shan Y. & Rui JA. (2011). Overexpression of LAPTM4B-35 attenuates epirubucin-induced apoptosis of gallbladder carcinoma GBC-SD cells. *Surgery,* Vol. 150, No.1, pp.25-31

2

# Novel Therapeutic Targets for Hepatocellular Carcinoma Treatment

Yangchao Chen and Chi Han Li
*School of Biomedical Sciences, Faculty of Medicine*
*The Chinese University of Hong Kong*
*Hong Kong SAR*

## 1. Introduction

Hepatocellular carcinoma (HCC) is one of the most common cancers worldwide. Surgery is a possible curative treatment, but most symptomatic HCC cases are in advanced stage where surgical resection is not possible. For this group of patients, the prognosis after any kind of therapy remains unsatisfactory due to high relapse rate (Llovet et al., 2003). Studies were rigorously conducted to tackle various obstacles in treating HCC, putting the focuses on targeting cancer cells that either disseminated from the tumor origin, or escaped from therapeutic effects. Recently, a multikinase inhibitor sorafenib was approved by FDA for the treatment of advanced HCC patients. It marks a major advance in the field as the first efficacious targeted therapy for HCC. The primary molecular targets of sorafenib include vascular endothelial factor receptor (VEGFR), platelet derived growth factor receptor (PDGFR) and Raf (Wilhelm et al., 2004). Although it significantly prolongs both patient survival and the time to progression, its overall survival benefit is modest (Llovet et al., 2008).

Other HCC associated targets, such as epidermal growth factor (EGF) signaling (Hampton, 2007), telomerase (Djojosubroto et al., 2005) and cyclooxygenase (Márquez-Rosado et al, 2005), were studied intensively with regard to their therapeutic effects. However, the benefits are far from satisfactory, so there is still a need to identify new therapeutic targets. The exploration of new targets against HCC involves multiple disciplines including hepatology, oncology, pathology and molecular studies. Increasing number of therapeutic targets which play crucial roles in HCC were identified. Identification of new targets not only improves the current HCC therapeutic modality, but also drives a deeper understanding of HCC that allows personalized treatment in the future. In this chapter, we will briefly review the novel molecular and cellular players that contribute to HCC tumorigenesis and progression, and evaluate their potential as additional therapeutic targets.

## 2. Growth receptor signaling

The studies of sorafenib administration and other growth signaling inhibitors demonstrated the prowess of targeting growth signalings such as epidermal growth factor (EGF), VEGF and PDGF pathways. In HCC, many other growth signalings were identified that markedly contributes to tumorigenesis and pathogenesis. They include insulin-like growth factor signaling and mTOR pathway, and numerous studies suggested these pathways can be the targets against HCC.

### 2.1 Insulin-like growth factor signaling

The insulin-like growth factor (IGF) signaling pathway is frequently dysregulated in HCC. The activation of IGF signaling can be established in malignant cells through an autocrinal route when the activated signaling is induced by an overexpressed IGF ligand in HCC cells (Nussbaum et al., 2008). Insulin-like growth factor 2 (IGF-2) is increased after an inflammatory response to liver damage or viral transactivation (Feitelson et al., 2004), and it is the major ligand contributing to the increased IGF activity in HCC. IGF-2-mediated induction of IGF signaling is prevalent in human HCC, where IGF-2 is overexpressed in 16-40%, whilst the level of competitive receptor for IGF-2 is decreased in around 80% (Whittaker et al., 2010). As such, IGF receptor-ligand binding is enhanced, and subsequent downstream signaling is activated in cancer cells. Activation of IGF signaling in HCC cells is associated with increase of cell proliferation rate (Schirmacher et al, 1992). While RNAi-mediated knockdown of IGF-2 could reduce the cell proliferation and induce apoptosis in HCC cells, small molecule inhibiting IGF-2-dependent IGF signaling was able to impair the growth of HCC cells and retard tumour growth in mice xenograft (Lund et al., 2004).

Altered IGF-2 bioavailability is another reason for the hyperactivation of IGF signaling in HCC. Normally, circulating IGF-2 is bound by IGF-binding protein (IGFBP) so that the efficiency of ligand-receptor binding is lowered. In HCC, members of IGFBPs are downregulated so that less IGF-2 is sequestrated which allow uncontrolled IGF-2-receptor interaction (Hanafusa et al, 2002). Hence, reducing the level of IGF-2 in circulation is another valid approach to abrogate the IGF signaling. Re-introduction of recombinant human IGFBP-3 was tested and showed potent effect in lowering the activity of IGF-2 (Aishima et al., 2006). IGFBP-3 was able to inhibit cancer cell growth and attenuate mitogenic activity of HCC cells. It is also reported that IGFBP-3 decreased the phosphorylation and activity of numerous pro-tumorigenic proteins such as IRS-1, MAPK, Elk-1, Akt-1 and phosphatidylinositol 3'-kinase (Huynh et al., 2002).

In addition, inhibition of IGF signaling can also be achieved by disrupting other players along the IGF signaling axis. IGF signal transduction is mediated by the Insulin receptor, IGF-IR and a hybrid of both receptors. In HCC, there is detectable level of IGF receptors ready for the signal generation stimulated by the overexpressed IGF-2. Studies showed that blocking of the receptors was able to give antitumoral effect in HCC cells (Nussbaum et al., 2008). Selective blockage of IGF-IR by monoclonal antibody effectively disrupted IGF signaling, reduced cell viability and proliferation. The inhibition of IGF-IR signal initiation was able to delay tumor growth and prolonged survival in vivo (Tovar et al., 2010). With understanding of IGF signaling mechanism in HCC, it is possible to employ various strategies to effectively inhibit IGF signaling, and in turn suppress cell proliferation and increase apoptosis in HCC.

### 2.2 mTOR pathway

mTOR pathway is a downstream growth signal induced by EGF and IGF signaling, and is coupled with PI3K/AKT pathway. mTOR pathway has an important role in the pathogenesis of HCC, where aberration of mTOR pathway was seen in 15% to 41% of HCC cases ranged from 15% to 41% (Hu et al., 2003). In HCC, the commonly hyperactive EGF and IGF signaling is responsible for the induction of PI3K/AKT/mTOR pathway, promoting tumor progression. The mTOR signaling is mediated by mTOR complex 1 and 2 (mTORC1 and mTORC2). mTORC1 is comprised of mTOR, regulatory associated protein of mTOR (RAPTOR), and mammalian LST8/G-protein β-subunit-like protein. mTORC1 is a downstream signal of AKT, and has a pivotal role in regulating cell growth and proliferation. mTORC1 activates S6 kinase to regulate protein synthesis and induces cell cycle to proceed from G1 to S phase (Bjornsti and Houghton, 2004).

Besides, mTOR is also the subunit of mTORC2 which consists of a protein RAPTOR-independent companion of mTOR (RICTOR), and proline-rich protein 5/G-protein β-subunit-like protein. Unlike mTORC1 which is inducible by AKT, mTORC2 plays a critical role in the phosphorylation and activation of AKT (Sarbassov et al., 2005). The serine/threonine kinase AKT acts as a cytoplasmic regulator of numerous signals. It is shown that AKT is frequently amplified and overexpressed in various cancers, and it demonstrates significant oncogenic properties in diverse cancer types. In homeostasis condition, AKT is negatively regulated by the tumor-suppressor PTEN. However, increased activation of AKT is often observed, because PTEN is frequently lost in cancers including HCC. Other than mTORC1, AKT regulates a wide-spectrum of targets such as cyclin D1 and MDM2/p53 (Vivanco & Sawyers, 2002). In HCC, aberration of mTORC2 enhances AKT activity, induces downstream AKT targets and promotes tumorigenesis. One can see that the AKT regulating effect of mTORC2 is as important as mTORC1 within the PI3K/AKT/mTOR pathway.

Recently, it is suggested that the PI3K/AKT/mTOR pathway can be a major molecular target in cancer remedy. As a critical player in the mTOR signaling, the activity of mTOR often increases in HCC. Blockage of mTOR-mediated signaling showed antineoplastic activity in different experimental models of HCC. The use of mTOR inhibitors could reduce cell proliferation in vitro, and decrease tumor growth in xenografted mouse model (Villanueva et al., 2008). mTOR inhibitors such as sirolimus and everolimus demonstrated potent antitumor properties. Encouraging results were obtained when both mTOR inhibitors were studied in clinical trials, either as a single agent or as adjuvant. Furthermore, components in the mTOR complexes can also be the therapeutic targets. High level of RICTOR is correlated to early recurrence in HCC, and siRNA knockdown of RICTOR reduces HCC cells viability (Villanueva et al., 2008). Disruption of mTOR complexes might have additive benefit along with mTOR inhibition to abrogate mTOR pathway in treating HCC.

## 3. Cell-surface protein

### 3.1 Glypican-3

Glypican-3 (GPC3) is a protein anchored to the cell surface by a glycosyl-phosphatidylinositol link. Glypican-3 is highly expressed in HCC, and plays a role in stimulating various tumorigenic signaling pathways. GPC3 is specifically expressed in HCC, but not in cholangiocarcinoma or normal liver tissue. More than 70% of HCC tumors were observed with high GPC3 level compared to normal liver tissues (Hsu et al., 1997). Consistent with the high GPC3 protein expression found in clinical samples, numerous

HCC cell lines have high expression level of GPC3 (Midorikawa et al., 2003). In addition, GPC3 expression is correlated with the prognosis of HCC, where GPC3-positive HCC patients have a significantly lower 5-year survival rate than patients who are GPC3-negative (Shirakawa et al., 2009).

One of the GPC3 tumorigenic roles is the activation of Wnt/β-catenin signaling. It is shown that GPC3 is able to interact with Wnt ligands, and induces canonical Wnt-signaling to trigger the stabilization of β-catenin and induction of cyclin D1 (Capurro et al., 2005). The heparin sulfate chain of GPC3 is reported to bind with basic growth factors such as FGF-2. The interaction between GPC3 and FGF-2 is frequently observed in HCC cells, and is responsible for phosphorylation of ERK and AKT (Midorikawa et al., 2003). This interaction plays a role in the increase of HCC cell proliferation, and growth of tumor in nude mouse model. Additionally, GPC3 interplays with hedgehog signaling in regulating developmental growth (Capurro et al., 2008). Though yet to be elucidated, the GPC3-hedgehog signaling is suggested to contribute to HCC development.

Targeting GPC3 and its related growth signaling is a relevant approach to inhibit HCC growth. Inhibition of the interaction between GPC3 and Wnt or FGF-2 should theoretically reduce HCC growth (Capurro et al., 2005; Midorikawa et al., 2003). GPC3 is also a useful target in immunotherapy against HCC. The therapeutic monoclonal antibody against GPC3 has been developed which could induce antibody-dependent HCC cytotoxicity. Targeting GPC3 is able to inhibit tumor growth of HCC cell line xenograft (Ishiguro et al., 2008). Study also showed the concomitant treatment with GPC3 monoclonal antibody and sorafenib was more potent in preventing tumor growth than sorafenib alone in the HepG2 xenograft model (Ishiguro et al., 2008). It is likely that targeting GPC3 could provide great clinical benefit during HCC management.

### 3.2 Cadherin 17

Cadherins are important cell adhesion molecules strongly associated with cancer progression. Downregulation of E-cadherin (Du et al., 2009) and overexpression of P-cadherin are often observed in advanced tumor which processes crucial cellular event like epithelial-mesenchymal transition (Sun et al., 2011). Cadherin 17 (CDH17) is another adhesion molecule upregulated in HCC, and it is linked to the tumorigenesis in various gastrointestinal regions (Wang et al., 2005). The upregulation of CDH17 is capable of transforming premalignant liver progenitor cells into liver carcinomas in mice. While forced expression of CDH17 promoted tumor growth from hepatic progenitor cells, silencing of CDH17 reduced the aggressiveness of metastatic HCC cells (Liu et al., 2009). Knockdown of CDH17 by RNA-interference decreased the proliferation rate of HCC cell lines despite their metastatic potential in vitro and in vivo. It is shown that targeting CDH17 can concurrently inactivate Wnt/β-catenin signaling and reduce cyclin D1 level, leading to both growth inhibition and cell death. Inhibition of CDH17 results in the re-localization of nuclear β-catenin to the cytoplasm so as to attenuate the Wnt/β-catentin signaling (Liu et al., 2009).

Multiple isoforms of CDH17 protein are present in the HCC samples, and it is found that the isoform lacking exon 7 is the most abundant in HCC samples (Wang et al., 2005). CDH17 isoform lacking exon 7 cannot be found in normal liver tissue whereas it is present in about 50% of human HCC and 30% of premalignant tissues. Detection of this CDH17 isoform was strongly correlated with the prognosis of HCC patients, predicting a shorter overall survival rate as well as higher relapse rate and venous infiltration after surgery (Wang et al., 2005). This CDH17 isoform, together with others that are exclusively expressed in HCC, might contribute to the pathogenesis of HCC. Strategy to target the isoforms of CDH17 allows specifically aiming malignant cells rather than the normal hepatocytes. All available evidences suggested that targeting CDH17 might be a prospective molecular-based therapy in HCC.

## 4. Metabolic pathway

### 4.1 Arginine metabolism

Arginine content is well-known to affect transplanted tumor in mice. Enhanced in vivo tumor growth is observed when mice were fed with diet rich in arginine. On the other hand, depletion of arginine from their diet inhibits the growth of metastatic tumor (Gonzalez & Byus, 1991). It is later proved that arginine is essential for the survival of cancer cells. Cancer cells are dependent on exogenous arginine for growth because most of them cannot synthesize their own and become auxotropic for arginine (Dillon et al., 2004). There are various explanations for the acquisition of arginine auxotropic phenotype in various cancer cells, but generally it is associated with the downregulation of argininosuccinate synthase (ASS) (Dillon et al., 2004). Arginine auxotrophy is also a common phenomenon in HCC cells due to their lackage of ASS (Ensor et al., 2002).

In somatic cells, deficiency of arginine puts cell cycle on hold, and cells enter the quiescence $G_0$ phase. They can tolerate the depletion of arginine for weeks and return to normal condition once the arginine content is resumed. On the other hand, arginine deficiency is not sustainable in cancer cells (Delage et al., 2010). Defect in cell cycle checkpoint drives continuous cell proliferation even with insufficient arginine, but arginine is necessary for metabolic and enzymatic pathways in malignant cells. In essence, cancer cells with shortage of ASS rely heavily on exogenous arginine. If the uptake of arginine is disrupted, or the stability of arginine is lowered, cell death will occur due to a loss of gross balance (Delage et al., 2010). This physiological difference between normal and cancer cell makes the arginine metabolic pathway a potent target in treatment to distinguish HCC cells from normal cells.

Reducing arginine stability is one of the strategies against malignant cells, and arginine-degrading enzyme is the major group of enzymes that can serve the purpose in depleting internal arginine. Arginase belongs to such group of enzyme which is responsible for arginine degradation in the urea cycle, and its anticancer effect is well documented (Bach et al., 1963). In addition to arginase, the enzyme arginine deiminas is proved to efficiently deplete cellular arginine in vitro and in vivo (Cheng et al., 2007). Recombinant arginine-degrading enzymes were developed, and their anticancer effect was investigated in HCC. Satisfactory result was obtained using recombinant arginase and arginine deiminas to combat ASS-deficient tumors (Izzo et al., 2004). Studies are conducted to improve the efficacy of these arginine-degrading enzymes. Modification such as pygelation can increase the half-life of the enzyme and prolong its activity. Phase III trial deploying a pegylated form of recombinant ADI is undertaken in HCC patients who have failed prior systemic treatment. It is also reported that a modified recombinant human arginase is able to inhibit ASS-positive HCC, and inhibit tumor cell growth (Cheng et al., 2007).

### 4.2 GLUT1-mediated anaerobic glycolysis

Due to the high proliferation rate and cell motility rate, the energy requirement of malignant cells is immense. It is suggested that malignant cells have their metabolic rate accelerated in order to accommodate the excess energy consumption, and glucose is the basic unit necessary. Like most cancers, HCC has high glucose requirement and is observed with an increase of glucose metabolism. While glucose metabolism in eukaryotic cells has multiple levels of control, transport of glucose across the cell membrane is the first rate limiting step. Indeed, accelerated glucose metabolism in cancer cells has been associated with increased expression of glucose transporter proteins. In HCC, increase uptake of glucose is mediated by glucose transporter GLUT1. GLUT1 expression is elevated in hypoxic conditions, and this elevates the rate of anaerobic glycolysis which is a metabolic event frequently observed in HCC (Amann et al., 2009). Level of GLUT1 determines the rate of anaerobic glycolysis, affects glucose uptake and utilization, and plays a role in metastasis, chemoresistance and immunity evasion.

Increased GLUT1 expression is observed in all HCC cell lines compared with primary hepatocytes, and this increase could be found in a subset of HCC patients (Amann et al., 2009). It is demonstrated that suppression of GLUT1 expression by siRNA significantly impaired the tumorigenicity of HCC cells. Inhibition of GLUT1 could decelerate anaerobic glcolysis, implied by the reduction of both glucose uptake and lactate secretion (Amann et al., 2009). RNAi-mediated targeting of GLUT1 is a potent way to combat cancer cells as shown in the study of gastric cancer and laryngeal cancer. GLUT1 is possibly a druggable target as it is shown that the ATP-binding site is important for the conformation and transporter affinity (Liu et al., 2001). Several substances have demonstrated the ability to inhibit GLUT1 and cause cancer cell death (Martin et al., 2003). To increase the GLUT1 targeting specificity, derivatives of the GLUT1 inhibitors were generated and showed promising anticancer effect (Morris et al., 1991).

Glucose analogues or glucose conjugates also serve to inhibit anaerobic glycolysis. Glucose analog such as 2-Deoxyglucose reduced the proliferation rate of many hepatoma cells (Ingram et al., 2006), and showed enhanced anticancer effects in combination with conventional chemotherapeutic drugs such as adriamycin or paclitaxel in xenografted mice (Maschek et al., 2004). The use of ketogenic diets is an alternative strategy to target the anaerobic metabolism, which is based on a high fat and low carbohydrate diet and mimic the metabolic state of fasting (Zhou et al., 2007). As a result, a reduction of carbohydrate intake occurs which allows ketones as an alternative fuel for normal tissue. All in all, disruption of critical metabolic pathways in HCC cells or targeting the main components of the pathways might become alternative therapeutic strategies.

## 5. Protein folding and turnover

### 5.1 Heat shock protein 90

Heat shock protein 90 (HSP90) belongs to a highly conserved family of molecular chaperones. It plays a role in protein homeostasis by controlling the stabilization and activation processes of different proteins (Pearl et al., 2008). HSP90 level is often increased in various tumors, which is associated with the continuous protein translation and cell proliferation during stress condition (Workman et la., 2007). Upregulation of HSP90 is often associated with increased cyclin-dependent kinase 4 activity, and both were believed to contribute to HCC development (Pascale et al., 2005). HSP90 is involved in the folding and activity of many bona fide oncoproteins in tumor cells, maintaining their dysregulated expression and mutational status. Subsequently, tumor cells become sustainable for cell growth and survival, and equip with crucial aberrations required for metastasis (Whitesell & Lindquist, 2005).

HSP90 is proved to be an efficacious therapeutic target in HCC. Inhibition of a broad-spectrum tumorigenic mechanism is resulted when HSP90 is targeted in vitro and in vivo. Independent of the etiological background, all HCC cell lines responded to HSP90 inhibition similarly with increased cell cycle arrest and apoptosis (Breinig et al., 2009). It might due to the fact that HSP90 inhibition triggered a simultaneous degradation of various hepatocarcinogenesis driving factors. In vivo studies showed that inhibitor of HSP90 is tumor-cell specific, and is able to efficiently reduce HCC tumor growth. Newly developed HSP90 inhibitor showed a lack of significant hepatotoxicity and is more tolerated, which become more practical in therapeutic treatment (Breinig et al., 2009). HSP90 inhibition further prevents tumor growth by disruption of tumor angiogenesis, as demonstrated by blocking PDGFR-β expression in vascular smooth muscle cells and VEGF2 expression on endothelial cells (Lang et al., 2009). Moreover, the combinatory use of HSP90 inhibitor and other anticancer agents is proved to be beneficial. Blockage of HSP90 is able to enhance the antitumor effect of mTOR inhibitor rapamycin by blocking the alternative AKT signaling induced by rapamycin (Lang et al., 2009). Inhibition of HSP90 can be invaluable clinically during HCC treatment, either by targeting HSP90 alone or in combination with other anticancer agent.

### 5.2 Ubiquitin-proteasome system

The ubiquitin-proteasome system plays a crucial role in maintaining cellular homeostasis such as regulation of the cell cycle, apoptosis, receptor signaling and endocytosis. Aberration in different ubiquitin-proteasome systems is recognized as the fundamental cause of various human diseases including cancer. The dysregulation of NF-κB in HCC is one of the oncogenic events induced upon defect in ubiquitin-proteasome system. It is also observed proteins expressed by HBV (Hu et al., 1999) and HCV (Munakata et al., 2005) are reported to cause the alteration of different ubiquitin-proteasome systems, contributing to viral replication, hepatotumorigenesis and impairment of host immunity. These findings demonstrate the importance of an intact ubiquitin-proteasome system in preventing HCC development (Chen, 2005). In the United States, a proteasome inhibitor bortezomib is used clinically to manage late-stage multiple myeloma (Chauhan et al., 2008). Studying the mechanisms of various ubiquitin-proteasome systems not only enable a better understanding of cancers, but also help to explore new strategies to cancer management.

#### 5.2.1 Gankyrin

In human HCC, a small proteasome regulatory subunit called gankyrin is frequently over-expressed at both mRNA and protein levels. A study showed gankyrin expression levels were highly upregulated in hepatoma cell lines, and its level was higher in HCC samples compared to normal livers, and premalignant or cirrhotic livers (Higashitsuji et al., 2000). Gankyrin is found to interact with retinoblastoma, increasing its phosphorylation level so as to reduce cellular retinoblastoma stability (Li et al., 2005). In addition, gankyrin increases both the association and activity of MDM2 for p53. This inactivates p53 by increasing the ubiquitylation level of p53 and in turn driving proteasomal degradation of p53 (Higashitsuji et al., 2005). Gankyrin also promotes HCC growth through the activation of oncoprotein D cyclin-dependent kinase 4 (CDK4). The activity of the kinase is negatively regulated by p16 during stress condition, but this inhibitory effect is removed when gankyrin competes with p16 for the binding of CDK4 and thus allows the activation of CDK4 (Dawson et al., 2002). Other than tumor promoting effect, gankyrin contributes to cancer drug resistance. It desensitizes cancer cells to the effect of DNA-damaging chemical agents by preventing p53-dependent apoptosis (Higashitsuji et al., 2005).

The use of RNAi to knock down gankyrin in HCC resulted in a decrease of cell growth, as well as reduction in observed levels of hyperphosphorylated retinoblastoma (Li et al., 2005) and restoration of caspase 8/9-dependent apoptosis (Higashitsuji et al., 2005). Silencing of gankyrin expression also reportedly attenuated epithelial to mesenchymal transition together with cell migration and invasion. The inhibition of gankyrin also reduced the level of nuclear β-catenin (Dong et al., 2011), c-myc, cyclin D1 (Fu et al., 2011) and insulin-like growth factor binding protein 5 (Umemura et al., 2008). The close relationship with several pro-tumorgenic events makes gankyrin a rationale target during HCC treatment.

### 5.2.2 X-linked inhibitor of apoptosis

X-linked inhibitor of apoptosis (XIAP) belongs to the inhibitor of apoptosis (IAP) domain-containing family, and is famous of its anti-apoptotic ability. They are induced by NF-κB signaling to circumvent the pro-apoptotic effect induced by JNK pathway (Kaur et al., 2005), by inhibiting caspase-mediated apoptosis. Apart from this, XIAP participates in the regulation of transforming growth factor β (TGF-β) -induced apoptosis through an ubiqutin-proteasomal regulating machine. XIAP is able to complex with TGF-β activated kinase 1 (TAK1), as such this negatively regulates the TGF-β signaling (Chen, 2005). The RING domain of XIAP is responsible for the poly-ubiquitylation of TAK1, resulting the proteasome-mediated degradation of TAK1. Subsequently, it disrupts the activation of JNK signaling and halts apoptosis. It is speculated that the involvement of XIAP in HCC is common given that most HCCs acquire resistance to TGF-β-mediated cell killing (Chen, 2005). Moreover, TAK1 is important for the phosphorylation and activation of the IKK complex. Increased activity of IKK leads to the degradation of the IκB-α inhibitor of NF-κB and subsequent activation of classical NF-κB signaling. Activation of IKK also causes the degradation of MKK7, the upstream kinase essential for activation of JNK signaling. Reduction of MKK7 level could ablate the JNK signaling and inhibit apoptosis (Kaur et al., 2005).

Inhibition of XIAP sensitizes HCC cells to apoptotic signal owing to retaining of TAK1. In doing so, persistent activation of JNK signaling is resulted whenever the TGF-β-mediated apoptotic signal is induced. Stabilized TAK1 also potentially attenuate the influence of NF-κB signals (Chen, 2005). Besides, it is reported XIAP inhibition in HCC enhanced TRAIL-mediated cell killing. The combination of XIAP silencing shRNA and tumor-necrosis factor-related apoptosis TRAIL is reported to generate potent antitumor effect in HCC cells and tumors in animal models (Pan et al., 2008). Targeting XIAP further renders HCC cells vulnerable to other therapeutic effect by releasing the break for caspase-mediated apoptosis

(Deveraux et al., 1997). All in all, inhibition of XIAP or blockage of interaction between XIAP and TAK1 may be one of the best HCC management strategies.

## 6. HCC tumor microenvironment

It is gradually accepted that the progression and aggressiveness of cancer cells are defined by the tumor-stromal interaction. In HCC, the tumor microenvironment plays a pivotal role in affecting cancer development. Through paracrine and autocrine mechanisms, the stromal components communicate with the tumor, promoting the HCC cell proliferation, survival, and allowing them to invade and metastasize. In the past, majority of targeting therapies are derived from the research focusing on intracellular events of cancer cells. However, limited studies are able to be translated into effective therapies, because they ignored the influence from the surrounding components. Although the field is still in its embryonic stage waiting to be explored, targeting the interaction between tumor-stromal may be a more logical approach against HCC.

### 6.1 Hepatic stellate cells

Stromal remodeling occurs routinely during the development of hepatic fibrosis, cirrhosis and HCC, featured with the infiltration of activated hepatic stellate cells (HSC). Upon hepatic injury, HSCs is stimulated and transformed to acquire an activated myofibroblast-like phenotype that is responsible for the excessive hepatic matrix deposition in chronically damaged livers. They are densely located in tumor sinusoids, fibrous septa and HCC-generated capsule. Activation of HSC is recognized as a key event during hepatotumorigenesis (Zhao et al., 2011).

Activated HSCs considerably increase the activity of NF-κB and ERK in HCC. It is known that both NF-κB and MAP kinase/ERK pathways are involved in the progression of human HCC, and they induce the proliferation of HCC cells, and protect HCC cells from apoptosis (Amann et al., 2009). The paracrinal communication between HSC and HCC forms the major linkage for the induction of HCC development. Several soluble factors secreted by activated HSC are identified to be responsible for the tumorigenic effects. HSC released a substantial amount of protumorigenic factors, including the hepatic growth factor (HGF), which enhances the invasiveness of HCC cells. The growth and the migration capability of HCC were impaired once the binding of HGF to HCC cells was disrupted (Barnaeva et al., 2007). Other studies demonstrated that TGF-β secreted by HSC accelerated tumor progression in neoplastic hepatocyte (Sano et al., 2005). TGF-β was able to induce epithelial to mesenchymal transition and augment PDGF signaling in oncogenic Ras-transformed hepatocyte. It is believed that a combination of HSC-released growth factors consisting of FGF-1 and -2, PDGF and IGF are responsible for promoting HCC tumorigenesis (Bataller & Brenner, 2005). The emerging evidences support that the activated HSC/myofibroblasts in tumor microenvironment have huge impact on HCC development and progression, and this stromal components should be regarded as one of the primary targets in HCC therapy.

### 6.2 Heparan sulfate proteoglycan modulating enzymes

Heparan sulfate proteoglycans (HSPG) play important biological roles in both cellular and extracellular context, contributing to the proper communication between cells and their surrounding components. While extracellular HSPGs function to maintain extracellular matrix (ECM) self assembly and integrity with other ECM molecules, cell surface HSPGs are responsible for the binding of growth factors, chemokines, cytokines and enzymes. In addition to normal biological process, HSPGs also influence a number of pathological events including inflammation, tumor growth, metastasis and angiogenesis.

### 6.2.1 Heparanase

Evidences suggested that the expression of heparanase, an enzyme that degrade the side chain heparin sulfate, is closely related to tumor invasion, angiogenesis and metastasis in HCC (El-Assal et al., 2001). Heparanase level is high both in HCC patient serum and tumor tissues. Heparanase level in serum is linked with the aggressiveness of HCC (Wang et al., 2010), and that in tumors is positively correlated with tumor size, staging and portal vein invasiveness (El-Assal et al., 2001). It is speculated that the major pro-tumorigenic effect of heparanase is derived from the ability to cleave HSPG, resulting in the release of HS-bound molecules such as ECM digesting enzymes and angiogenic factors. Consequent ECM degradation and angiogenic factor released combine to construct a microenvironment favorable for HCC cell migration and invasion (Zhang et al., 2007).

Extensive cleavage of heparin sulfate might release other cell surface bound factors such as growth factors and chemokines that potentially generate diverse biological effects in both autocrine and paracine manners. Upregulation of heparanase is associated with increased releasing of basic fibroblast growth factor (bFGF). bFGF released in this way contributes to tumor progression through the activation of oncogenic signaling and construction of a favourable tumor niche (Zhao et al., 2006).

Targeting heparanase provides a novel perspective in managing HCC by modulating the tumor-stromal communication. Knocking down of heparanase can significantly inhibit the invasiveness, metastasis, and angiogenesis of HCC cell both in vitro and in vivo (Zhang et al., 2007). Several molecule inhibitors of heparanase can also attenuate the progression of hepatoma cells. The antitumor effect is possibly generated by preventing the degradation of ECM and basal membrane. Another study showed inhibiting heparanase could effectively stop the release of bFGF so as to inactivate the bFGF signaling effect and suppress subsequent angiogenesis (Zhao et al., 2006). These findings have gradually switched the attention in cancer therapy research, from focusing solely in intracellular targets to the interplay between cancer cells and the surrounding microenvironment.

### 6.2.2 Sulfatase 2

Another important feature of heparin sulfate chains is related to its substrate binding capacity. 6-O-sulfation, a type of heparin sulfate modification, is known to play a specific role in modulating ligand binding. The enzyme SULF2 is a member of the sulfatase family that modulates critical cellular signaling pathways by the removal of 6-O-sulfation (Morimoto-Tomita et al., 2002). In contrast to another sulfatase member tumor suppressor SULF1, SULF2 has an oncogenic role in cancer, and its expression is elevated in HCC. Upregulation of SULF2 is observed in 57% HCC tissues and 73% HCC cell lines. Level of SULF2 is positively correlated with a more aggressive tumor phenotype and poorer patient survival (Lai et al., 2008). Ectopic expression of SULF2 promoted cell proliferation and migration in various HCC cell lines, and enhanced tumor growth in vivo. The tumorigenic effect of SULF2 is partially brought by the induction of the aforementioned pro-cancerous glypican-3 expression. It was found that SULF2 enhanced the binding of FGF2 to the cancer cell and activated FGF signaling in a glypican-3 dependent manner (Lai et al., 2008). In addition, SULF2 increased cell surface glypican-3 and Wnt3a level in HCC, leading to the increase of glypican-3-dependent Wnt/β-catenin signaling (Lai et al., 2010).

SULF2 is a rational target in HCC therapy as suggested by several SULF2 knockdown studies. RNAi-induced suppression of SULF2 reduced the cell growth and migration in cell lines with high SULF2 expression (Lai et al., 2010) in vivo and in vitro. Knockdown of SULF2 was able to reduce the expression of GPC3, as well as the activity of FGF signaling by blocking FGF2 binding (Lai et al., 2008). Reduction of GPC3 also downregulates Wnt3a expression, and attenuates the Wnt/β-catenin signaling with reduced phosphorylated GSK3-β and β-catenin. Given the relationship between SULF2 and GPC3, it is worthwhile to investigate the clinical benefit in targeting SULF2 in HCC treatment. Furthemore, SULF2 protects against caspase 3 and 7 mediated apoptosis induced by PI3K, ERK and JNK inhibitor. Inhibition of SULF2 re-sensitized HCC cells to the drug-induced apoptosis by reducing phosphorylation of AKT, downregulation of cyclin D1 and anti-apoptotic BCL-2, as well as upregulation of pro-apoptotic BAD (Lai et al., 2010). The findings might have implication to develop combinatory treatment against drug-resistant HCC.

## 7. Epigenetic modulator

Abnormal epigenetic events are frequently observed in HCC, which can alter gene expression through modification of histone tails or DNA. The major players contributing to these aberrations such as DNA methyltransferase and histone deacetylase are under intensive investigations. In fact, there are many other players involved during the establishment of aberrant epigenetic status. Among them, polycomb repressive complexes (PRC) are catching more attention recently due to their significant roles during cancer development via suppression of various tumor suppressor genes (Steele et al., 2006). In human, there are two polycomb repressive complexes namely PRC1 and PRC2. Despite their unique gene repression mechanism, both of them are frequently involved in the oncogenesis of HCC. Targeting of epigenetic modulators in theory generates persistent effects on tumors as heritable changes are induced. Such an approach is superior to targeting other molecular players that only bring out transient effects.

### 7.1 BMI1

PRC aroused increasing attention recently as they are shown to contribute heavily in the maintenance of stem cell and the determination of cell fate. BMI1 is a critical component of PRC1 in mediating the ubiquitination of histone in order to regulate local gene expression. BMI1 is not detected in normal hepatocyte but is overexpressed in HCC. Dysregulation of BMI1 is speculated to promote activation of cancer stem cell in HCC. BMI1 has a higher basal level in the side-population (SP) cell where such a subgroup of cancer cells is characterized by the ability to exclude Hoechst 33342 dye via the ABC cassette transporter. This subpopulation is believed to harbor stem cell properties, and BMI1 is shown to play a crucial role in their self-renewal process (Chiba et al., 2008).

BMI1 mediates stemness features in HCC cells. In HCC, SP cells expressing BMI1 showed enhanced tumorigenic potential compared to the corresponding non-SP cells. Knockdown of BMI1 markedly abolished the tumor-initiating ability of SP cells in non-obese diabetic/severe combined immunodeficiency mice, leading to a 100 fold decrease of tumorigenic activity (Chiba et al., 2008). Such decrease in tumorigenic activity was accompanied with a reduction of SP cell number in different HCC cell lines. It is shown that BMI1 mediates the suppression of INK4A/ARF and drives self-renewal. Inhibition of BMI1 resulted in the derepression of INK4A/ARF, and in turn disrupted self-renewal in SP cells, hence suppressed SP cells survival upon long time culture. BMI1 additionally regulates diverse cellular processes including cell cycle, apoptosis and senescence by the repression of the INK4A/ARF expression (Xu et al., 2009).

Since there are numerous targets of BMI1 in human genome, it is predictable that the oncogenic effect of BMI1 should not simply depend on INK4A and ARF repression. BMI1 was able to cooperate with activated RAS to transform hepatocytes into malignant cells (Xu et al., 2009). Furthermore, BMI1 expression in HCC is significantly associated with the expression of ABC transporter B1 (ABCB1) which was consistently reported to generate the multiple drug-resistant phenotype (Effendi et al., 2010). It is possible that one of the downstream targets of BMI1 is ABCB1. The ability to eliminate cancer progenitor cell in HCC by BMI1 inhibition is a potent anticancer mediation, and potentially provides a cure for HCC patients.

### 7.2 EZH2

Polycomb repressive complex 2 (PRC2) is another modifier of the chromatin structure, which determines the activity of gene expression. PRC2 primarily regulates gene expression by inducing the methylation on lysine 9 and lysine 27 of histone 3, and plays important roles during development and tumorigenesis. In this complex, EZH2 is the catalytic subunit directly involves in transferring methyl-group to the histone tails (Kirmizis et al., 2004). The level of EZH2 is important in determining the PRC2 activity in cells. EZH2 regulates cell proliferation, and its expression is often augmented during tumorigenesis. EZH2 overexpression can be observed in many cancers, including prostate, breast and pancreas cancer, and most often high level of EZH2 is correlated to aggressiveness of the malignancies (Tsang et al., 2011). EZH2 is rarely detected in normal hepatocytes, but is frequently detected in HCC cell lines and HCC tissues (Chen et al., 2007).

EZH2 is involved in numerous cellular processes and signaling pathways and evidences suggested that EZH2 promotes cancer development by repressing diverse tumor-suppressors. Recently, EZH2 reportedly activated Wnt signaling in HCC. Concurrent overexpression of EZH2 and β-catenin was observed in more than 30% of human HCC, which is associated with tumor progression (Cheng et al., 2011). In HCC cells, EZH2 is found to frequently occupy the promoter of numerous Wnt pathway antagonists. As such, these antagonists are silenced, relieving the inhibitory effect on Wnt/β-catenin signaling. In immortalized hepatocytes, ectopic expression of EZH2 activated Wnt/β-catenin signaling and triggered cell proliferation (Cheng et al., 2011). Conversely, downregulation of EZH2 inhibited β-catenin signaling, resulting in the retardation of HCC cell growth. Study showed that knockdown of EZH2 by lentivirus-based shRNA inhibited tumor growth in vivo (Chen et al., 2007), demonstrating a potent effect against HCC by targeting EZH2. The significance of EZH2 role in HCC suggested that strategies built around EZH2 is definitely advantageous.

EZH2 is theoretically suitable for pharmalogical targeting as it contains a SET domain responsible for the histone methyltransferase activity. Targeting of the enzymatic domain is proved to reduce histone methylation and de-repress expression of tumor suppressor genes. In addition to the catalytic domain, there are two N-terminal domains mediating protein-protein interactions and promoting nuclear localization within EZH protein, which are druggable targets in ablating EZH2 activity. Disruption of the PRC2 is also effective to attenuate the tumorigenic effect of EZH2. The formation of functional PRC2 requires other protein subunits such as EED and SUZ12. Report revealed that the use of agent disrupting PRC2 subunits is a relevant way to affect PRC2 function (Tan et al., 2007). Although currently there is no EZH2 specific inhibitor, but agent such as DZnep is also able to deplete the cellular EZH2, inhibit EZH2 functions and lower the H3K27 trimethylation level (Chiba et al., 2011). This fundamental knowledge surely enables researchers to design potent agents to target EZH2 in HCC.

## 8. Non-coding RNA

### 8.1 MicroRNA

MicroRNAs are small non-coding RNAs that regulate the translation of many genes. They not only regulate normal cell development but also play important roles in cancer development and progression by affecting cell survival, angiogenesis and metastasis. Many studies illustrated the potential of manipulating microRNA expression in cancer therapy. It is believed that microRNA-based remedy can have a huge impact on cancer cells, as they regulate whole programs of gene expression via suppressing hundreds of genes simultaneously (Farazi et al., 2011). In human HCC, numerous microRNAs are identified to give major contributions, either having oncogenic or tumor suppressing ability. Here, those microRNAs having great potential as HCC therapeutic targets will be discussed.

OncomiR is a novel term coined for microRNAs possessing proto-oncogenic effects in cancers. In HCC, a number of oncomiRs are identified and their roles are characterized. Among them, the roles of microRNA-21 (miR-21) in HCC development were well-documented (Liu et al., 2010). miR-21 is universally overexpressed in majority of cancers and is phenomenally involved in approximately all tumorigenic processes. miR-21 is able to induce cell transformation, mediate cancer cell growth, cell cycle and self-renewal, prevent apoptosis, promote metastasis and generate drug-resistance (Liu et al., 2010). High expression of miR-21 is correlated with advanced tumor stage, frequent metastasis and poor patient prognosis. In HCC, miR-21 is overexpressed, and has been proved to promote malignant cell growth and spreading by targeting tumor suppressor PTEN and inducing FAK phosphorylation (Meng et al., 2007). Furthermore, miR-21 induces resistance to anticancer effect of interferon-α and 5-fluorouracil in HCC (Tomimaru et al., 2010). Importantly, inhibition of miR-21 is able to reduce the aggressiveness in HCC, and relieves the suppressive effect to several tumor suppressor genes targeted. Besides miR-21, targeting other oncomiRs such as miR-29 (Xiong et al., 2010) and miR-221 (Pineau et al., 2010) is also robust in reversing the malignant phenotypes in HCC.

On the other hand, various microRNAs with tumor suppressing capacity are lost or underexpressed in HCC. Restoration of their expression in HCC is another effective approach against HCC. Previous studies suggested a strong association between low miR-26 expression and both prognosis and response to interferon therapy in patients with HCC (Ji et al., 2009). Low miR-26 expression is highly associated with tumor formation in vivo, and replenishing miR-26 in liver tumors with the use of gene therapy could generate potent antitumor effects. miR-26a in particular is substantially reduced in MYC-induced HCC (Ji et al., 2009). The replacement therapy of miR-26 is considered safe, because miR-26 is expressed by most normal cells and is unlikely to be toxic. Other than miR-26, miR-122 is significantly downregulated in liver cancer with intrahepatic metastasis. Restoration of miR-122 reduced cell migration, invasion and colony formation ability in vitro, and tumorigenesis, angiogenesis and metastasis in vivo (Coulouarn et al., 2009). Currently, more microRNAs with antitumor effect including miR-199a/b-3p were identified and potentially play a pivotal role in the combat against HCC (Hou et al., 2011).

To note, increased activity of RNA-induced silencing complex (RISC) was observed in HCC (Yoo et al., 2011). The role of RISC is critical in facilitating activity of RNAi including microRNA-mediated target silencing. The components of RISC including AEG-1 and SND1 were both overexpressed in HCC, which leads to the hyperactivity of RISC. Increased RISC activity resulted in an accelerated degradation of numerous tumor suppressor genes that are the target of various oncomiRs. Report showed that inhibition of RISC activity by knocking down SND1 abrogated cell growth in HCC cells in vitro and in vivo (Yoo et al., 2011). It not only unveils a new microRNA associated pro-tumorigenic mechanism, but also provides an additional approach to disrupt microRNA-mediated tumorigenic effect during HCC remedy.

### 8.2 Long non-coding RNA

In eukaryotes, there are abundant amount of transcripts which are long in length and lack any substantial open reading frame as well as protein coding capacity. Increasing evidences suggested that these long non-coding RNAs (lncRNA) play critical role in cellular processes such as development, via the modulation of chromatin structure. Some of them possess the ability to modulate cancer epigenome and contribute to different pathological conditions such as tumor invasion and metastasis. A better understanding in the oncogenic mechanisms of lncRNA will unveil a new direction in cancer therapy.

Highly upregulated in liver cancer (HULC) is an lncRNA that is frequently overexpressed in HCC. siRNA knockdown of HULC in HCC cell lines was able to alter the expression of genes described in the context of HCC (Panzitt et al., 2007). Reduction of cellular HULC upregulated genes participates in diverse biological processes including cell differentiation, cell adhesion, protein phosphorylation and tumor suppression. Another study reported that HULC was also expressed in metastasized tumor nodules in liver originated from colorectal cancer, but not in primary colorectal cancer (Matouk et al., 2009). It suggested that expression of HULC might be a pre-requisite for any tumor formed in liver. The importance of HULC in HCC is further supported by the observation that HULC expression is strongly linked to HBV infection (Matouk et al., 2009). Due to the high specificity of HULC for cancer located in liver, it is worthy of studying its potential role in managing HCC.

There are two other lncRNAs recently reported to be overexpressed in HCC cell lines and tissues, namely the metastasis associated lung adenocarcinoma transcript 1(MALAT-1) and HOX transcript antisense RNA (HOTAIR). Both of them have been previously implicated in other malignancies regarding their capacity to promote cancer metastasis. In HCC, their expression is correlated to the prognosis of the patients which predicts tumor recurrence after liver transplantation. Inhibition of MALAT-1 in vitro effectively reduced cell viability, motility, invasiveness, and HCC cells became sensitive to pro-apoptotic signal (Lai et al., 2011). Similarly, knockdown of HOTAIR decreased cell viability and cell invasiveness, as well as sensitized HCC cells to tumor necrosis factor- α induced apoptosis, and cytotoxic effect of doxorubicin and cisplatin (Yang et al., 2011). Their roles in HCC progression are important which provide a rational base to take into consideration during HCC therapy.

## 9. Liver cancer stem cell

Accumulating evidences support that the development of HCC is based on the cancer stem cell (CSC) model. In this hypothesis, there is only a subset of cells within a tumor or in the cell pool that sustains malignant growth. Such cellular subset is referred to as the cancer-initiating cells or cancer-propagating cells (Visvader, 2011). It provides the explanations for cancer initiation, local recurrence, metastasis and therapy resistance which raised enormous controversies in the past. CSCs have been identified in many cancer types including HCC (Mishra et al., 2009). In this regard, CSC should be the principal target of HCC therapy. However, conventional methods such as chemotherapy and radiotherapy are ineffective because of the CSC resistant properties, as well as their pro-angiogenic effect. Studies are vigorously conducted to develop effective methods to extinguish CSC in HCC.

### 9.1 Cancer stem cell markers

Numerous surface markers for HCC stem cells were identified, and they include CD133, CD90, CD44, CD13 and EpCAM. Although their roles in liver CSC are unclear, studies showed that targeting these markers can specifically harm CSC with high efficacy. It is reported that tumorigenicity and invasive capacity of liver CSC were impaired by targeting CSC surface marker EpCAM, leading to reduction of CSC pool (Yamashita et al., 2009). Besides, inhibition of CD44 in HCC cells could enhance apoptosis, reduce tumorigenicity and invasion. Interestingly, isoforms of CD44 are differentially expressed between HCC and normal hepatocytes. Targeting of the CD44 isoforms prevalent in HCC was able to selectively deplete HCC cells without harming normal cells (Miletti-González et al., 2005). Therefore, direct targeting of CSC-specific markers may also be a promising therapeutic strategy to eradicate liver CSC.

### 9.2 Stemness signaling

Cancer stem cells share various common characters with somatic and embryonic stem cells. Many signaling pathways observed exclusively in stem cells can also be detected in cancer stem cells. These signalings include Wnt/β-catenin, Hedgehog and Notch signaling (Mishra et al., 2009). Disturbing the signalings involved in normal stem cell fate reportedly decreased the self-renewal and proliferating capabilities of CSCs. For example, small molecule inhibitor of hedgehog pathway could reduce the likely CSC with progenitor marker aldehyde dehydrogenase in pancreatic cancer (Feldmann et al., 2007); Targeting Notch pathway was able to inhibit cancer stem cell self-renewal and decreases tumor growth (Cheng et al., 2004); The Wnt pathway can be inhibited by blocking the β-catenin interaction with TCF gene, and as such there was a reduction of CSC cells and spheroid formation (Lepourcelet et al., 2004). Apart from tumor promoting effects, stem cell signalings could induce resistances and recurrences to different cancer therapies in HCC. HCC cells survived through radiation, and acquired radioresistance was found to have Wnt/β-catenin signaling activated (Woodward et al., 2007). Relapse of HCC after radiation was also associated with the induction of Notch and Hedgehog signaling pathways which sustained HCC cell self-renewal and tumorigenicity (Clement et al., 2007).

Recently, the STAT3/IL-6 signaling is revealed as another pathway activated in liver CSC and plays an important role in maintaining the liver CSC. Activation of IL-6 pathway is suggested to be a consequence of TGF-β signaling defects (Tang et al., 2008). Impaired TGF-β signaling is a piece of useful information to distinguish liver CSC from normal stem cells. Hence, targeting IL-6 pathway might be a specific way to target liver CSC without affecting somatic stem cells. STAT3/IL-6 pathway inhibition by small inhibitor is also effective in HCC with lesion of TGF-β signaling, attenuating tumorigensis of HCC (He et al., 2004).

### 9.3 Differentiation pathway

Like other cancer types, HCC cells are highly heterogenous. It is believed that liver cancer stem cells are the initiator in establishing the heterogenous background of the tumor, whilst liver CSC themselves remains undifferentiated (Visvader, 2011). Forced differentiation of the CSC in HCC is a relevant approach to deplete the CSC in the cancer cell pool. Differentiation of cancer cells into less aggressive forms has been a successful strategy as demonstrated in the treatment of acute promyelocytic leukemia. The application of all-trans retinoic acid after normal chemotherapy resulted in a 90% remission and 70% cure rate in acute promyelocytic leukemia. Differentiation therapy can be an appealing and effective treatment against HCC (Massard et al., 2006).

It is reported that force expression of hepatocyte nuclear factor 4-α (HNF4-α) could promote the differentiation of hepatoma cells to normal hepatocytes. Most importantly, there is a reduction of stemness genes and a decrease of $CD133^+$ /$CD90^+$ subpopulation during the differentiation. HNF4-α is able to induce cell cycle arrest, cell senescense in HCC cells as well as the tumorigenic ability in mice (Yin et al., 2008). Systemic and intratumoral administration of HNF4-α carrying adenovirus could respectively prevent tumor metastasis and exhibit antitumor effect. Understanding the differentiation pathways in liver CSC allows identification of key differentiating factors (Yin et al., 2008). Identification of valid differentiation pathways in CSC enables scientists to explore a new avenue in countering liver CSC.

### 9.4 Cancer stem cell niche

Other novel ideas for stem cell targeting therapy include the disruption of the tumor niche essential for CSC homeostasis (Gokmen-Polar et al., 2008). The specified microenvironment where stem cells reside often dictates self-renewal and reproduction. Alteration of stem cell niche components can effectively change stem cell fate, as in the case of experimental parathyroid hormone induction. Furthermore, human embryonic stem cell-derived fibroblast-like cells provide a supportive environment for stem cells through insulin-like growth factor 2 (Martínez-Iglesias et al., 2008). Targeting insulin like growth factor 2 therefore can manipulate the stem cell microenvironment. Apart from the molecular content surrounding liver CSC, there is accumulating evidence that the physical environment is a critical mediator of HCC tumor behaviour. The stiffness of matrix is a strong predictor of HCC development. Increasing stiffness was found to promote HCC cell proliferation. On the other hand, a soft environment induces reversible stem cell characteristics in HCC (Schrader et al., 2011). With understanding of critical factors influencing liver CSC, comprehensive approach will be developed to eradicate these primary targets in HCC.

## 10. References

Aishima S, Basaki Y, Oda Y, Kuroda Y, Nishihara Y, Taguchi K, Taketomi A, Maehara Y, Hosoi F, Maruyama Y, Fotovati A, Oie S, Ono M, Ueno T, Sata M, Yano H, Kojiro M, Kuwano M, Tsuneyoshi M. (2006) High expression of insulin-like growth factor binding protein-3 is correlated with lower portal invasion and better prognosis in human hepatocellular carcinoma. Cancer Sci. Nov;97(11):1182-90.

Alexia C, Fallot G, Lasfer M, Schweizer-Groyer G, Groyer A. (2004) An evaluation of the role of insulin-like growth factors (IGF) and of type-I IGF receptor signalling in hepatocarcinogenesis and in the resistance of hepatocarcinoma cells against drug-induced apoptosis. Biochem Pharmacol. Sep 15;68(6):1003-15.

Amann T, Bataille F, Spruss T, Mühlbauer M, Gäbele E, Schölmerich J, Kiefer P, Bosserhoff AK, Hellerbrand C. (2009) Activated hepatic stellate cells promote tumorigenicity of hepatocellular carcinoma. Cancer Sci. Apr;100(4):646-53.

Amann T, Maegdefrau U, Hartmann A, Agaimy A, Marienhagen J, Weiss TS, Stoeltzing O, Warnecke C, Schölmerich J, Oefner PJ, Kreutz M, Bosserhoff AK, Hellerbrand C. (2009) GLUT1 expression is increased in hepatocellular carcinoma and promotes tumorigenesis. Am J Pathol. Apr;174(4):1544-52.

Bach SJ, Hawkins RA, Swaine D. (1963) A short method for the purification of arginase from ox liver. Biochem J. Nov;89:263-5.

Barnaeva E, Nadezhda A, Hannappel E, Sjogren MH, Rojkind M. (2007) Thymosin beta4 upregulates the expression of hepatocyte growth factor and downregulates the expression of PDGF-beta receptor in human hepatic stellate cells. Ann N Y Acad Sci. Sep;1112:154-60.

Bataller R, Brenner DA. (2005) Liver fibrosis. J Clin Invest. Feb;115(2):209-18. Review

Bjornsti MA, Houghton PJ. (2004) The TOR pathway: a target for cancer therapy. Nat Rev Cancer. May;4(5):335-48.

Breinig M, Caldas-Lopes E, Goeppert B, Malz M, Rieker R, Bergmann F, Schirmacher P, Mayer M, Chiosis G, Kern MA. (2009) Targeting heat shock protein 90 with non-quinone inhibitors: a novel chemotherapeutic approach in human hepatocellular carcinoma. Hepatology. Jul;50(1):102-12.

Breuhahn K, Vreden S, Haddad R, Beckebaum S, Stippel D, Flemming P, Nussbaum T, Caselmann WH, Haab BB, Schirmacher P. (2004) Molecular profiling of human hepatocellular carcinoma defines mutually exclusive interferon regulation and insulin-like growth factor II overexpression. Cancer Res. Sep 1;64(17):6058-64.

Capurro MI, Xiang YY, Lobe C, Filmus J. (2005) Glypican-3 promotes the growth of hepatocellular carcinoma by stimulating canonical Wnt signaling. Cancer Res. Jul 15;65(14):6245-54.

Capurro MI, Xu P, Shi W, Li F, Jia A, Filmus J. (2008) Glypican-3 inhibits Hedgehog signaling during development by competing with patched for Hedgehog binding. Dev Cell. May;14(5):700-11.

Chauhan D, Hideshima T, Anderson KC. (2008) Targeting proteasomes as therapy in multiple myeloma. Adv Exp Med Biol.;615:251-60.

Cheng AS. (2011) Epigenetic regulation of signaling pathways in cancer: role of the histone methyltransferase EZH2. J Gastroenterol Hepatol. Jan;26(1):19-27.

Cheng AS, Lau SS, Chen Y, Kondo Y, Li MS, Feng H, Ching AK, Cheung KF, Wong HK, Tong JH, Jin H, Choy KW, Yu J, To KF, Wong N, Huang TH, Sung JJ. (2011) EZH2-Mediated Concordant Repression of Wnt Antagonists Promotes {beta}-Catenin-Dependent Hepatocarcinogenesis. Cancer Res. Jun 1;71(11):4028-4039.

Cheng PN, Lam TL, Lam WM, Tsui SM, Cheng AW, Lo WH, Leung YC. (2007) Pegylated recombinant human arginase (rhArg-peg5,000mw) inhibits the in vitro and in vivo proliferation of human hepatocellular carcinoma through arginine depletion. Cancer Res. Jan 1;67(1):309-17.

Cheng T. (2004) Cell cycle inhibitors in normal and tumor stem cells. Oncogene. Sep 20;23(43):7256-66. Review.

Chen Y, Lin MC, Yao H, Wang H, Zhang AQ, Yu J, Hui CK, Lau GK, He ML, Sung J, Kung HF. (2007) Lentivirus-mediated RNA interference targeting enhancer of zeste homolog 2 inhibits hepatocellular carcinoma growth through down-regulation of stathmin. Hepatology. Jul;46(1):200-8.

Chen ZJ. (2005) Ubiquitin signalling in the NF-kappaB pathway. Nat Cell Biol. Aug;7(8):758-65. Review.

Chiba T, Suzuki E, Negishi M, Saraya A, Miyagi S, Konuma T, Tanaka S, Tada M, Kanai F, Imazeki F, Iwama A, Yokosuka O. (2011) 3-deazaneplanocin A is a promising therapeutic agent for the eradication of tumor-initiating hepatocellular carcinoma cells. Int J Cancer. Jun 29.

Chiba T, Miyagi S, Saraya A, Aoki R, Seki A, Morita Y, Yonemitsu Y, Yokosuka O, Taniguchi H, Nakauchi H, Iwama A. (2008) The polycomb gene product BMI1 contributes to the maintenance of tumor-initiating side population cells in hepatocellular carcinoma. Cancer Res. Oct 1;68(19):7742-9.

Clement V, Sanchez P, de Tribolet N, Radovanovic I, Ruiz i Altaba A. (2007) HEDGEHOG-GLI1 signaling regulates human glioma growth, cancer stem cell self-renewal, and tumorigenicity. Curr Biol. Jan 23;17(2):165-72.

Coulouarn C, Factor VM, Andersen JB, Durkin ME, Thorgeirsson SS. (2009) Loss of miR-122 expression in liver cancer correlates with suppression of the hepatic phenotype and gain of metastatic properties. Oncogene. Oct 8;28(40):3526-36. Epub 2009 Jul 20.

Dawson S, Apcher S, Mee M, Higashitsuji H, Baker R, Uhle S, Dubiel W, Fujita J, Mayer RJ. (2002) Gankyrin is an ankyrin-repeat oncoprotein that interacts with CDK4 kinase and the S6 ATPase of the 26 S proteasome. J Biol Chem. Mar 29;277(13):10893-902.

Delage B, Fennell DA, Nicholson L, McNeish I, Lemoine NR, Crook T, Szlosarek PW. (2010) Arginine deprivation and argininosuccinate synthetase expression in the treatment of cancer. Int J Cancer. Jun 15;126(12):2762-72. Review.

Deveraux QL, Takahashi R, Salvesen GS, Reed JC. (1997) X-linked IAP is a direct inhibitor of cell-death proteases. Nature. Jul 17;388(6639):300-4.

Dillon BJ, Prieto VG, Curley SA, Ensor CM, Holtsberg FW, Bomalaski JS, Clark MA. (2004) Incidence and distribution of argininosuccinate synthetase deficiency in human cancers: a method for identifying cancers sensitive to arginine deprivation. Cancer. Feb 15;100(4):826-33.

Djojosubroto MW, Chin AC, Go N, Schaetzlein S, Manns MP, Gryaznov S, Harley CB, Rudolph KL. (2005) Telomerase antagonists GRN163 and GRN163L inhibit tumor growth and increase chemosensitivity of human hepatoma. Hepatology. Nov;42(5):1127-36.

Dong LW, Yang GZ, Pan YF, Chen Y, Tan YX, Dai RY, Ren YB, Fu J, Wang HY. (2011) The oncoprotein p28(GANK) establishes a positive feedback loop in β-catenin signaling. Cell Res. Jun 21.

Dong S, Wu XZ. (2010) Heparanase and hepatocellular carcinoma: promoter or inhibitor? World J Gastroenterol. Jan 21;16(3):306-11.

Du GS, Wang JM, Lu JX, Li Q, Ma CQ, Du JT, Zou SQ. (2009) Expression of P-aPKC-iota, E-cadherin, and beta-catenin related to invasion and metastasis in hepatocellular carcinoma. Ann Surg Oncol. Jun;16(6):1578-86.

Effendi K, Mori T, Komuta M, Masugi Y, Du W, Sakamoto M. (2010) Bmi-1 gene is upregulated in early-stage hepatocellular carcinoma and correlates with ATP-binding cassette transporter B1 expression. Cancer Sci. Mar;101(3):666-72.

El-Assal ON, Yamanoi A, Ono T, Kohno H, Nagasue N. (2001) The clinicopathological significance of heparanase and basic fibroblast growth factor expressions in hepatocellular carcinoma. Clin Cancer Res. May;7(5):1299-305.

Ensor CM, Holtsberg FW, Bomalaski JS, Clark MA. (2002) Pegylated arginine deiminase (ADI-SS PEG20,000 mw) inhibits human melanomas and hepatocellular carcinomas in vitro and in vivo. Cancer Res. Oct 1;62(19):5443-50.

Farazi TA, Spitzer JI, Morozov P, Tuschl T. (2011) miRNAs in human cancer. J Pathol. Jan;223(2):102-15.

Feldmann G, Dhara S, Fendrich V, Bedja D, Beaty R, Mullendore M, Karikari C, Alvarez H, Iacobuzio-Donahue C, Jimeno A, Gabrielson KL, Matsui W, Maitra A. (2007) Blockade of hedgehog signaling inhibits pancreatic cancer invasion and metastases: a new paradigm for combination therapy in solid cancers. Cancer Res. Mar 1;67(5):2187-96.

Feitelson MA, Pan J, Lian Z. (2004) Early molecular and genetic determinants of primary liver malignancy. Surg Clin North Am. Apr;84(2):339-54. Review.

Fu J, Chen Y, Cao J, Luo T, Qian YW, Yang W, Ren YB, Su B, Cao GW, Yang Y, Yan YQ, Shen F, Wu MC, Feng GS, Wang HY. (2011) p28GANK overexpression accelerates hepatocellular carcinoma invasiveness and metastasis via phosphoinositol 3-kinase/AKT/hypoxia-inducible factor-1α pathways. Hepatology. Jan;53(1):181-92.

Gokmen-Polar Y, Miller KD. (2008) Redefining the target again: chemotherapeutics as vascular disrupting agents? Cancer Cell. Sep 9;14(3):195-6.

Gonzalez GG, Byus CV. (1991) Effect of dietary arginine restriction upon ornithine and polyamine metabolism during two-stage epidermal carcinogenesis in the mouse. Cancer Res. Jun 1;51(11):2932-9.

Hampton T. (2007)Cancer drug trials show modest benefit: drugs target liver, gastric, head and neck cancers. JAMA. Jul 18;298(3):273-5.

Hanafusa T, Yumoto Y, Nouso K, Nakatsukasa H, Onishi T, Fujikawa T, Taniyama M, Nakamura S, Uemura M, Takuma Y, Yumoto E, Higashi T, Tsuji T. (2002) Reduced expression of insulin-like growth factor binding protein-3 and its promoter hypermethylation in human hepatocellular carcinoma. Cancer Lett. Feb 25;176(2):149-58.

He XC, Zhang J, Tong WG, Tawfik O, Ross J, Scoville DH, Tian Q, Zeng X, He X, Wiedemann LM, Mishina Y, Li L. (2004) BMP signaling inhibits intestinal stem cell self-renewal through suppression of Wnt-beta-catenin signaling. Nat Genet. Oct;36(10):1117-21.

Higashitsuji H, Itoh K, Nagao T, Dawson S, Nonoguchi K, Kido T, Mayer RJ, Arii S, Fujita J. (2000) Reduced stability of retinoblastoma protein by gankyrin, an oncogenic ankyrin-repeat protein overexpressed in hepatomas. Nat Med. Jan;6(1):96-9.

Higashitsuji H, Higashitsuji H, Itoh K, Sakurai T, Nagao T, Sumitomo Y, Masuda T, Dawson S, Shimada Y, Mayer RJ, Fujita J. (2005)The oncoprotein gankyrin binds to MDM2/HDM2, enhancing ubiquitylation and degradation of p53. Cancer Cell. Jul;8(1):75-87.

Hou J, Lin L, Zhou W, Wang Z, Ding G, Dong Q, Qin L, Wu X, Zheng Y, Yang Y, Tian W, Zhang Q, Wang C, Zhang Q, Zhuang SM, Zheng L, Liang A, Tao W, Cao X. (2011) Identification of miRNomes in human liver and hepatocellular carcinoma reveals miR-199a/b-3p as therapeutic target for hepatocellular carcinoma. Cancer Cell. Feb 15;19(2):232-43.

Hsu HC, Cheng W, Lai PL. (1997) Cloning and expression of a developmentally regulated transcript MXR7 in hepatocellular carcinoma: biological significance and temporospatial distribution. Cancer Res. Nov 15;57(22):5179-84

Hu TH, Huang CC, Lin PR, Chang HW, Ger LP, Lin YW, Changchien CS, Lee CM, Tai MH. (2003) Expression and prognostic role of tumor suppressor gene PTEN/MMAC1/TEP1 in hepatocellular carcinoma. Cancer. Apr 15;97(8):1929-40.

Hu Z, Zhang Z, Doo E, Coux O, Goldberg AL, Liang TJ. (1999) Hepatitis B virus X protein is both a substrate and a potential inhibitor of the proteasome complex. J Virol. Sep;73(9):7231-40.

Huynh H, Chow PK, Ooi LL, Soo KC. (2002) A possible role for insulin-like growth factor-binding protein-3 autocrine/paracrine loops in controlling hepatocellular carcinoma cell proliferation. Cell Growth Differ. Mar;13(3):115-22.

Ingram DK, Zhu M, Mamczarz J, Zou S, Lane MA, Roth GS, deCabo R. (2006) Calorie restriction mimetics: an emerging research field. Aging Cell. Apr;5(2):97-108. Review.

Ishiguro T, Sugimoto M, Kinoshita Y, Miyazaki Y, Nakano K, Tsunoda H, Sugo I, Ohizumi I, Aburatani H, Hamakubo T, Kodama T, Tsuchiya M, Yamada-Okabe H. (2008) Anti-glypican 3 antibody as a potential antitumor agent for human liver cancer. Cancer Res. Dec 1;68(23):9832-8.

Izzo F, Marra P, Beneduce G, Castello G, Vallone P, De Rosa V, Cremona F, Ensor CM, Holtsberg FW, Bomalaski JS, Clark MA, Ng C, Curley SA. (2004) Pegylated arginine deiminase treatment of patients with unresectable hepatocellular carcinoma: results from phase I/II studies. J Clin Oncol. May 15;22(10):1815-22.

Ji J, Shi J, Budhu A, Yu Z, Forgues M, Roessler S, Ambs S, Chen Y, Meltzer PS, Croce CM, Qin LX, Man K, Lo CM, Lee J, Ng IO, Fan J, Tang ZY, Sun HC, Wang XW. (2009) MicroRNA expression, survival, and response to interferon in liver cancer. N Engl J Med. Oct 8;361(15):1437-47.

Kaur S, Wang F, Venkatraman M, Arsura M. (2005) X-linked inhibitor of apoptosis (XIAP) inhibits c-Jun N-terminal kinase 1 (JNK1) activation by transforming growth factor beta1 (TGF-beta1) through ubiquitin-mediated proteosomal degradation of the TGF-beta1-activated kinase 1 (TAK1). J Biol Chem. Nov 18;280(46):38599-608.

Kirmizis A, Bartley SM, Kuzmichev A, Margueron R, Reinberg D, Green R, Farnham PJ. (2004) Silencing of human polycomb target genes is associated with methylation of histone H3 Lys 27. Genes Dev. Jul 1;18(13):1592-605.

Lai JP, Sandhu DS, Yu C, Han T, Moser CD, Jackson KK, Guerrero RB, Aderca I, Isomoto H, Garrity-Park MM, Zou H, Shire AM, Nagorney DM, Sanderson SO, Adjei AA, Lee JS, Thorgeirsson SS, Roberts LR. (2008) Sulfatase 2 up-regulates glypican 3, promotes fibroblast growth factor signaling, and decreases survival in hepatocellular carcinoma. Hepatology. Apr;47(4):1211-22.

Lai JP, Oseini AM, Moser CD, Yu C, Elsawa SF, Hu C, Nakamura I, Han T, Aderca I, Isomoto H, Garrity-Park MM, Shire AM, Li J, Sanderson SO, Adjei AA, Fernandez-Zapico ME, Roberts LR. (2010) The oncogenic effect of sulfatase 2 in human hepatocellular carcinoma is mediated in part by glypican 3-dependent Wnt activation. Hepatology. Nov;52(5):1680-9.

Lai JP, Sandhu DS, Yu C, Moser CD, Hu C, Shire AM, Aderca I, Murphy LM, Adjei AA, Sanderson S, Roberts LR. (2010) Sulfatase 2 protects hepatocellular carcinoma cells against apoptosis induced by the PI3K inhibitor LY294002 and ERK and JNK kinase inhibitors. Liver Int. Nov;30(10):1522-8.

Lai MC, Yang Z, Zhou L, Zhu QQ, Xie HY, Zhang F, Wu LM, Chen LM, Zheng SS. (2011) Long non-coding RNA MALAT-1 overexpression predicts tumor recurrence of hepatocellular carcinoma after liver transplantation. Med Oncol. Jun 16.

Lang SA, Moser C, Fichnter-Feigl S, Schachtschneider P, Hellerbrand C, Schmitz V, Schlitt HJ, Geissler EK, Stoeltzing O. (2009) Targeting heat-shock protein 90 improves efficacy of rapamycin in a model of hepatocellular carcinoma in mice. Hepatology. Feb;49(2):523-32.

Lepourcelet M, Chen YN, France DS, Wang H, Crews P, Petersen F, Bruseo C, Wood AW, Shivdasani RA. (2004) Small-molecule antagonists of the oncogenic Tcf/beta-catenin protein complex. Cancer Cell. Jan;5(1):91-102.

Li H, Fu X, Chen Y, Hong Y, Tan Y, Cao H, Wu M, Wang H. (2005) Use of adenovirus-delivered siRNA to target oncoprotein p28GANK in hepatocellular carcinoma. Gastroenterology. Jun;128(7):2029-41.

Liu C, Yu J, Yu S, Lavker RM, Cai L, Liu W, Yang K, He X, Chen S. (2010) MicroRNA-21 acts as an oncomir through multiple targets in human hepatocellular carcinoma. J Hepatol. Jul;53(1):98-107.

Liu LX, Lee NP, Chan VW, Xue W, Zender L, Zhang C, Mao M, Dai H, Wang XL, Xu MZ, Lee TK, Ng IO, Chen Y, Kung HF, Lowe SW, Poon RT, Wang JH, Luk JM. (2009) Targeting cadherin-17 inactivates Wnt signaling and inhibits tumor growth in liver carcinoma. Hepatology. Nov;50(5):1453-63.

Liu Q, Vera JC, Peng H, Golde DW. (2001) The predicted ATP-binding domains in the hexose transporter GLUT1 critically affect transporter activity. Biochemistry. Jul 3;40(26):7874-81.

Llovet JM, Burroughs A, Bruix J. (2003) Hepatocellular carcinoma. Lancet. Dec 6;362(9399):1907-17. Review.

Llovet JM, Ricci S, Mazzaferro V, Hilgard P, Gane E, Blanc JF, de Oliveira AC, Santoro A, Raoul JL, Forner A, Schwartz M, Porta C, Zeuzem S, Bolondi L, Greten TF, Galle PR, Seitz JF, Borbath I, Häussinger D, Giannaris T, Shan M, Moscovici M, Voliotis D, Bruix J; SHARP Investigators Study Group. (2008) Sorafenib in advanced hepatocellular carcinoma. N Engl J Med. Jul 24;359(4):378-90.

Lund P, Schubert D, Niketeghad F, Schirmacher P. (2004) Autocrine inhibition of chemotherapy response in human liver tumor cells by insulin-like growth factor-II. Cancer Lett. Mar 31;206(1):85-96.

Márquez-Rosado L, Trejo-Solís MC, García-Cuéllar CM, Villa-Treviño S. (2005) Celecoxib, a cyclooxygenase-2 inhibitor, prevents induction of liver preneoplastic lesions in rats. J Hepatol. Oct;43(4):653-60.

Martin HJ, Kornmann F, Fuhrmann GF. (2003) The inhibitory effects of flavonoids and antiestrogens on the Glut1 glucose transporter in human erythrocytes. Chem Biol Interact. Dec 15;146(3):225-35. PubMed PMID: 14642735.

Martínez-Iglesias O, Ruiz-Llorente L, Sánchez-Martínez R, García L, Zambrano A, Aranda A. (2008) Histone deacetylase inhibitors: mechanism of action and therapeutic use in cancer. Clin Transl Oncol. Jul;10(7):395-8. Review.

Maschek G, Savaraj N, Priebe W, Braunschweiger P, Hamilton K, Tidmarsh GF, De Young LR, Lampidis TJ. (2004) 2-deoxy-D-glucose increases the efficacy of adriamycin and paclitaxel in human osteosarcoma and non-small cell lung cancers in vivo. Cancer Res. Jan 1;64(1):31-4.

Massard C, Deutsch E, Soria JC. (2006) Tumour stem cell-targeted treatment: elimination or differentiation. Ann Oncol. Nov;17(11):1620-4. Review.

Matouk IJ, Abbasi I, Hochberg A, Galun E, Dweik H, Akkawi M. (2009) Highly upregulated in liver cancer noncoding RNA is overexpressed in hepatic colorectal metastasis. Eur J Gastroenterol Hepatol. Jun;21(6):688-92.

Meng F, Henson R, Wehbe-Janek H, Ghoshal K, Jacob ST, Patel T. (2007) MicroRNA-21 regulates expression of the PTEN tumor suppressor gene in human hepatocellular cancer. Gastroenterology. Aug;133(2):647-58. Epub 2007 May 21.

Midorikawa Y, Ishikawa S, Iwanari H, Imamura T, Sakamoto H, Miyazono K, Kodama T, Makuuchi M, Aburatani H. (2003) Glypican-3, overexpressed in hepatocellular carcinoma, modulates FGF2 and BMP-7 signaling. Int J Cancer. Feb 10;103(4):455-65.

Miletti-González KE, Chen S, Muthukumaran N, Saglimbeni GN, Wu X, Yang J, Apolito K, Shih WJ, Hait WN, Rodríguez-Rodríguez L. (2005) The CD44 receptor interacts with P-glycoprotein to promote cell migration and invasion in cancer. Cancer Res. Aug 1;65(15):6660-7.

Mishra L, Banker T, Murray J, Byers S, Thenappan A, He AR, Shetty K, Johnson L, Reddy EP. (2009) Liver stem cells and hepatocellular carcinoma. Hepatology. Jan;49(1):318-29.

Morimoto-Tomita M, Uchimura K, Werb Z, Hemmerich S, Rosen SD. (2002) Cloning and characterization of two extracellular heparin-degrading endosulfatases in mice and humans. J Biol Chem. Dec 20;277(51):49175-85. Epub 2002 Oct 3.

Morris DI, Robbins JD, Ruoho AE, Sutkowski EM, Seamon KB. (1991) Forskolin photoaffinity labels with specificity for adenylyl cyclase and the glucose transporter. J Biol Chem. Jul 15;266(20):13377-84.

Munakata T, Nakamura M, Liang Y, Li K, Lemon SM. (2005) Down-regulation of the retinoblastoma tumor suppressor by the hepatitis C virus NS5B RNA-dependent RNA polymerase. Proc Natl Acad Sci U S A. Dec 13;102(50):18159-64.

Nussbaum T, Samarin J, Ehemann V, Bissinger M, Ryschich E, Khamidjanov A, Yu X, Gretz N, Schirmacher P, Breuhahn K. (2008) Autocrine insulin-like growth factor-II stimulation of tumor cell migration is a progression step in human hepatocarcinogenesis. Hepatology. Jul;48(1):146-56.

Pan Q, Liu B, Liu J, Cai R, Liu X, Qian C. (2008) Synergistic antitumor activity of XIAP-shRNA and TRAIL expressed by oncolytic adenoviruses in experimental HCC. Acta Oncol. 47(1):135-44.

Panzitt K, Tschernatsch MM, Guelly C, Moustafa T, Stradner M, Strohmaier HM, Buck CR, Denk H, Schroeder R, Trauner M, Zatloukal K. (2007) Characterization of HULC, a novel gene with striking up-regulation in hepatocellular carcinoma, as noncoding RNA. Gastroenterology. Jan;132(1):330-42.

Pascale RM, Simile MM, Calvisi DF, Frau M, Muroni MR, Seddaiu MA, Daino L, Muntoni MD, De Miglio MR, Thorgeirsson SS, Feo F. (2005) Role of HSP90, CDC37, and CRM1 as modulators of P16(INK4A) activity in rat liver carcinogenesis and human liver cancer. Hepatology. Dec;42(6):1310-9.

Pearl LH, Prodromou C, Workman P. (2008) The Hsp90 molecular chaperone: an open and shut case for treatment. Biochem J. Mar 15;410(3):439-53.

Pineau P, Volinia S, McJunkin K, Marchio A, Battiston C, Terris B, Mazzaferro V, Lowe SW, Croce CM, Dejean A. (2010) miR-221 overexpression contributes to liver tumorigenesis. Proc Natl Acad Sci U S A. Jan 5;107(1):264-9.

Sano T, Kagawa M, Okuno M, Ishibashi N, Hashimoto M, Yamamoto M, Suzuki R, Kohno H, Matsushima-Nishiwaki R, Takano Y, Tsurumi H, Kojima S, Friedman SL, Moriwaki H, Tanaka T. (2005) Prevention of rat hepatocarcinogenesis by acyclic retinoid is accompanied by reduction in emergence of both TGF-alpha-expressing oval-like cells and activated hepatic stellate cells. Nutr Cancer. 51(2):197-206.

Sarbassov DD, Guertin DA, Ali SM, Sabatini DM. (2005) Phosphorylation and regulation of Akt/PKB by the rictor-mTOR complex. Science. Feb 18;307(5712):1098-101.

Scharf JG, Braulke T. (2003) The role of the IGF axis in hepatocarcinogenesis. Horm Metab Res. Nov-Dec;35(11-12):685-93.

Schirmacher P, Held WA, Yang D, Chisari FV, Rustum Y, Rogler CE. (1992) Reactivation of insulin-like growth factor II during hepatocarcinogenesis in transgenic mice suggests a role in malignant growth. Cancer Res. May 1;52(9):2549-56.

Schrader J, Gordon-Walker TT, Aucott RL, van Deemter M, Quaas A, Walsh S, Benten D, Forbes SJ, Wells RG, Iredale JP. (2011) Matrix stiffness modulates proliferation, chemotherapeutic response, and dormancy in hepatocellular carcinoma cells. Hepatology. Apr;53(4):1192-205.

Shirakawa H, Suzuki H, Shimomura M, Kojima M, Gotohda N, Takahashi S, Nakagohri T, Konishi M, Kobayashi N, Kinoshita T, Nakatsura T. (2009) Glypican-3 expression is correlated with poor prognosis in hepatocellular carcinoma. Cancer Sci. Aug;100(8):1403-7.

Steele JC, Torr EE, Noakes KL, Kalk E, Moss PA, Reynolds GM, Hubscher SG, van Lohuizen M, Adams DH, Young LS. (2006) The polycomb group proteins, BMI-1 and EZH2, are tumour-associated antigens. Br J Cancer. Nov 6;95(9):1202-11.

Sun L, Hu H, Peng L, Zhou Z, Zhao X, Pan J, Sun L, Yang Z, Ran Y. (2011) P-cadherin promotes liver metastasis and is associated with poor prognosis in colon cancer. Am J Pathol. Jul;179(1):380-90.

Tan J, Yang X, Zhuang L, Jiang X, Chen W, Lee PL, Karuturi RK, Tan PB, Liu ET, Yu Q. (2007) Pharmacologic disruption of Polycomb-repressive complex 2-mediated gene repression selectively induces apoptosis in cancer cells. Genes Dev. May 1;21(9):1050-63.

Tang Y, Kitisin K, Jogunoori W, Li C, Deng CX, Mueller SC, Ressom HW, Rashid A, He AR, Mendelson JS, Jessup JM, Shetty K, Zasloff M, Mishra B, Reddy EP, Johnson L, Mishra L. (2008) Progenitor/stem cells give rise to liver cancer due to aberrant TGF-beta and IL-6 signaling. Proc Natl Acad Sci U S A. Feb 19;105(7):2445-50.

Tomimaru Y, Eguchi H, Nagano H, Wada H, Tomokuni A, Kobayashi S, Marubashi S, Takeda Y, Tanemura M, Umeshita K, Doki Y, Mori M. (2010) MicroRNA-21 induces resistance to the anti-tumour effect of interferon-α/5-fluorouracil in hepatocellular carcinoma cells. Br J Cancer. Nov 9;103(10):1617-26.

Tovar V, Alsinet C, Villanueva A, Hoshida Y, Chiang DY, Solé M, Thung S, Moyano S, Toffanin S, Mínguez B, Cabellos L, Peix J, Schwartz M, Mazzaferro V, Bruix J, Llovet JM. (2010) IGF activation in a molecular subclass of hepatocellular carcinoma and pre-clinical efficacy of IGF-1R blockage. J Hepatol. Apr;52(4):550-9. Tsang DP,

Umemura A, Itoh Y, Itoh K, Yamaguchi K, Nakajima T, Higashitsuji H, Onoue H, Fukumoto M, Okanoue T, Fujita J. (2008) Association of gankyrin protein expression with early clinical stages and insulin-like growth factor-binding protein 5 expression in human hepatocellular carcinoma. Hepatology. Feb;47(2):493-502.

Villanueva A, Chiang DY, Newell P, Peix J, Thung S, Alsinet C, Tovar V, Roayaie S, Minguez B, Sole M, Battiston C, Van Laarhoven S, Fiel MI, Di Feo A, Hoshida Y, Yea S, Toffanin S, Ramos A, Martignetti JA, Mazzaferro V, Bruix J, Waxman S, Schwartz M, Meyerson M, Friedman SL, Llovet JM. (2008) Pivotal role of mTOR signaling in hepatocellular carcinoma. Gastroenterology. Dec;135(6):1972-83, 1983.e1-11.

Visvader JE. (2011) Cells of origin in cancer. Nature. Jan 20;469(7330):314-22.

Vivanco I, Sawyers CL. (2002) The phosphatidylinositol 3-Kinase AKT pathway in human cancer. Nat Rev Cancer. Jul;2(7):489-501.

Wang GB, Zhou XY, Wang XQ. (2010) Relationship between serum heparanase and microscopic venous invasion in patients with hepatocellular carcinoma. Am J Clin Pathol. Aug;134(2):242-8.

Wang XQ, Luk JM, Leung PP, Wong BW, Stanbridge EJ, Fan ST. (2005) Alternative mRNA splicing of liver intestine-cadherin in hepatocellular carcinoma. Clin Cancer Res. Jan 15;11(2 Pt 1):483-9.

Whitesell L, Lindquist SL. (2005) HSP90 and the chaperoning of cancer. Nat Rev Cancer. Oct;5(10):761-72.

Whittaker S, Marais R, Zhu AX. (2010) The role of signaling pathways in the development and treatment of hepatocellular carcinoma. Oncogene. Sep 9;29(36):4989-5005.

Wilhelm SM, Carter C, Tang L, Wilkie D, McNabola A, Rong H, Chen C, Zhang X, Vincent P, McHugh M, Cao Y, Shujath J, Gawlak S, Eveleigh D, Rowley B, Liu L, Adnane L, Lynch M, Auclair D, Taylor I, Gedrich R, Voznesensky A, Riedl B, Post LE, Bollag G, Trail PA. (2004) BAY 43-9006 exhibits broad spectrum oral antitumor activity and targets the RAF/MEK/ERK pathway and receptor tyrosine kinases involved in tumor progression and angiogenesis. Cancer Res. Oct 1;64(19):7099-109

Woodward WA, Chen MS, Behbod F, Alfaro MP, Buchholz TA, Rosen JM. (2007) WNT/beta-catenin mediates radiation resistance of mouse mammary progenitor cells. Proc Natl Acad Sci U S A. Jan 9;104(2):618-23.

Workman P, Burrows F, Neckers L, Rosen N. (2007) Drugging the cancer chaperone HSP90: combinatorial therapeutic exploitation of oncogene addiction and tumor stress. Ann N Y Acad Sci. Oct;1113:202-16.

Xiong Y, Fang JH, Yun JP, Yang J, Zhang Y, Jia WH, Zhuang SM. (2010) Effects of microRNA-29 on apoptosis, tumorigenicity, and prognosis of hepatocellular carcinoma. Hepatology. Mar;51(3):836-45.

Xu CR, Lee S, Ho C, Bommi P, Huang SA, Cheung ST, Dimri GP, Chen X. (2009) Bmi1 functions as an oncogene independent of Ink4A/Arf repression in hepatic carcinogenesis. Mol Cancer Res. Dec;7(12):1937-45.

Yamashita T, Ji J, Budhu A, Forgues M, Yang W, Wang HY, Jia H, Ye Q, Qin LX, Wauthier E, Reid LM, Minato H, Honda M, Kaneko S, Tang ZY, Wang XW. (2009) EpCAM-positive hepatocellular carcinoma cells are tumor-initiating cells with stem/progenitor cell features. Gastroenterology. Mar;136(3):1012-24.

Yang Z, Zhou L, Wu LM, Lai MC, Xie HY, Zhang F, Zheng SS. (2011) Overexpression of long non-coding RNA HOTAIR predicts tumor recurrence in hepatocellular carcinoma patients following liver transplantation. Ann Surg Oncol. May;18(5):1243-50.

Yin C, Lin Y, Zhang X, Chen YX, Zeng X, Yue HY, Hou JL, Deng X, Zhang JP, Han ZG, Xie WF. (2008) Differentiation therapy of hepatocellular carcinoma in mice with recombinant adenovirus carrying hepatocyte nuclear factor-4alpha gene. Hepatology. Nov;48(5):1528-39.

Yoo BK, Santhekadur PK, Gredler R, Chen D, Emdad L, Bhutia S, Pannell L, Fisher PB, Sarkar D. (2011) Increased RNA-induced silencing complex (RISC) activity contributes to hepatocellular carcinoma. Hepatology. May;53(5):1538-48.

Zhang Y, Li L, Wang Y, Zhang J, Wei G, Sun Y, Shen F. (2007) Downregulating the expression of heparanase inhibits the invasion, angiogenesis and metastasis of human hepatocellular carcinoma. Biochem Biophys Res Commun. Jun 22;358(1):124-9..

Zhou W, Mukherjee P, Kiebish MA, Markis WT, Mantis JG, Seyfried TN. (2007) The calorically restricted ketogenic diet, an effective alternative therapy for malignant brain cancer. Nutr Metab (Lond). Feb 21;4:5.

Zimmerman RL, Fogt F, Burke M, Murakata LA. (2002)Assessment of Glut-1 expression in cholangiocarcinoma, benign biliary lesions and hepatocellular carcinoma. Oncol Rep. Jul-Aug;9(4):689-92.

Zhao W, Zhang L, Yin Z, Su W, Ren G, Zhou C, You J, Fan J, Wang X. (2011) Activated hepatic stellate cells promote hepatocellular carcinoma development in immunocompetent mice. Int J Cancer. Jan 6.

Zhao H, Liu H, Chen Y, Xin X, Li J, Hou Y, Zhang Z, Zhang X, Xie C, Geng M, Ding J. (2006) Oligomannurarate sulfate, a novel heparanase inhibitor simultaneously targeting basic fibroblast growth factor, combats tumor angiogenesis and metastasis. Cancer Res. Sep 1;66(17):8779-87.

3

# Clinical Significance of Serum Ornithine Carbamoyltransferase in Liver Diseases – Is the Ratio of OCT/ALT a New Tumor Marker?

Katsutoshi Tokushige[1], Etsuko Hashimoto[1*], Noriko Matsushita[1,2], Nobuyuki Torii[1], Makiko Taniai[1], Keiko Shiratori[1] and Hiroshi Maruyama[3]
[1]*Tokyo Women's Medical University, Department of Medicine and Gastroenterology*
[2]*Tokyo Women's Medical University, Support Center for Women Health Care Professionals and Researchers Tokyo*
[3]*YAMASA Corporation, Chiba*
*Japan*

## 1. Introduction

Hepatocellular carcinoma (HCC) is the fifth most common cancer worldwide and the third most common cause of cancer-related mortality (World Health Organization. Mortality database, 2010). According to the most recent nationwide Japanese registration data, primary liver cancer ranks fourth for men and sixth for women as cause of death from malignant neoplasm (Journal of Health and Welfare Statistics. Health and Welfare Statistics Association, 2009).

The leading major causes of HCC in Japan are viruses, hepatitis C accounting for 70% and hepatitis B for 16% of all cases of HCC. Recently, the incidence of HCC in cases of non-viral liver disease has gradually increased (Ikai et al., 2010). According to our hospital database, increasing numbers of HCC cases arising from non-alcoholic steatohepatitis (NASH) have been seen, with such cases accounting for 4% of all cases of HCC each year since 2000. Together with the recent increase the metabolic syndrome population in Japan, cases of NASH have increased dramatically, and it is logical that the incidence of HCC in these patients can be expected to increase as well (Tokushige et al., 2010).

Since evaluation of viable HCC is important for monitoring and deciding therapeutic strategies, the serum tumor markers alpha-fetoprotein (AFP) and des-gamma-carboxy prothrombin (DCP), the protein induced by vitamin K absence, as well as imaging provide useful information. However, a recent report demonstrated that AFP is not sensitive in NASH-related HCC (Hashimoto & Tokushige, 2011). Although DCP is highly specific for HCC, its sensitivity is reported to be no more than 50% in patients with HCC measuring 3cm or less in diameter (Okuda H et al., 2000). Moreover, DCP can be affected by some

* Corresponding Author

medicines such as warfarin, or by the condition of patients with severe liver failure or bile acid outflow obstruction. There are still some problems about tumor markers of HCC.

Histological analysis via liver biopsy is one of the most accurate methods for evaluating liver status, but the method is too invasive for frequent use. Especially, liver biopsy is only method for the diagnosis of NASH and the evaluation of progression. Hence, minimally invasive, impervious and reliable markers are still required for early diagnosis and optimal treatment. Ornithine carbamoyltransferase (OCT), a mitochondrion-derived protein, has been reported as a useful marker superior to cytosol-derived markers in the detection of liver injury in murine model (Maruyama et al., 2008). Murayama et al. also reported that OCT is highly liver-specific for the evaluation of hepatocellular damage, whereas alanine aminotransferase (AST) and aspartate aminotransferase (ALT) are useful but not liver-specific, existing in a variety of organs such as heart, muscle, and kidney. Since mitochondrial dysfunction is regarded as a pathogenesis of NASH, we thought that OCT might be a useful marker to detect the progression of NASH and NASH-caused HCC. In our previous study, we demonstrated that serum OCT levels and the ratios of OCT/ALT and OCT/AST were markedly increased in NASH with HCC. Importantly, the amount of serum OCT and the ratio of OCT/AST were significantly higher in patients with NASH-HCC than in those with NASH-liver cirrhosis (NASH-LC) (Tokushige et al., 2009). Therefore, in this study, we investigated the clinical significance of OCT in several chronic liver diseases, including HCC and OCT compared with the histological stage. To confirm whether OCT is a useful tumor marker for HCC, we measured serum OCT and OCT/ALT ratios before and after therapy, and then compared the results with other tumor markers such as AFP and DCP.

AFP, alpha-fetoprotein; ALT, alanine aminotransferase; AST, aspartate aminotransferase; AUC, area under the ROC curve; CH, chronic hepatitis; ELISA, enzyme-linked immunosorbent assay; HCC, hepatocellular carcinoma; HBV, hepatitis B virus; HCV, hepatitis C virus; LC, liver cirrhosis; OCT, ornithine carbamoyltransferase; DCP, des-gamma-carboxy prothrombin

## 2. Patients and method

### 2.1 Patients

One hundred eighty-nine patients with biopsy-proven NASH (including 24 LC and 12 HCC), 27 patients with alcoholic liver diseases (ALD) according to the diagnostic criteria of ALD in Japan (Takada & Tsutsumi, 1995), and 70 patients with chronic liver diseases by hepatitis C virus (HCV) (including 16 LC and 14 HCC), at Tokyo Women's Medical University between 1995 and 2011 were evaluated along with 80 healthy subjects serving as controls (Table 1).

Diagnosis of NASH was based on the following criteria: (1) detection of steatohepatitis on liver biospy, (2) intake of <100g of ethanol per week, and (3) approriate exclusion of other liver diseases (Brunt et al., 1999; Neuschwander-Tetri & Cadwell, 2003). All liver biopsy specimens were examined using hematoxylin-eosin, Mallory, and silver reticulin as stains. Fibrosis was scored using a 5-grade scale: F0, normal connective tissue; F1, foci of perivenular fibrosis in zone 3; F2, perivenular or percicellular fibrosis confined to zone 3 and 2, with or without portal/periportal fibrosis; F3, bridging fibrosis or septal fibrosis; F4, cirrhosis. Patients in the HCV group were shown to be positive for HCV-RNA by a quantitative polymerase chain reaction assay.

We collected serum samples from 10 patients with HCC both pre-treatment and post-treatment, 4 patients with hepatitis C and 6 patients with non-virus diseases including NASH and ALD. Nine patients with HCC underwent transcatheter arterial chemoembolization (TACE). Partial hepatectomy was selected for 1 patient. Post-treatment samples were collected at 3 months after each therapy.

All patients underwent liver tests for measurement of the following laboratory parameters: AST, ALT, platelet count, hepatitis B serology (hepatitis B surface antigen, antibody to hepatitis B surface antigen, and antibody to hepatitis B core antigen), hepatitis C virus (HCV) serology (antibody to HCV and HCV-RNA polymerase chain reaction), and autoantibodies (antinuclear antibody (ANA), anti-smooth muscle antibody, and anti-mitochondrial antibody). Written informed consent was obtained from each patient, and the study protocol conformed to the ethical guidelines of the 1975 Declaration of Helsinki and was approved by our institution's research committee.

### 2.2 Method

Serum OCT levels were measured by ELISA as reported previously (Murayama et al., 2006). Briefly, 50 μL of the HRP-conjugated F(ab') fraction of anti-OCT monoclonal IgG (secondary antibody, Mo5B11), and 50 μL of standard solution or sample diluted 10-fold with assay buffer (250 mmol/L glycine-buffer pH 9.4, containing 0.1% bovine serum albumin, 50 mmol/L NaCl and 0.1% ProClin950) were added to an antibody-coated dish (first antibody, Mo3B11). After mixing, the dish was incubated for 2 h and then washed with washing solution (10 mmol/L phosphate-buffer pH 7.4, containing 0.1% BSA, 150 mmol/L NaCl and 0.1% ProClin950). Then, a substrate solution (200 μg/mL 3, 3', 5, 5'-teramethylbenzidine containing 0.001% $H_2O_2$) was added. After the coloring reaction (20 min) was terminated by adding a stop solution (0.5 mol/L $H_2SO_4$), absorbance at 450 nm was measured with a microplate reader.

The serum AFP levels were determined by enzyme-linked immunosorbent assay with a commercially available kit (ELISA-AFP, International Reagents, Kobe, Japan; cut-off level 10ng/ml). The serum DCP levels were determined by sensitive enzyme-linked immunoassay (Eitest PIVKA-II kit, Eisai Co., Tokyo, Japan; cut-off level 40 mAU/ml) according to the manufacturer's instructions.

### 2.3 Statistical analysis

Data were expressed as mean ± standard deviation (SD). Statistical comparison among the groups was conducted using Dunn's test, with $P < 0.05$ considered statistically significant. The comparison between pre-treatment and post-treatment of patients with HCC was performed by paired-t-test. The correlations between serum OCT levels and serum ALT and AST levels or platelet count were confirmed by Spearman's correlation test.

## 3. Results

### 3.1 Serum OCT levels and ratios of OCT/AST and OCT/ALT

Table 1 shows the mean serum AST, ALT, OCT levels, platelet counts, and the ratios of AST/ALT, OCT/AST and OCT/ALT in 153 NASH patients without HCC and LC, 24 NASH-LC patients, 12 NASH-HCC patients, 27 ALD patients, 40 chronic hepatitis with HCV<CH(C)> patients, 16 LC with HCV<LC(C)> patients without HCC, and 14 LC(C)-HCC patients. Significant associations between serum OCT levels and serum AST levels or ALT levels were noted (ALT, R=0.784 p<0.01; AST, r=0.853 p<0.01).

The AST and ALT levels of NASH-HCC were increased compared to those of NASH-LC. The ALT level of NASH-LC was slightly decreased compared to those of NASH. However, regarding AST and ALT, the differences between NASH and NASH-LC were not significant. In contrast, the serum OCT levels in NASH were higher than those of controls, and gradually increased with the development of liver disease from NASH to LC and HCC. In addition, the ratios of OCT/ALT and OCT/AST were significantly increased in parallel with the progression of NASH, LC and HCC. Especially, serum OCT levels and the ratios of OCT/ALT and OCT/AST were markedly increased in HCC.

Concerning CH(C), serum OCT levels were increased, but the ratios of OCT/ALT and OCT/AST were not significantly different from those of NASH patients. The ratio of OCT/ALT was slightly increased in LC(C) patients, compared with CH(C). Furthermore, in HCC with LC(C), both the ratios of OCT/ALT and OCT/AST were significantly increased.

As for comparison with several liver diseases without LC and HCC, serum OCT levels, OCT/ALT and OCT/AST ratios in ALD were significantly higher than those of other liver diseases (Figure 1).

### 3.2 Association with fibrosis grade in NASH patients

Figure 2 shows the association between liver fibrosis grade and serum OCT levels and the ratios of OCT/AST and OCT/ALT in NASH patients on the basis of liver biopsies. Serum OCT levels and OCT/ALT ratios were significantly increased in parallel with fibrosis grade (mean OCT levels: 50.8 ng/mL in F0-1, 68.7 ng/mL in F2, 108.3 ng/mL in F3, 156.4 ng/mL in F4)(mean OCT/ALT ratio: 1.43 in F0-1, 1.05 in F2, 1.69 in F3, 2.58 in F4). Regarding the relationship between OCT or ratios and platelet counts, there was a significant association between the ratio of OCT/ALT and platelet counts (r=-0.285 p<0.01)(Figure 3).

### 3.3 OCT in NASH patients with a normal range of ALT

Among all NASH patients, 42 patients had a normal range of ALT, among these 42 patients, 13 (31%) had OCT over 43ng/mL (mean ± 1.96 SD in control=43.2ng/mL). Of these 13 patients, eight had F3 or F4 fibrosis (Figure 4).

### 3.4 Change of OCT and ratio of OCT/ALT after therapy

Serum level of OCT and OCT/ALT ratio were significantly decreased in HCC after a therapeutic procedure, TACE or surgery (p<0.05). Out of 10 patients received therapy, serum OCT levels were decreased in 8 patients. The ratio of OCT/ALT was decreased in 7 patients (Figure 5). On the contrast, in 9 patients DCP was decreased, in 7 patients AFP was decreased. The tendencies were almost same among 4 tumor markers.

| Disease | OCT (ng/mL) | AST (U/L) | ALT (U/L) | OCT /ALT | OCT /AST | AST /ALT | Plt (×10⁴/μL) |
|---|---|---|---|---|---|---|---|
| **Control** (n=80) | 20.6 ± 12.6 | 18.4 ± 4.3 | 16.3 ± 7.0 | 1.30 ± 0.87 | 1.09 ± 0.62 | 1.22 ± 0.33 | N.D. |
| **NASH** (n=153) | 73.3 [a] ± 73.2 | 41.2 [a] ± 33.9 | 63.9 [a] ± 80.9 | 1.34 ± 0.95 | 1.68 [a,d] ± 0.84 | 0.8 [a] ± 0.27 | 21.7 ± 6.39 |
| **NASH-LC** (n=24) | 102.7 [a,b] ± 107.2 | 38.0 ± 16.2 | 35.5 ± 20.7 | 2.27 [a,b] ± 1.26 | 1.93 [a,b] ± 0.93 | 1.19 [b] ± 0.45 | 12.8 [b] ± 6.21 |
| **NASH-HCC** (n=12) | 375.9 [a,b,c] ± 574.9 | 80.25 [a,c] ± 38.4 | 88.3 [a,c] ± 101.2 | 4.95 [a,b,c] ± 4.73 | 3.74 [a,b,c] ± 0.153 | 1.27 [b] ± 0.9 | 12.9 [b] ± 4.1 |
| **ALD** (n=27) | 114.8 [a,b,d] ± 106.5 | 40.2 ± 26.0 | 35.6 ± 30.2 | 4.30 [a,b,d] ± 6.19 | 3.19 [a,b,d] ± 4.31 | 1.35 [b] ± 0.49 | 19.1 ± 8.65 |
| **CH(C)** (n=40) | 53.3 [a] ± 41.3 | 43.9 ± 23.3 | 49.9 ± 35.3 | 1.19 ± 0.98 | 1.14 ± 0.67 | 1.06 ± 0.43 | 17.8 ± 3.91 |
| **LC(C)** (n=16) | 51.7 [a] ±28.9 | 42.2 ± 22.2 | 33.1 ± 21.1 | 1.94 ± 1.25 | 1.29 ± 0.52 | 1.49 ± 0.73 | 4.95 [b,c,d] ± 1.87 |
| **LC(C)-HCC** (n=14) | 142.5 [a,d,e] ± 12.6 | 57.9 ± 18.0 | 51.6 ± 21.2 | 2.98 [d,e] ± 4.38 | 2.25 [d] ± 2.77 | 1.19 ± 0.26 | 4.06 [b,c,d] ± 4.66 |

1. Data are expressed as mean ± standard deviation (SD). [a], $P < 0.05$ versus control. [b], $P < 0.05$ versus NASH. [c], $P < 0.05$ versus NASH-LC. [d], $P < 0.05$ versus CH(C). [e], $P < 0.05$ versus LC(C).
2. NASH, non-alcoholic steatohepatitis; NASH-HCC, non-alcoholic steatohepatitis with hepatocellular carcinoma; NASH-LC, liver cirrhosis induced by NASH; ALD, alcoholic liver disease without liver cirrhosis and hepatocellular carcinoma; CH(C), chronic hepatitis C; LC(C), liver cirrhosis due to hepatitis C virus; LC(C)-HCC, liver cirrhosis due to hepatitis C virus with hepatocellular carcinoma;

Table 1. Serum levels of liver specific markers and their ratios in chronic liver disease

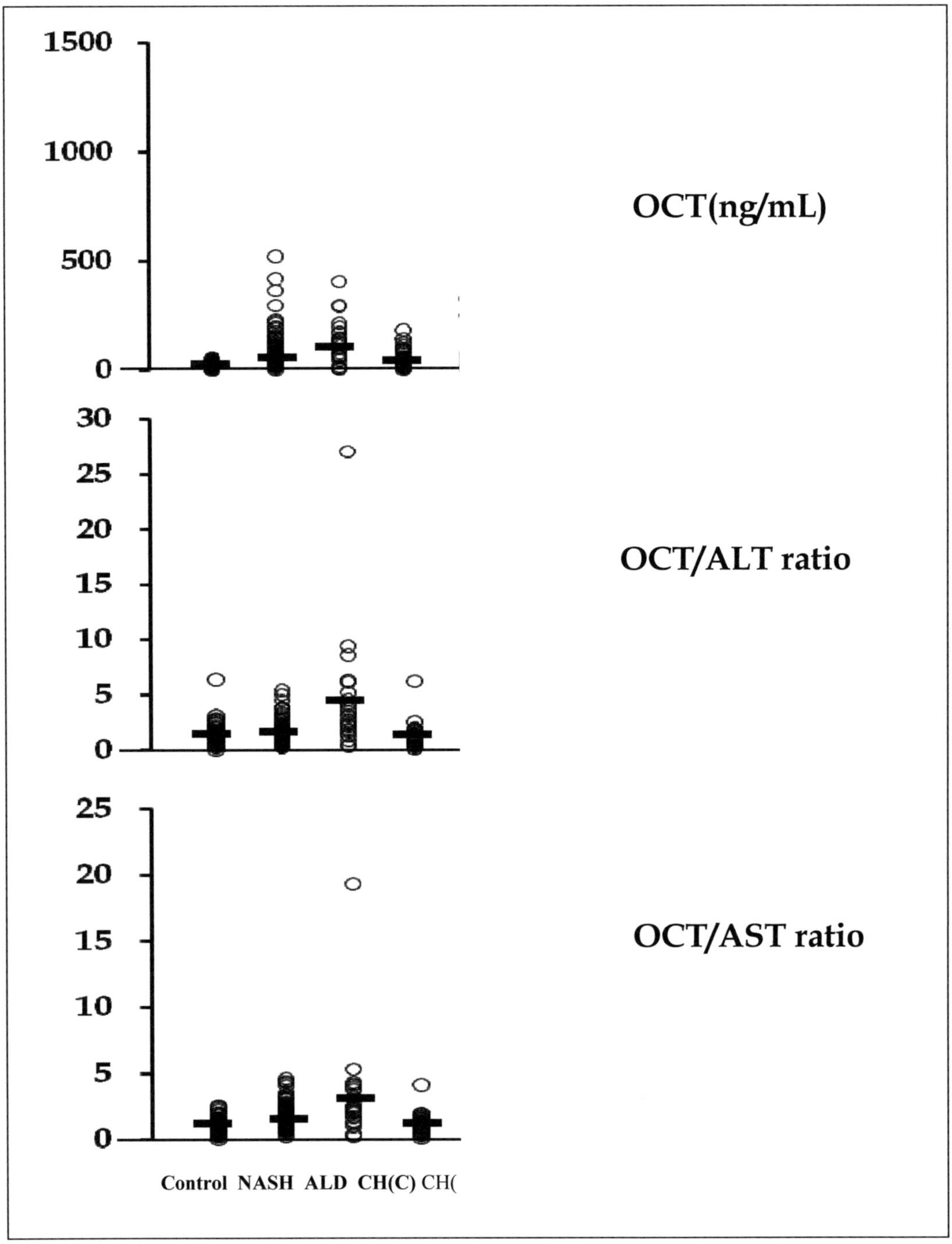


Fig. 1. Comparison of OCT and ratios of OCT/ALT, OCT/AST in various liver diseases without LC and HCC. Serum OCT levels, OCT/ALT and OCT/AST ratios in ALD were significantly higher.

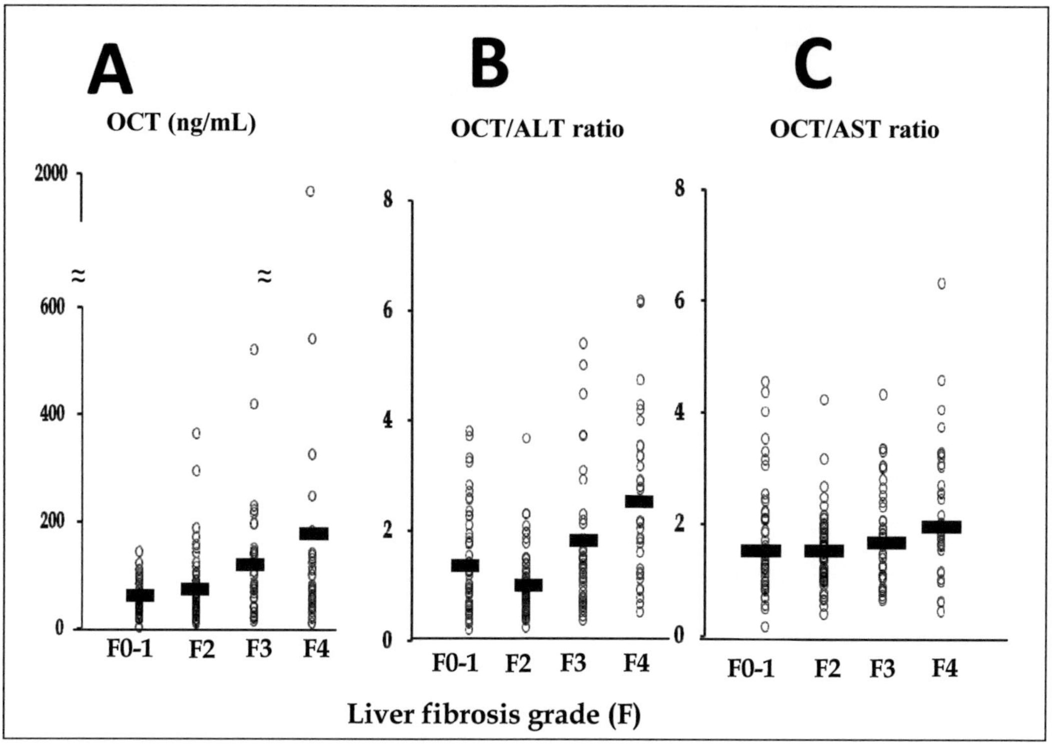


Fig. 2. The relationship between liver fibrosis grade (F) and OCT levels (A), OCT/ALT ratio (B), OCT/AST(C) ratio in NASH. The serum OCT levels and the ratio of OCT/ALT were increased in parallel with liver fibrosis.

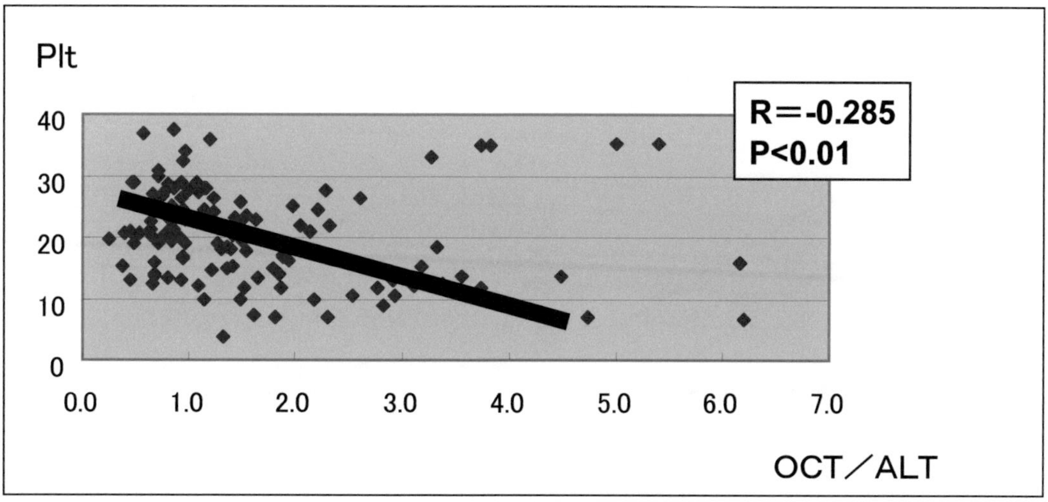


Fig. 3. The relationship between OCT / ALT ratio and platelet counts. There was a significant association between the ratio of OCT/ALT and platelet counts

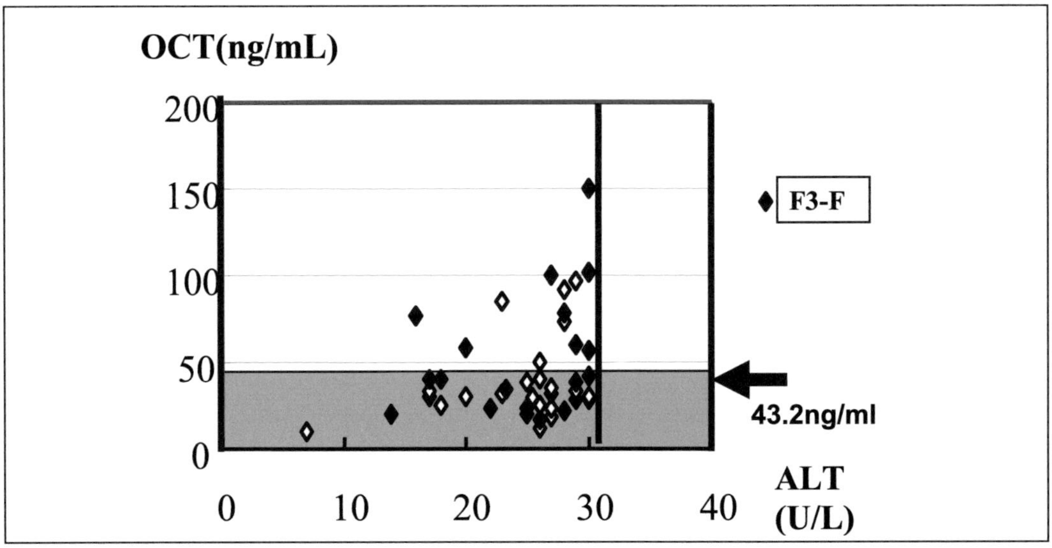


Fig. 4. OCT in NASH patients with a normal range of ALT. Forty-two patients had a normal rage of ALT, among these 42 patients, 13 (31%) had OCT over 43.2ng/mL. Of these 13 patients, eight had F3 or F4 fibrosis

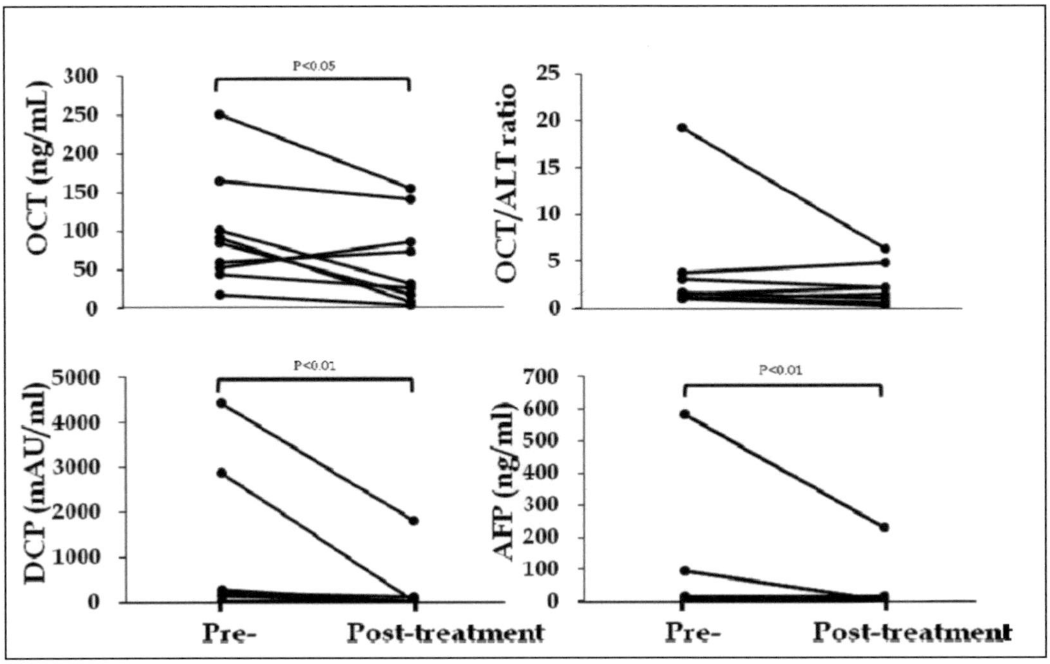


Fig. 5. Variations between the serum levels of OCT, OCT/ALT, DCP, and AFP in patients with HCC pre- and post-treatment. Serum level of OCT and OCT/ALT ratio were significantly decreased in HCC after a therapy

## 4. Discussion

An ideal biomarker should be simple, accurate, specific, inexpensive and readily available.

In this study, both the ratios of OCT/ALT and OCT/AST were increased in LC induced by NASH or HCV. Further, the significant association with fibrosis grade in NASH was confirmed. These data suggested that even without liver biopsy, we are able to speculate about the progression of various liver diseases by routine laboratory examinations. Concerning to the relationship between aminotransferase and the progression of liver diseases, serum AST and ALT levels do not necessarily reflect the activity and progression of NASH. It was reported that more than half of NASH patients with persistently normal ALT have a potentially progressive liver disease (Fracanzani et al., 2008). In our study, about 30% of NASH patients with a normal range of ALT show the elevation of OCT. In addition, the majority of these patients had severe fibrosis. It was reported that serum ALT levels in severe fibrosis of NASH were decreased (Hashimoto et al., 2009). Taken together, in NASH patients with normal range of ALT and severe fibrosis, OCT might be a normal useful marker. It is unclear why OCT is frequently elevated in NASH patients with a normal range of ALT and severe fibrosis.

In addition, serum OCT and both ratios were increased in HCC compared to LC. In the previous study, we reported that the ratios were increased in HCC with NASH (Tokushige et al., 2009). In the present study, the increase in the ratios was confirmed in HCC on chronic liver dieases infected by HCV. These data suggested that the ratios were common tumor markers in HCC based on various liver diseases. In addition, we confirmed that OCT and OCT/ALT ratio were decreased after therapy. These data suggested that OCT and OCT/ALT ratio might be useful for monitoring HCC during follow-up. Especially, in HCC with NASH, the positive percentage of DPC was higher than that of AFP. However, DCP can be affected by certain medications such as warfarin, or by the condition of the patients with severe liver failure or with bile acid outflow obstruction. As some of the NASH patients were complicated with cardiovascular diseases, they required warfarinization. Also, in about 25% of HCC patients, AFP and DCP were negative (Okuda et al.,, 2001). In these cases, OCT and OCT/ALT ratio might be useful as new HCC tumor markers for diagnosis and monitoring. We need to compare the sensitivity and specificity of these ratios and AFP or DCP in much greater numbers of samples. Recently, the association of DCP with tumor invasion and pathological grading was reported (Sakon et al., 1992; Koike et al., 2001). In the future, we need to investigate the association between OCT, OCT/ALT ratio and pathological grading or the condition of HCC.

The reason why the ratio of OCT/ALT was increased in HCC is still unclear. This increase could not be explained by the distribution of OCT and ALT, since both are located in the periportal region. One possibility is that cancer cells, expressing Fas-Ligand, might have induced apoptosis of hepatocytes (Shiraki et al., 1997). Then, in apoptotic cell death, mitochondoria-related proteins were released. Another possibility is that the expression of enzymes might change in HCC.

As for comparison with several liver diseases, serum OCT levels, OCT/ALT and OCT/AST ratios in ALD were significantly higher than those of other liver diseases. ALD is reported to be associated with mitochondrial dysfunction (Dey & Cederbaum, 2006). Therefore, it is reasonable that serum OCT levels are increased in ALD. In the future, we need to compare the sensitivity and specificity of serum OCT levels with those of serum γ-GTP levels in ALD.

## 5. Conclusion

Serum OCT levels and the ratios of OCT/ALT and OCT/AST are useful for monitoring the progression of liver diseases. Moreover, the possibility was suggested that serum OCT level and the OCT/ALT ratio might represent a new tumor marker of HCC and be a potent indicator for evaluation of the post-treatment HCC status. To confirm this possibility, we need validation study in much greater numbers of HCC samples.

## 6. References

Brunt, E.M., Janney, C.G., Di Biscrglie, A.M., Neuschwander Tetri, B.A. & Bacon, B.R. (1999). Nonalcoholic steatohepatitis: a proposal for grading and staining the histological lesions. *American Journal of Gastroenterology,* Vol.94, No.9, (September 1999), pp.2467-2474. ISSN 0002-9270

Dey, A. & Cederbaum, A.I. (2006). Alcohol and oxidative liver injury. *Hepatology,* Vol. 43, Suppl. 1, (February 2006), pp. 63-74. ISSN 1527-3350

Fracanzani, A.L., Valenti, L., Bugianesi, E., Andreoletti, M., Colli, A., Vanni, E., Bertelli, C., Fatta, E., Bignamini, D., Marchesini, G. & Fargion, S. (2008). Risk of severe liver disease in nonalcoholic fatty liver disease with normal aminotransferase levels: a role for insulin resistance and diabetes. *Hepatology,* Vol. 48, No.3, (September 2008), pp. 792-728. ISSN 1527-3350

Hashimoto, E. & Tokushige, K.(2011). Hepatocellular Carcinoma in Nonalcoholic Steatohepatitis; Growing Evidence of an Epidemic? *Hepatology Research,* In Press ISSN 1872-034X

Hahimoto, E., Yatsuji, S., Tobari, M. Taniai, M., Torii, N., Tokushige, K. & Shiratori, K. (2009). Hepatocellular carcinoma in patients with nonalcoholic steatohepatitis. *Journal of Gastroentrology,* Vol. 44, Suppl. 19, (January 2009), pp. 89-95. ISSN 0944-1174

Ikai, I., Kudo,M., Arii, S., Omata, M., Kojiro, M. & Sakamoto, M. Report of the 18th follow-up surver of promary liver cancer. *Hepatology Research,* Vol.40, No.9, (September 2010), pp.1045-1059. ISSN 1872-034X

Journal of Health and Welfare Statistics. Health and Welfare Statistics Association 2009 Japan (2009). Vol. 56, No.9, pp. 39-89.

Koike, Y., Shiratori, Y., Sato, S., Obi, S., Teratani, T., Imamura, M., Yoshida, H., Shiina, S. & Omata, M. Des-gamma-carboxy prothrombin as a useful predisposing factor for the development of portal venous invasion in patients with hepatocellular carcinoma: a prospective analysis of 227 patients. *Cancer.* Vol. 91, No. 3, (February 2001), pp. 561-9. ISSN 1097-0142

Murayama, H., Igarashi, M., Mori, M., Fukuda, Y., Ikemoto, M. & Nagata, A. (2006). A sensitive ELISA for serum ornithine carbamoyltransferase utilizing the enhancement of immunoreactivity at alkaline pH. *Clinca Chimca Acta,* Vol. 368, No.1-2, (June 2006), pp. 125-130. ISSN 0009-8981

Murayama, H., Ikemoto, M. , Fukuda, Y., & Nagata, A. (2008). Superiority of serum type-I arginase and ornithine carbamyltransferase in the detection of toxicant-induced acute hepatic injury in rats. *Clinca Chimca Acta,* Vol. 391, No. 1-2, (May 2008), pp.31-5. ISSN 0009-8981

Neuschwander-Tetri, B.A. & Caldwell, S.H.(2003). Nonalcoholic steatohepatitis: Summary of an AASLD Single Topic Conference. *Hepatology.* Vol.37, No.5, (May 2003), pp. 1202-1219. ISSN 1527-3350

Okuda, H., Nakanishi, T., Takatsu, K., Saito, A., Hayashi, N., Yamamoto, M., Takasaki, K & Nakano M.(2001) Comparison of clinicopathological features of patients with hepatocellular carcinoma seropositive for alpha-fetoprotein alone and those seropositive for des-gamma-carboxy prothrombin alone. *Journal of Gastroenterology and Hepatology.* Vol.16, No.11, (November 2001), pp.1290-1296. ISSN 1440-1746

Okuda, H., Nakanishi, T., Takatsu, K., Saito, A., Hayashi, N., Takasaki. K., Takenami, K., Yamamoto, M. & Nakano, M. (2000). Serum levels of des-gamma-carboxy prothrombin measured using the revised enzyme immunoassay kit with increased sensitivity in relation to clinicopathologic features of solitary hepatocellular carcinoma. *Cancer.* Vol. 88, No. 3, (February 2000), pp.544-549. ISSN 1097-0142

Sakon, M., Monden, M., Gotoh, M., Kanai, T., Umeshita, K., Nakano, Y., Mori, T., Sakurai, M. & Wakasa K. (1992). Relationship between pathologic prognostic factors and abnormal levels of des-gamma-carboxy prothrombin and alpha-fetoprotein in hepatocellular carcinoma. *American Journal of Surgery,* Vol. 163, No.2, (February 1992), pp. 251-256.

Shiraki, K, Tsuji, N, Shioda, T, Isselbacher, K.J . & Takahashi, H. (1997). Expression of Fas ligand in liver m &etastases of human colonic adenocarcinomas. *Proceedings of the National Academy of Sciences of the United States of America,* Vol.97, No.12, (Jun 1997), pp.6420–6425. ISSN 1091-6490

Takada ,A. & Tsutsumi M. (1995). National survey of alcoholic liver disease in Japan (1968-91). *Journal of Gastroenterol ogy and Hepatology,* Vol.10, No. 5, (September 1995 ), pp.509-516. ISSN 1440-1746

Tokushige, K., Hshimoto, E., Noto, H., Yatsuji, S., Tobari, M., Torii, N., Shiratori, K. & Murayama, H. (2009). Clinical significance of serum ornithine carbamoyltransferase in patients with non-alcoholic steatohepatitis. *Hepatology Research,* Vol.39, No.9, (September 2009), pp.939-43. ISSN 1872-034X

Tokushige, K., Hashimoto, E., Yatsuji, S., Tobari, M., Taniai, M.., Torii, N. & Shoratori, K. (2009). Prospective study of hepatocellular carcinoma in nonalcoholic steatohepatitis in comparison with hepatocellulacarcinoma cause by chronic hepatitis C. *Journal of Gastroentelorogy,* Vol.45, No.9, (September 2010) pp.960-7. ISSN 0944-1174

World Health Organization. Mortality database. (2010) www.who.int/whosis/en. Accessed February 2010

4

# New Molecular Biomarkers Candidates for the Development of Multiparametric Platforms for Hepatocellular Carcinoma Diagnosis, Prognosis and Personalised Therapy

Annalucia Serafino and Pasquale Pierimarchi
*Institute of Translational Pharmacology,*
*National Research of Council of Italy (CNR), Rome*
*Italy*

## 1. Introduction

Hepatocellular carcinoma (HCC) is one of the most common cancers in the world, showing a rapid progressive clinical course, poor response to pharmacological treatment and a severe prognosis (Colombo, 2003; Sherlock & Dooley, 2002). HCC generally develops from chronic liver injury, which leads to inflammation, hepatocyte regeneration, liver matrix remodeling, fibrosis, and finally, cirrhosis. The main risk factors for HCC are hepatitis B (HBV) or C virus (HCV) infection, alcohol-induced liver disease (ALD), non-alcoholic fatty liver disease (NAFLD), primary biliary cirrhosis and exposure to environmental carcinogens (particularly aflatoxin), and genetic metabolic diseases. (Chuang et al., 2009; Di Bisceglie, 1995; Kato et al, 1994; Malaguarnera et al., 2006; Malaguarnera et al., 2009; Seitz & Becker, 2007; Takano et al., 1995). Obesity has also been identified as an independent risk factor for developing HCC in patients with alcoholic or cryptogenic cirrhosis (Nair et al, 2002). Actually, HCV-related cirrhosis is considered the major risk factor since many HCV chronically infected patients remain asymptomatic for a long period, with liver cirrhosis developing after approximately 30 years (Yano et al., 1996; Poynard et al., 1997). The lack of predictive markers that makes unforeseeable the insurgence of liver cirrhosis in chronic HCV patients may also contribute to HCC late diagnosis, progression and poor prognosis. Currently, alpha-fetoprotein (AFP) is the most common marker for early malignancy used in clinical practice, in combination with hepatic echography, to detect HCC in patients suffering from cirrhosis. Nevertheless, most episodes of AFP elevation were transient and closely correlated with the presence of bridging hepatic necrosis, without subsequent development of HCC (Liaw et al., 1986). Since an early diagnosis of HCC is extremely important in improving the survival of patients, the identification of new and more reliable biological markers of HCC insurgence, recurrence and metastasis is essential for the proper management of this malignancy. Once hepatic cancer develops, one of the main reasons for the high mortality rate in patients with HCC is the lack of effective treatment options, especially for those with advanced disease. Although surgery and percutaneous ablation can achieve long-term control in some patients with early HCC, recurrence rates are high, approximately 50% at 3 years (Mulcahy, 2005). Furthermore, due to the asymptomatic nature of early HCC, lack of awareness and poorly defined screening strategies, approximately 80% of patients present with advanced or unresectable disease (Thomas & Abbruzzese, 2005). These patients generally have a very poor prognosis and treatments, such as transarterial chemoembolization, intra-arterial or systemic chemotherapy, radiotherapy, immunotherapy or hormonal therapy, are mainly used as palliative, with a 5-year relative survival rate of only 7% (Bosch et al., 2004).

The lack of effective and well-tolerated treatments for advanced HCC highlights the need for innovative approaches for diagnosis, prognosis and therapy for hepatic cancer. In this context, multiparametric platforms allowing simultaneous detection of multiple serological and immunohistochemical markers for HCC insurgence, recurrence and metastasis would represent a high-performance technological tools useful not only for diagnosis and prognosis, but also for improving the clinical management of HCC patients, allowing us, in the near future, to design therapies adapted to the aggressiveness of each individual tumor.

Starting from this background, in this chapter will be collected some of the data existing in literature on the main serological and immunohistochemical biomarkers for HCC diagnosis, prognosis and target therapy, also focusing on new molecules which might be attractive candidates for improvement of the diagnostic/therapeutic approaches. In particular will be covered the following topics : 1) Some new candidates recently proposed as potential biological markers of HCC insurgence, recurrence and metastasis, that could be useful for early diagnosis of this malignancy and improve patient's prognosis; 2) Some signaling pathways which deregulation or constitutive activation have been demonstrated to have a role in HCC insurgence and progression and that could be of interest for therapeutic perspectives, since targeting them may contribute to prevent tumorigenesis or achieve tumor reversion; 3) Molecules over-expressed in late stages of cancer or in the metastatic diseases that should be considered a good targets for therapy and drug delivery.

## 2. Biological markers useful for early diagnosis of HCC insurgence, recurrence and metastasis

Currently, the diagnosis of HCC is mainly based on the atypical histopathology of bioptic liver tissues, combined with the laboratory screening including the index of hepatic damage (alanine aminotransferase and aspartate aminotransferase), the index of hepatic synthesis (albumin, prothrombin time, bilirubin), the index of cholestasis (alkaline phosphatase and gamma-glutamyl transpeptidase), and finally, tumor markers and instrumental analyses, including hepatic ultrasonography, computed tomography, nuclear magnetic resonance. Some of the tumor markers for HCC diagnosis, such as alpha-fetoprotein (AFP), *lens culinaris* agglutinin-reactive AFP (AFP-L3) and des-γ-carboxyprothrombin (DCP) have now been incorporated into HCC staging classification (Marrero et al., 2010) and are routinely taken into account for the screening for early malignancy (**Table 1**). Other biomarkers, including some growth factors, such as Vascular Endothelial Growth Factor (VEGF), Transforming Growth Factor β1 (TGF-β1), Hepatocyte Growth Factor EGF), Epidermal

Growth Factor receptor (EGFR), and numerous other molecules (**Table 1**), are used as diagnostic/prognostic aid for HCC and for staging (Malaguarnera et al., 2010; Mann et al., 2007; Qin & Tang, 2004). Nevertheless, each existing marker alone is poorly specific to predict the disease and most markers are not related to each other. Currently the absolute positive and negative serological and/or immunohistochemical markers for HCC are still lacking, and even those selected for high sensitivity and specificity do not exhibit an universal diagnostic/prognostic value. Therefore, in the last years, a great number of studies has been dedicated to the discovery and validation of more specific biomarkers for HCC, driven by the idea that the simultaneous screening for multiple markers should greatly reduce errors from false-negative results, which significantly contribute to an incorrect diagnosis.

### 2.1 Main markers used for the screening for early malignancy

Alpha-fetoprotein (AFP) is a 70 kDa glycoprotein that is physiologically synthesized by the embryonic liver cells of the yolk sac and fetal intestinal tract. The AFP is expressed in hepatocytes and endodermal cells of the yolk sac during fetal life and its expression is reduced after birth, with very low levels in adults. The AFP levels rise in hepatocyte regeneration, hepatocarcinogenesis, and embryonic carcinomas. Its biological function in embryo- and carcinogenesis and in adult organisms is still not well identified, but, due to its structural similarity with albumin, a function as a carrier for several ligands, including bilirubin, steroids, fatty acids and various drugs has been proposed (Mizejewski, 2002; Terentiev & Moldogazieva, 2006). Recognized as a tumor-associated fetal protein, AFP has long been considered the 'gold-standard' among tumor markers, and, it has been purified, characterized, cloned and sequenced for use in the clinical diagnostic. It is principally used: i) for the screening and diagnosis of hepatocarcinoma in patients at risk of developing HCC, in combination with hepatic ultrasonography; ii) as a marker of tumor progression in HCC patients with high levels of AFP; iii) for monitoring the response to treatment during the follow-up of HCC patients, with a prognostic value; iv) in HCC staging.

*Lens culinaris* agglutinin-reactive AFP (AFP-L3) is one of the AFP isoform which exhibits an elevated affinity for *Lens culinaris* agglutinin (LCA). This AFP isoform, that has $\alpha 1 \rightarrow 6$ fucose residues on N-acetylglucosamine at reducing end, seems to be exclusively expressed by cancer cells, and is considered a more specific marker for HCC (Oka et al., 2001; Sato et al., 1993). AFP-L3 should be used as a supplemental test in patients with elevated total AFP. It has been reported as a potential indicator of a poor prognosis, since increasing AFP-L3 levels seem to correlate with progression from moderately differentiated to poorly differentiated tumors (Miyaaki et al., 2007).

Des-c-carboxy prothrombin (DCP) or prothrombin induced by vitamin K absence (PIVKA) is an abnormal prothrombin derived by an acquired defect in the post-translational carboxylation of the prothrombin precursor in HCC cells (Ono et al., 1990). DCP derives by a reduced activity of gamma-glutamyl carboxylase, highly expressed in the liver; this reduced activity is attributed to defective gene expression in HCC patients (Grizzi et al., 2007). DCP is a HCC marker more specific than AFP since other liver diseases are not associated to an increase of DCP serum levels. Apart its diagnostic significance, increased DCP levels may also have a prognostic value, being often related to early portal vein invasion and metastatization by cancer cells.

### 2.2 Some growth factors used as diagnostic/prognostic aid

Vascular Endothelial Growth Factor (VEGF), plays an crucial role in angiogenesis and is highly expressed in various human cancers (Brown et al., 1993; Mattern et al., 1996; Toi et al., 1994), including HCC (Mise et al., 1996; Suzuki et al., 1996). Specifically, VEGF levels are higher in HCC patients than in patients suffering from chronic hepatitis, and its expression is more elevated in advanced HCC as compared to early HCC. High serum VEGF levels are associated with tumors with portal vein emboli, poor-encapsulated tumors, microscopic vein invasion, and recurrence in HCC patients (Li et al., 1999). It is considered as a possible marker for predicting invasion and metastatization of HCC, and in general, of tumor aggressiveness.

Transforming Growth Factor β1 (TGF-β1), is a polypeptide member of the transforming growth factor beta superfamily of cytokines. It is an important mediator of control of liver cell proliferation and replication. In normal liver tissues, TGF-β1 is produced by non-parenchymal cells (Kupffer cells, storing cells, and endothelial cells), but not by hepatocytes. Conversely, transcription of TGF-β1 gene is activated in human HCC tissues and is higher in patients with advancing histological aggressiveness (Ito et al., 1990). Moreover, TGF-β1 serum levels are reported to be increased in HCC patients (Grizzi et al., 2007). TGF-β1 has been proposed as a possible prognostic factor for reduced survival in patients with HCC (Mann et al., 2007; Okumoto et al., 2004; Tsai et al., 1997)

Hepatocyte growth factor (HGF) is a cytokine with a wide range of effects, including liver regeneration for protection and/or repair of different organs, including kidney, lung, and cardiovascular system (Birchmeier et al., 1998). It promotes proliferation in normal hepatocyte and in hepatocellular carcinoma cells (Breuhan et al., 2006) through expression of its high-affinity tyrosine kinase receptor (Met/*HGF*-R). HGF is detected in the serum from patients suffering from hepatic chronic disease and its serum values seems to be correlated with a worsening of liver disease (Breuhan et al., 2006). Increased HGF serum levels in cirrhotic patients is an indicator of HCC development (Yamagamim et al., 2002). It is considered a prognostic marker since elevated HGF serum levels, are predictive of HCC recurrence and metastasis after hepatic resection (Wu et al., 2006).

Epidermal growth factor receptor (EGFR) is a member of the ErbB family of receptors, a subfamily of four closely related receptor tyrosine kinases, EGFR (ErbB-1), HER2/c-neu (ErbB-2), Her 3 (ErbB-3) and Her 4 (ErbB-4). These receptors bind ligands of the EGF family, including EGF, TGF-α and heparin-binding EGF. EGFR has been found to be overexpressed in poorly differentiated HCC and primarily in patients with early tumor recurrence (Daveau et al., 2003; Ito et al., 2001) EGFR tissue overexpression is also correlated with high proliferating activity, advanced stage, the presence of intrahepatic metastasis and poor disease-free survival following resection (Ito et al., 2001). EGFR strongly reflects the biological aggressiveness of HCC and might be considered a possible prognostic factor of reduced survival of HCC patients.

| HCC biomarker | Biological material mainly analyzed | Main use/s | References |
|---|---|---|---|
| Alpha-fetoprotein (AFP) | Serum | Early diagnosis; HCC staging; monitoring the response to treatment during the follow-up of patients with HCC | Terentiev & Moldogazieva, 2006; Mizejewski, 2002; Malaguarnera et al., 2010; Marrero et al., 2010 |
| *Lens culinaris* agglutinin-reactive AFP (AFP-L3) | Serum | Early diagnosis and prognosis; progression from moderately differentiated to poorly differentiated tumors | Oka et al., 2001; Sato et al., 1993; Malaguarnera et al., 2010; Marrero et al., 2004 |
| Des-c-carboxy prothrombin (DCP) | Serum | Early diagnosis and prognosis (more specific than AFP); related to early portal vein invasion and metastasis | Grizzi et al., 2007; Malaguarnera et al., 2010; Marrero et al., 2004 |
| Golgi protein-73 | Serum | HCC early diagnosis | Malaguarnera et al., 2010 |
| Squamous cell carcinoma antigen (SCCA) | Tissue/Serum | Early diagnosis; detection of micro-metastasis in tissues; large-scale screening of serum in patients at risk | Malaguarnera et al., 2010 |
| Glypican-3 | Tissue/Serum | HCC early diagnosis; useful for discriminating malignant from benign hepatic lesions | Malaguarnera et al., 2010 |
| Vascular Endothelial Growth Factor (VEGF) | Tissue/Serum | HCC prognosis; predictive of invasion and metastatization of HCC cells | Suzuki et al., 1996; Mise et al., 1996; Li et al., 1999; Qin &Tang, 2004; Mann et al., 2007; Malaguarnera et al., 2010 |
| Transforming Growth Factor β1 (TGF-β1) | Tissue/Serum | HCC progression; prognostic factor for reduced survival in patients with HCC | Ito et al., 1990; Grizzi et al., 2007; Mann et al., 2007; Okumoto et al., 2004; Tsai et al., 1997 |
| Hepatocyte Growth Factor (HGF) | Serum | HCC prognosis; predictive of HCC recurrence and metastasis after hepatic resection | Breuhan et al., 2006; Yamagamim et al., 2002; Wu et al., 2006; Malaguarnera et al., 2010 |
| Epidermal Growth Factor Receptor (EGFR) | Tissue | HCC prognosis; predictive of reduced survival of HCC patients | Daveau et al., 2003; Ito et al., 2001; Mann et al., 2007 |
| p53 antibodies | Serum | HCC prognosis (poor differentiation); associated with a poor prognosis of HCC patients | Malaguarnera et al., 2010 |
| Survivine | Tissue | HCC prognosis; poor prognosis following resection of HCC; associated with reduced disease-free survival. | Fields et al., 2004; Mann et al., 2007 |
| Nerve Growth Factor (NGF) and its high-affinity receptor $trkA^{NGF}$ | Tissue/Serum | HCC prognosis and progression; predictive of progression of liver fibrosis towards HCC | Rasi et al, 2007; Malaguarnera et al., 2010 |

Table 1. List of the main biomarkers useful for HCC diagnosis/prognosis

### 2.3 The Nerve Growth Factor (NGF): A new candidate proposed as potential histological/serum marker for HCC diagnosis and prognosis

In the last years, some new candidates have been proposed as potential biological markers of HCC insurgence, recurrence and metastasis, that could be therefore useful for early diagnosis of this malignancy and improve patient's prognosis. In particular we focus on our recently published data that suggested an involvement of Nerve Growth Factor (NGF) in liver tissue remodelling processes and HCC progression, describing the correlation between NGF tissue distribution and serum levels in patients suffering from cirrhosis and/or HCC (Rasi et al, 2007).

NGF is a prototypical member of neurotrophin family essential for survival, differentiation, and maintenance of neuronal cells in the central and peripheral nervous system (Levi-Montalcini, 1987). In recent years, many findings have indicated that NGF could also have a role outside the central and peripheral nervous system. In particular, it may be involved in lung and skin tissue repair (Micera et al., 2001) as well as in allergic inflammation and fibrosis (Micera et al., 2003). Increased levels of circulating NGF were observed in several autoimmune, chronic inflammatory and fibrotic disorders (Aloe & Tuveri, 1997; Bonini et al., 1999). Numerous data also indicate that NGF is involved in tumor growth, invasion and metastasis (Bold et al., 1995; Descamps et al., 1998; Djakiew et al., 1991; Koizumi et al., 1998; McGregor et al., 1999; Oelmann et al., 1995; Pflug et al., 1992; Revoltella & Butler, 1980; Sortino et al., 2000).The NGF effects are mediated by two types of receptor: the high-affinity receptor $trkA^{NGF}$, specific for NGF, and the low-affinity glycoprotein receptor $p75^{NTR}$, also binding other neurotrophins (Meakin & Shooter, 1992). Most of the biological activities elicited by NGF are mediated by binding to the $trkA^{NGF}$ receptor (Sofroniew et al., 2001).

In the 2007 (Rasi et al., 2007), we provided immunohistochemical evidence that NGF and its high-affinity receptor $trkA^{NGF}$ are over expressed in patients suffering from HCC (**Fig. 1**) and to a greater extent from HCC with cirrhosis (**Fig. 2B, C**). Specifically, in HCC tissues NGF was detectable in a high number of cells (**Table 2**), at different levels of intensities depending on the patient, but never in normal liver tissue. Interestingly NGF and $trkA^{NGF}$ were negative in liver specimens from patients with cirrhosis undergoing transplantation (Child-C) but without HCC (**Fig. 2A**), while they were markedly positive in patients with cirrhosis that had evolved into HCC, already at early staging (Child- Pugh A, **Fig. 2B**).

Transmission electron microscopy, after immunogold labeling, showed that in hepatocytes of HCC tissue and, at higher extent, of cirrhotic tissue from the same liver, NGF mainly localized on cytoplasmic vesicles, free in the cytoplasm and along endoplasmic reticulum (**Fig. 3**), indicating that it might be actively produced by the hepatocytes constituting the cirrhotic/HCC tissues. The evidence that hepatocytes in HCC and cirrhotic tissues from the same liver produce NGF and express its receptor suggested that NGF may act by both autocrine and paracrine mechanisms, as a messenger molecule in the cross-talk between different cell types. Moreover, in sera obtained from patients with documented cirrhosis, HCC, or both, circulating NGF levels elevated 25-fold over the normal (range 73-520pg/ml, compared to a mean of 20pg/ml in healthy donors) were recorded (**Fig. 4**). These elevated circulating NGF levels, as well as the tissue distribution of NGF and its receptor strongly support a correlation between NGF activity and the progression of liver fibrosis towards HCC. This open up an interesting perspective for the possible use of NGF, not only as a marker of progression and transformation, but also as an attractive target for a new therapeutic approach.

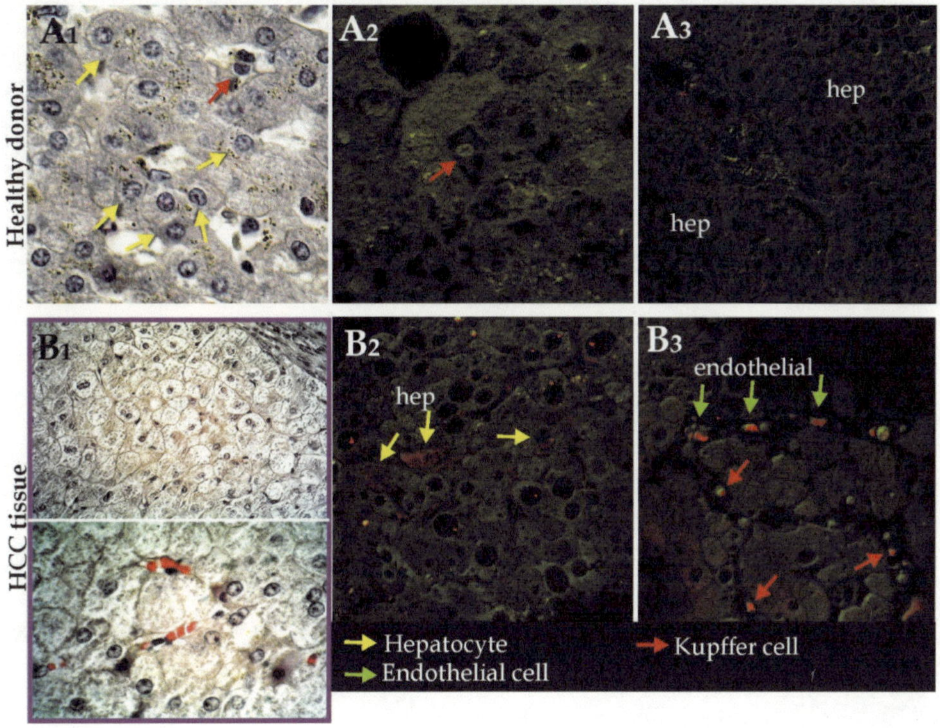


Fig. 1. NGF distribution (red hue) in tissues from healthy donors (**A**) and from patients suffering from HCC (**B**). Green hue represents the auto-fluorescence used to visualize liver tissue morphology. **A1** and **B1**: Images of H&E stained sections close to that used for immunohistochemistry. Differently coloured arrows indicate the different cell types (see legend). hep: hepatocytes.

| | Marker | Hep | Bec | Ec | Ssc | Lymph | Kpf |
|---|---|---|---|---|---|---|---|
| **Health** | NGF | - | - | - | nd | + | - |
| | trkA | - | - | - | nd | nd | - |
| **HCC** | NGF | +* | ± | + | nd | + | + |
| | trkA | ± | ± | ± | nd | nd | ± |
| **CIRR** | NGF | ++* | ++** | ++ | + | + | ± |
| | trkA | ++ | ++** | + | + | + | + |

IF: immunofluorescence labelling; IG: immunogold labelling; nd: not determined.
*Immunoreaction mainly localized on cytoplasmic vesicles and endoplasmic reticulum.
**Immunoreaction mainly localized in the portion of cells near the ductal lumen.

Table 2. Expression of NGF and $trkA^{NGF}$ in liver cell types from healthy donors and from patients with cirrhosis and HCC. Hep: Hepatocyte; Bec, Biliary epithelial cells; Ec, Endothelial cells; Ssc, Spindle-shaped cells; Lymph, Lymphocytes; Kpf, Kupffer cells.

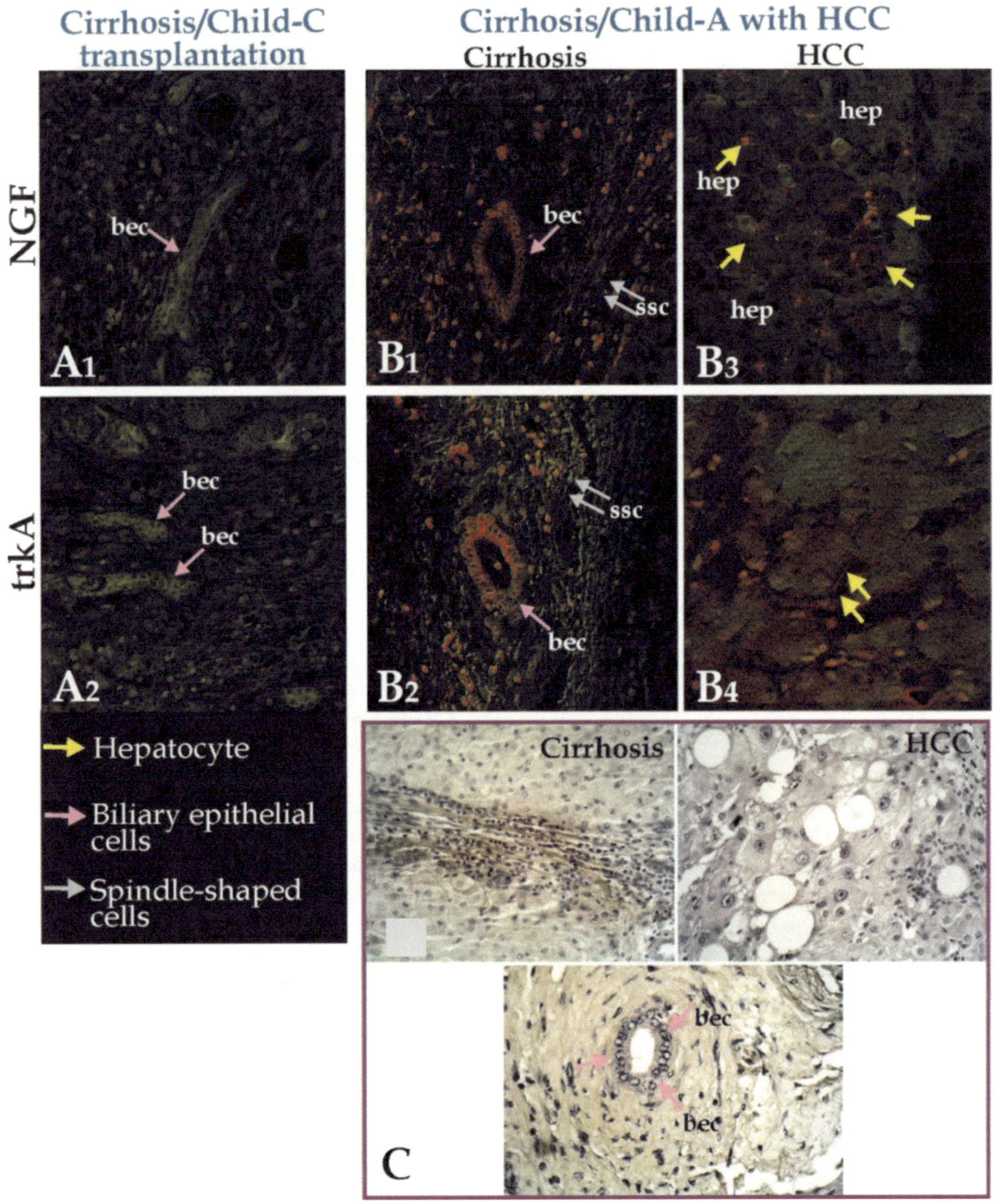


Fig. 2. NGF and trkA$^{NGF}$ distribution in liver specimens. **A**: tissues obtained before transplantation from patients with cirrhosis but without HCC (Child-Pugh C). **B:** tissue from patient also suffering from cirrhosis with HCC. Red hue represents the NGF or trkA immunostaining; green hue represents the auto-fluorescence used to visualize liver tissue morphology. **C**: Images of H&E stained sections close to that used for immunohistochemistry. Differently coloured arrows indicate the different cell types (see legend). hep: hepatocytes; bec: biliary epithelial cells; ssc: spindle-shaped cells

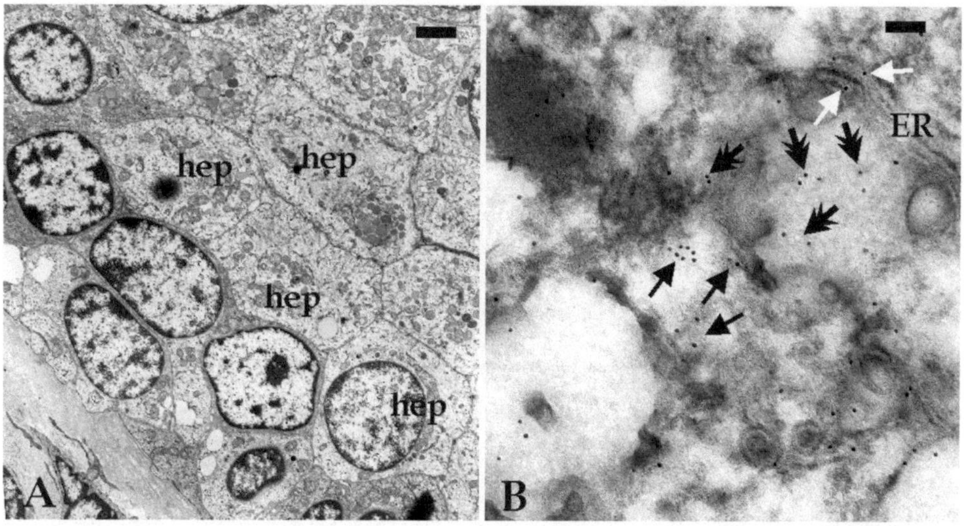


Fig. 3. NGF distribution in cirrhotic tissue from patient with HCC by immunogold labelling. Transmission electron micrographs of hepatocytes showing positive immunogold reaction on cytoplasmic vesicles (black arrows), free in the cytoplasm (double pointed arrows) and along endoplasmic reticulum (white arrows). hep: hepatocytes; ER: endoplasmic reticulum. Scale bars = **A**: 2*μm*; **B**: 100*nm*.

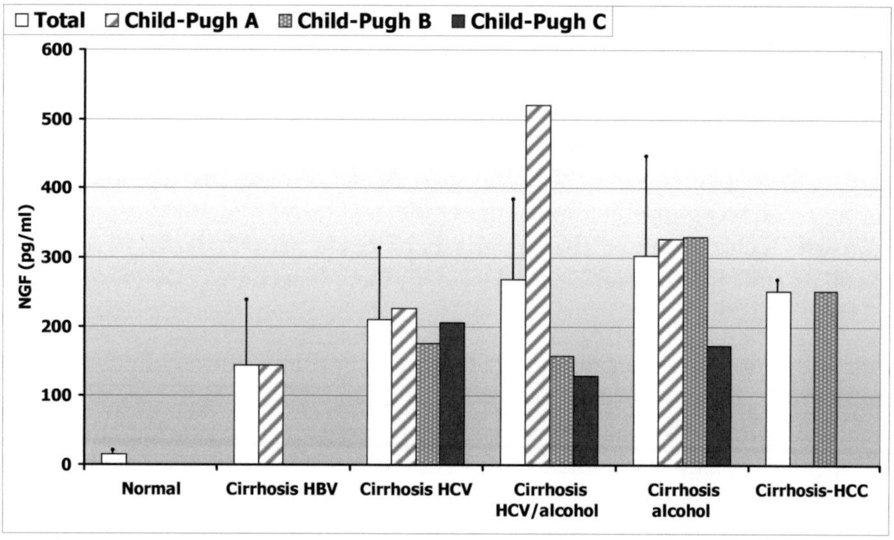


Fig. 4. Bar diagram illustrating the circulating NGF levels, determined by ELISA test , in patients with documented cirrhosis/HCC. NGF amounts, reported with regard to the etiology, is calculated either as total mean values ± SD (all patients examined) or as mean values for Child-Pugh class A (score = 5-6), for Child-Pugh class B (score = 7-9) and for Child-Pugh class C (score = 10-15). As a control, mean value ± SD of circulating NGF levels from some healthy individuals is also reported

## 3. Components of signaling pathways involved in HCC insurgence and progression as innovative biomarkers for diagnosis, prognosis and drug targeting

In the last years, great attention has been given to some signaling pathways which deregulation or constitutive activation have been demonstrated to have a role in cancer insurgence and progression. These pathways could be of interest for therapeutic perspectives, because targeting them may contribute to prevent tumorigenesis or achieve tumor reversion. Drugs directly acting on components of the signaling pathways implicated in tumorigenesis have exhibited clinical benefit in patients with various tumor types, including colorectal, renal, breast and lung cancers, and more recently, HCC (Whittaker et al., 2010). Thus, deepening of knowledge on the molecular pathways actively involved in HCC insurgence and progression could potentially provide new targets for drug delivery and therapy, allowing to overcome the poor response to the current therapeutic strategies. Moreover, owing the role of these pathways in the carcinogenetic process, crucial molecules of this signaling should be validate as new HCC-related biomarkers for the improvement of the current diagnostic/prognostic tools.

### 3.1 Main signaling pathways implicated in HCC

During hepatocarcinogenesis, two main pathogenic mechanisms predominate: 1) cirrhosis associated with hepatic regeneration after tissue damage caused by hepatitis infection, toxins such as alcohol or aflatoxin, or metabolic syndromes such as insulin resistance, obesity, type 2 diabetes or dyslipidemia in non-alcoholic steatohepatitis (Bugianesi, 2005); 2) mutations occurring in single or multiple oncogenes or tumor suppressor genes (Thorgeirsson & Grisham, 2002; Villanueva et al., 2007; Wang et al., 2002). These two mechanisms have been related to aberrations in various critical molecular signaling pathways that participate to the carcinogenic process. The most important of these pathways include the growth factor-mediated angiogenic signaling (mainly the VEGF receptor signaling), the epidermal growth factor receptor (EGFR), the insulin growth factor receptor (IGFR), the hepatocyte growth factor receptor HGF/c-MET signaling, and the platelet-derived growth factor receptor (PDGFR) signaling (**Fig. 5**) (Whittaker et al., 2010).

Since liver is a highly vascular organ, HCC growth and invasion is highly dependent on dysregualtion of angiogenensis (Semela & Dufour, 2004), and targeting molecular components of pathway signaling involved in the angiogenetic process are currently the main therapeutic strategy exploited for HCC treatment. Actually, targeted drug selectively hitting the VEGF/VEGFR and PDGFR signaling (Sunitinib, Bevacizumab, Cediranib and Vatalanib) or the EGF/EGFR and IGFR signaling (Lapatinib, Cetuximab, Erlotinib Gefitinib, Everolimus, Sirolimus) (Fig. 5) are under evaluation in phase I-III clinical trials as monotherapy or in combination with other chemotherapeutics (see for review, Whittaker et al., 2010). Sorafenib (Nexavar; Bayer HealthCare Pharmaceuticals Inc., Wayne, NJ, USA), a potent inhibitor of VEGFR and PDGFR, has been approved for treatment of HCC and is the only option of effective systemic treatment currently available for management of the advanced malignancy (Llovet et al., 2008).

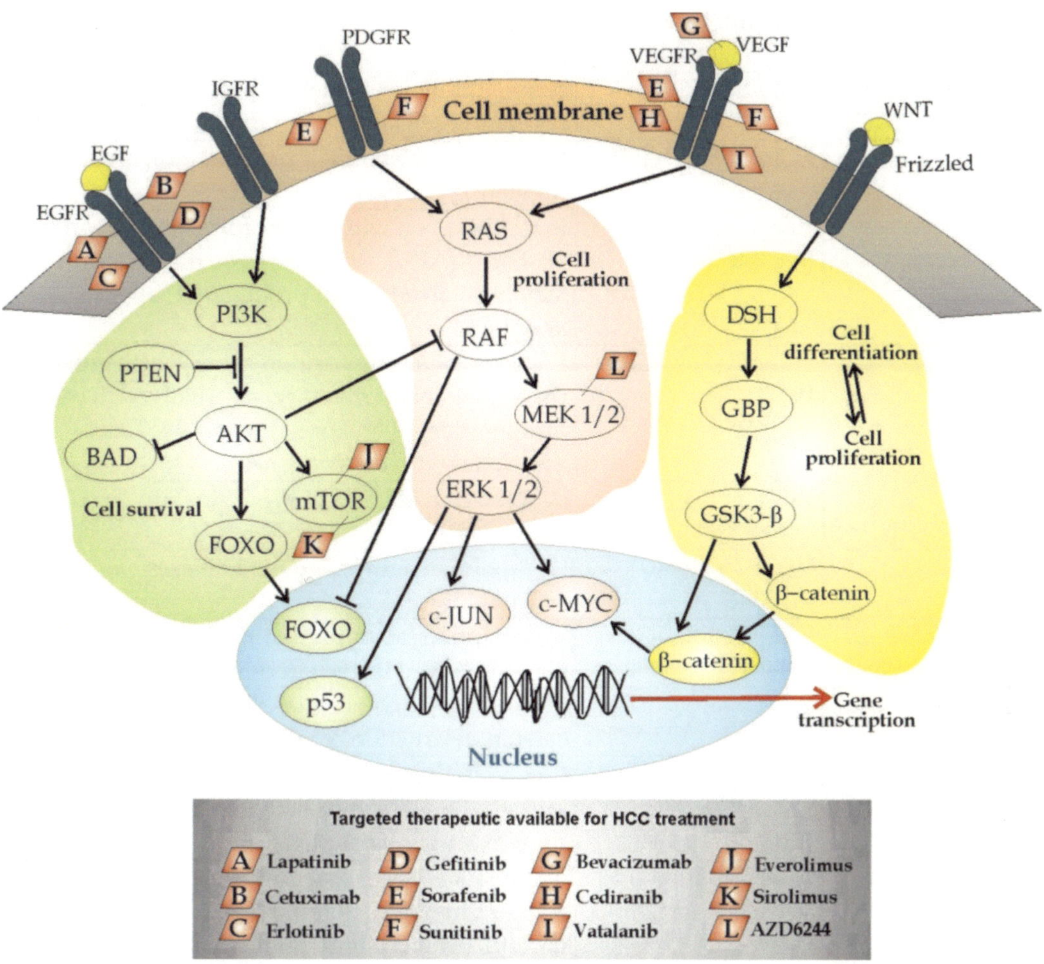


Fig. 5. Cellular signaling pathways implicated in the pathogenesis of HCC and therapeutics targeting molecular components of these pathway, useful for HCC treatment. EGF, epidermal growth factor; EGFR, EGF receptor; IGFR, insulin-like growth factor receptor; PDGFR, platelet-derived growth factor receptor; WNT, family of secreted glycoproteins that act as ligands of the Frizzled receptor; VEGF, vascular endothelial growth factor; VEGFR, VEGF receptor. Details and main function/s of AKT, BAD, c-JUN, c-MYC, DSH, ERK 1/2, FOXO, GSK-3β, GBP, MEK 1/2, mTOR, PI3K, PTEN, p53, RAF, RAS, β-catenin, are reported in **Table 3**. Adapted from Whittaker et al., 2010

Besides the mentioned pathways, directly or indirectly involved in the angiogenic signaling, in the last years numerous studies demonstrated that the WNT/β-catenin pathway is actively involved in initiation and progression of several kinds of human cancers, including HCC (De La et al., 1998; Polakis, 1999; Waltzer & Bienz, 1999) and growing attention has been given to new anti-tumor therapeutic approaches targeting components of this signaling pathway (Gonsalves et al., 2011; Luu et al., 2004; Moon et al., 2004).

| Molecular components | Main Cellular signaling | Main role and function |
|---|---|---|
| AKT | EGF/EGFR, IGFR | serine/threonine protein kinase involved in regulating cell survival |
| BAD | EGF/EGFR, IGFR | BCL-2-associated death promoter, involved in regulating apoptosis |
| c-JUN | VEGF/VEGFR, PDGFR | in combination with c-FOS, forms the activator protein-1 (AP-1) early-response transcription factor; involved in cell proliferation and apoptosis. |
| c-MYC | EGF/EGFR , IGFR, WNT | Encodes for a transcription factor that regulates the expression of many genes involved in cell proliferation; overexpression of c-MYC is associated with carcinogenesis. |
| DSH (Dishevelled) | WNT | downstream effector of WNT sinaling |
| ERK 1/2 | VEGF/VEGFR, PDGFR | extracellular signal-regulated kinases |
| FOXO (Forkhead box subclass O) | EGF/EGFR , IGFR | transcription factor regulating the expression of genes involved in cell survival and proliferation |
| GSK-3β | WNT | glycogen synthase kinase-3β, component of β-catenin destruction complex |
| GBP | WNT | GSK3-binding protein |
| MEK 1/2 | VEGF/VEGFR, PDGFR | kinases that phosphorylate mitogen-activated protein (MAP) kinase (MAPK) |
| mTOR | EGF/EGFR , IGFR | mammalian target of rapamycin, a serine/threonine protein kinase that regulates cell growth, proliferation, motility, and survival |
| PI3K | EGF/EGFR , IGFR | phosphatidylinositol-3-kinase |
| PTEN | EGF/EGFR , IGFR | phosphatase and tensin homolog that regulates cell-survival pathway |
| p53 | VEGF/VEGFR, PDGFR, EGF/EGFR, IGFR | tumor suppressor protein, regulates the cell cycle |
| RAF | VEGF/VEGFR, PDGFR | MAP kinase kinase kinase (MAP3K); functions in the MAPK/ERK signal transduction pathway |
| RAS | | prototypical member of the RAS superfamily of proteins; RAS signaling causes cell growth, differentiation and survival |
| β-catenin | WNT | integral component of the WNT/β-catenin signaling |

Table 3. List of the main molecular component of cellular signaling pathways implicated in the pathogenesis of HCC.

### 3.2 Molecular component of the WNT/β-catenin signaling as innovative diagnostic biomarkers and therapeutic targets

Wnts are secreted glycoproteins that act as ligands to stimulate receptor-mediated signal transduction pathways in both vertebrates and invertebrates. Activation of Wnt pathways can modulate cell proliferation, survival, cell behavior, and cell fate in both embryos and adults. Wnt signaling pathway, and its signaling cascade is one of the core signal transduction pathway driving tissue morphogenesis during both development and progression of human cancers (see for reviews on Wnt: Moon et al., 2004; Nelson et al., 2004). Wnt signaling also plays a critical role in regulating liver cell proliferation during development (Monga et al., 2003; Suksaweang et al., 2004) and in controlling crucial functions of the adult liver (Sekine et al., 2006).

β-catenin was originally identified as a protein interacting with the cell adhesion molecule E-cadherin (E-cad) at the cell-cell junction (Ozawa et al., 1989; Vestweber & Kemler, 1984), but in the last few years has gained growing interest as one of the most important mediators of the Wnt signaling pathway (Moon et al., 2004; Nelson et al., 2004), specifically in respect to the role of this pathway in tumorigenesis (**Fig. 6**). In non normal condition, β-catenin exists in a cadherin-bound form that regulates adhesion, and the β-catenin excess, not segregated by E-cad on the cell membrane, is rapidly phosphorylated by glycogen synthetase kinase-3β(GSK-3β) in the adenomatous polyposis coli (APC)/axin/GSK-3β complex (destruction complex) and is subsequently degraded by the ubiquitin-proteosome pathway. Conversely, in tumor cells, Wnt signaling, through the Frizzled serpentine receptor and the low-density lipoprotein receptor-related protein-5 or -6 (LRP5 or 6) coreceptors, activates the cytoplasmic phosphoprotein Dishevelled, which blocks the degradation of β-catenin that accumulates in the cytosol and is translocated into the nuclei. Here, through the binding with transcription factors, T-cell factor (TCF)/lymphoid enhancer factor (LEF), β-catenin activates transcription of genes such as cyclinD1 and c-MYC, thus modulating cell proliferation and invasion.

Many of the molecular component of the WNT/β-catenin signaling have been reported to be modified in HCC, and are proposed as HCC diagnostic/prognostic markers or as therapeutic target for treatment of the primary or metastatic malignancy (**Table 4**).

Mutations of Axin or stabilizing mutations of β-catenin genes, leading to constitutive activation of the Wnt/β-catenin pathway, have been recovered in various cancers, including hepatoblastoma and HCC (Buendia, 2000; De La et al., 1998; Whittaker et al., 2010).

Conversely, inactivating mutations of the APC gene, frequently implicated in other tumor and particularly in colorectal cancer, have not been described in HCC. However, loss of APC function activating the WNT/β-catenin signaling seems to be implicated in liver carcinogenesis (Colnot et al., 2004). Moreover, aberrant reactivation of Wnt signaling due to accumulation of β-catenin is evident in many different tumors of the liver (Colnot et al., 2004). Frequent overexpression of the Wnt receptor Frizzled-7 has been detected in HCC and mainly in hepatitis B virus–related HCCs, and this overexpression seems to be an early event in hepatocarcinogenesis (Merle et al., 2004). It has been recently reported that serum β-catenin levels were significantly elevated in patients with HCC compared to those with chronic hepatitis or healthy controls, and it has been proposed as a potential marker for early diagnosis of HCC in HCV infected patients (Zekri et al., 2011). Moreover, in human

HCC tissues, higher levels of β-catenin expression was found in the tumor area compared to the non-tumor area and the level of expression and nuclear translocation of β-catenin was increased in HCC late-stage. Thus, β-catenin have been proposed as a suitable diagnostic marker of metastasis in human HCC (Lai et al., 2011).

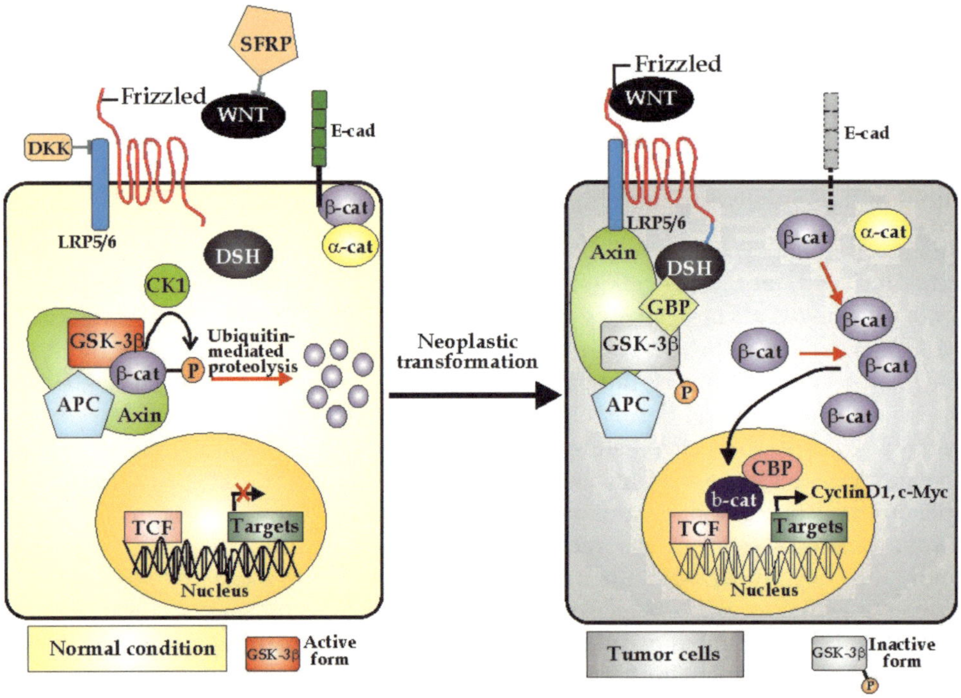


Fig. 6. Schematic representation of the Wnt/β-catenin signaling activation. APC, adenomatous polyposis coli; β-cat, β-catenin; CBP, CREB-binding protein; CK, casein kinase; DKK, Dickkopf; DSH, Dishevelled; GBP, GSK3-binding protein; GSK-3β, glycogen synthase kinase 3β; LRP, LDL receptor-related protein; P, phosphorylation; sFRP, secreted Frizzled-related protein; TCF, T-cell factor.

Finally, due to the tight interaction of β-catenin with E-cad at the cell-cell junction, activation of WNT signaling has also been related to dysregulation of cadherin expression, which is often associated with dysplasia, tumor formation, and metastasis. This causal relationship between E-cad and Wnt signaling makes E-cad an additional molecular marker that should be taken into account in the setting up a multiparametric diagnostic/prognostic platform for HCC. The E-cad expression levels have been reported to inversely correlate with histological grade and prognosis, and might be a prognostic marker of early recurrence of HCC after hepatic resection (Huang et al. 1999; Matsumura et al. 2001). Since E-cad expression is higher in well-differentiated tumors compared to poorly differentiated cancers, that exhibit lost of the intercellular junction integrity and development of metastasis (Shiozaki et al., 1996; Wijnhoven et al., 2000), it may also be predictive of invasion and metastatization of HCC cells.

While several drugs targeting the VEGF/VEGFR, PDGFR , EGF/EGFR and IGFR signaling have been approved or are in late-stage clinical trials (**Fig. 5**), clinically useful agents that specifically inhibit Wnt signaling cascade are not currently available. However, owing the crucial role in cancer ascribed to this pathway, in the last years the researches on the molecular mechanisms driving this signaling are in increasing and conspicuous funds are invested by several pharmaceutical and biotech companies for the development of innovative drugs targeting its molecular components. The main therapeutic strategies currently explored include:

1. The use of small-molecules able to regulate the catenin responsive transcription (Chen et al., 2009a; Lepourcelet et al., 2004; Thorne et al., 2010; Vo & Goodman, 2001).
2. Compounds that inhibit Wnt signaling by influencing the stability and expression levels of β-catenin (Chen et al., 2009a; Huang et al., 2009; Thorne et al., 2010)
3. Molecules that inhibit Wnt signaling by acting on events upstream of the axin/APC/GSK-3β complex, such as the secretion or reception of Wnt ligands at the plasma membrane (Chen et al., 2009a; Chen et al., 2009b) or transduction of the Wnt signal by Dishevelled (Dvl) (Chen et al., 2009b, Shan et al., 2005)

| Molecular component of the WNT signaling | Biological material analyzed | Trends found in HCC | Main possible use/s |
|---|---|---|---|
| β-catenin | Tissue | Gene mutation recovered in pre-cancerous lesion and increased in tumor; increased mRNA expression compared to normal liver; nuclear translocation in the early stages; increased protein expression in the late stage | Indicative of WNT signaling activation (early diagnosis); diagnostic marker of metastasis ; therapeutic target |
| β-catenin | Serum | Elevated in patients with HCC compared to those with chronic hepatitis (CH) and healthy controls | Early diagnosis of HCV-associated HCC |
| APC | Tissue | Gene mutation not frequently evidenced; loss of function implicated in liver carcinogenesis; | Early diagnosis; therapeutic target |
| Frizzled receptor | Tissue | Overexpressed in HCC compared to normal liver, already at early stages | Early diagnosis; therapeutic target |
| E-cadherin | Tissue | Expression increased in well-differentiated tumors compared to poorly differentiated cancers; Expression levels inversely correlated with histological grade and prognosis | Predictive of early recurrence after hepatic resection and metastatization of HCC cells; marker of tumor differentiation |

Table 4. List of the main molecular component of the WNT signaling useful for HCC diagnosis/therapy

Moreover, it has been recently reported that microRNA-181s (miR-181s) are transcriptionally activated by the Wnt/β-catenin signaling in HCC and these miRs have been proposed as attractive molecular target to eradicate liver cancer stem cells (Ji et al., 2011)

## 4. CD44 as a multifunctional marker of HCC late stages and metastatic disease, also useful for targeted therapy and drug delivery

The high mortality rate in patients with HCC is mainly due the lack of effective treatment options, especially for those with advanced or unresectable disease. These patients generally have a very poor prognosis and treatments, such as transarterial chemo-embolization, intra-arterial or systemic chemotherapy, radiotherapy, immunotherapy or hormonal therapy, are mainly used as palliative. Thus, the development of more effective therapeutic tools and strategies is much needed. The conventional chemotherapy, implying the use of systemic administration or non-targeted distribution of the drug, has numerous drawback such as the limited accessibility of drug to the tumor tissue, that reduces its therapeutic efficacy, the requirement of high doses, and undesirable side effects, primarily the high mielotoxicity and the development of multidrug resistance. To overcome these problems, in the last decades numerous researches focused on developing cancer-specific drugs or systems of antitumor drug delivery (Allen, 2002; Gabizon, 2002; Gabizon et al., 2003; Mohanty et al., 2011; Sapra & Allen, 2003). This therapeutic strategy may allow a controlled release of the drug and a high targeting selectivity on tumor cells, increasing drug cytotoxicity and decreasing its undesirable side effects. In this context, targeted drug delivery involving the use of drugs covalently conjugated to macromolecular carriers, that are able to specifically link to over-expressed molecules on tumor cells, is one the most promising approach in developing innovative therapies against cancer.

CD44, the receptor for hyaluronic acid-mediated cell motility, is a highly glycosylated transmembrane protein involved in cell–cell and cell–matrix interactions. The standard isoform (CD44s), participates to several functions including lymphocyte homing, tissue regeneration, signal transmission involved in cell proliferation, migration and apoptosis (Goodison et al., 1999; Ponta et al., 2003). Besides its involvement in physiological activities of normal cells, CD44 is associated with pathologic functions of tumor cells. Increased expression of CD44 (the standard isoform CD44s and the splice variant CD44v) has been associated to advanced stages not only of hepatocellular carcinoma (Endo & Terada, 2000) but also of breast cancer, colorectal cancer, thyroid carcinoma, lung cancer, renal cell carcinoma, gallbladder carcinoma, ovarian carcinoma, endometrial cancer and melanoma (Akisik et al., 2002; Bendardaf et al., 2006; Jothy , 2003; Naor et al., 2002; Seiter et al., 1996). For this reason, CD44 is emerging as a valuable metastatic tumor marker, also associated with an unfavorable prognosis for a variety of cancers, including HCC (Beckebaum et al., 2008). Therefore, agents specifically targeting CD44 should be promising drug for inhibiting tumor spread and for treatment of metastatic disease. It has been demonstrated that targeting CD44 with specific anti-CD44 monoclonal antibodies is able to inhibit proliferation and to induce terminal differentiation or apoptosis in leukemic cell lines (Charrad et al., 2002; Jin et al., 2006). Furthermore, inhibition of CD44 expression by CD44 antisense oligonucleotide significantly induced apoptosis, decreased tumorigenesis and invasion, and increased chemosensitivity in a CD44 over-expressing human HCC cell line (Xie et al., 2008).

The described overexpression of CD44 in advanced stages of several kinds of cancer including HCC, makes hyaluronic acid (HA), the well-known component of the extracellular matrix to which CD44 binds for driving the cell motility, an excellent macromolecular carrier for anticancer drug delivery. HA is a natural and biodegradable polysaccharide formed by D-glucuronic acid and *N*-acetyl-D-glucosamine repetitive units **(Fig. 7A)**, used for the development of pharmaceutical carriers and biomedical systems. HA plays crucial roles in cell adhesion, growth, and migration, by interacting with specific cellular receptors (CD44, RHAMM, ICAM), and acts as a signaling molecule in cell motility, inflammation, wound healing, and cancer metastasis (Marhaba & Zoller, 2004; Nedvetzkiet al., 2004; Toole, 2004; Weigel et al., 2003). In this context, HA-drug bioconjugates inherently show a marked selectivity for cancer cells, also providing advantages in drug solubilization, stabilization, localization, and controlled release. Bioconjugates of hyaluronic acid with different antineoplastic drugs, such as paclitaxel, doxorubicin and SN-38 (the active metabolite of Irinotecan) have been reported to posses promising anti-tumor effects both *in vitro* and *in vivo* (Banzato et al., 2008; Luo & Prestwich, 1999; Luo et al., 2000; Luo et al., 2002; Rosato et al., 2006; Serafino et al., 2011).

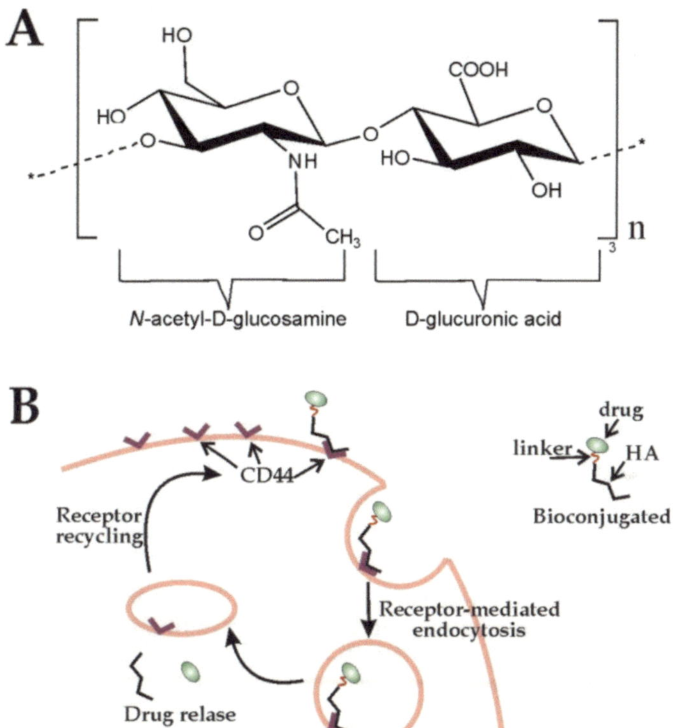


Fig. 7. **A**: Molecular structure of hyaluronic acid. **B**: mechanism of HA-drug biocojugate internalization by cancer cells.

In our recent paper (Serafino et al., 2011) we showed that the HA-drug bioconjugates, after interaction of the HA backbone with CD44, enter the tumor cells through a receptor-mediated endocytosis, followed by release of the active drug in the cytosol, where it directly reach its site of action. The internalized bioconjugate/CD44 complex has been recovered on cytoplasmic vesicles-like and lysosome-like structures, suggesting that processing of the HA-drug molecules might be coupled with a recycling of the CD44 receptor (**Fig. 7B**). We have also demonstrated that, using this drug delivery strategy, the delivered drug exerts a strong and irreversible *in vitro* inhibitory effect on growth of CD44 over-expressing cancer cells, higher than that exerted by free drug.

As mentioned above, the effectiveness of the drug delivery strategy using HA as a carrier targeting its CD44 receptor has been demonstrated in several kinds of CD44 over-expressing tumors, including colorectal, ovarian, bladder, gastric, breast, oesophageal and lung cancers, not only *in vitro* but also *in vivo* (Banzato et al., 2008; Luo & Prestwich, 1999; Luo et al., 2000; Luo et al., 2002; Rosato et al., 2006; Serafino et al., 2011). Due the association of increased expression of CD44 to advanced stages of hepatocellular carcinoma, this therapeutic approach might be also applicable for treatment of metastatic HCC. In addition, the growing evidences concerning the CD44 expression on liver cancer stem cells (Liu et al., 2011) not only improve the prognostic significance of CD44 but also make the drug delivery strategy through CD44/HA binding interaction useful for eradicating hepatic cancer stem cells.

## 5. Conclusion

Hepatocellular carcinoma is a malignancy having multifactorial etiology and a very complex pathogenesis, that make difficult the clinical management of HCC patients. Similarly to the other kinds of cancer, HCC insurgence, progression and recurrence involve gene mutations, that might be different depending on the individual genotype profiling and tumor stage, and different signaling pathways, which often share some crucial molecules/steps and are subjected to additional post-transductional regulation. To overcome the complex network of signaling pathways and gene mutations underlying hepatic cancer, innovative diagnostic, prognostic and therapeutic strategies are needed. Nowadays, each existing biomarker used or proposed for HCC early diagnosis, staging and prognosis alone is poorly specific and the absolute positive and negative serological and/or immunohistochemical markers are still lacking. Even those markers selected for high sensitivity and specificity do not exhibit an universal diagnostic/prognostic value, also due to the individual genotype variability. The more promising approach for developing more specific diagnostic/prognostic tools might be to combine several positive or negative indicators in multiparametric platforms, that allow simultaneous detection of multiple serological or immunohistochemical markers for HCC. These platforms might be used to design "specific maps" for HCC early diagnosis, staging and prognosis, also taking into account the individual variability of each patient. Detecting expression patterns of combined biomarkers may also be a new method useful for identifying new and unique markers.

Moreover, since target-specific cancer therapy has remarkably improved the outcomes of patients and represents the frontline approach for cancer treatment, the development of such multiparametric platforms would also represent a high-performance technological tools useful for designing personalized therapies, adapted to the aggressiveness of each individual tumor. The final goal should be to discriminate, for each target-specific therapy and on the basis of the "biomarker profiling" of each patient, the "responder" to the "not responder", thus increasing the therapeutic effectiveness, improving patient outcomes, and resulting in saving healthcare costs. Thus, the discovery and validation of new HCC biomarkers useful for early diagnosis and prognosis, such as the NGF, and for target therapy and drug delivery, such as the CD44, as well as the deepening of knowledge on pathways actively involved in hepatocarcinogenesis, helpful for HCC staging and target-specific cancer therapy, such as the WNT/β-catenin signaling, are essential steps to achieve this goal.

## 6. Acknowledgment

We would like to thank Federica Andreola, Noemi Moroni and Manuela Zonfrillo, for their valuable contribution to the researches carried out in our laboratory on NGF and on CD44 and to the ongoing study on the role of WNT/β-catenin signaling in cancer. We are also grateful to Dr. Giuseppe Nicotera for his scientific secretariat support.

## 7. References

Allen, T. M. (2002) Ligand-targeted therapeutics in anticancer therapy. *Nature Reviews Cancer*, Vol.2, No.10, (October 2002), pp. 750-763, ISSN 1474-175X

Aloe, L & Tuveri, M.A. (1997). Nerve growth factor and autoimmune rheumatic diseases. *Clinical and Experimental Rheumatology*, Vol.15, No.4, (August 1997), pp. 433-438, ISSN 0392-856X

Akisik, E., Bavbek, S. & Dalay, N. (2002). CD44 variant exons in leukemia and lymphoma. *Pathology Oncology Research*, Vol.8, No.1, (March 2002), pp. 36–40, ISSN 1219-4956

Banzato, A., Bobisse, S., Rondina, M., Renier, D., Bettella, F., Esposito, G., Quintieri, L., Meléndez-Alafort, L., Mazzi, U., Zanovello, P. & Rosato, A. (2008). A paclitaxel-hyaluronan bioconjugate targeting ovarian cancer affords a potent in vivo therapeutic activity. *Clinical Cancer Rresearch*, , Vol.14, No.11, (June 2008), pp. 3598-3606, ISSN 1078-0432

Beckebaum, S., Chen, X., Sotiropoulos, G.C., Radtke, A., Daoudaki, M., Baba, HA., Wohlschlaeger, J., Broelsch, C.E., Gerken, G. & Cicinnati, V.R. (2008) Role of osteopontin and CD44s expression for patients with hepatocellular carcinoma undergoing liver transplantation or resection. *Transplantation Proceedings*, Vol.40, No.9, ( November 2008), pp. 3182-3184, ISSN 0041-1345

Bendardaf, R., Algars, A., Elzagheid, A., Korkeila, E., Ristamäki, R., Lamlum, H., Collan, Y., Syrjänen, K. & Pyrhönen, S. (2006). Comparison of CD44 expression in primary tumours and metastases of colorectal cancer. *Oncology Reports*, Vol.16, No.4, (October 2006), pp. 741-746, ISSN 1021-335X

Birchmeier, C. & Gherardi, E. (1998). Development roles of HGF/SF and its receptor c-Met tyrosine kinase. *Trends in Cell Biology*, Vol.8, No.10, (October 1998), pp. 404–410, ISSN 0962-8924

Bold, R.J., Ishizuka, J., Rajaraman, S., Perez-Polo, J.R., Townsend, C.M. Jr. & Thompson, J.C. (1995). Nerve growth factor as a mitogen for a pancreatic carcinoid cell line. *Journal of Neurochemistry*, Vol.64, No. 6, (June 1995), pp. 2622-2628, ISSN 0022-3042

Bonini, S., Lambiase, A., Bonini, S., Levi-Schaffer, F. & Aloe, L. (1999). Nerve growth factor: an important molecule in allergic inflammation and tissue remodelling. *International Archives of Allergy and Immunology*, Vol.118, No.2-4, (April 1999), pp. 159-162, ISSN 1018-2438

Bosch, F.X., Ribes, J., Diaz, M. & Cleries, R. (2004). Primary liver cancer: worldwide incidence and trends. *Gastroenterology*, Vol.127, No. 5 Suppl.1, (November 2004), pp. S5–S16, ISSN 0016-5085

Breuhan, K., Longerich, T. & Schirmacher, P. (2006). Dysregulation of growth factor signalling in human hepatocellular carcinoma. *Oncogene*, Vol.25, No.27, (June 2006), pp. 3787–3800, ISSN 0950-9232

Brown, L.F., Berse, B., Jackman, R.W., Tognazzi, K., Manseau, E.J., Senger, D.R. & Dvorak, H.F. (1993). Expression of vascular permeability factor (vascular endothelial growth factor) and its receptors in adenocarcinoma of gastrointestinal tract. *Cancer Research*, Vol.53, No.19, (October 1993), pp. 4727–4735, ISSN 0008-5472

Buendia, M.A. (2000). Genetics of hepatocellular carcinoma. *Seminars in Cancer Biology*, Vol.10, No.3, (June 2000), pp. 185–200, ISSN 1044-579X

Bugianesi, E. (2005). Review article: steatosis, the metabolic syndrome and cancer. *Alimentary Pharmacology & Therapeutics*, Vol.22, Suppl 2, (November 2005), pp. 40–43, ISSN 0269-2813

Charrad, R.S., Gadhoum, Z., Qi, J., Glachant, A., Allouche, M., Jasmin, C., Chomienne, C. & Smadja-Joffe, F. (2002). Effects of anti-CD44 monoclonal antibodies on differentiation and apoptosis of human myeloid leukemia cell lines. *Blood*, Vol.99, No.1, (January 2002), pp. 290–299, ISSN 0006-4971

Chen, B., Dodge, M.E., Tang, W., Lu, J., Ma, Z., Fan, C.W., Wei, S., Hao, W., Kilgore, J., Williams, N.S., Roth, M.G., Amatruda, J.F., Chen, C. & Lum, L. (2009a) Small molecule-mediated disruption of Wnt-dependent signaling in tissue regeneration and cancer. *Nature Chemical Biology*, Vol.5, No.2, (February 2009), pp., 100–107, ISSN 1552-4450

Chen M, Wang, J., Lu, J., Bond, M.C., Ren, X.R., Lyerly, H.K., Barak, L.S. & Chen, W. (2009b) The anti-helminthic niclosamide inhibits Wnt/Frizzled1 signaling. *Biochemistry*, Vol.48, No.43, (November 2009), pp. 10267–10274, ISSN 0006-2960

Chuang, S.C., La Vecchia, C. & Boffetta, P. (2009). Liver cancer: descriptive epidemiology and risk factors other than HBV and HCV infection. *Cancer Letters*, Vol.286, No.1, (December 2009), pp. 9-14, ISSN 0304-3835

Colnot, S., Decaens, T., Niwa-Kawakita, M., Godard, C., Hamard, G., Kahn, A., Giovannini, M. & Perret, C. (2004). Liver-targeted disruption of APC in mice activates β-catenin signaling and leads to hepatocellular carcinomas. *Proceedings of the National Academy of Sciences of the United States of America*, Vol.101, No.49, (December 2004), pp. 17216–17221, ISSN 0027-8424

Colombo, M. (2003). Malignant neoplasm of the liver. In: *Schiff's Disease of the Liver*, E.R. Schiff, M.F. Sorrell & W.C. Maddrey, (Eds.), Lippincott William & Wilkins, pp. 1377-404, ISBN 978-0-7817-6040-9, Philadelphia

Daveau, M., Scotte, M., Francois, A., Coulouarn, C., Ros, G., Tallet, Y., Hiron, M., Hellot, M.F. & Salier, J.P. (2003). Hepatocyte growth factor, transforming growth factor a, and their receptors as combined markers of prognosis in hepatocellular carcinoma. *Molecular Carcinogenesis*, Vol.36, No.3, (March 2003), pp. 130–41, ISSN 0899-1987

De La, C.A., Romagnolo, B., Billuart, P., Renard, C.A., Buendia, M.A., Soubrane, O., Fabre, M., Chelly, J., Beldjord, C., Kahn, A. & Perret, C. (1998). Somatic mutations of the beta-catenin gene are frequent in mouse and human hepatocellular carcinomas. *Proceedings of the National Academy of Sciences of the United States of America*, Vol.95, No.15, (July 1998), pp. 8847–8851, ISSN 0027-8424

Descamps, S., Lebourhis, X., Delehedde, M., Boilly, B. & Hondermarck, H. (1998), Nerve growth factor is mitogenic for cancerous but not normal human breast epithelial cells. *Journal Biological Chemistry*, Vol.273, No.27, (July 1998), pp. 16659-16662, ISSN 0021-9258

Di Bisceglie AM. (1995). Hepatitis C and hepatocellular carcinoma. *Seminars in Liver Disease*, Vol.15, No.1, (February 1995), pp. 64-69, ISSN 0272-8087

Djakiew, D., Delsite, R., Pflug, B., Wrathall, J., Lynch, J.H. & Onoda, M. (1991). Regulation of growth by a nerve growth factor-like protein which modulates paracrine interactions between a neoplastic epithelial cell line and stromal cells of the human prostate. *Cancer Research*, Vol.51, No.12, (June 1991), pp. 3304-3310, ISSN 0008-5472

Endo, K. & Terada, T. (2000) Protein expression of CD44 (standard and variant isoforms) in hepatocellular carcinoma: relationships with tumor grade, clinicopathologic parameters, p53 expression, and patient survival. *Journal of Hepatology*, Vol.32, No.1, (January 2000), pp. 78–84, ISSN 0168-8278

Fields, A.C., Cotsonis, G., Sexton, D., Santoianni, R. & Cohen, C. (2004). Survivin expression in hepatocellular carcinoma: correlation, with proliferation, prognostic parameters, and outcome. *Modern Pathology*, Vol.17, No.11, (November 2004), pp. 1378–85, ISSN 0893-3952

Gabizon, A.A. (2002). Liposomal drug carrier systems in cancer chemotherapy: current status and future prospects. *Journal of Drug Targeting*, Vol.10, No.7, (November 2002), pp. 535-538, ISSN 1061-186X

Gabizon, A., Shmeeda, H. & Barenholz, Y. (2003). Pharmacokinetics of pegylated liposomal Doxorubicin: review of animal and human studies. *Clinical Pharmacokinetics*, Vol.42, No.5, (December 2003), pp. 419-436, ISSN 0312-5963

Gonsalves, F.C., Klein, K., Carson, B.B., Katz, S., Ekas, L.A., Evans, S., Nagourney, R., Cardozo, T., Brown, A.M. & Dasgupta, R. (2011). An RNAi-based chemical genetic screen identifies three small-molecule inhibitors of the Wnt/wingless signaling pathway. *Proceedings of the National Academy of Sciences of the United States of America*, Vol.108, No.15, (April 2011), pp. 5954-5963, ISSN 0027-8424

Goodison, S., Urquidi, V. & Tarin, D. (1999). CD44 cell adhesion molecules. *Molecular pathology*, Vol.52, No.4, (August 1999), pp. 189-196, ISSN 1366-8714

Grizzi, F., Franceschini, B., Hamrick, C., Frezza, E.E., Cobos, E. & Chiriva-Internati, M. (January 2007). Usefulness of cancer-testis antigens as biomarkers for the diagnosis and treatment of hepatocellular carcinoma. In: *Journal of Translational Medicine*, 23.01.2007, Available from
http://www.translational-medicine.com/content/5/1/3

Huang, G.T., Lee, H.S., Chen, C.H., Sheu, J.C., Chiou, L.L., Chen, D.S. (1999) Correlation of E-cadherin expression and recurrence of hepatocellular carcinoma. *Hepatogastroenterology*, Vol.46, No.27, (June 1999), pp. 1923–1927, ISSN 0172-6390

Huang, S.M., Mishina, Y.M., Liu, S., Cheung, A., Stegmeier, F., Michaud, G.A., Charlat, O., Wiellette, E., Zhang, Y., Wiessner, S., Hild, M., Shi, X., Wilson, C.J., Mickanin, C., Myer, V., Fazal, A., Tomlinson, R., Serluca, F., Shao, W., Cheng, H., Shultz, M., Rau, C., Schirle, M., Schlegl, J., Ghidelli, S., Fawell, S., Lu, C., Curtis, D., Kirschner, M.W., Lengauer, C., Finan, P.M., Tallarico, J.A., Bouwmeester, T., Porter, J.A., Bauer, A. & Cong, F. (2009) Tankyrase inhibition stabilizes axin and antagonizes Wnt signalling. *Nature*, Vol. 461, No.7264, (October 2009), pp. 614–620, ISSN 0028-0836

Ito, N., Kawata, S., Tamura, S., Takaishi, K., Yabuuchi, I., Matsuda, Y., Nishioka, M. & Tarui, S. (1990). Expression of transforming growth factor b1 mRNA in human hepatocellular carcinoma. *Japanese Journal of Cancer Research*, Vol.81, No.12, (December 1990), pp. 1202–1205, ISSN 0910-5050

Ito, Y., Takeda, T., Sakon, M., Tsujimoto, M., Higashiyama, S., Noda, K., Miyoshi, E., Monden, M. & Matsuura, N. (2001). Expression and clinical significance of the erb-B receptor family in hepatocellular carcinoma. *British Journal of Cancer*, Vol.84, No.10, (May 2001), pp. 1377–83, ISSN 0007-0920

Ji, J., Yamashita, T. & Wang, XW. (January 2011). Wnt/beta-catenin signaling activates microRNA-181 expression in hepatocellular carcinoma. In: *Cell and Bioscience*, 18.01.2011, Available from http://www.cellandbioscience.com/content/1/1/4

Jin, L., Hope, K.J., Zhai, Q., Smadja-JoVe, F. & Dick, J.E. (2006) Targeting of CD44 eradicates human acute myeloid leukemic stem cells. *Nature Medicine*, Vol.12, No.10, (October 2006), pp. 1167–1174, ISSN 1078-8956

Jothy, S. (2003). CD44 and its partners in metastasis. *Clinical and experimental metastasis*, Vol.20, No.3, (July 2003), pp. 195–201, ISSN 0262-0898

Kato, Y., Nakata, K., Omagari, K. Furukawa, R., Kusumoto, Y., Mori, I,, Tajima, H., Tanioka, H., Yano, M. & Nagataki, S. (1994). Risk of hepatocellular carcinoma in patients with cirrhosis in Japan. Analysis of infectious hepatitis viruses. Cancer, Vol.74, No.8, (October 1994), pp. 2234-8, ISSN 0008-543X

Koizumi, H., Morita, M., Mikami, S., Shibayama, E. & Uchikoshi, T. (1998). Immunohistochemical analysis of TrkA neurotrophin receptor expression in human non-neuronal carcinomas. *Pathology International*, Vol.48, No.2, (February 1998), pp. 93-101, ISSN 1320-5463

Lai, T.Y., Su, C.C., Kuo, W.W., Yeh, Y.L., Ku,o W.H., Tsai, F.J., Tsai, C.H., Weng, Y.J., Huang, C.Y. & Chen, L.M. (2011). β-catenin plays a key role in metastasis of human hepatocellular carcinoma. *Oncology Reports*, Vol.26, No.2, (August 2011), pp. 415-22, ISSN 1021-335X

Lepourcelet, M., Chen, Y.N., France, D.S., Wang, H., Crews, P., Petersen, F., Bruseo, C., Wood, A.W. & Shivdasani, R.A. (2004) Small-molecule antagonists of the oncogenic Tcf/betacatenin protein complex. *Cancer Cell*, Vol.5, No.1, (January 2004), pp. 91–102. ISSN 1535-6108

Levi-Montalcini, R. (1987). The nerve growth factor 35 years later. *Science*, Vol.237, No.4819, (September 1987), pp. 1154-1162, ISSN 0036-8075

Liaw, Y.F., Tai, D.I., Chen, T.J., Chu, C.M. & Huang, M.J. (1986). Alpha-fetoprotein changes in the course of chronic hepatitis: relation to bridging hepatic necrosis and hepatocellular carcinoma. *Liver*, Vol.6, No.3, (June 1986), pp. 133–137, ISSN 0106-9543

Li, X.M., Tang, Z.Y., Qin, L.X., Zhou, J. & Sun, H.C. (1999). Serum vascular endothelial growth factor is a predictor of invasion and metastasis in hepatocellular carcinoma. *Journal of Experimental & Clinical Cancer Research*, Vol.18, No.4, (December 1999), pp. 511–517, ISSN 0392-9078

Llovet, J.M., Ricci, S., Mazzaferro, V., Hilgard, P., Gane, E., Blanc, J.F., de Oliveira, A.C., Santoro, A., Raoul, J.L., Forner, A., Schwartz, M., Porta, C., Zeuzem, S., Bolondi, L., Greten, T.F,. Galle, P.R., Seitz, J.F., Borbath, I., Häussinger, D., Giannaris, T., Shan, M., Moscovici, M., Voliotis, D., Bruix, J. & SHARP Investigators Study Group. (2008). Sorafenib in advanced hepatocellular carcinoma. *The New England Journal of Medicine*, Vol.359, No.4, (July 2008), pp. 378–390, ISSN 0028-4793

Luo, Y. & Prestwich, G. D. (1999). Synthesis and selective cytotoxicity of a hyaluronic acid-antitumor bioconjugate. *Bioconjugate Chemistry*, Vol.10, No.5, (October 1999), pp. 755–763, ISSN 1043-1802

Luo, Y., Ziebell, M. R. & Prestwich, G. D. (2000). A hyaluronic acid-taxol antitumor bioconjugate targeted to cancer cells. *Biomacromolecules*, Vol.1, No.2, (Summer 2000), pp. 208–218, ISSN 1525-7797

Luo, Y., Bernshaw, N. J., Lu, Z. R., Kopecek, J. & Prestwich, G. D. (2002). Targeted delivery of doxorubicin by HPMA copolymer-hyaluronan bioconjugates. *Pharmaceutical Research*, Vol.19, No.4, (April 2002), pp. 396–402, ISSN 0724-8741

Liu, L.L., Fu, D., Ma, Y., Shen, X. (2011) The Power and the Promise of Liver Cancer Stem Cell Markers. Stem Cells and Development, Epub ahead of print (Jun 2011), ISSN 1547-3287

Luu, H.H., Zhang, R., Haydon, R.C., Rayburn, E., Kang, Q., Si, W., Park, J.K., Wang, H., Peng, Y., Jiang, W., and He, T.C. (2004) Wnt/beta-catenin signaling pathway as a novel cancer drug target. *Current Cancer Drug Targets*, Vol.4, No.8, (December 2004), pp. 653-667, ISSN 1568-0096

Malaguarnera, L., Rosa, M.D., Zambito, A.M., dell'Ombra, N., Marco, R.D. & Malaguarnera, M. (2006). Potential role of chitotriosidase gene in non-alcoholic fatty liver disease evolution. *The American Journal of Gastroenterology*, Vol.101, No.9, (September 2006), pp. 2060–2069, ISSN 0002-9270

Malaguarnera, M., Di Rosa, M., Nicoletti, F. & Malaguarnera, L. (2009). Molecular mechanisms involved in NAFLD progression. *Journal of Molecular Medicine*, Vol.87, No.7, (July 2009), pp. 679–695. ISSN 0946-2716

Malaguarnera, G., Giordano, M., Paladina, I., Berretta, M., Cappellani, A. & Malaguarnera, M. (2010). Serum markers of hepatocellular carcinoma. *Digestive Diseases and Sciences*, Vol.55, No.10, (October 2010), pp. 2744-55, ISSN 0163-2116

Mann, C.D., Neal, C.P., Garcea, G., Manson, M.M., Dennison, A.R. & Berry, D.P. (2007). Prognostic molecular markers in hepatocellular carcinoma: a systematic review. *European Journal of Cancer*, Vol.43, No.6, (April 2007), pp. 979-92. ISSN 0959-8049

Marhaba, R. & Zoller, M. (2004). CD44 in cancer progression: Adhesion, migration and growth regulation. *Journal of Molecular Histology*, Vol.35, No.3, (March 2004), pp. 211–231, ISSN 1567-2379

Marrero, J.A., Kudo, M. & Bronowicki, J.P. (2010). The Challenge of Prognosis and Staging for Hepatocellular Carcinoma. *The Oncologist*, Vol.15, No.11 suppl 4, (November 2010), pp. 23–33, ISSN 1083-7159

Matsumura, T., Makino, R. & Mitamura, K. (2001). Frequent downregulation of E-cadherin by genetic and epigenetic changes in the malignant progression of hepatocellular carcinomas. *Clinical Cancer Research*, Vol.7, No.3, (March 2001), pp. 594–599, ISSN 1078-0432

Mattern, J., Koomagi, R. & Volm, M. (1996). Association of vascular endothelial growth factor expression with intratumoural microvessel density and tumor cell proliferation in human epidermoid lung carcinoma. *British Journal of Cancer*, Vol.73, No.7, (April 1996), pp. 931–934, ISSN 0007-0920

McGregor, L.M., McCune, B.K., Graf,f J.R., McDowell, P.R., Romans, K.E., Yancopoulos, G.D., Ball, D.W., Baylin, S.B. & Nelkin, B.D. (1999). Roles of trk family neurotrophin receptors in medullary thyroid carcinoma development and progression. *Proceedings of the National Academy of Sciences of the United States of America*, Vol.96, No.8, (April 1999), pp. 4540-4545, ISSN 0027-8424

Meakin, S.O. & Shooter, E.M. (1992). The nerve growth factor family of receptors. *Trends in Neurosciences*, Vol.15, No.9, (September 1992), pp. 323-331 ISSN 0166-2236

Merle, P., de la Monte, S., Kim, M., Herrmann, M., Tanaka, S., Von Dem Bussche, A., Kew, M.C., Trepo, C. & Wands, J.R. (2004). Functional consequences of frizzled-7 receptor overexpression in human hepatocellular carcinoma. *Gastroenterology*, Vol.127, No.4, (October 2004), pp. 1110–1122, ISSN 0016-5085

Micera, A., Vigneti, E., Pickholtz, D., Reich, R., Pappo, O., Bonini, S., Maquart, F.X., Aloe, L. & Levi-Schaffer, F. (2001). Nerve growth factor displays stimulatory effects on human skin and lung fibroblasts, demonstrating a direct role for this factor in tissue repair. *Proceedings of the National Academy of Sciences of the United States of America*, Vol.98, No.11, (May 2001), pp. 6162-6167, ISSN 0027-8424

Micera, A., Puxeddu, I., Aloe, L. & Levi-Schaffer, F. (2003). New insights on the involvement of Nerve Growth Factor in allergic inflammation and fibrosis. Cytokine and Growth Factor Reviews, Vol.14, No.5, (October 2003), pp. 369-374, ISSN 1359-6101

Mise, M., Arii, S., Higashituji, H., Furutani, M, Niwano, M., Harada, T., Ishigami, S., Toda, Y., Nakayama, H., Fukumoto, M., Fujita, J. & Imamura, M. (1996). Clinical significance of vascular endothelial growth factor and basic fibroblast growth factor gene expression in liver tumor. *Hepatology*, Vol.23, No.3, (March 1996), pp. 455–464, ISSN 0270-9139

Miyaaki, H., Nakashima, O., Kurogi, M., Eguchi, K. & Kojiro, M. (2007). Lens culinaris agglutinin-reactive alpha-fetoprotein and protein induced by vitamin K absence II are potential indicators of a poor prognosis: a histopathological study of surgically resected hepatocellular carcinoma. *Journal of Gastroenterology*, Vol.42, No.12, (December 2007), pp. 962–968, ISSN 0944-1174

Mizejewski, G.J. (2002). Biological role of alpha-fetoprotein in cancer: prospects for anticancer therapy. *Expert Review of Anticancer Therapy*, Vol.2, No.6, (December 2002), pp. 709–735, ISSN 1473-7140

Mohanty, C., Das, M., Kanwar, J.R. & Sahoo, S.K. (2011). Receptor mediated tumor targeting: an emerging approach for cancer therapy. *Current Drug Delivery*, Vol.8, No.1 (January 2011), 45-58, ISSN 1567-2018

Monga, S.P., Monga, H.K., Tan, X., Mule, K., Pediaditaki,s P. & Michalopoulos, G.K. (2003). β-catenin antisense studies in embryonic liver cultures: role in proliferation, apoptosis, and lineage specification. *Gastroenterology*, Vol.124, No.1, (January 2003), pp. 202–216, ISSN 0016-5085

Moon, R.T., Kohn, A.D., De Ferrari, G.V. & Kaykas, A. (2004) WNT and beta-catenin signalling: diseases and therapies. *Nature Reviews. Genetics*, Vol.5, No.9, (September 2004), pp. 691-701, ISSN 1471-0056

Mulcahy, M.F. (2005) Management of hepatocellular cancer. *Current Treatment Options in Oncology*, Vol.6, No.5, (September 2005), pp. 423–435, ISSN 1527-2729

Nair, S., Mason, A., Eason, J., Loss, G. & Perrillo, R.P. (2002). Is obesity an independent risk factor for hepatocellular carcinoma in cirrhosis? *Hepatology*, Vol.36, No.1, (July 2002), pp. 150-155, ISSN 0270-9139

Naor, D., Nedvetzki, S., Golan, I., Melnik, L. & Faitelson, Y. (2002) CD44 in cancer. *Critical Reviews in Clinical Laboratory Sciences*, Vol.39, No.6, (November 2002), pp. 527–579, ISSN 1040-8363

Nedvetzki, S., Gonen, E., Assayag, N., Reich, R., Williams, R.O., Thurmond, R.L., Huang, J.F., Neudecker, B.A., Wang, F.S., Turley, E.A. & Naor, D. (2004). RHAMM, a receptor for hyaluronan-mediated motility, compensates for CD44 in inflamed

CD44-knockout mice: A different interpretation of redundancy. *Proceedings of the National Academy of Sciences of the United States of America*, Vol.101, No.52, (December 2004), pp. 18081–18086, ISSN 0027-8424.

Nelson, W.J. & Nusse, R. (2004). Convergence of Wnt, β-Catenin, and Cadherin Pathways. *Science*, Vol.303, No.5663, (March 2004), pp. 1483-1487, ISSN 0036-8075

Oelmann, E., Sreter, L., Schuller, I., Serve, H., Koenigsmann, M., Wiedenmann, B., Oberberg, D., Reufi, B., Thiel, E. & Berdel, W.E. (1995). Nerve growth factor stimulates clonal growth of human lung cancer cell lines and a human glioblastoma cell line expressing high-affinity nerve growth factor binding sites involving tyrosine kinase signaling. *Cancer Research*, Vol.55, No.10, (May 1995), pp. 2212-2219, ISSN 0008-5472

Oka, H., Saito, A., Ito, K., Kumada, T., Satomura, S., Kasugai, H., Osaki, Y., Seki, T., Kudo, M., Tanaka, M. & Collaborative Hepato-Oncology Study Group of Japan. (2001). Multicenter prospective analysis of newly diagnosed hepatocellular carcinoma with respect to the percentage of Lens culinaris agglutinin-reactive alpha-fetoprotein. *Journal of Gastroenterology and Hepatology*, Vol.16, No.12, (December 2001), pp. 1378–1383, ISSN 0815-9319

Okumoto, K., Hattori, E., Tamura, K., Kiso, S., Watanabe, H., Saito, K., Saito, T., Togashi, H. & Kawata, S. (2004). Possible contribution of circulating transforming growth factor-b1 to immunity and prognosis in unresectable hepatocellular carcinoma. *Liver International*, Vol.24, No.1, (February 2004), pp. 21–28, ISSN 1478-3223

Ono, M., Ohat, H., Ohhira, M., Sekiya, C. & Namiki, M. (1990). Measurement of immunoreactive prothrombin precursor and vitamin-K-dependent gammacarboxylation in human hepatocellular tissues: decreased carboxylation of prothrombin precursor as a cause of des-gamma-carboxyprothrombin synthesis. *Tumour Biology*, Vol.11, No.6, (December 1990), pp. 319–326, ISSN 1010-4283

Ozawa, M., Baribault, H. & Kemler, R. (1989). The cytoplasmic domain of the cell adhesion molecule uvomorulin associates with three independent proteins structurally related in different species. *The EMBO Journal*, Vol.8, No.6, (June 1989), pp. 1711-1717, ISSN 0261-4189

Pflug, B.R., Onoda, M., Lynch, J.H. & Djakiew, D. (1992). Reduced expression of the low affinity nerve growth factor receptor in benign and malignant human prostate tissue and loss of expression in four human metastatic prostate tumor cell lines. *Cancer Research*, Vol.52, No.19, (October 1992), pp. 5403-540, ISSN 0008-5472

Polakis, P. (1999). The oncogenic activation of beta-catenin. *Current Opinion in Genetics & Development*, Vol.9, No.1, (Febraury 1999), pp. 15-21, ISSN 0959-437X

Ponta, H., Sherman, L. & Herrlich, P.A. (2003) CD44: from adhesion molecules to signaling regulators. *Nature Reviews. Molecular Cell Biology*, Vol.4, No.1, (January 2003), pp. 33–45, ISSN 1471-0072

Poynard, T., Bedossa, P. & Opolon, P. (1997). Natural history of liver fibrosis progression in patients with chronic hepatitis C. The OBSVIRC, METAVIR, CLINIVIR, and DOSVIRC groups. *Lancet*, Vol.349, No.9055, (March 1997), pp. 825-832, ISSN 0140-6736

Qin, L.X. & Tang, Z.Y. (2004). Recent progress in predictive biomarkers for metastatic recurrence of human hepatocellular carcinoma: a review of the literature. *Journal of Cancer Research and Clinical Oncology*, Vol.130, No.9, (September 2004), pp. 497–513, ISSN 0171-5216

Rasi, G., Serafino, A., Bellis, L., Lonardo, M.T., Andreola, F., Zonfrillo, M., Vennarecci, G., Pierimarchi, P., Sinibaldi Vallebona, P., Ettorre, G.M., Santoro, E. & Puoti, C. (2007)

Nerve Growth Factor (NGF) involvement in liver cirrhosis and hepatocellular carcinoma. *World Journal of Gastroenterology*, Vol.13, No.37, (October 2007), pp. 4986-4995, ISSN 1007-9327

Revoltella, R.P. & Butler, R.H. (1980). Nerve growth factor may stimulate either division or differentiation of cloned C1300 neuroblastoma cells in serum-free cultures. *Journal of Cellular Physiology*, Vol.104, No.1, (July 1980), pp. 27-33, ISSN0021-9541

Rosato, A., Banzato, A., De Luca, G., Renier, D., Bettella, F., Pagano, C., Esposito, G., Zanovello, P. & Bassi, P. (2006). HYTAD1-p20: a new paclitaxel-hyaluronic acid hydrosoluble bioconjugate for treatment of superficial bladder cancer. *Urologic Oncology*, Vol.24, No.3, (June 2006), pp. 207-215, ISSN 1078-1439

Sapra, P. & Allen, T. M. (2003). Ligand-targeted liposomal anticancer drugs. *Progress in Lipid Research*, Vol.42, No.5, (September 2003), pp. 439-462, ISSN 0163-7827

Sato, Y., Nakata, K., Kato, Y., et al. (1993). Early recognition of hepatocellular carcinoma based on altered profiles of alpha-fetoprotein. *The New England Journal of Medicine*, Vol.328, No.25, (June 1993), pp. 1802–1806, ISSN 0028-4793

Seiter, S., Schadendorf, D., Herrmann, K., Schneider, M., Rosel, M., Arch, R. Tilgen, W. & Zöller, M. (1996) Expression of CD44 variant isoforms in malignant melanoma. *Clinical Cancer Research*, Vol.2, No.3, (March 1996), pp. 447–456, ISSN 1078-0432

Seitz, H.K. & Becker, P. (2007). Alcohol metabolism and cancer risk. *Alcohol Research & Health*, Vol.30, No.1, (December 2007), pp. 38-41 44-47, ISSN 1535-7414

Sekine, S., Lan, B.Y., Bedolli, M., Feng, S. & Hebrok, M. (2006). Liver-specific loss of β-catenin blocks glutamine synthesis pathway activity and cytochrome p450 expression in mice. *Hepatology*, Vol.43, No.4, (April 2006), pp. 817–825, ISSN 0270-9139

Semela, D. & Dufour JF. (2004). Angiogenesis and hepatocellular carcinoma. *Journal of Hepatology*, Vol.41, No.5, (November 2004), pp. 864–880, ISSN 0168-8278

Serafino, A., Zonfrillo, M., Andreola, F., Psaila, R., Mercuri, L., Moroni, N., Renier, D., Campisi, M., Secchieri, C. & Pierimarchi, P. CD44-Targeting for Antitumor Drug Delivery: a New SN-38-Hyaluronan Bioconjugate for Locoregional Treatment of Peritoneal Carcinomatosis. (2011). *Current Cancer Drug Targets*, Vol.11, No.5, (June 2011), pp. 572-585, ISSN1568-0096

Shan, J., Shi, D.L., Wang, J. & Zheng, J. (2005). Identification of a specific inhibitor of the dishevelled PDZ domain. *Biochemistry*, Vol.44, No.47, (November 2005), pp. 15495–15503, ISSN 0006-2960

Sherlock, S. & Dooley, J. (2002). Malignant liver tumors, In: *Diseases of the Liver and Biliary System*, S. Sherlock & J. Dooley (eds.), pp. 537-562, Blackwell Publishing Company ISBN 0-632-05582-0, Oxford, UK

Shiozaki, H., Oka, H., Inoue, M., Tamura, S. & Monden, M. (1996). E-cadherin mediated adhesion system in cancer cells. *Cancer*, Vol.77, No.8 Suppl, (April 1996), pp. 1605–1613, ISSN 0008-543X

Sofroniew, M.V., Howe, C.L. & Mobley, W.C. (2001). Nerve growth factor signaling, neuroprotection, and neural repair. *Annual Review of Neuroscience*, Vol.24, (March 2001), pp. 1217-1281, ISSN 0147-006X

Sortino, M.A., Condorelli, F., Vancheri, C., Chiarenza, A., Bernardini, R., Consoli, U. & Canonico, P.L. (2000). Mitogenic effect of nerve growth factor (NGF) in LNCaP prostate adenocarcinoma cells: role of the high- and low-affinity NGF receptors. *Molecular Endocrinology*, Vol.14, No, (January 2000), pp, 124-136, ISSN 0888-8809

Suksaweang, S., Lin, C.M., Jiang, T.X., Hughes, M.W., Widelitz, R.B. & Chuong, C.M. (2004). Morphogenesis of chicken liver: identification of localized growth zones and the role of β-catenin/Wnt in size regulation. *Developmental Biology*, Vol.266, No.1, (February 2004), pp. 109–122, ISSN 0012-1606

Suzuki, K., Hayashi, M., Miyamaoto; Y., Yamamoto, M., Ohkawa, K., Ito, Y., Sasaki, Y., Yamaguchi, Y., Nakase, H., Noda, K., Enomoto, N., Arai, K., Yamada, Y., Yoshihara, H., Tujimura, T., Kawano, K., Yoshikawa, K. & Kamada, T. (1996). Expression of vascular permeability factor/vascular endothelial growth factor in human hepatocellular carcinoma. *Cancer Research*, Vol.56, No.13, (July 1996), pp. 3004–3009. ISSN 0008-5472

Takano, S., Yokosuka, O., Imazeki, F., Tagawa, M. & Omata, M. (1995). Incidence of hepatocellular carcinoma in chronic hepatitis B and C: a prospective study of 251 patients. *Hepatology*, Vol.21, No.3, (march 1995), pp. 650-655, ISSN 0270-9139

Terentiev, A.A. & Moldogazieva, N.T. (2006). Structural and functional mapping of alpha-fetoprotein. *Biochemistry (Moscow)*, Vol.71, No.2, (February 2006), pp. 120–132, ISSN 0006-2979

Thomas, M.B. & Abbruzzese, J.L. (2005). Opportunities for targeted therapies in hepatocellular carcinoma. *Journal of Clinical Oncology*, Vol.23, No.31, (November 2005), pp. 8093–8108, ISSN 0732-183X

Thorgeirsson, S.S. & Grisham, J.W. (2002). Molecular pathogenesis of human hepatocellular carcinoma. *Nature Genetics*, Vol.31, No.4, (August 2002), pp. 339–346, ISSN 1061-4036

Thorne, C.A., Hanson, A.J., Schneider, J., Tahinci, E., Orton, D., Cselenyi, C.S., Jernigan, K.K., Meyers, K.C., Hang, B.I., Waterson, A.G., Kim, K., Melancon, B., Ghidu, V.P., Sulikowski ,G.A., LaFleur, B., Salic, A., Lee, L.A., Miller, D.M. 3rd, & Lee, E. (2010) Small-molecule inhibition of Wnt signaling through activation of casein kinase 1α. *Nature Chemical Biology*, Vol.6, No.11, (November 2010), pp. 829–836, ISSN 1552-4450

Toi, M., Hoshina, S., Takayanagi, T. & Tominaga, T. (1994). Association of vascular endothelial growth factor expression with tumour angiogenesis and early relapse in primary breast cancer. *Japanese Journal of Cancer Research*, Vol.85, No.10, (October 1994), pp. 1045-1049, ISSN 0910-5050

Toole, B.P. (2004). Hyaluronan: From extracellular glue to pericellular cue. Nature Reviews. Cancer, Vol.4, No.7, (July 2004), pp. 528–539, ISSN 1474-175X

Tsai, J.F., Jeng, J.E., Chuang, L.Y., Yang, M.L., Ho, M.S., Chang, W.Y., Hsieh, M.Y., Lin, Z.Y. &Tsai, J.H. (1997). Elevated urinary transforming growth factor-beta1 level as a tumour marker and predictor of poor survival in cirrhotic hepatocellular carcinoma. *British Journal of Cancer*, Vol.76, No.2, (June 1997), pp. 244–250 ISSN 0007-0920

Vestweber, D. & Kemler, R. (1984). Some structural and functional aspects of the cell adhesion molecule uvomorulin. *Cell Differentiation*, Vol.15, No.2-4, (December 1984), pp. 269-73, ISSN 0045-6039

Villanueva, A., Newell, P., Chiang, D.Y., Friedman, S.L. & Llovet, J.M. (2007). Genomics and signaling pathways in hepatocellular carcinoma. *Seminars in Liver Disease*, Vol.27, No.1, (February 2007), pp. 55–76, ISSN 0272-8087

Vo, N. & Goodman, R.H. (2001) CREB-binding protein and p300 in transcriptional regulation. *The Journal of Biological Chemistry*, Vol.276, No.17, (April 2001), pp. 13505–13508, ISSN 0021-9258

Waltzer, L. & Bienz, M. (1999). The control of beta-catenin and TCF during embryonic development and cancer. *Cancer and Metastasis Reviews*,Vol.18, No.2, (June 1999), pp. 231-246, ISSN 0167-7659

Wang, X.W., Hussain, S.P., Huo, T.I., Wu, C.G., Forgues, M., Hofseth, L.J. Brechot, C. & Harris, C.C. (2002). Molecular pathogenesis of human hepatocellular carcinoma. *Toxicology*, Vol.181–182, (December 2002), pp. 43–47, ISSN 0300-483X

Weigel, J.A., Raymond, R.C., McGary, C., Singh, A. & Weigel, P.H. (2003). A blocking antibody to the hyaluronan receptor for endocytosis (HARE) inhibits hyaluronan clearance by perfused liver. *The Journal of Biological Chemistry*, Vol.278, No.11, (March 2003), pp. 9808–9812, ISSN 0021-9258

Whittaker, S., Marais, R. & Zhu, A.X. (2010). The role of signaling pathways in the development and treatment of hepatocellular carcinoma. *Oncogene*, Vol.29, No.36, (September 2010 ), pp. 4989-5005, ISSN 0950-9232

Wijnhoven, B.P., Dinjens, W.N. & Pignatelli, M. (2000). E-cadherin-catenin cell-cell adhesion complex and human cancer. *The British Journal of Surgery*, Vol.87, No.8, (August 2000), pp. 992–1005, ISSN 0007-1323

Wu, F.S., Zheng, S.S., Wu, L.J., Ding, W., Ma, Z.M., Wang, Z.M., Teng, L.S. & Zhao, W.H. (2006). Study on the prognostic value of hepatocyte growth factor and c-met for patients with hepatocellular carcinoma. *Zhongua Wai Ke Za Zhi.*, Vol. 44, No.9, (May 2006), pp. 603–608, ISSN 0529-5815

Xie, Z., Choong, P.F., Poon, L.F., Zhou, J., Khng, J., Jasinghe, V.J., Palaniyandi, S. & Chen, C.S. (2008). Inhibition of CD44 expression in hepatocellular carcinoma cells enhances apoptosis, chemosensitivity, and reduces tumorigenesis and invasion. *Cancer Chemotherapy and Pharmacology*, Vol.62, No.6, (November 2008), pp. 949-957, ISSN 0344-5704

Yamagamim, H., Moriyana, M., Matsumura, H., Aoki, H., Shimizu, T., Saito, T., Kaneko, M., Shioda, A., Tanaka, N. & Arakawa, Y. (2002). Serum concentrations of human hepatocyte growth factor is a usefulindicator for predicting the occurrence of hepatocellular carcinomas in C-viral chronic liver diseases. *Cancer*, Vol.95, No.4, (August 2002), pp. 824–834, ISSN 0008-543X

Yano, M., Kumada, H., Kage, M. Ikeda, K., Shimamatsu, K., Inoue, O., Hashimoto, E., Lefkowitch, J.H., Ludwig, J., Okuda, K. (1996). The long-term pathological evolution of chronic hepatitis C. *Hepatology*, Vol.23, No.6, (June 1996), pp. 1334-1340, ISSN 0270-9139

Zekri, A.R., Bahnassy, A.A., Alam El-Din, H.M., Morsy, H.M., Shaarawy, S., Moharram, N.Z. & Daoud, S.S. (2011). Serum levels of β-catenin as a potential marker for genotype 4/hepatitis C-associated hepatocellular carcinoma. *Oncology Reports*, (no date Epub ahead of print) doi: 10.3892/or.2011.1355, ISSN 1021-335X

# Part 2

## Carcinogenesis / Invasion / Metastasis

5

# Modulation of Cell Proliferation Pathways by the Hepatitis B Virus X Protein: A Potential Contributor to the Development of Hepatocellular Carcinoma

Jessica C. Casciano[1*], Sumedha Bagga[1*], Bei Yang[1] and Michael J. Bouchard[2]
[1]*Graduate Program in Molecular and Cellular Biology*
[2]*Department of Biochemistry and Molecular Biology,*
*Drexel University College of Medicine, Philadelphia PA*
*U.S.A.*

## 1. Introduction

Globally, hepatocellular carcinoma (HCC) is the fifth most common cancer and the third highest cause of cancer-associated deaths. Although the development of HCC has been linked to exposure to various toxins or infectious agents, the majority of HCC cases are associated with chronic hepatitis B virus (HBV) infections [reviewed in (Block et al, 2003; Seeger et al, 2007)]. Worldwide, there are an estimated 350 million cases of chronic HBV infections, and approximately 25% of chronically HBV-infected individuals will eventually develop HCC [(Beasley et al, 1981); reviewed in (Seeger et al, 2007)]. The high global incidence of chronic HBV infections, high mortality rate of individuals with HCC, increased prevalence of HCC, and the close association between chronic HBV infections and HCC development have generated intense interest in understanding the molecular mechanisms that underlie the development of HBV-induced HCC. In this chapter, we provide a review of HBV biology and potential mechanisms that link a chronic HBV infection to the development of HCC. We specifically focus on activities of the HBV X protein (HBx), a multifunctional HBV protein that can alter hepatocyte physiology and stimulate HBV replication. While a brief survey of HBx activities that could influence HCC development is provided, we emphasize HBx regulation of intracellular calcium signaling and cell proliferation pathways as HBx activities that could potentially influence hepatocyte transformation.

## 2. Hepatitis B virus

HBV is a member of the *Hepadnaviridae,* a family of hepatotropic viruses that predominately infect hepatocytes in their respective hosts; similar viruses have been isolated from apes, woodchucks, squirrels, ducks, geese, and cranes [reviewed in (Seeger et al, 2007)]. HBV has a highly compact DNA genome of about 3200 nucleotides in length that contains four overlapping open reading frames (ORFs); every nucleotide of the genome is in at least one

---

* Co-first authors

open reading frame (Figure 1). The four overlapping ORFs of the HBV genome encode seven proteins: the reverse transcriptase/polymerase, the pre-core (E antigen) and core (capsid) proteins, three envelope (large, middle, and small hepatitis B surface antigens) proteins, and the nonstructural X protein (HBx) [reviewed in (Seeger et al, 2007)]. The cell-surface receptor of HBV that facilitates HBV infection of hepatocytes has not been conclusively identified, and the mechanism by which HBV enters hepatocytes is not clear. Upon infection of hepatocytes, the encapsidated, partially double-stranded DNA genome is transported to the nucleus, where it is converted into a covalently closed, double-stranded, circular DNA (cccDNA). cccDNA is the template for all HBV RNA transcripts; the transcripts are exported out of the nucleus into the cytoplasm and are translated to form the HBV pre-core, core, envelope, reverse transcriptase/polymerase, and HBx proteins. The largest HBV RNA transcript, the pregenomic RNA (pgRNA), is packaged with the reverse transcriptase into viral capsids in the cytosol and is reverse transcribed to generate the partially double-stranded HBV DNA genome [reviewed in (Seeger et al, 2007)]. HBV viral capsids containing the replicating genome bud into the endoplasmic reticulum by envelopment within the HBV envelope proteins and are secreted from the infected hepatocyte [reviewed in (Nguyen et al, 2008; Seeger et al, 2007)].

### 2.1 Model systems for studying HBV infections

Each member of the hepadnavirus family has a narrow host range that is thought to be defined primarily by the interaction between the virus and a specific receptor that is present on the surface of host hepatocytes [reviewed in (Seeger et al, 2007)]. Available cell culture systems for studying the life cycle of the *Hepadnaviridae* are limited. Typically, members of the hepadnavirus family can only directly infect hepatocytes within the liver of their respective avian or mammalian hosts or cultured, well-differentiated primary hepatocytes that are derived from these hosts; this has hampered the capabilities of researchers to study a natural HBV infection [reviewed in (Koike, 2009; Seeger et al, 2007)]. Chimpanzees are the most relevant animal model for studying the consequences of an HBV infection; however, due to cost and ethical reasons, studies in chimpanzees are limited (Prince & Brotman, 2001). HBV infections in chimpanzees also do not completely mimic all aspects of an HBV infection in humans; chimpanzees chronically infected with HBV usually do not develop liver cirrhosis or HCC (Prince & Brotman, 2001). HBV-transgenic mice have served as an important small animal model for studying *in vivo* HBV replication and immune-mediated HBV clearance from hepatocytes [(Guidotti et al, 1995); reviewed in (Guidotti & Chisari, 2006)]. However, because HBV-transgenic mice contain a copy of the HBV genome that is integrated into the genome of all hepatocytes in these mice, the consequences of chronic inflammation for the development of HBV-associated HCC cannot be studied in this model [reviewed in (Bouchard & Navas-Martin, 2011)]. More recently, human hepatocyte chimeric mice, which were generated by the replacement of the majority of the mouse hepatocytes with implanted human hepatocytes, have been used to study HBV infections in what may become a more experimentally tractable and relevant model than other currently available small animal model systems (Tsuge et al, 2005). Mice with humanized-livers that were inoculated with HBV had high levels of HBV viremia that lasted for up to 22 weeks (Tsuge et al, 2005). Hydrodynamic transfection of the HBV genome into mouse livers has also been used as a method for studying HBV replication in hepatocytes; however, due to rapid clearance of the virus, persistent HBV infection cannot be studied in this system (Keasler et al, 2007). The paucity of *in vivo* models for studying direct HBV infections, and the limited availability of cultured primary human hepatocytes, has lead many researchers to study HBV replication and the activities of HBV-encoded proteins in immortalized or transformed liver cell lines and in cultured primary hepatocytes derived from small animal models such as rats or mice [reviewed in (Bouchard & Navas-Martin, 2011; Seeger et al, 2007)]. Use of these systems necessitates the bypass of the initial receptor-mediated infection of the cell by direct transfection of the HBV DNA genome. Although studies in immortalized or transformed cells have served as powerful models for studying various aspects of HBV replication and the functions of HBV-encoded proteins, these studies have also demonstrated that the activities of HBV proteins may vary in different cellular contexts [reviewed in (Bouchard & Navas-Martin, 2011; Neuveut et al, 2010)]. Studies in cultured primary hepatocytes have begun to clarify HBV replication strategies and the function of HBV proteins in a more relevant context [reviewed in (Bouchard & Navas-Martin, 2011)]. Recently, cultured primary rat hepatocytes have been used to study HBV replication and functions of the HBx protein (Clippinger & Bouchard, 2008; Clippinger et al, 2009; Gearhart & Bouchard, 2010a; Gearhart & Bouchard, 2010b); HBx activities in cultured primary rat hepatocytes were similar to HBx activities in cultured primary human hepatocytes, supporting the use of cultured primary rat hepatocytes as a good model system for studying the impact of HBV on hepatocyte physiology (Gearhart & Bouchard, 2011).

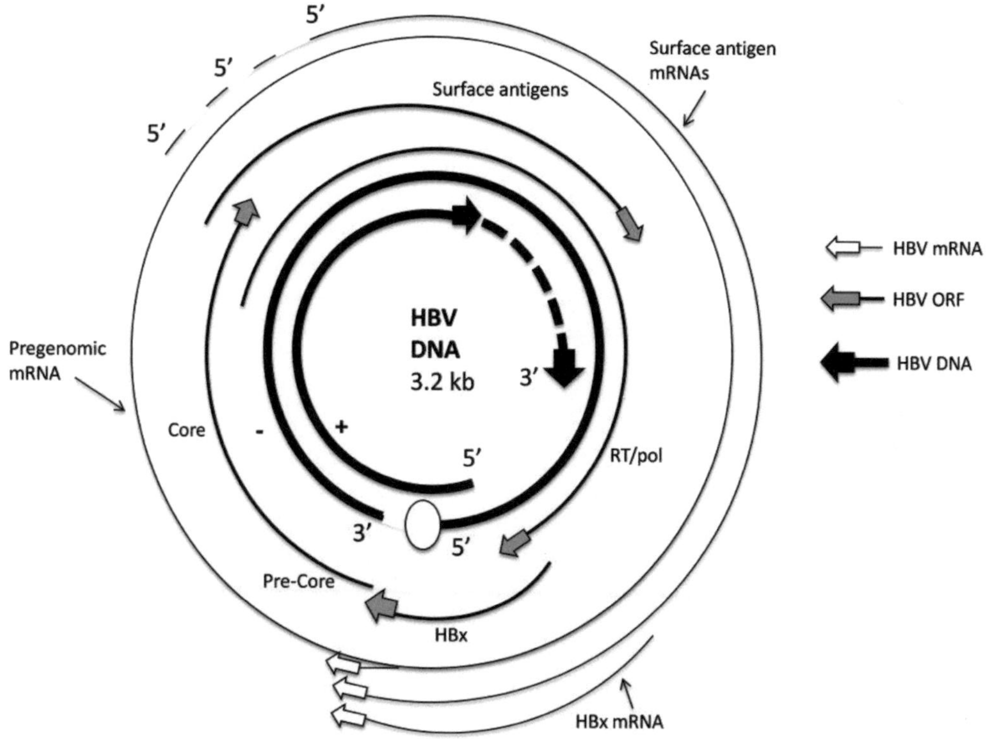


Fig. 1. Schematic depiction of the HBV genome. HBV DNA is denoted by bold lines with black arrows, HBV open reading frames (ORFs) are represented by inner arrows shown in gray, and HBV mRNAs are represented by outer arrows shown in white. See text for detailed description.

### 2.2 HBV and hepatocellular carcinoma

Common modes of HBV transmission include exposure to HBV-contaminated blood, unsafe injection practices, sexual contact with an HBV-infected individual, and perinatal transmission from an HBV-infected mother to her child (WHO, 2008). HBV infections are classified as acute, chronic, or occult. In most people with acute or short-term HBV infections, the infection is resolved by immune-mediated viral clearance. The inflammatory response to the HBV infection causes many of the symptoms that have been associated with hepatitis; these symptoms include jaundice, fatigue, nausea, vomiting, and abdominal pain [(WHO, 2008); reviewed in (Seeger et al, 2007)]. Chronic HBV infections are characterized by the continued presence of detectable levels of the HBV small envelope protein in the blood of an HBV-infected individual for more than six months [reviewed in (Lok & McMahon, 2001)]. Chronic infections with either HBV or the hepatitis C virus (HCV) are estimated to account for more than 80% of primary liver cancers; approximately 60% of these liver cancers are attributed to chronic HBV infections and 40% to chronic HCV infections [reviewed in (El-Serag & Rudolph, 2007; Koike, 2009)]. Currently, the geographic locations with the highest incidence of HCC are areas where HBV infection is highly endemic [reviewed in (Pang et al, 2006)]. There are eight known genotypes of HBV, and mounting evidence suggests that increased persistence of an HBV infection and a greater risk for HCC development may be influenced by the HBV genotype in the infected individual [reviewed in (Chemin & Zoulim, 2009)]. Environmental factors such as alcohol consumption, aflatoxin exposure, and tobacco use increase the risk for developing HCC in HBV-infected individuals [reviewed in (Chemin & Zoulim, 2009)].

Although the association between chronic HBV infections and HCC development is clear, the mechanisms that link a chronic HBV infection to HCC development are incompletely understood. Three potential mechanisms have been commonly invoked as consequences of an HBV infection that could contribute to HCC development. The first mechanism that may contribute to the development of HBV-associated HCC is persistent liver inflammation and hepatocyte proliferation that is caused by recurrent immune-mediated destruction of HBV-infected hepatocytes and concomitant liver regeneration in chronically HBV-infected individuals [reviewed in (Bouchard & Navas-Martin, 2011; Guidotti & Chisari, 2006)]. Persistent liver inflammation can cause fibrosis and cirrhosis and may eventually select for hepatocytes that have accumulated tumorigenic properties [reviewed in (Bouchard & Navas-Martin, 2011; Chemin & Zoulim, 2009)]. Chronic liver inflammation, the associated elevation of reactive oxygen species (ROS), and the potential for ROS to cause DNA damage may also produce a more cancer-prone environment [reviewed in (Chemin & Zoulim, 2009)]. The second mechanism that has been proposed to contribute to the development of HBV-associated HCC is the possible consequence of HBV genome integration into the host genome, which could cause genetic or epigenetic changes and genomic instability [reviewed in (Chemin & Zoulim, 2009; Neuveut et al, 2010)]. Integration of the HBV genome into the host genome could potentially result in the loss of tumor suppressive functions and/or the gain of tumor-promoting activities [reviewed in (Chemin & Zoulim, 2009)]. The third mechanism that has been proposed to be involved in the development of HBV-associated HCC, and the primary focus of this chapter, is the alteration of hepatocyte physiology and stimulation of HBV replication that is linked to expression of the HBV HBx protein [reviewed in (Bouchard & Navas-Martin, 2011; Koike, 2009; Neuveut et al, 2010)]. The multifunctional HBx protein has been shown to affect numerous cellular signaling pathways that could influence HBV replication, hepatocyte transformation, and HCC development [reviewed in (Benhenda et al, 2009; Koike, 2009; Neuveut et al, 2010)]. Although this chapter focuses on HBx activities, it is important to note that in the context of an HBV infection, multiple mechanisms are likely to influence HCC development.

## 3. HBx

HBx is a 154 amino acid, 17 kDa, multifunctional protein that is encoded by the smallest open reading frame of the HBV genome. HBx can stimulate HBV replication and modulate intracellular calcium signaling, cell proliferation and apoptotic pathways, signal transduction pathways, and the activity of various transcription factors and the proteasome (Figure 2) [reviewed in (Benhenda et al, 2009; Bouchard & Schneider, 2004; Koike, 2009)]. Because HBx activities appear to be influenced by the cell type and the method of HBx expression used in a study, not all HBx functions in normal hepatocytes and in the context of HBV replication are completely understood. Most studies that have assessed the effects of HBx have been performed in immortalized or transformed cells, when HBx was expressed at higher levels than observed during HBV replication, and when HBx was expressed outside of the context of HBV replication. Because HBx is expressed at low levels during HBV replication, it has been difficult to establish systems in which HBx interacting partners or HBx activities can be easily studied in the context of HBV replication. Consequently, the use of various cellular model systems to study HBx has sometimes identified seemingly discrepant HBx activities. It is important to note however, that many studies that have analyzed HBx activities in systems where HBx is expressed in the context of HBV replication and in normal hepatocytes have confirmed HBx activities that were identified when HBx

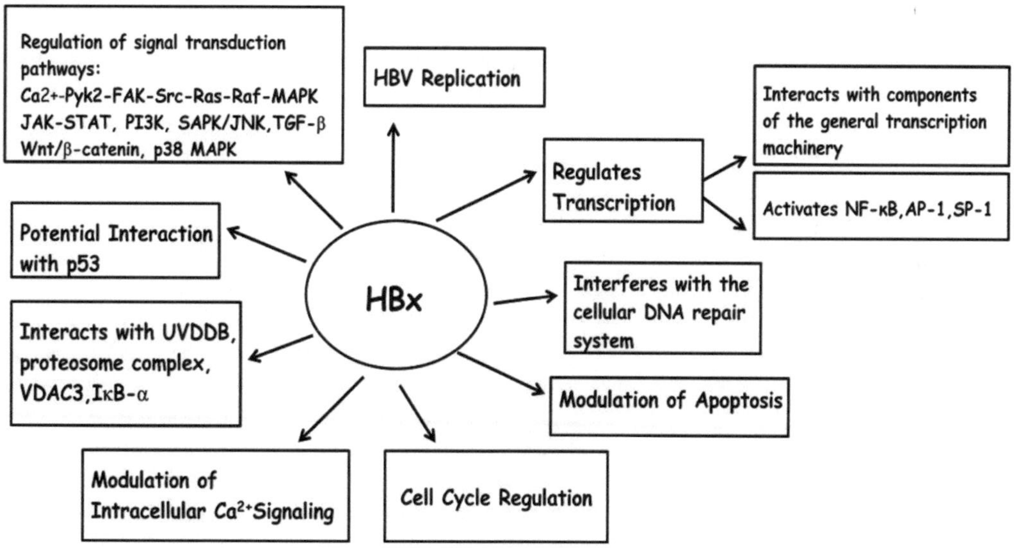


Fig. 2. Schematic representation of HBx activities. HBx is a multifunctional protein known to regulate HBV replication, numerous signal transduction pathways, the cell cycle, apoptosis, and transcription. HBx can also bind multiple cellular proteins. One or more of these HBx activities could contribute to the development of HBV-associated HCC. See text for references and details.

was overexpressed out of the context of HBV replication, suggesting that studies in various cellular systems can provide valuable insights into HBx activities [reviewed in (Benhenda et al, 2009; Bouchard & Schneider, 2004; Koike, 2009)]. Moreover, because HBx is often expressed in HBV-associated liver tumor cells even when expression of other HBV proteins is not detectable (Wang et al, 2004b; Wollersheim et al, 1988), studies in immortalized or transformed cells may help identify HBx activities that could be present in transformed cells but absent in normal hepatocytes. Overall, it is likely that studies in immortalized or transformed cells, in cultured primary hepatocytes, in the livers of available animal models, and when HBx is expressed in the absence of other HBV proteins and in the context of HBV replication each contribute important information regarding the various activities of this protein. Considering the compact nature of the HBV genome, the limited number of proteins encoded by the HBV genome, and the necessity for these proteins to perform their functions in an environment that may not favor viral replication, it is not surprising that HBV proteins such as HBx, which is the only regulatory protein encoded by the HBV genome, have multiple functions that impact HBV replication and cellular physiology.

### 3.1 HBx and HBV replication

Many studies have indicated that replication of mammalian hepadnaviruses is stimulated by their respective X proteins. Two different studies performed in woodchucks showed that the woodchuck hepatitis virus (WHV) X protein (WHx) is absolutely required for WHV replication in the livers of woodchucks (Chen et al, 1993; Zoulim et al, 1994); however, in one dissenting study, another group detected a very low level of WHV replication in woodchucks infected with an WHx-deficient WHV mutant (Zhang et al, 2001). Evidence that HBx stimulates HBV replication has been generated from studies in various mouse models and cell culture systems. Transgenic mice were generated with either a wild-type HBV genome or a mutant form of the HBV genome that did not express HBx; HBV replication was detected in both the wildtype HBV and mutant HBV-transgenic mice (Xu et al, 2002). However, when the HBx-deficient HBV-transgenic mice were bred with HBx-transgenic mice, higher levels of circulating HBV viremia and higher levels of HBV core and envelope proteins were detected in the double transgenic mice than in their HBx-deficient, HBV-transgenic counterparts (Xu et al, 2002). These studies suggest that although HBx may not be absolutely required for HBV replication in this model system, HBx does enhance HBV replication in the livers of these mice. An important caveat to the studies in HBV-transgenic mice is that these mice do not produce nuclear HBV cccDNA and may not recapitulate all aspects of authentic HBV replication (Guidotti et al, 1995). Additional evidence that HBx stimulates HBV replication has come from a study where mice were hydrodynamically injected with a plasmid encoding the wild-type HBV genome or a mutant HBx-deficient HBV genome (Keasler et al, 2007). The results of these studies demonstrated that although HBx was not absolutely required for HBV replication, there was a very significant decrease in HBV replication in mice injected with the HBx-deficient HBV as compared to mice injected with the wildtype HBV genome (Keasler et al, 2007). Interestingly, when a plasmid encoding HBx was co-injected with a plasmid encoding the mutant HBx-deficient HBV genome, HBV replication levels were restored to those seen in mice injected with the plasmid encoding wild-type HBV (Keasler et al, 2007). Finally, studies in mice with humanized livers showed that after direct infection with wild-type HBV or an HBx-deficient HBV, HBV replication was only seen in the livers of mice that were infected with wild-type HBV (Tsuge et al, 2010; Tsuge et al, 2005). HBx expression also stimulates HBV replication in HepG2 cells, a human hepatoblastoma cell line, and in cultured primary rat hepatocytes [reviewed in (Bouchard & Schneider, 2004)]. Although most studies indicate that HBV replication in Huh7 cells, a human hepatoma cell line, is not regulated by HBx expression, a recent study demonstrated that HBx can also stimulate HBV replication in Huh7 cells (Lim et al, 2010). Many of the signaling pathways that are modulated by HBx, and will be discussed in the following sections of this chapter, have also been shown to influence HBV replication. HBx modulation of intracellular calcium signaling, activation of the Proline-rich tyrosine kinase 2 (Pyk2)/Focal adhesion kinase (FAK)-Src-Ras-Raf-MAPK signaling pathway, regulation of transcription pathways, interaction with ultraviolet DNA damage binding protein 1 (UVDDB1), and association with proteasome factors affect HBx regulation of HBV replication (Bouchard et al, 2001b; Gearhart & Bouchard, 2010b; Klein et al, 1999; Leupin et al, 2005; Tan et al, 2009; Tang et al, 2005; Zhang et al, 2004). Overall, studies in various model systems suggest that the X proteins of mammalian hepadnaviruses have an important stimulatory role during replication of mammalian hepadnaviruses.

### 3.2 HBx and hepatocellular carcinoma

HBx expression and activities are thought to be major contributing factors in the development of HBV-associated HCC; however, the exact contribution of HBx to HCC development is unknown. One important clue that implicates HBx in the development of HBV-associated HCC is that chronic infections of birds with avian hepadnaviruses are not associated with the development of HCC [reviewed in (Seeger et al, 2007)]. The avian hepadnaviruses either do not encode an X protein or encode an X protein that is highly divergent from the X proteins of mammalian hepadnaviruses (Mandart et al, 1984; Sprengel et al, 1988). The mammalian hepadnaviruses all encode an X protein, and only infections with mammalian hepadnaviruses are associated with the development of HCC in their respective hosts [reviewed in (Seeger et al, 2007)]. Additional evidence for the involvement of HBx in HCC development has come from studies in HBx-transgenic mice. Some studies have shown that HBx expression can directly cause HCC in HBx-transgenic mice (Kim et al, 1991; Yu et al, 1999). In contrast, other researchers have found that HBx expression alone is not sufficient for the development of liver tumors in HBx-transgenic mice but can sensitize these mice to chemical- or oncogene-induced HCC (Madden et al, 2001; Slagle et al, 1996; Terradillos et al, 1997; Zhu et al, 2004). While the reason for the observed differences in tumor development in the various HBx-transgenic mice has not been completely explored and may be related to the genetic background of the mice and/or the level of HBx expression, studies in these HBx-transgenic mice strongly support the notion that HBx can have at least a co-factor role in the development of HCC. Importantly, a co-factor role for HBx in the development of HBV-associated HCC is more consistent with the biology of HCC development in chronically HBV-infected individuals; development of HCC in chronically HBV-infected individuals can take decades to arise [reviewed in (Seeger et al, 2007)]. The observation that HBV-associated HCC requires decades to arise suggests that HBV does not encode a strongly oncogenic protein but instead encodes proteins that can cause subtle changes to hepatocyte physiology that could sensitize hepatocytes to other oncogenic signals [reviewed in (Bouchard & Navas-Martin, 2011; Neuveut et al, 2010)]. The activities of HBx that could influence HCC development are discussed below.

### 3.3 Intracellular localization of HBx

The primary intracellular location of HBx is the cytoplasm, although a small fraction of HBx can be found in the nucleus of cells (Doria et al, 1995; Haviv et al, 1998b; Henkler et al, 2001; Siddiqui et al, 1987; Urban et al, 1997; Vitvitski-Trepo et al, 1990). The localization of HBx is dependent on its level of expression. When HBx is expressed at very low levels, it is mainly localized to the nucleus, and when HBx is expressed at high levels, its localization is mainly cytoplasmic (Henkler et al, 2001). Many studies have also shown that a fraction of cytosolic HBx localizes to the mitochondria and can interact with the voltage-dependent anion channel (VDAC) 3, a component of the mitochondrial permeability transition pore (MPTP) (Clippinger & Bouchard, 2008; Henkler et al, 2001; Huh & Siddiqui, 2002; Kim et al, 2007; Rahmani et al, 2000; Shirakata & Koike, 2003; Takada et al, 1999). Cytoplasmic, nuclear, and mitochondrial HBx localization have been directly linked to HBx activities that regulate specific cellular signal transduction or transcription pathways [reviewed in (Ma et al, 2011)].

### 3.4 HBx interacts with multiple cellular proteins

HBx has been reported to interact with various cellular proteins, such as components of the proteasome complex (Fischer et al, 1995; Huang et al, 1996), UVDDB1 and 2 (Becker et al, 1998; Lee et al, 1995; Sitterlin et al, 2000)), the cell cycle regulatory protein p53 (Elmore et al, 1997; Feitelson et al, 1993; Wang et al, 1994), the NF-κB inhibitory protein IκB-α (Weil et al, 1999), and VDAC3 (Rahmani et al, 2000; Rahmani et al, 1998), to name a few. HBx can also interact with components of the general transcription machinery such as the TATA-binding protein (TBP), the RBP5 subunit of RNA polymerase, and the general transcription factors TFIIB and TFIIH [(Aufiero & Schneider, 1990; Barnabas et al, 1997; Cheong et al, 1995; Haviv et al, 1998a; Haviv et al, 1998b; Maguire et al, 1991; Williams & Andrisani, 1995; Yang et al, 1999); reviewed in (Bouchard & Schneider, 2004)]. While the potential association of HBx with many cellular proteins could explain the multifunctional nature of HBx, because many studies that have analyzed HBx-interacting proteins were conducted in systems in which both HBx and these proteins were overexpressed, whether all of these interactions exist in normal hepatocytes when HBx is expressed during HBV replication remains to be determined. Due to space limitations, the following sections will focus on the interaction of HBx with UVDDB1 and 2 and p53; these interactions have been studied by various groups and may play an important role in HBV-induced HCC (Feitelson et al, 1993; Lee et al, 1995; Sitterlin et al, 2000; Wang et al, 1994). A more extensive discussion of proteins that may interact with HBx can be found in recently published reviews of this topic (Arbuthnot et al, 2000; Benhenda et al, 2009; Wei et al, 2010; Zhang et al, 2006).

#### 3.4.1 HBx and UVDDB1 and 2

UVDDB1 associates with UVDDB2 to form the UV-DDB complex, which functions in nucleotide excision repair. The UVDDB complex also interacts with the transcription factor E2F1, indicating a role for the UVDDB complex in both DNA repair and cell cycle control [(Datta et al, 2001; Hayes et al, 1998); reviewed in (Butel et al, 1996)]. Results from yeast-2-hybrid screens indicated that HBx can directly interact with UVDDB1 (Lee et al, 1995; Lin-Marq et al, 2001; Sitterlin et al, 2000). Further evidence for an interaction between hepadnavirus X proteins and the UVDDB complex was provided from studies performed with WHV; these studies confirmed an interaction between WHx and UVDDB1 (Bergametti et al, 2002). Disruption of the WHx-UVDDB1 interaction inhibited WHV replication in woodchucks, indicating that WHx and UVDDB1 must associate in order for WHV replication to occur *in vivo* (Sitterlin et al, 2000). WHx was also shown to interact with UVDDB2. The interaction between WHx and UVDDB1 stabilized WHx by protecting it from proteasomal degradation, but the interaction between UVDDB1 and UVDDB2 and between HBx and UVDDB2 counteracted this protection (Bergametti et al, 2002). In one study, HBx altered UVDDB1 activity, resulting in decreased cell viability (Lin-Marq et al, 2001). Similar to the required interaction of WHx and UVDDB1 for WHV replication, HBx association with UVDDB1 was also shown to be required for HBV replication (Sitterlin et al, 2000). HBx expression diminished the innate ability of cells to repair DNA damage, and the results of a study in HepG2 cells suggested that the binding of HBx to UVDDB1 inhibits normal UVDDB1 functions and can result in chromosome segregation defects (Becker et al, 1998; Martin-Lluesma et al, 2008). Results from studies in HBx-transgenic mice, however, indicated that the expression of HBx did not significantly increase the accumulation of spontaneous mutations, implying that although the interaction between HBx and UVDDB1 may inhibit the ability of cells to repair DNA damage, this interaction is not directly mutagenic (Madden et al, 2000). Interestingly, it has been suggested that the interaction between HBx and UVDDB1 may be involved in the HBx-related cell cycle arrest at the G1/S phase border [reviewed in (Bouchard & Schneider, 2004)]. Overall, a decreased ability to repair DNA damage caused by the interaction of HBx with the UVDDB complex, combined with modulation of cell proliferation pathways, could be important factors in the development of HBV-associated HCC.

### 3.4.2 HBx and p53

The results of various studies suggest that HBx may interact with the tumor suppressor p53 both *in vivo* and *in vitro*. HBx that was tagged with glutathione S-transferase (GST-HBx) was shown to interact with *in vitro* translated p53; a reciprocal interaction between GST-p53 and *in vitro* translated HBx was also observed (Wang et al, 1994). p53 and HBx produced by *in vitro* translation and subsequently co-immunoprecipitated with either anti-HBx or anti-p53 antibodies also confirmed an interaction between p53 and HBx (Feitelson et al, 1993). Several reports indicate that HBx can alter the sequence-specific DNA binding and transcriptional regulatory capacity of p53 as well as p53 stimulation of apoptotic pathways (Elmore et al, 1997; Lee & Rho, 2000; Wang et al, 1994; Wang et al, 1995). The results of one study suggested that HBx can interact with the carboxy-terminal domain of p53 and that this interaction leads to inhibition of p53-induced apoptosis in normal primary human fibroblasts (Wang et al, 1995). Results of another study suggested that p53 can be sequestered in the cytoplasm by HBx, thus leading to the inhibition of p53-mediated apoptosis (Elmore et al, 1997). Interestingly, there are varying results regarding the role of p53 in the regulation of apoptosis by HBx; both p53-dependent (Wang et al, 2008) and p53-independent regulation of apoptosis by HBx have been observed (Shintani et al, 1999; Terradillos et al, 1998). Studies have also interrogated the influence of p53 on HBx regulation of the cyclin-dependent kinase inhibitor, p21; HBx increased the level of p21 in NIH3T3 cells in the presence of p53 but did not increase the level of p21 when p53 was knocked down (Ahn et al, 2002). However, in a different study, HBx increased p21 levels in Hep3B cells, a p53 mutant HCC cell line (Park et al, 2000). Since activities of HBx that were linked to p53-dependent pathways were also observed in the absence of p53, the functional importance of the putative interaction between p53 and HBx has been questioned (Groisman et al, 1999; Terradillos et al, 1998). In one study, an *in vivo* interaction between HBx and p53 was observed in liver tissues of HBV-infected patients with HCC; however, contradictory results were obtained in a different study where p53 was found to be present only in the nucleus and HBx predominantly in the cytoplasm of liver tissues of HBV-infected patients (Feitelson et al, 1993; Su et al, 2000). The effect of HBx on the activities of p53 could directly influence the development of HBV-associated HCC; deregulation of p53 activities, such as its ability to regulate the cell cycle and apoptotic pathways, could favor processes that cause hepatocyte transformation. Overall, studies that have addressed a potential interaction between HBx and p53 suggest that this may occur in a cell-specific context; additional studies are required to examine whether HBx and p53 interact in the context of HBV replication in normal hepatocytes.

### 3.5 HBx activates transcription

Although HBx does not bind directly to DNA, it can function as a modest transcriptional activator [reviewed in (Benhenda et al, 2009; Bouchard & Schneider, 2004; Koike, 2009)]. HBx can activate multiple viral and cellular transcription promoters and enhancers [reviewed in (Benhenda et al, 2009; Murakami, 2001; Yen, 1996)]. HBx can activate promoters that contain DNA binding sites for transcription factors such as nuclear factor-kappa-B (NF-κB), activating protein-1 (AP-1), nuclear factor of activated T cells (NFAT), cAMP response element-binding transcription factor (CREB)/activating transcription factor (ATF)-2, CCAAT/enhancer binding protein (C/EBP), and stimulating protein 1 (Sp1), to name a few (Carretero et al, 2002; Chirillo et al, 1996; Cougot et al, 2007; Doria et al, 1995; Lara-Pezzi et al, 1999; Lee et al, 1998; Lucito & Schneider, 1992; Maguire et al, 1991; Mahe et al, 1991; Natoli et al, 1994a; Purcell et al, 2001; Spandau & C., 1988; Su & Schneider, 1996; Waris et al, 2001; Williams & Andrisani, 1995). HBx can activate transcription factors directly, through interactions with specific transcription regulatory proteins, or indirectly, by activation of cytosolic signal transduction pathways [(reviewed in (Bouchard & Schneider, 2004)]. HBx can directly interact with components of the basal transcription machinery, such as TBP, RBP5, TFIIB, and TFIIH; in addition, it also interacts with CREB and c-AMP dependent transcription factor (ATF)-3, a member of the basic leucine zipper (b-Zip) family of transcription factors (Aufiero & Schneider, 1990; Barnabas et al, 1997; Cheong et al, 1995; Cougot et al, 2007; Haviv et al, 1998a; Haviv et al, 1998b; Lin et al, 1997; Maguire et al, 1991; Williams & Andrisani, 1995; Yang et al, 1999). Interestingly, some studies suggest that HBx can activate its own promoter through an X responsive element (XRE) and can also activate HBV enhancers (Doria et al, 1995; Faktor & Shaul, 1990; Spandau & C., 1988). Whether the transcriptional activation functions of HBx in normal hepatocytes and in the context of HBV replication completely overlap with activities identified in established cell lines awaits a comprehensive analysis of HBx activities during a natural HBV infection.

### 3.6 HBx activates multiple signal transduction pathways

HBx can regulate numerous signal transduction pathways, including the Ras-Raf-Mitogen activated protein kinase (MAPK) pathway, the Janus-kinase signal transducer and activator of transcription pathway (JAK-STAT pathway), the phosphoinositide 3-kinase (PI3K) pathway, the stress-activated protein kinase/NH2-terminal-Jun kinase (SAPK/JNK) pathway, the transforming growth factor-β (TGF-β) pathway, the protein kinase C (PKC) and the p38 mitogen-activated protein kinase (p38MAPK) pathway (Benn & Schneider, 1994; Benn et al, 1996; Bouchard et al, 2003; Bouchard et al, 2001b; Chung et al, 2004; Cong et al, 1997; Cross et al, 1993; Johnson et al, 2000; Kekule et al, 1993; Klein et al, 1999; Klein & Schneider, 1997; Lara-Pezzi et al, 1999; Lee & Yun, 1998; Lucito & Schneider, 1992; Natoli et al, 1994a; Natoli et al, 1994b; Purcell et al, 2001; Tarn et al, 1999; Tarn et al, 2001; Tarn et al, 2002; Wang et al, 1998). The results of various studies suggest that HBx regulation of cytosolic signal transduction pathways could play a role in activation of transcription factors, HBx modulation of HBV replication, and HBx modulation of apoptotic and cell proliferation pathways [reviewed in (Benhenda et al, 2009; Bouchard & Schneider, 2004)].

The various signaling pathways that are stimulated by HBx have also been linked to mechanisms that are associated with cell transformation. For example, the Ras-Raf-MAPK signaling cascade has been implicated in the regulation of cell cycle progression, cellular differentiation, and cellular transcription pathways [reviewed in (Boguski & McCormick, 1993; McCubrey et al, 2007)]. HBx can activate the Ras/Raf kinase pathway in HeLa cells, a human cervical carcinoma cell line, and F9 cells, a mouse teratocarcinoma cell line; dominant negative mutants of Ras and the kinase Raf, an effector of the Ras-Raf-MAPK signaling cascade, blocked HBx activation of AP-1 (Natoli et al, 1994b). HBx activation of the Ras-Raf-MAPK signaling cascade was also observed in Chang cells, a human liver cell line, and directly in mouse livers (Benn & Schneider, 1994; Nijhara et al, 2001). Chang cells that expressed HBx had increased levels of Ras-GTP as compared to control cells, suggesting that HBx can increase the exchange of GDP for GTP (Benn & Schneider, 1994). Various reports indicate that the activation of Ras by HBx is indirect; HBx was not associated with Ras, Ras-GAP, the GTP exchange factor sons of sevenless (Sos), or the Ras adapter proteins Grb2 or Shc (Benn et al, 1996; Klein & Schneider, 1997). Instead, HBx was shown to constitutively activate non-receptor tyrosine kinases of the Src family (Src and Fyn), which can signal to Ras; inhibition of Src in Chang cells blocked HBx-induced Ras signaling and activation of the MAPK, ERK-2 (Klein et al, 1999; Klein & Schneider, 1997). HBx activation of Src kinases has been linked to the HBx-induced elevation of cytosolic calcium levels and activation of Pyk2 and FAK (Bouchard et al, 2006; Bouchard et al, 2001b). HBx stimulation of Src kinases promoted cycling of growth-arrested HepG2 and Chang cells; HBx induced arrested cells to exit G0 but stall at the G1/S border of the cell cycle, an activity that is thought to be important for HBV replication (Bouchard et al, 2001a). Importantly, active Src kinases are required for WHV replication, and HBx activation of Pyk2 and FAK, which is required for HBx activation of Src kinases, is also important for HBV replication (Bouchard et al, 2006; Bouchard et al, 2001b; Klein et al, 1999; Klein & Schneider, 1997). Finally, HBx-induced activation of Src kinases has been shown to be required for the stimulation of p38 MAPK, STAT3, and AP-1; activation of these proteins have been linked to various cell transformation processes and could contribute to processes that link chronic HBV infections to HCC development (Klein et al, 1999; Klein & Schneider, 1997; Lee & Yun, 1998; Tarn et al, 2002).

### 3.7 HBx regulates apoptotic pathways

Whether HBx is anti- or pro-apoptotic has been the subject of considerable debate. HBx has been reported to induce apoptosis (Bergametti et al, 1999; Chami et al, 2003; Chirillo et al,

1997; Kim et al, 1998; Kim et al, 2008; Kim & Seong, 2003; Koike et al, 1998; Lee et al, 2004; Liang et al, 2007; Liu et al, 2007; Lu & Chen, 2005; Miao et al, 2006; Shintani et al, 1999; Su & Schneider, 1997; Su et al, 2001; Takada et al, 1999; Tanaka et al, 2004; Terradillos et al, 2002; Terradillos et al, 1998; Wang et al, 2004a), sensitize cells to pro-apoptotic stimuli (Lee et al, 2004; Su & Schneider, 1997; Wang et al, 2004a), inhibit apoptosis (Clippinger et al, 2009; Diao et al, 2001; Elmore et al, 1997; Gottlob et al, 1998; Kang-Park et al, 2006; Lee et al, 2001; Pan et al, 2001; Shih et al, 2000), or have no impact on apoptosis (Klein et al, 2003; Madden et al, 2000; Yun et al, 2002). Interestingly, the effect of HBx on apoptosis was found to differ depending on the differentiation status of hepatocytes; HBx sensitized dedifferentiated hepatocytes, but not differentiated hepatocytes, to apoptotic signals (Wang et al, 2004a). The differing effects of HBx expression on apoptotic pathways that have been reported are likely attributed to the use of numerous cell types and experimental conditions for studying HBx apoptotic activities, and it is now apparent that HBx activities can vary in different cellular environments. Few studies have analyzed the impact of HBx expression on apoptosis in the context of HBV replication. Recent studies in cultured primary rat hepatocytes demonstrated that HBx has both pro- and anti-apoptotic activities in normal hepatocytes; similar HBx effects were observed when HBx was expressed in the absence of other HBV proteins or in the context of HBV replication. The anti-apoptotic activity of HBx in cultured primary rat hepatocytes was linked to HBx activation of NF-κB; however, when activation of NF-κB was blocked, HBx was found to induce apoptosis through a mechanism that was dependent on activities of the MPTP (Clippinger et al, 2009). The exact nature of HBx regulation of the MPTP is currently unknown. Whether HBx regulates apoptosis to affect HBV replication or the spread of HBV within the infected liver is not known. It is possible that HBx inhibits apoptosis during early stages of an HBV infection and later induces apoptosis to assist in viral spread [reviewed in (Benhenda et al, 2009; Ng & Lee, 2011)]. Although the pro-apoptotic effects of HBx might facilitate HBV replication and spread and lead to evasion of host cell-mediated immunity [reviewed in (Arbuthnot et al, 2000)], a recent study has provided evidence that modulation of apoptosis during an HBV infection is unlikely to affect viral spread (Arzberger et al, 2010). It is possible that the ability of HBx to induce or inhibit apoptosis might change during the course of an HBV infection as the liver is undergoing regeneration, or when the hepatocytes undergo transformation or respond to cytokines such as TNFα [reviewed in (Benhenda et al, 2009; Brenner, 1998; FitzGerald et al, 1995)]; both the activation and inactivation of apoptosis by HBx could contribute to HCC development. Enhanced compensatory hepatocyte regeneration that is induced by an HBx pro-apoptotic effect could lead to selection of hepatocytes that are resistant to apoptotic signals, thus leading to HCC (Koike et al, 1998). Alternatively, inhibition of apoptosis by HBx may increase the accumulation of potentially transforming mutations, leading to the development of liver cancer [reviewed in (Arbuthnot et al, 2000)]. Although the precise mechanisms that underlie HBx regulation of apoptosis in naturally infected hepatocytes remain incompletely understood, HBx modulation of hepatocyte apoptotic pathways is a potential mechanism that could influence the development of HBV-associated HCC.

## 4. HBx and the cell cycle

### 4.1 Cell cycle overview

The process of cellular replication and division is known as the cell cycle. The cell cycle is a highly regulated series of events and can be controlled by intracellular and extracellular factors [reviewed in (Harper & Brooks, 2005)]. Differentiated cells, such as hepatocytes, are typically maintained in a non-dividing, resting state, known as quiescence [reviewed in (Taub, 2004)]. When cells are quiescent, also known as the G0 phase, they must receive a signal in order to exit the G0 phase and enter the cell cycle [reviewed in (Cook et al, 2000; Harper & Brooks, 2005; Vermeulen et al, 2003)]. If they receive this signal, they will enter into the first phase of the cell cycle, known as the Gap 1 (G1) phase. During G1 phase, cells are preparing to replicate their DNA, and as long as the first major checkpoint of the cell cycle, the restriction point (R) at the G1/S border, is not activated and the growth signal is still present, cells will proceed into the Synthesis (S) phase. During S phase, the cells undergo DNA replication; once cells enter into this phase, DNA replication is completed regardless of removal of the growth signal or the presence of DNA damage. After DNA replication is completed, cells enter into the Gap 2 (G2) phase where the cellular machinery checks for DNA damage that may have accumulated during DNA replication and prepares for the Mitosis (M) phase. Once the proper signals are in place for cell cycle progression, cells will enter into M phase, during which mitosis occurs [reviewed in (Harper & Brooks, 2005; Vermeulen et al, 2003)]. A third checkpoint, the spindle checkpoint, exists after metaphase and prior to anaphase; at this checkpoint the cell employs methods to detect improper alignment of chromosomes on the mitotic spindle (Amon, 1999; Fang et al, 1998). If improper alignment is not detected, cells will continue into anaphase, at which point, the cells will complete the cell cycle, generating two daughter cells [reviewed in (Vermeulen et al, 2003)].

### 4.1.1 Positive regulators of cell cycle progression: Cyclins and cyclin-dependent kinases

Transition from one phase of the cell cycle to the next is tightly regulated and progressive. Key regulatory proteins that control cell cycle progression are cyclins and cyclin-dependent kinases (CDKs). CDKs are a family of serine/threonine protein kinases that are only activated at certain points in the cell cycle, although their expression levels remain constant throughout the entire cell cycle [reviewed in (Vermeulen et al, 2003)]. Currently, there are five CDKs that are associated with cell cycle progression in mammalian cells: CDKs 4 and 6, which are active during early G1 phase, CDK2, which is active in late G1 and S phase, CDK1, which is active during G2 and M phase, and CDK7, which can act in combination with cyclin H as a CDK-activating kinase (CAK) [(Fisher & Morgan, 1994); reviewed in (Harper & Brooks, 2005)]. CDK activity is highly regulated and requires both the expression of activating proteins, cyclins, and phosphorylation of the cyclin-CDK complex [reviewed in (Harper & Brooks, 2005; Vermeulen et al, 2003)]. The expression of cyclins is highly regulated, and their levels rise and fall depending on the cell cycle phase (Evans et al, 1983; Pines & Hunter, 1991). There are three D type cyclins, cyclin D1, cyclin D2, and cyclin D3, which bind to CDK4 and CDK6, resulting in activation of these CDKs; activation of CDK4 and CDK6 is required for entry into the cell cycle [reviewed in (Sherr, 1993; Sherr, 1994)]. Unlike the other cyclins, cyclin D expression is maintained as long as growth factor stimulation is present (Assoian & Zhu, 1997). Cyclin E binds to CDK2 and regulates cell cycle progression from G1 into S phase (Ohtsubo et al, 1995). Cyclin A binds to CDK2 to regulate S phase progression and also binds to CDK1 during late G2 and M phase to promote entry into M phase (Arellano & Moreno, 1997; Girard et al, 1991; King et al, 1994;

Walker & Maller, 1991). During mitosis, an additional cyclin, cyclin B, is expressed; cyclin B binds to CDK1 to regulate the remainder of mitosis (Arellano & Moreno, 1997; King et al, 1994). In accordance with the dynamic nature of the induction of cyclin expression, cyclins are rapidly degraded when the cell cycle has progressed beyond the phase during which their expression is required. Cyclins D and E contain a PEST sequence, a segment rich in proline (P), glutamic acid (E), serine (S), and threonine (T) residues, and cyclins A and B contain destruction boxes. The PEST sequence and destruction boxes facilitate ubiquitin-mediated proteasomal degradation of the cyclins (Glotzer et al, 1991; Rechsteiner & Rogers, 1996).

Full CDK activity is dependent upon proper cyclin expression and binding and phosphorylation of the cyclin-CDK complex. Phosphorylation of the cyclin-CDK complex occurs on conserved threonine and tyrosine residues and induces conformational changes, which can enhance cyclin binding and CDK activity (Jeffrey et al, 1995; Paulovich & Hartwell, 1995). Activation of CDK4 requires phosphorylation of threonine 172, activation of CDK2 requires phosphorylation of threonine 160, and activation of CDK1 requires phosphorylation of threonine 161 by the CDK7-cyclin H complex, CAK [reviewed in (Vermeulen et al, 2003)]. Alternatively, phosphorylation of cyclin-CDK complexes can also inhibit CDK activity when the cyclin-CDK complex is primed by cyclin binding to its partner CDK, but the cell does not yet require full activation of the CDK. For example, the cyclin A-CDK1 complex can be inhibited by phosphorylation at tyrosine 15 and/or threonine 14 by the kinases Wee1 and Myt1. The inhibitory phosphate can be removed by the Cdc25 phosphatase; this dephosphorylation is required for the full activation of CDK1 and subsequent progression through the cell cycle (Lew & Kornbluth, 1996). Once fully activated, the CDKs induce downstream signaling events by phosphorylating select substrates that regulate cell cycle progression (Morgan, 1997; Pines & Hunter, 1991). One such event is the phosphorylation of the retinoblastoma tumor suppressor gene (Rb) by the CDK4/6-cyclin D complex. In its active, dephosphorylated state, Rb is in a complex with the histone deacetylase protein HDAC and the transcription factors E2F-1 and DP-1. Upon phosphorylation in G1 phase, Rb is inactivated, resulting in the release of E2F-1 and DP-1, which then activate transcription of genes which are required for S phase progression, including those encoding cyclin E, cyclin A, and Cdc25 (Brehm et al, 1998; Buchkovich et al, 1989; Kato et al, 1993). Rb remains hyperphosphorylated for the remainder of the cell cycle; the cyclin E-CDK2 complex stabilizes this hyperphosphorylated state. The cyclin E-CDK2 complex can also phosphorylate its negative regulator p27, resulting in proteasomal degradation of p27 (Hinds et al, 1992; Montagnoli et al, 1999).

### 4.1.2 Negative regulators of cell cycle progression: CDK inhibitors

CDK activity can also be negatively regulated by interaction with various cellular proteins that are generically named CDK inhibitors, or CKIs. CKIs can bind to isolated CDKs or to the CDK-cyclin complex to prevent the full activation of CDKs [reviewed in (Harper & Brooks, 2005)]. There are two families of CKIs, the INK4 (inhibitor of CDK4) family and the Cip (CDK-interacting protein)/Kip (kinase inhibitor protein) family [reviewed in (Sherr & Roberts, 1995)]. The INK4 family includes p15 (INK4b), p16 (INK4a), p18 (INK4c), and p19 (INK4d) [reviewed in (Carnero & Hannon, 1998)]. Members of the INK4 family inactivate CDK4 and CDK6 by forming stable complexes with the CDK prior to cyclin binding; this blocks association of CDK4 and CDK6 with cyclin D and prevents entry into G1 phase [reviewed in (Harper & Brooks, 2005)]. Members of the Cip/Kip family include p21 (Waf1, Cip1), p27 (Cip2), and p57 (Kip2); these proteins contain a conserved region that is involved in cyclin binding and kinase inhibition [(Polyak et al, 1994a; Polyak et al, 1994b); reviewed in (Harper & Brooks, 2005; Roberts et al, 1994)]. Unlike members of the INK4 family, members of the Cip/Kip family bind to and inhibit the activity of the entire cyclin-CDK complex. Additionally, this CKI family displays a broader specificity than the INK4 family, as its members can bind and inhibit the activities of many cyclin-CDK complexes, including cyclin E-CDK2, cyclin A- CDK2, and cyclin B-CDK1 [(Hengst et al, 1998; Hengst & Reed, 1998); reviewed in (Harper & Brooks, 2005)]. Interestingly, the Cip/Kip family of CKI proteins can coordinate the assembly of the cyclin D-CDK4/6 complexes in the early G1 phase and stabilize this complex throughout G1 [(Cheng et al, 1999); reviewed in (Sherr & Roberts, 1999)].

### 4.2 The cell cycle and HCC

Deregulation of the cell cycle and alteration in the expression of cyclins and the activities of CDKs are frequently observed in transformed cells; consequently, disruption of normal mechanisms that regulate the cell cycle is thought to contribute to the development of many cancers [reviewed in (Hanahan & Weinberg, 2000)]. The expression of many cell cycle regulatory proteins is altered during the onset of HCC and is continually deregulated throughout the progression of liver cancer. For example, the transcription promoters of the *p15* and *p16* genes are frequently hypermethylated (Csepregi et al, 2010; Matsuda et al, 1999; Shim et al, 2003a; Shim et al, 2003b; Wong et al, 2000a; Wong et al, 2000b) and a significant percentage of HCCs are associated with decreased expression of p16, which occurs via hypermethylation, deletion, or mutation of the *p16* gene (Biden et al, 1997; Chaubert et al, 1997; Csepregi et al, 2010; Hui et al, 1996; Liew et al, 1999; Matsuda et al, 1999; Shen et al, 1998). Expression of DNA methyltransferase I, which methylates the *p16* promoter to inhibit transcription, is frequently upregulated in HCC (Huang et al, 2010; Oh et al, 2007). Decreased expression of p18, a potential tumor suppressor, is associated with poorly differentiated HCCs (Morishita et al, 2004). Interestingly, an increase in the phosphorylation of Rb has also been observed in HCCs that were negative for p18 expression (Morishita et al, 2004). Rb, a known tumor suppressor, is frequently inactivated (hyperphosphorylated) in HCC; approximately 15-30% of advanced HCCs display mutations in Rb [reviewed in (Burkhart & Sage, 2008)]. In addition to alterations in the INK4 family of CKIs, variations in the expression levels of the Cip/Kip family have also been found in HCC. Although a number of studies have demonstrated that the downregulation of p21 and p27 occurs in HCC, some other reports have suggested that the expression of p21 and p27 is increased in HCC (Gramantieri et al, 2003; Qin & Ng, 2001; Ren, 1991). Overexpression of cyclin D1 in mice has been linked to the development of hyperplasia and ultimately liver cancer (Deane et al, 2001). Importantly, the tumor suppressor p53 is frequently lost or mutated in many cancers, including in liver tumors [reviewed in (Hollstein et al, 1991)]. It is possible that p53 mutations could lead to the alteration of the cell cycle profile of hepatocytes and contribute to the development of liver cancer. Overall, it is evident that alterations in the expression levels or activities of cell cycle regulatory proteins and protein complexes could play a major role in hepatocarcinogenesis.

### 4.3 HBV replication and the cell cycle

DNA viruses have evolved different strategies to deregulate cell cycle checkpoint controls and modulate cell proliferation pathways. Because many DNA viruses primarily infect differentiated, quiescent cells, it is thought these viruses must induce cells to exit G0 and enter the cell cycle to create an environment that generates factors, such as nucleotides, that are required for viral replication [reviewed in (Mukherji & Kumar, 2008; Swanton & Jones, 2001)]. An unfortunate consequence of virus-mediated alterations in normal cell cycle control mechanisms is that these viral effects may ultimately generate an environment that also favors cell transformation and cancer development [reviewed in (Bouchard & Navas-Martin, 2011; Mukherji & Kumar, 2008)].

HBV replication has been associated with modulation of cell cycle progression, and HBV replication has been shown to be cell cycle dependent in certain experimental systems [reviewed in (Madden & Slagle, 2001)]. HBV replication in Huh7 cells, a human hepatoma cell line, and in primary marmoset hepatocytes, was shown to regulate the cell cycle (Chin et al, 2007). Huh7 cells infected with HBV were found to stall in the G2 phase of the cell cycle; HBV replication in these cells increased activation of both MAPK and Akt pathways. Interestingly, p53, p21, cdc2 and intranuclear cyclin B1 levels were elevated in primary marmoset hepatocytes that were infected with HBV, which also suggested features consistent with a G2 arrest (Chin et al, 2007). Alternatively, the results of studies in HepG2.2.15 cells, human hepatoblastoma HepG2 cells that contain an integrated HBV genome and replicating HBV, and Huh7 cells that were transiently transfected with the HBV genome showed that expression of the HBV genome caused these cells to progress through the G1 phase while inhibiting entry into S phase (Friedrich et al, 2005). The results of a different study in HepG2.2.15 cells also showed decreased proliferation of HepG2.2.15 cells as compared to HepG2 cells; this study also demonstrated that HBV can modulate the expression levels of cell cycle regulatory proteins, which resulted in a G1 phase arrest (Wang et al, 2011). Cumulatively, it can be concluded that HBV infection can influence cell cycle progression; however, the exact consequence of HBV infection on cell proliferation pathways is likely influenced by the characteristics of the cell type used for a particular study.

Several studies have analyzed the impact of the cell cycle phase on HBV replication. HBV replication in HepG2.2.15 cells varied depending on the phase of the cell cycle. Arresting HepG2.2.15 cells in either G1 or G2 resulted in an increase in the levels of HBV DNA and mRNA, while cell entry into S phase increased cellular DNA synthesis and decreased levels of HBV replication (Huang et al, 2004; Ozer et al, 1996). Studies in liver specimens from HBV-infected patients demonstrated that hepatocytes expressing proliferating cell nuclear antigen (PCNA), which is expressed during S phase and required for DNA replication [reviewed in (Harper & Brooks, 2005)], contained negligible amounts of HBV-specific DNA (Ozer et al, 1996). Cumulatively, the results of these studies suggest that HBV replication is decreased when cells are actively proliferating. The results from a recent study suggested, although did not definitively show, that microRNA (miRNA) regulation of cell proliferation pathways could affect HBV replication; over-expression of miRNA-1 (miR-1) arrested HepG2.2.15 cells in the G1 phase and promoted differentiation, which could be beneficial for HBV replication (Zhang et al, 2011). In contrast to studies that demonstrated that HBV replication is affected by the phase of the cell cycle, one group demonstrated that HBV replication is independent of cell cycle status in HBV-transgenic mice (Guidotti et al, 1997). However, because HBV-transgenic mice do not produce cccDNA and do not recapitulate every step of an authentic HBV infection, it is unclear whether results in this system accurately reflect all mechanisms that can regulate HBV replication (Guidotti et al, 1995).

Overall, the results of most studies suggest that cell proliferation pathways are altered in cells with replicating HBV and that the status of the cell cycle can influence HBV replication. The effect of cell cycle phase on HBV replication in cultured primary rat and human hepatocytes will be discussed in a separate section of this chapter.

### 4.4 HBx modulation of cell cycle

HBx expression has been linked to modulation of cell cycle progression, although the effect of HBx on cell proliferation pathways has varied depending on the cell type used and the experimental conditions of the study [reviewed in (Madden & Slagle, 2001)]. In this section, we summarize published studies that have analyzed the impact of HBx on cell cycle progression in immortalized or transformed cells; more recent studies in cultured primary hepatocytes will be discussed in a separate section. Overall, studies in various immortalized or transformed cells have shown that HBx can induce cells to enter the cell cycle, enter the cell cycle but stall at G1/S border of the cell cycle, or progress more rapidly through the cell cycle (Benn & Schneider, 1994; Benn & Schneider, 1995; Bouchard et al, 2001a; Chen et al, 2008; Koike et al, 1994; Lee et al, 2002; Mukherji et al, 2007; Singh et al, 2011; Zhang et al, 2005). It is likely that the observed variations in HBx effects reflect the use of different cell lines, different methods of HBx expression, and whether or not the studies were performed in the presence of growth factors. It is important to note that some seemingly discrepant results that have been reported may reflect a different interpretation of similar data. For example, HBx expression can cause cells in G0 to exit G0 but stall at the G1/S phase; this could be interpreted as stimulation of cell progression beyond G0 or inhibition of cell progression into S phase [reviewed in (Bouchard & Schneider, 2004)]. Additionally, most of the studies that analyzed the impact of HBx on cell cycle proliferation and cell cycle regulatory proteins were conducted when HBx was expressed in the absence of other HBV proteins, and it is unclear whether all the reported HBx activities that were associated with regulation of cell proliferation pathways are also present in the context of HBV replication.

Serum deprivation of cultured cells is a commonly used method for arresting cells in G0 or at the G0-G1 junction. When serum-starved Chang liver cells were infected with HBx-expressing recombinant adenoviruses, HBx increased cellular DNA synthesis and stimulated cell proliferation (Benn & Schneider, 1994). HBx eliminated the requirement for serum in cell cycle activation in Chang cells, and HBx-expressing Chang cells that were stimulated with serum entered S phase and progressed through the G2/M checkpoint more rapidly than control cells (Benn & Schneider, 1995). Additionally, HBx activation of Ras was necessary for HBx-dependent activation of cell cycling in Chang cells (Benn & Schneider, 1995). HBx activation of Src kinases was linked with the ability of HBx to cause serum-starved, quiescent Chang cells to transit through the G1 phase but stall at the G1/S phase of the cell cycle (Bouchard et al, 2001a). HBx expression in HepG2 cells increased cellular proliferation, as demonstrated in a 3-(4,5-Dimethylthiazol-2-yl)-2,5-diphenyltetrazolium bromide (MTT) cell proliferation assay (Zhang et al, 2005). Furthermore, an increase in DNA synthesis, as demonstrated by bromo-deoxyuridine (BrdU) incorporation, was observed in serum starved, HBx-expressing NIH3T3 cells, a mouse embryonic fibroblast cell line (Koike et al, 1994). Additional analysis of cell cycle progression in NIH3T3 cells indicated that expression of HBx caused cells to move from the G0/G1 phase to the S and G2/M phase (Koike et al, 1994). Alternatively, studies in HL-7702 cells, a normal human liver cell line, showed that the expression of HBx in these cells caused an increased accumulation of cells in S phase (Chen et al, 2008). The results from another study in Huh7 and human embryonic kidney 293 (HEK 293) cells suggested that HBx can cause these cells to transit through the G0 and G1/S checkpoints of the cell cycle even in the absence of serum (Mukherji et al, 2007). Additionally, HBx expression was found to increase the rate of entry of cells into S phase, thus causing rapid cycling of these cells; constitutive activation of Src kinases was shown to be required for HBx-mediated shortening of the cell cycle (Mukherji et al, 2007). In a seminal study that may explain the reason for the different effects of HBx on the cell cycle that have been observed in various cellular contexts, HBx expression was shown to modulate cell cycle progression differently in cells that had characteristics of differentiated or dedifferentiated hepatocytes. In these studies, two HBx-expressing cell lines were derived from the same parental AML12 liver cell line. AML12 cells are immortalized mouse hepatocytes that were originally derived from TGFα-transgenic mice; these cells maintain many characteristics that are similar to normal hepatocytes in the liver (Wu et al, 1994a). One of the newly derived HBx-expressing AML12 cell lines showed characteristics similar to differentiated hepatocytes, whereas the other cell line displayed a more dedifferentiated phenotype (Tarn et al, 1999; Wu et al, 1994b). HBx expression in the more differentiated cells caused the cells to rapidly progress through the cell cycle; however, HBx expression in the more dedifferentiated cells caused these cells to enter the cell cycle but pause in S phase (Lee et al, 2002). These observations support the notion that the impact of HBx on cell proliferation pathways varies depending on the characteristics of the cells used for the study. Taken together, the results of these numerous studies suggest that HBx can modulate cell cycle progression, though the exact impact of HBx on cell proliferation pathways when HBx is expressed from replicating HBV in normal hepatocytes in the liver remains to be completely defined.

#### 4.4.1 HBx regulation of cyclins and CDKs

The results of multiple studies have demonstrated that HBx can regulate the levels of cyclins and the activities of CDKs, although these HBx activities have varied in different experimental conditions. In one study, both stable and transient expression of HBx was found to increase the level of cyclin D1 in HepG2 cells (Jung et al, 2007). The level of cyclin D1 was also elevated in Huh7 cells that contained replicating HBV; however, this observation could not be directly linked to HBx since the effects of HBV on cell cycle regulatory proteins was not compared to an HBx-deficient HBV (Chin et al, 2007). Studies from another group suggested that HBx activation of NF-κB may play a role in up-regulation of cyclin D1 levels in Chang cells (Park et al, 2006). Additional studies have shown that HBx can also regulate the expression levels of cyclins that are required during later stages of the cell cycle. HBx activated the cyclin A promoter, increased cyclin A protein levels, and promoted the formation of cyclin A-CDK2 complexes in ts13 cells (Bouchard et al, 2001a); these cells are derived from a hamster cell line containing a temperature-sensitive defect in TBP-associated factor 250 (TAFII 250). The TAFII 250 ts13 mutation has been shown to induce cell cycle arrest and apoptosis when these cells are shifted from the permissive temperature to the nonpermissive temperature (Hayashida et al, 1994; Talavera & Basilico, 1977). The ability of HBx to activate the endogenous cyclin A promoter and cyclin A-CDK2 complexes was linked to stimulation of Src kinase signaling pathways (Bouchard et al, 2001a). HBV replication in Huh7 cells increased the levels of cyclin A and intranuclear cyclin B, which is active during the G2/M phase. Whether the elevation of cyclin A or intranuclear cyclin B was caused by HBx in these studies is not entirely clear because the results were not compared to similar assays with an HBx-deficient HBV (Chin et al, 2007). HBx increased the activation of CDK2 and CDK1 in Chang liver cells; this HBx activity was blocked with a dominant-negative mutant of Ras (Benn & Schneider, 1995). Finally, the results of studies in Huh7 cells demonstrated that HBx expression increased the stability of cyclin E in these cells and significantly enhanced CDK2 activity (Mukherji et al, 2007). Moreover, HBx was able to bind to the cyclin E/A-CDK2 complex in Huh 7 cells; expression of c-terminal src kinase (CSK), a physiological inhibitor of Src kinases, abrogated the interaction of HBx with the cyclin E-CDK2 complex (Mukherji et al, 2007). Overall, the various studies in immortalized and transformed cells demonstrate that HBx can modulate the levels and activities of positive regulators of the cell cycle. Whether similar HBx activities are apparent in the context of an authentic HBV infection of hepatocytes in the liver awaits further investigation.

### 4.4.2 HBx regulation of CKIs

In addition to the influence of HBx on positive regulators of the cell cycle, the results of some studies have suggested that HBx can also affect negative cell cycle regulators. These studies have mainly focused on the effect of HBx expression on the expression levels of p16, p21, and p27. Studies in HBV-associated cirrhotic livers and HBV-producing HCC cell lines showed a correlation between the hypermethylation of the *p16* gene, decreased expression of p16, and the presence of HBV (Shim et al, 2003b). Although this study demonstrated that HBV replication may be associated with deregulation of p16, these findings were not directly linked to HBx expression. However, in a subsequent study in HBV-associated HCC liver sections, the methylation status of the *p16* promoter was analyzed; liver sections that contained high levels of methylated *p16* promoters also had high expression levels of HBx, indicating that HBx expression correlates with the methylation status of the *p16* promoter (Zhu et al, 2007). Studies in HepG2 cells stably transfected with an HBx-expression plasmid showed that HBx induced hypermethylation of the *p16* promoter and down-regulation of p16 protein levels, which resulted in the activation of the cyclin D1-CDK4/6 complex, phosphorylation of Rb, activation of E2F1, and transcriptional activation of DNA methyltransferase 1 (DNMT1) (Jung et al, 2007). Interestingly, this induction of DNMT1 expression was found to be required for the *p16* promoter methylation and also for the expression of DNMT1 itself, suggesting that there is communication between p16 and DNMT1 (Jung et al, 2007). The results of an additional study demonstrated that the HBx-mediated reduction in p16 expression enabled HBx-expressing HepG2 cells to evade $H_2O_2$-induced senescence (Kim et al, 2010). Studies in liver tissue samples from HBV-associated HCCs and corresponding HBV-infected non-cancerous liver sections showed that in the non-cancerous tissues, HBx expression correlated positively with DNMT1 expression and negatively with p16 protein expression (Zhu et al, 2010). Alternatively, in the HCC tissues, HBx expression still correlated positively with DNMT1 expression, but did not correlate with the hypermethylation of the *p16* promoter or with p16 expression, suggesting that HBx-mediated hypermethylation of *p16* may play a role in the early stages of HBV-related hepatocarcinogenesis (Zhu et al, 2010).

The results of various studies have also suggested that HBx can alter the expression of p21 and p27. In Huh7 cells that were infected with a recombinant HBV-encoding adenovirus, an increase in p21 was observed; however, these findings were not directly linked to HBx expression because the results were not compared to Huh7 cells infected with a recombinant adenovirus that contained an HBV mutant that lacked HBx expression (Chin et al, 2007). In another study in HBx-expressing NIH3T3 cells, a dose-dependent increase in the transcription of p21 was observed when p53 was functional (Ahn et al, 2002). Alternatively, in the absence or down-regulation of p53, a repression of p21 transcription by HBx was observed in NIH3T3 cells (Ahn et al, 2002). Moreover, HBx expression decreased the level of p21 RNA in NIH3T3 cells, which may be due to p53-independent transcriptional repression, resulting from an HBx-mediated Sp-1 inactivation (Ahn et al, 2001). Sp-1 is a transcription factor that can activate transcription of many target genes, including p21 (Pardali et al, 2000). Transcriptional repression of p21 was also observed in NIH3T3 cells co-transfected with plasmids encoding HBx and the hepatitis C virus (HCV) core protein (Han et al, 2002). While there have been many studies that have investigated the role of HBx in regulating p21, much less is known about the effect of HBx on p27. In Huh7 cells, HBx expression was found to increase proteasomal degradation of p27 (Mukherji et al, 2007). Overall, the precise impact of HBx expression on members of the Cip/Kip family seems to vary in different cellular contexts, and both upregulation and downregulation of the CIP/KIP family has been observed. Interestingly, the results of one study showed that the level of HBx expression influences its effects on p21 and p27 (Leach et al, 2003). When HBx was expressed at low levels in Chinese hamster ovary (CHO) cells, an increased activity of the p21 and p27 promoters was observed. Alternatively, when HBx was expressed at high levels in CHO cells, there was inhibition of the activity of the p21 and p27 promoters. This study suggests that the experimental conditions that are used to study HBx modulation of CKIs can influence the observed effect of HBx.

#### 4.4.3 HBx regulation of cell proliferation in primary hepatocytes

Although various studies have analyzed the impact of HBx on cell proliferation pathways, many of these studies have identified different HBx effects. Most of these studies were conducted in transformed or immortalized cell lines and when HBx was overexpressed in the absence of other HBV proteins, which could contribute to the different HBx activities that were observed. Because established cell lines often contain changes in pathways that control normal cell cycle progression, observations of HBx activities in these cells could reflect HBx activities that are apparent in a specific context but not necessarily present in normal hepatocytes during an HBV infection. Recent studies in cultured primary hepatocytes have begun to address the effect of HBx expression, both on its own and when expressed in the context of replicating HBV, on hepatocyte cell cycle regulatory pathways. These studies have provided important insights into HBx activities that regulate HBV replication and could influence the development of HBV associated HCC.

Cultured primary rat hepatocytes are a biologically relevant model system that can be used to characterize HBx activities in normal, untransformed hepatocytes. In a series of studies in cultured primary rat hepatocytes, the impact of HBx on cell cycle regulation and HBV replication in normal hepatocytes was analyzed (Figure 3). In cultured primary rat hepatocytes, HBx decreased the expression level of both p15 and p16 while increasing the expression of p21 and p27, demonstrating that HBx decreased the levels of factors that maintained the quiescent status of hepatocytes and elevated the levels of inhibitors of cell

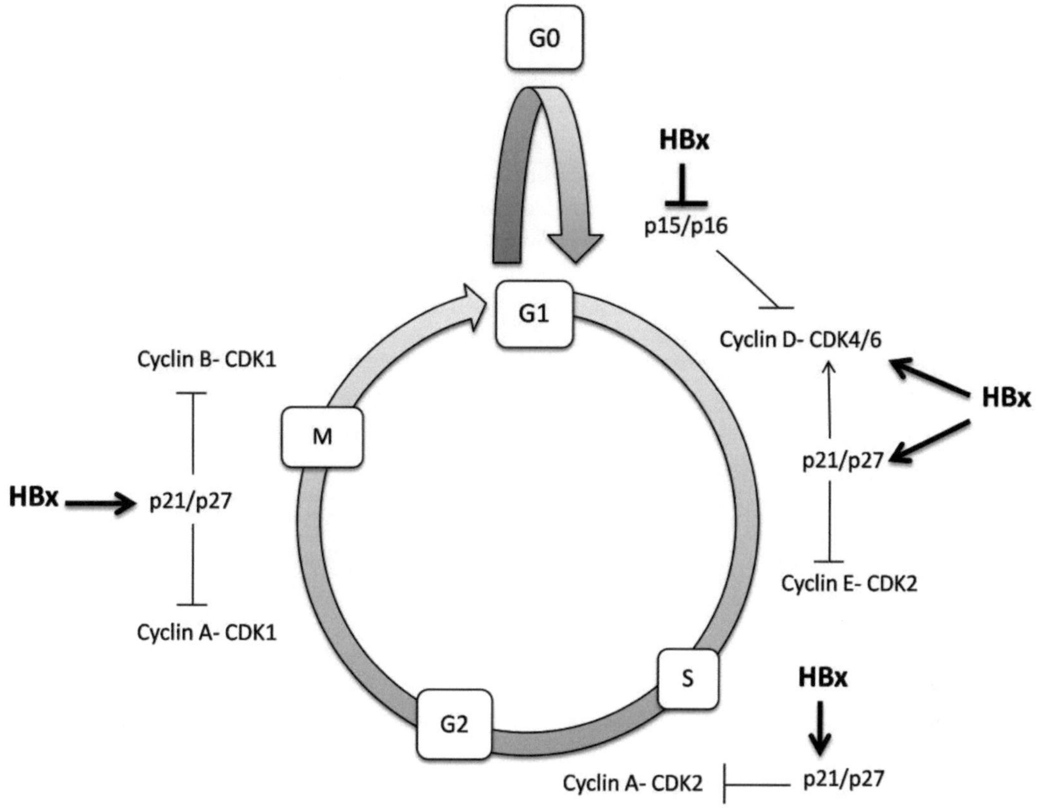


Fig. 3. Summary of HBx effects on the cell cycle in cultured primary hepatocytes. See text for details.

cycle progression past late G1 phase (Gearhart & Bouchard, 2010a). Similar studies in primary mouse hepatocytes that were infected with a recombinant HBx-expressing adenovirus also showed that HBx increased expression of both p21 and p27 and decreased DNA synthesis (Qiao et al, 2001). Finally, another study also identified an increase in p21 protein levels in primary mouse hepatocytes infected with a recombinant HBV-expressing adenovirus; however, these results were not directly linked to HBx expression because they were not compared to similar studies with an HBx-deficient HBV (Chin et al, 2007). In cultured primary rat hepatocytes, an increase in cyclin D1 and cyclin E expression in the presence of HBx was also observed; however, HBx-induced changes in S phase activating proteins, such as cyclin A and PCNA, were not observed, indicating that HBx expression did not cause entry into S phase (Gearhart & Bouchard, 2010a). Importantly, similar HBx activities were observed in cultured primary human hepatocytes that were infected with a recombinant HBx-expressing adenovirus (Gearhart & Bouchard, 2011) and in cultured primary rat hepatocytes infected with recombinant adenoviruses encoding the full HBV genome that was compared to a mutant HBV that did not produce HBx (Gearhart & Bouchard, 2010a). To determine the significance of the HBx-mediated elevation of cyclin D1 and cyclin E protein levels, the effect of HBx on the activities of CDK4 and CDK2 in cultured primary rat hepatocytes was also examined (Gearhart & Bouchard, 2010a). CDK4 and CDK2 activities were analyzed using standard kinase assays; the substrate for CDK4 phosphorylation was Rb and the substrate for CDK2 phosphorylation was histone H1. To analyze CDK2 activity, primary rat hepatocytes were plated at 50% confluency and stimulated with hepatocyte growth factor (HGF) to induce proliferation (Gearhart & Bouchard, 2010a). HBx, expressed either alone or in the context of HBV replication, increased the activity of CDK4 but decreased the activity of CDK2 (Gearhart & Bouchard, 2010a). The results of these studies confirmed that the HBx-mediated increase in cyclin D1 correlated with increased CDK4 activity; however, the increase in cyclin E expression was not coupled to an increase in CDK2 activity, confirming that HBx prevents cell cycle progression past G1 phase in normal hepatocytes. It is likely that HBx elevation of p21 and p27 inhibits the activity of cyclinE-CDK2 complexes. In contrast, the CIP/KIP proteins are thought to stimulate cell cycle progression in early G1 phase, which may contribute to the ability of HBx to cause hepatocytes to exit G0 and enter G1 [(Cheng et al, 1999); reviewed in (Harper & Brooks, 2005; Sherr & Roberts, 1999)]. Overall, these studies suggest that HBx causes quiescent hepatocytes to exit G0 but stall in G1.

Studies in primary rat hepatocytes were also conducted to examine the effect of cell cycle progression on HBV replication. Downregulation of p16 is required for cells to exit quiescence and enter the cell cycle [reviewed in (Harper & Brooks, 2005)]; primary rat hepatocytes were transfected with a p16 overexpression plasmid, infected with an HBV-encoding recombinant adenovirus, and HBV replication was analyzed to determine if HBV replication requires quiescent hepatocytes to enter the cell cycle (Gearhart & Bouchard, 2010a). Interestingly, preventing hepatocytes from entering the cell cycle by the overexpression of p16, inhibited HBV replication (Gearhart & Bouchard, 2010a). Importantly, this study was the first to directly examine the effect of cell quiescence on HBV replication and indicated that the HBx-mediated exit from quiescence is critical for HBV replication in normal hepatocytes. While this study was consistent with previous reports which indicate that HBV replication is higher in G1 phase (Huang et al, 2004; Ozer et al, 1996), it is important to note that some studies indicate that HBV may replicate better in quiescent cells (Friedrich et al, 2005; Guidotti et al, 1997); however, in contrast to the described studies in cultured primary rat hepatocytes, the studies that suggested that HBV replicates better in quiescent cells did not distinguish between the G0 and G1 phase of the cell cycle. Studies in primary rat hepatocytes were also conducted to determine whether the HBx-mediated cell cycle arrest at the G1/S phase border was also required for HBV replication. When levels of HBV replication were measured in cultured primary rat hepatocytes that were transfected with siRNAs to decrease expression of p21, p27, or both p21 and p27, replication levels were considerably lower when both p21 and p27 levels were decreased, as compared to control samples or samples in which p21 or p27 levels were individually decreased (Gearhart & Bouchard, 2010b). Overall, the results of these studies showed that HBV replication in cultured primary rat hepatocytes is regulated by HBx-mediated G1 entry from G0 and cell cycle arrest at the G1/S phase border; HBV replication is inhibited when hepatocytes are in S phase.

Finally, to determine how HBx-mediated modulation of the cell cycle affects HBV replication, studies in cultured primary rat hepatocytes were conducted to define how cell cycle modulation influences the activity of the HBV reverse transcriptase/polymerase. The activity of the HBV polymerase was assessed in hepatocytes that were infected with recombinant HBV-expressing adenoviruses and transfected with a p16 overexpression plasmid or siRNAs to p21 or p27 or both p21 and p27 (Gearhart & Bouchard, 2010b). The results of these studies demonstrated that entry of quiescent, primary rat hepatocytes into the G1 phase of the cell cycle is required for the activation of the HBV polymerase while progression into S phase did not affect the activity of the HBV polymerase (Gearhart & Bouchard, 2010b). In contrast, progression into S phase may inhibit HBV replication by causing a competition between the cell and the HBV replication machinery for available deoxynucleotide triphosphates (dNTPs). The levels of dNTPs in quiescent cells is low, and HBx modulation of the cell cycle is thought to increase the levels of cellular dNTPs that are available to the HBV polymerase [reviewed in (Yamashita & Emerman, 2006)]. Ribonucleotide reductase is the rate-limiting enzyme of DNA synthesis and is responsible for the synthesis of dNTPs [reviewed in (Elledge et al, 1992; Reichard, 1987)]. This enzyme contains two subunits, R1 and R2; R1 is expressed constitutively; however, the synthesis of R2, the catalytic subunit of ribonucleotide reductase, peaks closer to S phase, when the cells prepare for replication (Chabes & Thelander, 2000). Interestingly, HBx expression increased the levels of R2 in cultured primary rat and human hepatocytes, which would lead to the activation of ribonucleotide reductase and a possible increase in the number of available dNTPs (Gearhart & Bouchard, 2010b; Gearhart & Bouchard, 2011). Additional studies demonstrated that HBx elevation of R2 is required for HBV replication in cultured primary rat hepatocytes. Hydroxyurea, an inhibitor of ribonucleotide reductase (Thelander & Reichard, 1979), blocked HBV replication, as did transfection of a siRNA that targeted R2 (Gearhart & Bouchard, 2010b). Importantly, both hydroxyurea and the siRNA targeting R2 did not affect the activity of the HBV polymerase (Gearhart & Bouchard, 2010b). Cumulatively, the studies in primary hepatocytes demonstrated that HBx stimulates HBV replication by inducing hepatocytes to exit G0 and enter G1 to activate the HBV polymerase and increase the level of the R2 subunit of ribonucleotide reductase. Additionally, these studies confirmed that cultured rodent hepatocytes can serve as a powerful model system for studying HBx activities that are present in normal human hepatocytes, which are not always readily available for similar types of studies. Since deregulation of cell cycle checkpoints have been linked to cancer development [reviewed in (Collins et al, 1997; Ford & Pardee, 1999)], HBx modulation of cell cycle proliferation might also contribute to processes that influence the development of HBV-associated liver transformation by stimulating HBV replication and altering normal cell cycle control mechanisms in hepatocytes (Gearhart & Bouchard, 2010b). Overall, these observations indicate that HBx regulates the expression of cell cycle regulatory factors in normal hepatocytes when it is expressed in the absence of other HBV proteins and in the context of replication.

### 4.4.4 HBx and liver regeneration

Several studies have examined the effect of HBx expression on liver regeneration. In one study, moderate expression levels of HBx resulted in an inhibition of liver regeneration following a partial hepatectomy in HBx-transgenic mice (Tralhao et al, 2002). Overall inhibition of liver regeneration was also observed after a partial hepatectomy in mice that were transplanted with HBx-expressing liver cells (Tralhao et al, 2002). HBx-mediated inhibition of liver regeneration in HBx-transgenic mice occurred at the G1/S phase transition (Wu et al, 2006). HBx also caused an increase in the levels of alanine aminotransferase and alpha-fetoprotein (AFP) that were detected after the partial hepatectomy, indicating that HBx expression made the hepatocytes more susceptible to damage during regeneration (Wu et al, 2006). HBx also caused abnormal apoptosis, fat accumulation, and impaired glycogen storage when HBx was expressed during periods of regeneration (Wu et al, 2006). In contrast, the results of one study suggested that HBx can increase cell cycle progression following a partial hepatectomy in HBx-transgenic mice; in this study the effect of HBx on regeneration was measured by BrdU incorporation, levels of PCNA, and reduced steady-state p21 protein levels (Hodgson et al, 2008). Finally, in another study in HBx-transgenic mice, hepatocytes in these mice had both increased proliferation capacity and increased apoptosis; whether increased hepatocyte proliferation was induced to compensate for the increased apoptosis, or whether increased apoptosis was in response to the increased hepatocyte proliferation was not directly addressed (Koike et al, 1998). Overall, these studies indicate that HBx can modulate liver regeneration; however, due to differences in the mouse strains and methods of analysis that were used to address the influence of HBx expression on liver regeneration, the exact impact of HBx on liver regeneration is not fully understood but could be a major contributor to the development of HBV-associated HCC.

### 4.5 HBx and calcium signaling

#### 4.5.1 Calcium signaling overview

Calcium ($Ca^{2+}$) signaling controls a diverse range of cellular processes including cell proliferation, signal transduction, transcription, and apoptotic pathways [reviewed in (Berridge et al, 2003; Berridge et al, 2000; Bootman et al, 2001; Parekh, 2011)]. Calcium signals typically take the form of oscillating calcium spikes, and differences in the amplitude, frequency and spatial patterns of calcium oscillations will initiate different cellular responses, leading to a paradoxical combination of specificity and versatility in calcium signaling [reviewed in (Berridge et al, 2003; Berridge et al, 2000; Bootman et al, 2001; Parekh, 2011)]. The signaling functions of $Ca^{2+}$ mainly depend on the calcium concentration in the cytosolic compartment. The cytosolic calcium level ($[Ca^{2+}]_c$) in most resting cells is maintained at around 100nM but can reach 1000nM upon stimulation [reviewed in (Berridge et al, 2000)]. The $[Ca^{2+}]_c$ is regulated by the dynamic interplay between calcium "ON" and "OFF" mechanisms that can increase or decrease $[Ca^{2+}]_c$ [reviewed in (Berridge et al, 2003; Berridge et al, 2000; Bootman et al, 2001)].

The calcium "ON" mechanism includes external calcium entry and internal calcium release from the endoplasmic reticulum (ER) [reviewed in (Berridge et al, 2003; Berridge et al, 2000; Bootman et al, 2001)]. A variety of plasma membrane calcium channels responsible for external calcium entry have been identified, including voltage-operated calcium (VOC) channels, receptor-operated calcium (ROC) channels, and store-operated calcium (SOC) channels [reviewed in (Berridge et al, 2003; Berridge et al, 2000; Bootman et al, 2001)]. The ER is the main internal calcium store, and inositol 1,4,5-triphosphate receptors (IP3R) and ryanodine receptors (RyR) are the best-characterized ER calcium-releasing channels [reviewed in (Berridge et al, 2003; Berridge et al, 2000; Bootman et al, 2001)]. In non-excitable cells, such as hepatocytes, cytosolic calcium signals mainly derive from ER calcium release. Extracellular agonists such as hormones or growth factors activate phospholipase C through plasma membrane associated G-protein-coupled receptors or receptor tyrosine kinases, resulting in the breakdown of phosphatidylinositol 4,5-bisphoshate to produce inositol 1,4,5-triphosphate (IP3). IP3 binds to IP3Rs on the ER membrane and stimulates calcium release from the ER [reviewed in (Berridge, 1993; Berridge, 2009)]. IP3-linked ER calcium release is followed by extracellular calcium influx to replenish the ER calcium store, which is referred to as store-operated calcium entry (SOCE) (Putney, 1986). SOCE is essential for maintaining IP3-induced cytosolic calcium oscillations and normal ER functions, and also helps sustain elevated levels of $[Ca^{2+}]_c$ [reviewed in (Burdakov et al, 2005; Putney & Bird, 2008; Smyth et al, 2006)]. The process of SOCE is mediated by SOC channels, and the best characterized SOC channel is the calcium-release-activated calcium (CRAC) channel, which is highly selective for calcium and only activated by ER calcium depletion [reviewed in (Parekh, 2010)]. Recently, the ER transmembrane stromal interaction molecule (Stim) 1 (Stim1) and the plasma membrane proteins Orai family (Orai1, 2, and 3) have been identified as key molecular components of mammalian CRAC channels [reviewed in (Parekh, 2010)].

Once calcium signals are generated by the calcium "ON" mechanisms, they will be decoded and translated into different cellular processes by numerous calcium sensors. Some of these sensors, such as protein kinase C, bind to $Ca^{2+}$ and are directly regulated in a $Ca^{2+}$-dependent manner. Other calcium sensors, such as calmodulin (CaM), act as intermediaries to couple calcium signals with distal targets and specific cellular responses. CaM is a versatile calcium sensor with two C-terminal and two N-terminal EF-hand $Ca^{2+}$-binding motifs; these motifs bind $Ca^{2+}$ and induce conformational changes in CaM that facilitate activation of various downstream effectors, including CaM kinases (CaMKs) and calcineurin [reviewed in (Berridge et al, 2000; Parekh, 2011)]. Calcium signals also communicate with other signaling molecules including cyclic AMP, nitric oxide, phosphatidylinositol-3-OH (PI3) kinase, and MAPK [reviewed in (Berridge et al, 2000)]. Communication between calcium signaling and other signaling pathways greatly enhances the diverse functions of a calcium signal.

After a calcium signal has been executed, excess calcium will be rapidly removed from the cytosol by calcium pumps and exchangers; these pumps and exchangers constitute the cellular calcium "OFF" mechanisms [reviewed in (Berridge et al, 2000)]. The plasma membrane $Ca^{2+}$-ATPase pumps (PMCA) and $Na+/Ca^{2+}$ exchangers can remove $Ca^{2+}$ from the cytosol and transport $Ca^{2+}$ to the extracellular environment. The sarco-endoplasmic reticulum ATPase (SERCA) pumps can pump $Ca^{2+}$ from the cytosol into the ER (Berridge et al, 2003; Berridge et al, 2000; Bootman et al, 2001). Mitochondria also function as an important "OFF" mechanism by rapidly sequestering cytosolic $Ca^{2+}$ during the rising phase of $Ca^{2+}$ signals and then slowly releasing the $Ca^{2+}$ back into the cytosol during the declining phase of $Ca^{2+}$ signals (Berridge et al, 2000). Mitochondrial $Ca^{2+}$ transport can buffer a harmful elevation of cytosolic $Ca^{2+}$ and also increase the duration of $Ca^{2+}$ signals in the cytosol. Mitochondria, therefore, have an important role in shaping both the amplitude and spatio-temporal patterns of $Ca^{2+}$ signals [reviewed in (Berridge et al, 2000; Bootman et al, 2001)]. The major mitochondrial $Ca^{2+}$ uptake mechanism is the mitochondrial $Ca^{2+}$ uniporter (MCU) [reviewed in (Bernardi, 1999)]. Although the MCU has low $Ca^{2+}$ affinity, a local high $Ca^{2+}$ concentration in the ER-mitochondria microdomain can overcome this limitation and facilitate rapid mitochondrial $Ca^{2+}$ uptake from the cytosol through the MCU during IP3-linked $Ca^{2+}$ signaling (Rizzuto et al, 1993; Rizzuto et al, 1998). Mitochondrial $Ca^{2+}$ efflux mechanisms mainly include the mitochondrial Na+/$Ca^{2+}$ exchanger and the MPTP; the MPTP is a mitochondrial protein complex that is thought to be composed of VDAC, the adenine nucleotide translocase (ANT) and cyclophilin D (CypD) [reviewed in (Bernardi, 1999)]. The MPTP has two conductance states: at the low conductance state, the MPTP can function as a mitochondrial $Ca^{2+}$ efflux channel; at an irreversible high conductance state, mitochondria permeability transition will be induced and lead to the release of cytochrome C and the initiation of apoptosis (Ichas et al, 1997; Zoratti & Szabo, 1995).

### 4.5.2 Calcium signaling and the cell cycle

It is well recognized that $Ca^{2+}$ signaling is involved at different stages of the cell cycle, especially during the early G1 phase as well as at the G1/S and G2/M transitions. Both extracellular $Ca^{2+}$ and intracellular $Ca^{2+}$ are required for cell proliferation. In one study, when the extracellular $Ca^{2+}$ concentration was reduced from 1mM to 0.1mM, the rate of cell proliferation was gradually decreased (Hickie et al, 1983). The results of another study demonstrated that when intracellular $Ca^{2+}$ stores were depleted with pharmacological agents, cell division was also blocked (Short et al, 1993). The role of $Ca^{2+}$ signaling in progression through G1 and the G1/S boundary is particularly important. $Ca^{2+}$ spikes have been observed in early G1 and near the G1/S boundary in cells [reviewed in (Kahl & Means, 2003)]. During the G1 phase, $Ca^{2+}$ affects the expression of cyclin D1 by regulating the expression or activity of transcription factors such as fos, jun, and myc [reviewed in (Roderick & Cook, 2008)]; $Ca^{2+}$ signals can also stimulate phosphorylation of Rb at the G1/S boundary (Takuwa et al, 1993).

CaM is a general $Ca^{2+}$ sensor and relays $Ca^{2+}$ signals to $Ca^{2+}$/CaM-dependent targets. The expression level of CaM is regulated during cell cycle progression, and a pronounced increase in CaM levels just before entering S phase has been observed in different cell types [reviewed in (Kahl & Means, 2003)]. Increased CaM levels accelerated the rate at which cells passed through the G1/S boundary, and a decrease in CaM levels prevented progression into S phase, indicating that CaM can control the rate of entering into S phase (Rasmussen & Means, 1989). The addition of CaM inhibitors early in the G1 phase could completely inhibit DNA synthesis, but CaM inhibitors did not affect DNA synthesis if the inhibitors were added later in G1 after Rb hyperphosphorylation, suggesting that the requirement for $Ca^{2+}$/CaM in late G1 phase is before Rb hyperphosphorylation (Takuwa et al, 1992; Takuwa et al, 1993). Although the detailed molecular mechanisms that underlie these $Ca^{2+}$/CaM effects remain unknown, it is evident that $Ca^{2+}$ signaling can affect multiple signaling pathways to regulate G1 progression.

Two $Ca^{2+}$/CaM-dependent targets, calcineurin and CaMKs, have been shown to play an important role in cell-cycle progression and cell proliferation [reviewed in (Kahl & Means, 2003)]. The multifunctional CaMKs are a family of serine/threonine protein kinases that includes CaMKI, CaMKII, and CaMKIV. The auto-inhibition of CaMKs is removed upon the binding of Ca2+/CaM, which stimulates CaMK kinase activity [reviewed in (Kahl & Means, 2003)]. CaMKs are also associated with different aspects of cell cycle progression. In both normal and transformed cells, inhibition of CaMKs prevented G1 progression, suggesting that CaMKs are required for G1 progression [reviewed in (Kahl & Means, 2003)]. *In vitro,* CaMKI and CaMKII phosphorylated and increased the activity of cdc25C, a phosphatase responsible for cdc2 activation at the G2/M transition (Patel et al, 1999). Calcineurin is a

$Ca^{2+}$/CaM-dependent phosphatase, and its enzyme activity is stimulated by binding of $Ca^{2+}$/CaM to its regulatory domain [reviewed in (Kahl & Means, 2003)]. Calcineurin can affect cyclin D1 expression and control G1 progression by regulating cAMP-responsive element binding protein (CREB), which binds to the cyclin D1 promoter (Schneider et al, 2002). NFAT activation by calcineurin can also induce the expression of c-myc and increase the expression of E2F and cyclin E [reviewed in (Roderick & Cook, 2008)]. Finally, inhibition of calcineurin suppresses CDK2 activity because of increased expression of p21 or reduced cyclin E levels (Khanna & Hosenpud, 1999; Tomono et al, 1998).

Because of the pivotal role of calcium signaling in cell proliferation, abnormal $Ca^{2+}$ signaling may contribute to the development of cancer [reviewed in (Parkash & Asotra, 2010; Roderick & Cook, 2008)]. The involvement of $Ca^{2+}$, CaM, calcineurin, and NFAT signaling in carcinogenesis has been implicated in many different human malignant tumors. NFAT-mediated signaling can affect the development of cancer by upregulation of VEGF to stimulate angiogenesis, by upregulation of c-Myc to prompt tumor cell proliferation, and by upregulation of Cox-2 to facilitate tumor cell migration (Buchholz & Ellenrieder, 2007). $Ca^{2+}$ signaling can also regulate oncogenic signaling pathways by contributing to the magnitude and duration of Ras and ERK activation [reviewed in (Roderick & Cook, 2008)]. Furthermore, deregulation of $Ca^{2+}$ signals that are involved in centrosome replication and separation can result in aberrant mitotic spindles and genetic instability, contributing to the development of cancer [reviewed in (Roderick & Cook, 2008)]. Taken together, remodeling of $Ca^{2+}$ signaling in cell proliferation may act as an oncogenic mechanism facilitating the development of cancer.

### 4.5.3 HBx modulation of the cell cycle requires calcium signaling

Various studies suggest that HBx modulates cytosolic $Ca^{2+}$ signaling, which likely acts as an initiator of other reported HBx activities (Bouchard et al, 2006; Bouchard et al, 2001b; Gearhart & Bouchard, 2010a; Gearhart & Bouchard, 2010b). This notion is supported by studies of regulation of cell cycle and cell proliferation in cultured primary rat hepatocytes (Gearhart & Bouchard, 2010a; Gearhart & Bouchard, 2010b). Studies in cultured primary rat hepatocytes have demonstrated that HBx induced quiescent hepatocytes to enter the G1 phase of cell cycle but not to proceed to S phase and that HBV replication was reduced when cultured primary rat hepatocytes entry into G1 phase was blocked or when cultured primary rat hepatocytes entered S phase (Gearhart & Bouchard, 2010a; Gearhart & Bouchard, 2010b). Of significance to the role of HBx modulation of $Ca^{2+}$ signals, these studies in cultured primary rat hepatocytes showed that treatment with BAPTA-AM, an intracellular $Ca^{2+}$ chelator, inhibited HBx modulation of cell cycle regulatory proteins and abolished HBV replication, suggesting that HBx regulation of cell proliferation to stimulate HBV replication requires $Ca^{2+}$ signaling (Gearhart & Bouchard, 2010a; Gearhart & Bouchard, 2010b). This conclusion is consistent with previous studies in HepG2 cells that showed that the modulation of $Ca^{2+}$ signaling by HBx is essential to stimulate HBV replication. In HepG2 cells, the replication of HBx-deficient HBV was significantly reduced and was rescued by co-transfecting with an HBx-expressing plasmid or by simply increasing cytosolic $Ca^{2+}$ levels; BAPTA-AM treatment inhibited HBV replication (Bouchard et al, 2001b). Furthermore, the activation of Pyk2/FAK and Src kinase pathway has been identified as one of the downstream pathways of HBx-regulated $Ca^{2+}$ signals that stimulates HBV replication in HepG2 cells. HBx activation of Pyk2/FAK and Src kinases was $Ca^{2+}$-dependent, and the inhibition of Pyk2/FAK and Src kinases blocked HBx-stimulated HBV replication in HepG2 cells (Bouchard et al, 2003; Bouchard et al, 2006; Bouchard et al, 2001b). Taken together, these studies suggest that HBx modulation of $Ca^{2+}$ signaling can stimulate HBV replication in both HepG2 cells and cultured primary rat hepatocytes. In addition, these studies show that HBx regulation of hepatocyte proliferation is directly linked to HBx stimulation of $Ca^{2+}$ signals.

An unanswered question is precisely how HBx modulates cellular $Ca^{2+}$ signals. The results of many studies suggest that HBx affects $Ca^{2+}$ signaling by regulating the MPTP. Because cyclosporin A (CsA) inhibits both the MPTP and calcineurin and FK506 is only a calcineurin inhibitor that does not affect MPTP, the combined use of these two inhibitors has helped to define whether MPTP is involved in a specific cellular process. Importantly, CsA treatment, but not FK506 exposure, blocked the effect of HBx on cell cycle regulatory proteins such as p15, p16, p21, and p27 and HBx stimulation of HBV replication in cultured primary rat hepatocytes, indicating that HBx modulation of cell cycle factors in cultured primary rat hepatocytes is MPTP-dependent (Gearhart & Bouchard, 2010b). Similar results were observed in HepG2 cells that were treated with CsA; CsA treatment blocked HBx stimulation of HBV replication and activation of Pyk2 and FAK (Bouchard et al, 2006; Bouchard et al, 2001b). Finally, the direct link between HBx modulation of $Ca^{2+}$ signaling

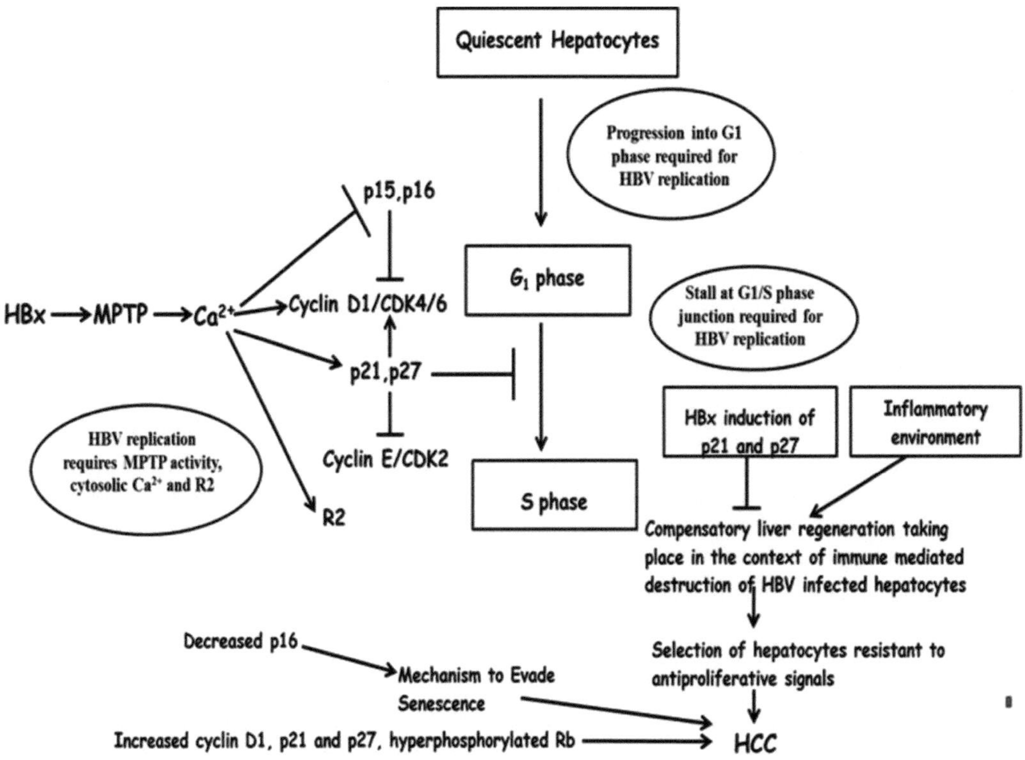


Fig. 4. HBx modulation of cell cycle in primary hepatocytes may lead to the development of HCC. Refer to Figure 2 for the other activities of HBx that could play a potential role in the development of HBV-induced HCC. See text and references for details.

and the MPTP was established in HepG2 cells. In these cells, HBx, both by itself and in the context of HBV replication, increased the basal cytosolic $Ca^{2+}$ level; this increase was blocked by CsA treatment, suggesting that MPTP is involved in the regulation of cytosolic calcium signals (McClain et al, 2007). Cumulatively, these studies suggest that HBx affects cellular $Ca^{2+}$ signaling in a manner that is dependent on the MPTP. Whether CaM acts a mediator of HBx-induced calcium signals remains to be investigated. Remodeling of $Ca^{2+}$ signals and the impact of this on cell proliferation could contribute to carcinogenesis, and HBx modulation of cellular $Ca^{2+}$ signals may contribute to the development of HBV-associated HCC. The precise mechanism used by HBx to regulate cellular $Ca^{2+}$ signals through the MPTP remains unclear, and a better understanding of this HBx activity may provide new targets for treatment of chronic HBV infections and prevention of the development of HBV-associated HCC.

### 4.6 Conclusions and future directions

#### 4.6.1 HBx modulation of calcium signaling and the cell cycle in hepatocarcinogenesis

HBx can influence a number of cellular activities that could alter normal hepatocyte physiology and predispose hepatocytes to transformation; these activities may include HBx regulation of cellular signal transduction, transcription, proliferation, and apoptotic pathways, as well as the direct interaction of HBx with cellular proteins such as UV-DDB and p53. In this chapter, we have focused on HBx modulation of hepatocyte proliferation pathways and cellular calcium signaling as HBx activities that could be major contributing factors to the development of HBV-associated HCC (Figure 4). Deregulation of calcium signaling can alter normal cellular physiology, thus potentially contributing to cancer development [reviewed in (Parkash & Asotra, 2010)]. As the upstream mediator of many HBx effects (Bouchard et al, 2006; Bouchard et al, 2001b; Gearhart & Bouchard, 2010a; Gearhart & Bouchard, 2010b), alterations in calcium signaling could play a major role in HBV-induced HCC. Many alterations of cell cycle regulatory proteins that have been identified in HCC are similar to alterations in cell cycle pathways that have been observed in primary hepatocytes when HBx is expressed in the absence of other proteins and in the context of HBV replication (Biden et al, 1997; Burkhart & Sage, 2008; Csepregi et al, 2010; Deane et al, 2001; Gearhart & Bouchard, 2010a). There are numerous ways in which HBx regulation of hepatocyte proliferation pathways could influence HCC development. For example, down-regulation of p16 by HBx enabled hepatocytes to evade senescence, a potent tumor suppressive mechanism (Kim et al, 2010). Overexpression of cyclin D1 promotes hepatocarcinogenesis (Deane et al, 2001), and HBx-mediated upregulation of cyclin D1 could affect the development of liver cancer. Stimulation of HBV replication by modulating the cell cycle could, in itself, generate a more inflammatory environment due to higher levels of HBV replication; increased inflammation could enhance the oncogenic environment in the liver. Overall, the HBx-mediated induction of cell cycle entry of quiescent primary hepatocytes during the course of a chronic HBV infection could alter the physiology of hepatocytes to favor carcinogenesis, and signal transduction pathways activated by HBx, including pathways involved in cell proliferation and survival, have been implicated in hepatocarcinogenesis [(Chen et al, 2010; Chung et al, 2004; Hsieh et al, 2011); reviewed in (Ierardi et al, 2010; Rodrigues & Barry, 2011; Thompson & Monga, 2007; Torbenson et al, 2004; Whittaker et al, 2010)]. In addition, in the context of an inflammatory environment where HBV-infected hepatocytes are being destroyed by inflammatory responses, any mechanisms that inhibit regeneration, such as HBx induction of p21 or p27, might eventually lead to compensatory mechanisms that select for cells that have become resistant to anti-proliferative signals. Repeated cycles of forced hepatocyte regeneration occurring in the context of the inflammatory environment of an HBV-infected liver could eventually contribute to HCC development.

### 4.6.2 Future directions

While recent studies are beginning to define the activities of HBx in normal hepatocytes, in the livers of small animal models, and in the context of HBV replication, the precise molecular mechanisms that underlie many HBx activities remain unknown and should be the focus of future studies. Although a bewildering array of functions have been linked to HBx expression, these activities may simply reflect the cell-specific consequence of a limited number of initiating events that are controlled by a small number of primary HBx activities. Due to the paucity of available model systems for studying direct HBV infections and the low level of HBx expression during HBV replication, identifying HBx activities during HBV replication in authentic normal human hepatocytes will likely remain a challenge. Studies in other model systems such as cultured primary rodent hepatocytes will provide valuable models for characterizing HBx activities in normal hepatocytes. The major focus of this chapter has been HBx regulation of calcium signaling and cell proliferation pathways and how these HBx activities regulated HBV replication and may influence the development of HCC; consequently, in the following section we will focus on potential future directions that are relevant to these HBx activities.

The role of the Pyk2/FAK-Src-Ras-Raf-MAPK pathway in HBx regulation of hepatocyte proliferation pathways remains unexplored and an important future area of investigation. HBx stimulation of the Pyk2/FAK-Src-Ras-Raf-MAPK pathway could profoundly affect hepatocyte physiology and modulate carcinogenic processes. Results from several studies have suggested that expression levels of p21, p27, and cyclin D1 can be regulated by MAPK signaling [(Bottazzi et al, 1999; Liu et al, 1996); reviewed in (Kerkhoff & Rapp, 1998)]. Importantly, the results of one study in mouse hepatocytes identified a role of prolonged MAPK signaling in HBx-induced elevation of p21 and p27 (Qiao et al, 2001). Whether the Pyk2/FAK-Src-Ras-Raf-MAPK pathway, which has been linked to HBx elevation of calcium, is directly responsible for HBx regulation of hepatocyte proliferation pathways and HBV replication in primary hepatocytes awaits further investigation. Additionally, the mechanism that underlies HBx regulation of cyclin D1 in normal hepatocytes is unknown. The cyclin D1 promoter contains several binding sites for the transcription factor NF-κB (Hinz et al, 1999), and studies have shown that HBx can activate NF-κB in cultured primary rat hepatocytes (Clippinger et al, 2009). One study in Chang liver cells suggested that the HBx-mediated increase in cyclin D1 expression was caused by HBx activation of NF-κB (Park et al, 2006); however, whether HBx upregulates expression of cyclin D1 through activation of NF-κB in a normal hepatocyte has yet to be determined and should be the subject of future studies. Activation of the Wnt pathway, inactivation of GSK3-β, and stabilization of β-catenin have also been linked to activation of the cyclin D1 transcription promoter [reviewed in (Monga, 2011)], and it was recently shown that HBx can activate the Wnt pathway (Cha et al, 2004; Hsieh et al, 2011), increase the phosphorylation and inactivation of GSK3-β (Cha et al, 2004; Yang et al, 2009), and increase β-catenin accumulation in some HCC cell lines (Cha et al, 2004; Hsieh et al, 2011). Whether HBx regulates cyclin D1 expression through activation of the Wnt signaling pathway in normal hepatocytes and in the context of HBV replication is unknown; inactive GSK3-β and increased β-catenin accumulation are associated with HCC development (Ban et al, 2003). An important HBx activity that could also affect cyclin D1 levels and requires further investigation is HBx stimulation of DNMT1 expression and the resulting elevation of methylation of the p16 promoter and decreased p16 expression; this HBx activity was linked to elevation of cyclin D1 and phosphorylation of Rb in HepG2 cells (Jung et al, 2007; Zhu et al, 2007). Although HBx regulation of p16 levels in cultured primary rat and human hepatocytes was linked to calcium signaling (Gearhart & Bouchard, 2010a), the possible role for DNMT1 in decreased expression of p16 was not assessed in these studies and could have important implications for HCC development.

The interaction of p53 and HBx, whether direct or indirect, remains a subject of considerable debate, and a comprehensive analysis of precisely how HBx or p53 each affects activities of the other protein could provide important insights into mechanisms that link HBV infections and HBx expression to HCC development. Although p53 stimulation of p21 expression has been extensively characterized (el-Deiry et al, 1993), whether p53 affects HBx regulation of p21 and hepatocyte proliferation pathways in normal hepatocytes and in the context of HBV replication remains to be determined. Interestingly, HBx was shown to induce p21 expression in a both a p53-dependent and independent manner (Ahn et al, 2002; Park et al, 2000). An important focus of future studies should be a comprehensive analysis of the interplay between HBx and p53 activities in normal hepatocytes and how this influences HBV replication and the development of HCC-associated HCC.

Although the future studies described above would address the impact of HBx expression on hepatocyte physiology, an equally important focus for future studies is to determine precisely how HBx modulation of the cell cycle directly affects HBV replication. Studies in primary rat hepatocytes have clearly shown that hepatocyte exit from G0 and subsequent arrest in G1 is required for HBV replication and for activation of the HBV polymerase (Gearhart & Bouchard, 2010a; Gearhart & Bouchard, 2010b); however, exactly how this HBx activity stimulates the polymerase remains unknown. Moreover, effects of cell cycle modulation on other HBV proteins that are required for HBV replication have not been investigated. The HBV core protein is phosphorylated on three serine residues; differential phosphorylation of these serines is required for various stages of HBV replication (Melegari et al, 2005). Whether HBx regulation of the cell cycle affects core phosphorylation in normal hepatocytes and whether this modulates HBV replication remains to be explored. The results of several studies have identified putative candidate kinases that are responsible for these phosphorylation events (Daub et al, 2002; Duclos-Vallee et al, 1998; Kann & Gerlich, 1994; Yeh et al, 1993); however, the events and kinase(s) that result in the phosphorylation of HBV core in hepatocytes are generally not well understood. It is possible that the kinase responsible for phosphorylation of the HBV core protein is activated by the HBx regulation of hepatocyte proliferation pathways, and specifically identifying this kinase(s) in HBV-infected hepatocytes will be an important focus of future studies. Finally, the upregulation of the R2 subunit of ribonucleotide reductase by HBx, and the dependence of HBV replication on upregulation of R2 expression suggest that HBx may cause cell cycle entry in order to increase the availability of dNTPs. Recently, it was shown that HBV can increase the cellular concentration of dNTPs in HepG2.2.15 cells, as compared to HepG2 cells (Cohen et al, 2010). Although these findings are intriguing, this increased pool of dNTPs was not directly linked to HBx and not confirmed in HBV-infected normal hepatocytes. Consequently, an important subject of future studies should be to determine whether an increase in dNTP concentration is the ultimate goal of the HBx-mediated cell cycle modulation and whether dNTPs are a limiting factor during HBV replication in hepatocytes. Ribonucleotide reductase could be a new drug target to inhibit HBV replication in HBV-infected individuals; recent studies have shown that inhibition of the R2 subunit of ribonucleotide reductase can reduce the growth potential of cancer cells (Heidel et al, 2007). Overall, the results of future studies that address HBx activities in authentic hepatocytes and in the context of HBV replication should focus on identifying primary HBx activities, thereby generating potential new therapeutic targets to inhibit HBV replication and the development of HBV-associated HCC.

## 5. References

Ahn JY, Chung EY, Kwun HJ, Jang KL (2001) Transcriptional repression of p21(waf1) promoter by hepatitis B virus X protein via a p53-independent pathway. *Gene* 275: 163-168

Ahn JY, Jung EY, Kwun HJ, Lee CW, Sung YC, Jang KL (2002) Dual effects of hepatitis B virus X protein on the regulation of cell-cycle control depending on the status of cellular p53. *J Gen Virol* 83: 2765-2772

Amon A (1999) The spindle checkpoint. *Curr Opin Genet Dev* 9: 69-75

Arbuthnot P, Capovilla A, Kew M (2000) Putative role of hepatitis B virus X protein in hepatocarcinogenesis: effects on apoptosis, DNA repair, mitogen-activated protein kinase and JAK/STAT pathways. *J Gastroenterol Hepatol* 15: 357-368

Arellano M, Moreno S (1997) Regulation of CDK/cyclin complexes during the cell cycle. *Int J Biochem Cell Biol* 29: 559-573

Arzberger S, Hösel M, Protzer U (2010) Apoptosis of hepatitis B virus-infected hepatocytes prevents release of infectious virus. *J Virol* 84: 11994-12001

Assoian RK, Zhu X (1997) Cell anchorage and the cytoskeleton as partners in growth factor dependent cell cycle progression. *Curr Opin Cell Biol* 9: 93-98

Aufiero B, Schneider RJ (1990) The hepatitis B virus X-gene product trans-activates both RNA polymerase II and III promoters. *Embo J* 9: 497-504

Ban KC, Singh H, Krishnan R, Seow HF (2003) GSK-3beta phosphorylation and alteration of beta-catenin in hepatocellular carcinoma. *Cancer Lett* 199: 201-208

Barnabas S, Hai T, Andrisani O (1997) The hepatitis B virus X protein enhances the DNA binding potential and transcription efficacy of bZip transcription factors. *J Biol Chem* 272: 20684-20690

Beasley R, Lin C-C, Hwang L-Y, Chien C-S (1981) Hepatocellular carcinoma and hepatitis B virus: a prospective study of 22 707 men in Taiwan. *Lancet*: 1129-1133

Becker S, Lee T-H, Butel J, Slagle B (1998) Hepatitis B virus X protein interferes with cellular DNA repair. *J Virol* 72: 266-272

Benhenda S, Cougot D, Buendia MA, Neuveut C (2009) Hepatitis B virus X protein molecular functions and its role in virus life cycle and pathogenesis. *Adv Cancer Res* 103: 75-109

Benn J, Schneider R (1994) Hepatitis B virus HBx protein activates Ras-GTP complex formation and establishes a Ras, Raf, MAP kinase signaling cascade. *Proc Natl Acad Sci USA* 91: 10350-10354

Benn J, Schneider R (1995) Hepatitis B virus HBx protein deregulates cell cycle checkpoint controls. *Proc Natl Acad Sci USA* 92: 11215-11219

Benn J, Su F, Doria M, Schneider R (1996) Hepatitis B virus HBx protein induces transcription factor AP-1 by activation of extracellular signal-regulated and c-Jun N-terminal mitogen-activated protein kinases. *J Virol* 70: 4978-4985

Bergametti F, Prigent S, Luber B, Benoit A, Tiollais P, Sarasin A, Transy C (1999) The proapoptotic effect of hepatitis B virus HBx protein correlates with transactivation activity in stably transfected cell lines. *Oncogene* 18: 2860-2871

Bergametti F, Sitterlin D, Transy C (2002) Turnover of hepatitis B virus X protein is regulated by damaged DNA-binding complex. *J Virol* 76: 6495-6501

Bernardi P (1999) Mitochondrial transport and cations: channels, exchangers, and permeability transition. *Physiol Rev* 79: 1127-1155

Berridge M (1993) Inositol trisphosphate and calcium signalling. *Nature* 361: 315-325

Berridge MJ. (2009) Inositol trisphosphate and calcium signalling mechanisms., Biochim Biophys Acta, Vol. 1793, pp. 933-940.

Berridge MJ, Bootman MD, Roderick HL (2003) Calcium signalling: dynamics, homeostasis and remodelling. *Nat Rev Mol Cell Biol* 4: 517-529

Berridge MJ, Lipp P, Bootman MD (2000) The versatility and universality of calcium signalling. *Nat Rev Mol Cell Biol* 1: 11-21

Biden K, Young J, Buttenshaw R, Searle J, Cooksley G, Xu DB, Leggett B (1997) Frequency of mutation and deletion of the tumor suppressor gene CDKN2A (MTS1/p16) in hepatocellular carcinoma from an Australian population. *Hepatology* 25: 593-597

Block TM, Mehta AS, Fimmel CJ, Jordan R (2003) Molecular viral oncology of hepatocellular carcinoma. *Oncogene* 22: 5093-5107

Boguski M, McCormick F (1993) Proteins regulating Ras and its relatives. *Nature* 366

Bootman MD, Collins TJ, Peppiatt CM, Prothero LS, MacKenzie L, De Smet P, Travers M, Tovey SC, Seo JT, Berridge MJ, Ciccolini F, Lipp P (2001) Calcium signalling--an overview. *Semin Cell Dev Biol* 12: 3-10

Bottazzi ME, Zhu X, Böhmer RM, Assoian RK (1999) Regulation of p21(cip1) expression by growth factors and the extracellular matrix reveals a role for transient ERK activity in G1 phase. *J Cell Biol* 146: 1255-1264

Bouchard M, Giannakopoulos S, Wang EH, Tanese N, Schneider RJ (2001a) Hepatitis B virus HBx protein activation of cyclin A-cyclin-dependent kinase 2 complexes and G1 transit via a Src kinase pathway. *J Virol* 75: 4247-4257

Bouchard MJ, Navas-Martin S (2011) Hepatitis B and C virus hepatocarcinogenesis: lessons learned and future challenges. *Cancer Lett* 305: 123-143

Bouchard MJ, Puro RJ, Wang L, Schneider RJ (2003) Activation and inhibition of cellular calcium and tyrosine kinase signaling pathways identify targets of the HBx protein involved in hepatitis B virus replication. *J Virol* 77: 7713-7719

Bouchard MJ, Schneider RJ (2004) The enigmatic X gene of hepatitis B virus. *J Virol* 78: 12725-12734

Bouchard MJ, Wang L, Schneider RJ (2006) Activation of focal adhesion kinase by hepatitis B virus HBx protein: multiple functions in viral replication. *J Virol* 80: 4406-4414

Bouchard MJ, Wang LH, Schneider RJ (2001b) Calcium signaling by HBx protein in hepatitis B virus DNA replication. *Science* 294: 2376-2378

Brehm A, Miska EA, McCance DJ, Reid JL, Bannister AJ, Kouzarides T (1998) Retinoblastoma protein recruits histone deacetylase to repress transcription. *Nature* 391: 597-601

Brenner DA (1998) Signal transduction during liver regeneration. *J Gastroenterol Hepatol* 13 Suppl: S93-95

Buchholz M, Ellenrieder V (2007) An emerging role for Ca2+/calcineurin/NFAT signaling in cancerogenesis. *Cell Cycle* 6: 16-19

Buchkovich K, Duffy LA, Harlow E (1989) The retinoblastoma protein is phosphorylated during specific phases of the cell cycle. *Cell* 58: 1097-1105

Burdakov D, Petersen OH, Verkhratsky A (2005) Intraluminal calcium as a primary regulator of endoplasmic reticulum function. *Cell Calcium* 38: 303-310

Burkhart DL, Sage J (2008) Cellular mechanisms of tumour suppression by the retinoblastoma gene. *Nat Rev Cancer* 8: 671-682

Butel J, Lee T-H, Slagle B (1996) Is the DNA repair system involved in hepatitis-B-virus-mediated hepatocellular carcinogenesis. *Trends in Micro* 4

Carnero A, Hannon GJ (1998) The INK4 family of CDK inhibitors. *Curr Top Microbiol Immunol* 227: 43-55

Carretero M, Gómez-Gonzalo M, Lara-Pezzi E, Benedicto I, Aramburu J, Martínez-Martínez S, Redondo JM, López-Cabrera M (2002) The hepatitis B virus X protein binds to and activates the NH(2)-terminal trans-activation domain of nuclear factor of activated T cells-1. *Virology* 299: 288-300

Cha MY, Kim CM, Park YM, Ryu WS (2004) Hepatitis B virus X protein is essential for the activation of Wnt/beta-catenin signaling in hepatoma cells. *Hepatology* 39: 1683-1693

Chabes A, Thelander L (2000) Controlled protein degradation regulates ribonucleotide reductase activity in proliferating mammalian cells during the normal cell cycle and in response to DNA damage and replication blocks. *J Biol Chem* 275: 17747-17753

Chami M, Ferrari D, Nicotera P, Paterlini-Brechot P, Rizzuto R (2003) Caspase-dependent alterations of Ca2+ signaling in the induction of apoptosis by hepatitis B virus X protein. *J Biol Chem* 278: 31745-31755

Chaubert P, Gayer R, Zimmermann A, Fontolliet C, Stamm B, Bosman F, Shaw P (1997) Germ-line mutations of the p16INK4(MTS1) gene occur in a subset of patients with hepatocellular carcinoma. *Hepatology* 25: 1376-1381

Chemin I, Zoulim F (2009) Hepatitis B virus induced hepatocellular carcinoma. *Cancer Lett* 286: 52-59

Chen H, Kaneko S, Girones R, Anderson R, Hornbuckle W, Tennant B, Cote P, Gerin J, Purcell R, Miller R (1993) The woodchuck helpatitis virus X gene is important for establishment of virus infection in woodchucks. *J Virol* 67: 1218-1226

Chen HY, Tang NH, Lin N, Chen ZX, Wang XZ (2008) Hepatitis B virus X protein induces apoptosis and cell cycle deregulation through interfering with DNA repair and checkpoint responses. *Hepatol Res* 38: 174-182

Chen L, Hu L, Li L, Liu Y, Tu QQ, Chang YX, Yan HX, Wu MC, Wang HY (2010) Dysregulation of beta-catenin by hepatitis B virus X protein in HBV-infected human hepatocellular carcinomas. *Front Med China* 4: 399-411

Cheng M, Olivier P, Diehl JA, Fero M, Roussel MF, Roberts JM, Sherr CJ (1999) The p21(Cip1) and p27(Kip1) CDK 'inhibitors' are essential activators of cyclin D-dependent kinases in murine fibroblasts. *Embo J* 18: 1571-1583

Cheong J, Yi M, Lin Y, Murakami S (1995) Human RPB5, a subunit shared by eukaryotic nuclear RNA polymerases, binds human hepatitis B virus X protein and may play a role in X transactivation. *EMBO* 14: 143-150

Chin R, Earnest-Silveira L, Koeberlein B, Franz S, Zentgraf H, Dong X, Gowans E, Bock CT, Torresi J (2007) Modulation of MAPK pathways and cell cycle by replicating hepatitis B virus: factors contributing to hepatocarcinogenesis. *J Hepatol* 47: 325-337

Chirillo P, Falco M, Puri PL, Artini M, Balsano C, Levrero M, Natoli G (1996) Hepatitis B virus pX activates NF-kappa B-dependent transcription through a Raf-independent pathway. *J Virol* 70: 641-646

Chirillo P, Pagano S, Natoli G, Puri P, Burgio V, Balsano C, Levrero M (1997) The hepatitis B virus X gene induces p53-mediated programmed cell death. *Proc Natl Acad Sci USA* 94: 8162-8167

Chung TW, Lee YC, Kim CH (2004) Hepatitis B viral HBx induces matrix metalloproteinase-9 gene expression through activation of ERK and PI-3K/AKT pathways: involvement of invasive potential. *Faseb J* 18: 1123-1125

Clippinger AJ, Bouchard MJ (2008) Hepatitis B virus HBx protein localizes to mitochondria in primary rat hepatocytes and modulates mitochondrial membrane potential. *J Virol* 82: 6798-6811

Clippinger AJ, Gearhart TL, Bouchard MJ (2009) Hepatitis B virus X protein modulates apoptosis in primary rat hepatocytes by regulating both NF-kappaB and the mitochondrial permeability transition pore. *J Virol* 83: 4718-4731

Cohen D, Adamovich Y, Reuven N, Shaul Y (2010) Hepatitis B virus activates deoxynucleotide synthesis in nondividing hepatocytes by targeting the R2 gene. *Hepatology* 51: 1538-1546

Collins K, Jacks T, Pavletich NP (1997) The cell cycle and cancer. *Proc Natl Acad Sci U S A* 94: 2776-2778

Cong Y-S, Yao Y-L, Yang W-M, Kuzhandaivelu N, Seto E (1997) The hepatitis B virus X-associated protein, XAP3, is a protein kinase C-binding protein. *J Biol Chem* 272: 16482-16489

Cook SJ, Balmanno K, Garner A, Millar T, Taverner C, Todd D (2000) Regulation of cell cycle re-entry by growth, survival and stress signalling pathways. *Biochem Soc Trans* 28: 233-240

Cougot D, Wu Y, Cairo S, Caramel J, Renard CA, Lévy L, Buendia MA, Neuveut C (2007) The hepatitis B virus X protein functionally interacts with CREB-binding protein/p300 in the regulation of CREB-mediated transcription. *J Biol Chem* 282: 4277-4287

Cross J, Wen P, Rutter W (1993) Transactivation by hepatitis B virus X protein is promiscuous and dependent on mitogen-activated cellular serine/threonine kinases. *Proc Natl Acad Sci USA* 90: 8078-8082

Csepregi A, Ebert MP, Röcken C, Schneider-Stock R, Hoffmann J, Schulz HU, Roessner A, Malfertheiner P (2010) Promoter methylation of CDKN2A and lack of p16 expression characterize patients with hepatocellular carcinoma. *BMC Cancer* 10: 317

Datta A, Bagchi S, Nag A, Shiyanov P, Adami GR, Yoon T, Raychaudhuri P (2001) The p48 subunit of the damaged-DNA binding protein DDB associates with the CBP/p300 family of histone acetyltransferase. *Mutat Res* 486: 89-97

Daub H, Blencke S, Habenberger P, Kurtenbach A, Dennenmoser J, Wissing J, Ullrich A, Cotten M (2002) Identification of SRPK1 and SRPK2 as the major cellular protein kinases phosphorylating hepatitis B virus core protein. *J Virol* 76: 8124-8137

Deane N, Parker M, Aramandla R, Diehl L, Lee W-J, Washington M, Nanney L, Shyr Y, Beauchamp R (2001) Hepatocellular carcinoma results in chronic cyclin D1 overexpression in transgenic mice. *cancer Res* 61: 5389-5395

Diao J, Khine AA, Sarangi F, Hsu E, Iorio C, Tibbles LA, Woodgett JR, Penninger J, Richardson CD (2001) X protein of hepatitis B virus inhibits Fas-mediated apoptosis and is associated with up-regulation of the SAPK/JNK pathway. *J Biol Chem* 276: 8328-8340

Doria M, Klein N, Lucito R, Schneider R (1995) The hepatitis B virus HBx protein is a dual specificity cytoplasmic activator of Ras and nuclear activator of transcription factors. *EMBO*: 4747-4757

Duclos-Vallee JC, Capel F, Mabit H, Petit MA (1998) Phosphorylation of the hepatitis B virus core protein by glyceraldehyde-3-phosphate dehydrogenase protein kinase activity. *J Gen Virol* 79 ( Pt 7): 1665-1670

el-Deiry WS, Tokino T, Velculescu VE, Levy DB, Parsons R, Trent JM, Lin D, Mercer WE, Kinzler KW, Vogelstein B (1993) WAF1, a potential mediator of p53 tumor suppression. *Cell* 75: 817-825

El-Serag HB, Rudolph KL (2007) Hepatocellular carcinoma: epidemiology and molecular carcinogenesis. *Gastroenterology* 132: 2557-2576

Elledge SJ, Zhou Z, Allen JB (1992) Ribonucleotide reductase: regulation, regulation, regulation. *Trends Biochem Sci* 17: 119-123

Elmore J, Hancock A, Chang S-F, Wang X, Chang S, Callahan C, Geller D, Will H, Harris C (1997) Hepatitis B virus X protein and p53 tumor suppressor interactions in the modulation of apoptosis. *Proc Natl Acad Sci USA* 94: 14707-14712

Evans T, Rosenthal ET, Youngblom J, Distel D, Hunt T (1983) Cyclin: a protein specified by maternal mRNA in sea urchin eggs that is destroyed at each cleavage division. *Cell* 33: 389-396

Faktor O, Shaul Y (1990) The identification of hepatitis B virus X gene responsive elements reveals funtional similarity of X and HTLV-I tax. *Oncogene* 5: 867-872

Fang G, Yu H, Kirschner MW (1998) The checkpoint protein MAD2 and the mitotic regulator CDC20 form a ternary complex with the anaphase-promoting complex to control anaphase initiation. *Genes Dev* 12: 1871-1883

Feitelson M, Zhu M, Duan L-X, London W (1993) Hepatitis B x antigen and p53 are associated *in vitro* and in liver tissues from patients with primary hepatocellular carcinoma. *Oncogene* 8: 1109-1117

Fischer M, Runkel L, Schaller H (1995) HBx protein of hepatitis B virus interacts with the C-terminal portion of a novel human proteasome alpha-subunit. *Virus Genes* 10: 99-102

Fisher RP, Morgan DO (1994) A novel cyclin associates with MO15/CDK7 to form the CDK-activating kinase. *Cell* 78: 713-724

FitzGerald MJ, Webber EM, Donovan JR, Fausto N (1995) Rapid DNA binding by nuclear factor kappa B in hepatocytes at the start of liver regeneration. *Cell Growth Differ* 6: 417-427

Ford HL, Pardee AB (1999) Cancer and the cell cycle. *J Cell Biochem* Suppl 32-33: 166-172

Friedrich B, Wollersheim M, Brandenburg B, Foerste R, Will H, Hildt E (2005) Induction of anti-proliferative mechanisms in hepatitis B virus producing cells. *J Hepatol* 43: 696-703

Gearhart TL, Bouchard MJ (2010a) The hepatitis B virus X protein modulates hepatocyte proliferation pathways to stimulate viral replication. *J Virol* 84: 2675-2686

Gearhart TL, Bouchard MJ (2010b) Replication of the hepatitis B virus requires a calcium-dependent HBx-induced G1 phase arrest of hepatocytes. *Virology* 407: 14-25

Gearhart TL, Bouchard MJ (2011) The hepatitis B virus HBx protein modulates cell cycle regulatory proteins in cultured primary human hepatocytes. *Virus Res* 155: 363-367

Girard F, Strausfeld U, Fernandez A, Lamb NJ (1991) Cyclin A is required for the onset of DNA replication in mammalian fibroblasts. *Cell* 67: 1169-1179

Glotzer M, Murray AW, Kirschner MW (1991) Cyclin is degraded by the ubiquitin pathway. *Nature* 349: 132-138

Gottlob K, Fulco M, Levrero M, Graessmann A (1998) The hepatitis B virus HBx protein inhibits caspase 3 activity. *J Biol Chem* 273: 33347-33353

Gramantieri L, Trerè D, Chieco P, Lacchini M, Giovannini C, Piscaglia F, Cavallari A, Bolondi L (2003) In human hepatocellular carcinoma in cirrhosis proliferating cell nuclear antigen (PCNA) is involved in cell proliferation and cooperates with P21 in DNA repair. *J Hepatol* 39: 997-1003

Groisman IJ, Koshy R, Henkler F, Groopman JD, Alaoui-Jamali MA (1999) Downregulation of DNA excision repair by the hepatitis B virus-x protein occurs in p53-proficient and p53-deficient cells. *Carcinogenesis* 20: 479-483

Guidotti L, Matze B, Chisari F (1997) Hepatitis B virus replication is cell cycle independent during liver regeneration in transgenic mice. *J Virol* 71: 4804-4808

Guidotti L, Matzke B, Schaller H, Chisari F (1995) High-level hepatitis B virus replication in transgenic mice. *J Virol* 69: 6158-6169

Guidotti LG, Chisari FV (2006) Immunobiology and pathogenesis of viral hepatitis. *Annu Rev Pathol* 1: 23-61

Han HJ, Jung EY, Lee WJ, Jang KL (2002) Cooperative repression of cyclin-dependent kinase inhibitor p21 gene expression by hepatitis B virus X protein and hepatitis C virus core protein. *FEBS Lett* 518: 169-172

Hanahan D, Weinberg R (2000) The hallmarks of cancer. *Cell* 100: 57-70

Harper JV, Brooks G (2005) The mammalian cell cycle: an overview. *Methods Mol Biol* 296: 113-153

Haviv I, Matza Y, Shaul Y (1998a) pX, the HBV-encoded coactivator, suppresses the phenotypes of TBP and $TAF_{II}250$ mutants. *Genes and Development*

Haviv I, Shamay M, Doitsh G, Shaul Y (1998b) Hepatitis B virus pX targets TFIIB in transcription coactivation. *Mol Cell Biol* 18: 1562-1569

Hayashida T, Sekiguchi T, Noguchi E, Sunamoto H, Ohba T, Nishimoto T (1994) The CCG1/TAFII250 gene is mutated in thermosensitive G1 mutants of the BHK21 cell line derived from golden hamster. *Gene* 141: 267-270

Hayes S, Shiyanov P, Chen X, Raychaudhuri P (1998) DDB, a putative DNA repair protein, can function as a trans riptional partner of E2F1. *Mol Cell Biol* 18: 240-249

Heidel JD, Liu JY, Yen Y, Zhou B, Heale BS, Rossi JJ, Bartlett DW, Davis ME (2007) Potent siRNA inhibitors of ribonucleotide reductase subunit RRM2 reduce cell proliferation in vitro and in vivo. *Clin Cancer Res* 13: 2207-2215

Hengst L, Göpfert U, Lashuel HA, Reed SI (1998) Complete inhibition of Cdk/cyclin by one molecule of p21(Cip1). *Genes Dev* 12: 3882-3888

Hengst L, Reed SI (1998) Inhibitors of the Cip/Kip family. *Curr Top Microbiol Immunol* 227: 25-41

Henkler F, Hoare J, Waseem N, Goldin R, McGarvey M, Koshy R, King I (2001) Intracellular localization of the hepatitis B virus HBx protein. *J Gen Virol* 82: 871-882

Hickie RA, Wei JW, Blyth LM, Wong DY, Klaassen DJ (1983) Cations and calmodulin in normal and neoplastic cell growth regulation. *Can J Biochem Cell Biol* 61: 934-941

Hinds PW, Mittnacht S, Dulic V, Arnold A, Reed SI, Weinberg RA (1992) Regulation of retinoblastoma protein functions by ectopic expression of human cyclins. *Cell* 70: 993-1006

Hinz M, Krappmann D, Eichten A, Heder A, Scheidereit C, Strauss M (1999) NF-kappaB function in growth control: regulation of cyclin D1 expression and G0/G1-to-S-phase transition. *Mol Cell Biol* 19: 2690-2698

Hodgson AJ, Keasler VV, Slagle BL (2008) Premature cell cycle entry induced by hepatitis B virus regulatory HBx protein during compensatory liver regeneration. *Cancer Res* 68: 10341-10348

Hollstein M, Sidransky D, Vogelstein B, Harris CC (1991) p53 mutations in human cancers. *Science* 253: 49-53

Hsieh A, Kim HS, Lim SO, Yu DY, Jung G (2011) Hepatitis B viral X protein interacts with tumor suppressor adenomatous polyposis coli to activate Wnt/beta-catenin signaling. *Cancer Lett* 300: 162-172

Huang J, Kwong J, Sun E, Liang T (1996) Proteosome complex as a potential cellular target of hepatitis B virus X protein. *J Virol* 70: 5582-5591

Huang J, Wang Y, Guo Y, Sun S (2010) Down-regulated microRNA-152 induces aberrant DNA methylation in hepatitis B virus-related hepatocellular carcinoma by targeting DNA methyltransferase 1. *Hepatology* 52: 60-70

Huang YQ, Wang LW, Yan SN, Gong ZJ (2004) Effects of cell cycle on telomerase activity and on hepatitis B virus replication in HepG2 2.2.15 cells. *Hepatobiliary Pancreat Dis Int* 3: 543-547

Huh KW, Siddiqui A (2002) Characterization of the mitochondrial association of hepatitis B virus X protein, HBx. *Mitochondrion* 1: 349-359

Hui AM, Sakamoto M, Kanai Y, Ino Y, Gotoh M, Yokota J, Hirohashi S (1996) Inactivation of p16INK4 in hepatocellular carcinoma. *Hepatology* 24: 575-579

Ichas F, Jouaville LS, Mazat JP (1997) Mitochondria are excitable organelles capable of generating and conveying electrical and calcium signals. *Cell* 89: 1145-1153

Ierardi E, Rosania R, Zotti M, Giorgio F, Prencipe S, Valle ND, Francesco VD, Panella C (2010) From chronic liver disorders to hepatocellular carcinoma: Molecular and genetic pathways. *World J Gastrointest Oncol* 2: 259-264

Jeffrey PD, Russo AA, Polyak K, Gibbs E, Hurwitz J, Massagué J, Pavletich NP (1995) Mechanism of CDK activation revealed by the structure of a cyclinA-CDK2 complex. *Nature* 376: 313-320

Johnson S, Mandavia N, Wang H-D, Johnson D (2000) Transcriptional regulation of the TATA-binding protein by Ras cellular signaling. *Mol Cell Biol* 20: 5000-5009

Jung JK, Arora P, Pagano JS, Jang KL (2007) Expression of DNA methyltransferase 1 is activated by hepatitis B virus X protein via a regulatory circuit involving the p16INK4a-cyclin D1-CDK 4/6-pRb-E2F1 pathway. *Cancer Res* 67: 5771-5778

Kahl CR, Means AR (2003) Regulation of cell cycle progression by calcium/calmodulin-dependent pathways. *Endocr Rev* 24: 719-736

Kang-Park S, Im JH, Lee JH, Lee YI (2006) PTEN modulates hepatitis B virus-X protein induced survival signaling in Chang liver cells. *Virus Res* 122: 53-60

Kann M, Gerlich W (1994) Effect of core protein phosphorylation by protein kinase C on encapsidation of RNA within core particles of hepatitis B virus. *J Virol*: 7993-8000

Kato J, Matsushime H, Hiebert SW, Ewen ME, Sherr CJ (1993) Direct binding of cyclin D to the retinoblastoma gene product (pRb) and pRb phosphorylation by the cyclin D-dependent kinase CDK4. *Genes Dev* 7: 331-342

Keasler VV, Hodgson AJ, Madden CR, Slagle BL (2007) Enhancement of hepatitis B virus replication by the regulatory X protein in vitro and in vivo. *J Virol* 81: 2656-2662

Kekule A, Lauer U, Weiss L, Luber B, Hofschneider P (1993) Hepatitis B virus transactivator HBx uses a tumour promoter signalling pathway. *Nature* 361: 742-745

Kerkhoff E, Rapp UR (1998) Cell cycle targets of Ras/Raf signalling. *Oncogene* 17: 1457-1462

Khanna AK, Hosenpud JD (1999) Cyclosporine induces the expression of the cyclin inhibitor p21. *Transplantation* 67: 1262-1268

Kim C, Koike K, Saito I, Miyamura T, Jay G (1991) HBx gene of hepatitis B virus induces liver cancer in transgenic mice. *Nature* 353: 317-320

Kim H, Lee H, Yun Y (1998) X-gene product of hepatitis B virus induces apoptosis in liver cells. *J Biol Chem* 273: 381-385

Kim HJ, Kim SY, Kim J, Lee H, Choi M, Kim JK, Ahn JK (2008) Hepatitis B virus X protein induces apoptosis by enhancing translocation of Bax to mitochondria. *IUBMB Life* 60: 473-480

Kim KH, Seong BL (2003) Pro-apoptotic function of HBV X protein is mediated by interaction with c-FLIP and enhancement of death-inducing signal. *Embo J* 22: 2104-2116

Kim S, Kim HY, Lee S, Kim SW, Sohn S, Kim K, Cho H (2007) Hepatitis B virus x protein induces perinuclear mitochondrial clustering in microtubule- and Dynein-dependent manners. *J Virol* 81: 1714-1726

Kim YJ, Jung JK, Lee SY, Jang KL (2010) Hepatitis B virus X protein overcomes stress-induced premature senescence by repressing p16(INK4a) expression via DNA methylation. *Cancer Lett* 288: 226-235

King R, Jackson P, Kirschner M (1994) Mitosis in transition. *Cell* 79

Klein A, Guhl E, Tzeng YJ, Fuhrhop J, Levrero M, Graessmann M, Graessmann A (2003) HBX causes cyclin D1 overexpression and development of breast cancer in transgenic animals that are heterozygous for p53. *Oncogene* 22: 2910-2919

Klein N, Bouchard M, Wang L-H, Kobarg C, Schneider R (1999) Src kinases involved in hepatitis B virus replication. *Embo J* 18: 5019-5027

Klein N, Schneider R (1997) Activation of Src family kinases by hepatitis B virus HBx protein and coupled signaling to Ras. *Mol Cell Biol* 17: 6427-6436

Koike K (2009) Hepatitis B virus X gene is implicated in liver carcinogenesis. *Cancer Lett* 286: 60-68

Koike K, Moriya K, Yotsuyanagi H, Iino S, Kurokawa K (1994) Induction of cell cycle progression by hepatitis B virus HBx gene expression in quiescent mouse fibroblasts. *J Clin Invest* 94: 44-49

Koike K, Moriya K, Yotsuyanagi H, Shintani Y, Fujie H, Tsutsumi T, Kimura S (1998) Compensatory apoptosis in preneoplastic liver of a transgenic mouse model for viral hepatocarcinogenesis. *Cancer Lett* 134: 181-186

Lara-Pezzi E, Armessila A, Majano P, Redondo J, Lopez-Cabrera M (1999) The hepatitis B virus X protein activates nuclear factor of activated T cells (NF-AT) by a cyclosporin A-sensitive pathway. *EMBO* 17: 7066-7077

Leach JK, Qiao L, Fang Y, Han SL, Gilfor D, Fisher PB, Grant S, Hylemon PB, Peterson D, Dent P (2003) Regulation of p21 and p27 expression by the hepatitis B virus X protein and the alternate initiation site X proteins, AUG2 and AUG3. *J Gastroenterol Hepatol* 18: 376-385

Lee S, Tarn C, Wang WH, Chen S, Hullinger RL, Andrisani OM (2002) Hepatitis B virus X protein differentially regulates cell cycle progression in X-transforming versus nontransforming hepatocyte (AML12) cell lines. *J Biol Chem* 277: 8730-8740

Lee SG, Rho HM (2000) Transcriptional repression of the human p53 gene by hepatitis B viral X protein. *Oncogene* 19: 468-471

Lee TH, Elledge SJ, Butel JS (1995) Hepatitis B virus X protein interacts with a probable cellular DNA repair protein. *J Virol* 69: 1107-1114

Lee YH, Yun Y (1998) HBx protein of hepatitis B virus activates Jak1-STAT signaling. *J Biol Chem* 273: 25510-25515

Lee YI, Hwang JM, Im JH, Kim NS, Kim DG, Yu DY, Moon HB, Park SK (2004) Human hepatitis B virus-X protein alters mitochondrial function and physiology in human liver cells. *J Biol Chem* 279: 15460-15471

Lee YI, Kang-Park S, Do SI (2001) The hepatitis B virus-X protein activates a phosphatidylinositol 3-kinase-dependent survival signaling cascade. *J Biol Chem* 276: 16969-16977

Lee YI, Lee S, Lee Y, Bong YS, Hyun SW, Yoo YD, Kim SJ, Kim YW, Poo HR (1998) The human hepatitis B virus transactivator X gene product regulates Sp1 mediated transcription of an insulin-like growth factor II promoter 4. *Oncogene* 16: 2367-2380

Leupin O, Bontron S, Schaeffer C, Strubin M (2005) Hepatitis B virus X protein stimulates viral genome replication via a DDB1-dependent pathway distinct from that leading to cell death. *J Virol* 79: 4238-4245

Lew DJ, Kornbluth S (1996) Regulatory roles of cyclin dependent kinase phosphorylation in cell cycle control. *Curr Opin Cell Biol* 8: 795-804

Liang X, Liu Y, Zhang Q, Gao L, Han L, Ma C, Zhang L, Chen YH, Sun W (2007) Hepatitis B virus sensitizes hepatocytes to TRAIL-induced apoptosis through Bax. *J Immunol* 178: 503-510

Liew CT, Li HM, Lo KW, Leow CK, Chan JY, Hin LY, Lau WY, Lai PB, Lim BK, Huang J, Leung WT, Wu S, Lee JC (1999) High frequency of p16INK4A gene alterations in hepatocellular carcinoma. *Oncogene* 18: 789-795

Lim W, Kwon SH, Cho H, Kim S, Lee S, Ryu WS (2010) HBx targeting to mitochondria and ROS generation are necessary but insufficient for HBV-induced cyclooxygenase-2 expression. *J Mol Med (Berl)* 88: 359-369

Lin Y, Nomura T, Cheong J, Dorjsuren D, Iida K, Murakami S (1997) Hepatitis B virus X protein is a transcriptional modulator that communicates with transcription factor IIB and the RNA polymerase II subunit 5. *J Biol Chem* 272: 7132-7139

Lin-Marq N, Bontron S, Leupin O, Strubin M (2001) Hepatitis B virus protein interferes with cell viability through interaction with the p127-kDa UV-damaged DNA-binding protein. *Virology* 287: 266-274

Liu Y, Martindale JL, Gorospe M, Holbrook NJ (1996) Regulation of p21WAF1/CIP1 expression through mitogen-activated protein kinase signaling pathway. *Cancer Res* 56: 31-35

Liu YG, Liu SX, Liang XH, Zhang Q, Gao LF, Han LH, Cao YL, Hou N, Du J, Sun WS (2007) Blockade of TRAIL pathway ameliorates HBV-induced hepatocyte apoptosis in an acute hepatitis model. *Biochem Biophys Res Commun* 352: 329-334

Lok A, McMahon B (2001) Chronic hepatitis B. *Hepatology* 34: 1225-1241

Lu YW, Chen WN (2005) Human hepatitis B virus X protein induces apoptosis in HepG2 cells: role of BH3 domain. *Biochem Biophys Res Commun* 338: 1551-1556

Lucito R, Schneider R (1992) Hepatitis B virus X protein activates transcription factor NF-kB without a requirement for protein kinase C. *J Virol* 66: 983-991

Ma J, Sun T, Park S, Shen G, Liu J (2011) The role of hepatitis B virus X protein is related to its differential intracellular localization. *Acta Biochim Biophys Sin (Shanghai)* 43: 583-588

Madden C, Finegold M, Slagle B (2001) Hepatitis B virus X protein acts a a tumor promoter in development of diethylnitrosamine-induced preneoplastic lesions. *J Virol* 75: 3851-3858

Madden CR, Finegold MJ, Slagle BL (2000) Expression of hepatitis B virus X protein does not alter the accumulation of spontaneous mutations in transgenic mice. *J Virol* 74: 5266-5272

Madden CR, Slagle BL (2001) Stimulation of cellular proliferation by hepatitis B virus X protein. *Dis Markers* 17: 153-157

Maguire H, Hoeffler J, Siddiqui A (1991) HBV X protein alters the DNA binding specificity of CREB and ATF-2 by protein-protein interactions. *Science* 252: 842-844

Mahe Y, Mukaida N, Kuno K, Akiyama M, Ikeda N, Matsushima K, Murakami S (1991) Hepatitis B virus X protein transactivates human interleukin-8 gene through acting on nuclear factor kB and CCAAT/enhancer-binding protein-like *cis*-elements. *J Biol Chem* 266: 13759-13763

Mandart E, Kay A, Galibert F (1984) Nucleotide sequence of a cloned duck hepatitis B virus genome: comparison with woodchuck and human hepatitis B virus sequences. *J Virol* 49: 782-792

Martin-Lluesma S, Schaeffer C, Robert EI, van Breugel PC, Leupin O, Hantz O, Strubin M (2008) Hepatitis B virus X protein affects S phase progression leading to chromosome segregation defects by binding to damaged DNA binding protein 1. *Hepatology* 48: 1467-1476

Matsuda Y, Ichida T, Matsuzawa J, Sugimura K, Asakura H (1999) p16(INK4) is inactivated by extensive CpG methylation in human hepatocellular carcinoma. *Gastroenterology* 116: 394-400

McClain SL, Clippinger AJ, Lizzano R, Bouchard MJ (2007) HBV replication is associated with an HBx-dependent mitochondrial regulated increase in cytosolic calcium levels. *J Virol*

McCubrey JA, Steelman LS, Chappell WH, Abrams SL, Wong EW, Chang F, Lehmann B, Terrian DM, Milella M, Tafuri A, Stivala F, Libra M, Basecke J, Evangelisti C, Martelli AM, Franklin RA (2007) Roles of the Raf/MEK/ERK pathway in cell growth, malignant transformation and drug resistance. *Biochim Biophys Acta* 1773: 1263-1284

Melegari M, Wolf SK, Schneider RJ (2005) Hepatitis B virus DNA replication is coordinated by core protein serine phosphorylation and HBx expression. *J Virol* 79: 9810-9820

Miao J, Chen GG, Chun SY, Lai PP (2006) Hepatitis B virus X protein induces apoptosis in hepatoma cells through inhibiting Bcl-xL expression. *Cancer Lett* 236: 115-124

Monga SP (2011) Role of Wnt/$\beta$-catenin signaling in liver metabolism and cancer. *Int J Biochem Cell Biol* 43: 1021-1029

Montagnoli A, Fiore F, Eytan E, Carrano AC, Draetta GF, Hershko A, Pagano M (1999) Ubiquitination of p27 is regulated by Cdk-dependent phosphorylation and trimeric complex formation. *Genes Dev* 13: 1181-1189

Morgan D (1997) Cyclin-dependent kinases: engines, clocks, and microprocessors. *Annu Rev Cell Dev Biol* 13: 261-291

Morishita A, Masaki T, Yoshiji H, Nakai S, Ogi T, Miyauchi Y, Yoshida S, Funaki T, Uchida N, Kita Y, Funakoshi F, Usuki H, Okada S, Izuishi K, Watanabe S, Kurokohchi K, Kuriyama S (2004) Reduced expression of cell cycle regulator p18(INK4C) in human hepatocellular carcinoma. *Hepatology* 40: 677-686

Mukherji A, Janbandhu VC, Kumar V (2007) HBx-dependent cell cycle deregulation involves interaction with cyclin E/A-cdk2 complex and destabilization of p27Kip1. *Biochem J* 401: 247-256

Mukherji A, Kumar V (2008) Regulation of the cell cycle by Hepatitis B Virus X protein. In *The Pleiotropic Functions of the Viral Protein HBx in Hepatitis B Virus Infection and the development of liver cancer.*, Kobarg J (ed). Research Signpost

Murakami S (2001) Hepatitis B virus X protein: a multifunctional viral regulator. *J Gastroenterol* 36: 651-660

Natoli G, Avantaggiati L, Chirillo P, Costanzo A, Artini M, Balsano C, Levrero M (1994a) Induction of the DNA-binding activity of c-Jun/c-Fos heterodimers by hepatitis B virus transactivator pX. *Mol Cell Biol* 14: 989-998

Natoli G, Avantaggiati L, Chirillo P, Puri P, Ianni A, Balsano C, Levrero M (1994b) Ras- and raf-dependent activation of c-jun transcriptonal activity by the hepatitis B virus transactivator pX. *Oncogene* 9: 2837-2843

Neuveut C, Wei Y, Buendia MA (2010) Mechanisms of HBV-related hepatocarcinogenesis. *J Hepatol* 52: 594-604

Ng SA, Lee C (2011) Hepatitis B virus X gene and hepatocarcinogenesis. *J Gastroenterol* 46: 974-990

Nguyen DH, Ludgate L, Hu J (2008) Hepatitis B virus-cell interactions and pathogenesis. *J Cell Physiol* 216: 289-294

Nijhara R, Jana S, Goswami S, Rana A, Majumdar S, Kumar V, Sarkar D (2001) Sustained activation of mitogen-activated protein kinases and activator protein 1 by the hepatitis B virus X protein in mouse hepatocytes in vivo. *J Virol* 75: 10348-10358

Oh BK, Kim H, Park HJ, Shim YH, Choi J, Park C, Park YN (2007) DNA methyltransferase expression and DNA methylation in human hepatocellular carcinoma and their clinicopathological correlation. *Int J Mol Med* 20: 65-73

Ohtsubo M, Theodoras AM, Schumacher J, Roberts JM, Pagano M (1995) Human cyclin E, a nuclear protein essential for the G1-to-S phase transition. *Mol Cell Biol* 15: 2612-2624

Ozer A, Khaoustov V, Mearns M, Lewis D, Genta R, Darlington G, Yoffe B (1996) Effect of hepatocyte proliferation and cellular DNA synthesis on hepatitis B virus replication. *Gastroenterology* 110: 1519-1528

Pan J, Duan LX, Sun BS, Feitelson MA (2001) Hepatitis B virus X protein protects against anti-Fas-mediated apoptosis in human liver cells by inducing NF-kappa B. *J Gen Virol* 82: 171-182

Pang R, Tse E, Poon RT (2006) Molecular pathways in hepatocellular carcinoma. *Cancer Lett* 240: 157-169

Pardali K, Kurisaki A, Morén A, ten Dijke P, Kardassis D, Moustakas A (2000) Role of Smad proteins and transcription factor Sp1 in p21(Waf1/Cip1) regulation by transforming growth factor-beta. *J Biol Chem* 275: 29244-29256

Parekh AB (2010) Store-operated CRAC channels: function in health and disease. *Nat Rev Drug Discov* 9: 399-410

Parekh AB (2011) Decoding cytosolic Ca2+ oscillations. *Trends Biochem Sci* 36: 78-87

Park SG, Chung C, Kang H, Kim JY, Jung G (2006) Up-regulation of cyclin D1 by HBx is mediated by NF-kappaB2/BCL3 complex through kappaB site of cyclin D1 promoter. *J Biol Chem* 281: 31770-31777

Park US, Park SK, Lee YI, Park JG (2000) Hepatitis B virus-X protein upregulates the expression of p21waf1/cip1 and prolongs G1-->S transition via a p53-independent pathway in human hepatoma cells. *Oncogene* 19: 3384-3394

Parkash J, Asotra K (2010) Calcium wave signaling in cancer cells. *Life Sci* 87: 587-595

Patel R, Holt M, Philipova R, Moss S, Schulman H, Hidaka H, Whitaker M (1999) Calcium/calmodulin-dependent phosphorylation and activation of human Cdc25-C at the G2/M phase transition in HeLa cells. *J Biol Chem* 274: 7958-7968

Paulovich AG, Hartwell LH (1995) A checkpoint regulates the rate of progression through S phase in S. cerevisiae in response to DNA damage. *Cell* 82: 841-847

Pines J, Hunter T (1991) Cyclin-dependent kinases: a new cell cycle motif? *Trends Cell Biol* 1: 117-121

Polyak K, Kato JY, Solomon MJ, Sherr CJ, Massague J, Roberts JM, Koff A (1994a) p27Kip1, a cyclin-Cdk inhibitor, links transforming growth factor-beta and contact inhibition to cell cycle arrest. *Genes Dev* 8: 9-22

Polyak K, Lee MH, Erdjument-Bromage H, Koff A, Roberts JM, Tempst P, Massagué J (1994b) Cloning of p27Kip1, a cyclin-dependent kinase inhibitor and a potential mediator of extracellular antimitogenic signals. *Cell* 78: 59-66

Prince AM, Brotman B (2001) Perspectives on hepatitis B studies with chimpanzees. *ILAR J* 42: 85-88

Purcell N, Yu C, He D, Xiang J, Paran N, DiDonato J, Yamaoka S, Shaul Y, Lin A (2001) Activation of NF-kB by hepatitis B virus X protein through an IkB kinase-independent mechansism. *Am J Physiol Gastointest Liver Physiol* 280: G669-G677

Putney JW (1986) A model for receptor-regulated calcium entry. *Cell Calcium* 7: 1-12

Putney JW, Bird GS (2008) Cytoplasmic calcium oscillations and store-operated calcium influx. *J Physiol* 586: 3055-3059

Qiao L, Leach K, McKinstry R, Gilfor D, Yacoub A, Park J-S, Grant S, Hylemon P, Fisher P, Dent P (2001) Hepatitis B virus X protein increases expression of $p21^{Cip-1/WAF1/MDA6}$ and $p27^{Kip-1}$ in primary mouse hepatocytes, leading to a reduced cell cycle progression. *Hepatology* 34: 906-917

Qin LF, Ng IO (2001) Expression of p27(KIP1) and p21(WAF1/CIP1) in primary hepatocellular carcinoma: clinicopathologic correlation and survival analysis. *Hum Pathol* 32: 778-784

Rahmani Z, Huh K-W, Lasher R, Siddiqui A (2000) Hepatitis B virus X protein colocalizes to mitochondria with human voltage -dependent anion channel, HVDAC3, and alters its transmembrane potential. *J Virol* 74: 2840-2846

Rahmani Z, Maunoury C, Siddiqui A (1998) Isolation of a novel human voltage-dependent anion channel gene. *Eur J Hum Genet* 6: 337-340

Rasmussen CD, Means AR (1989) Calmodulin is required for cell-cycle progression during G1 and mitosis. *Embo J* 8: 73-82

Rechsteiner M, Rogers SW (1996) PEST sequences and regulation by proteolysis. *Trends Biochem Sci* 21: 267-271

Reichard P (1987) Regulation of deoxyribotide synthesis. *Biochemistry* 26: 3245-3248

Ren CS (1991) [Expression of p21 in hepatocellular carcinoma and liver cirrhosis and its relation with HBV infection]. *Zhonghua Bing Li Xue Za Zhi* 20: 88-90

Rizzuto R, Brini M, Murgia M, Pozzan T (1993) Microdomains with high Ca2+ close to IP3-sensitive channels that are sensed by neighboring mitochondria. *Science* 262: 744-747

Rizzuto R, Pinton P, Carrington W, Fay FS, Fogarty KE, Lifshitz LM, Tuft RA, Pozzan T (1998) Close contacts with the endoplasmic reticulum as determinants of mitochondrial Ca2+ responses. *Science* 280: 1763-1766

Roberts JM, Koff A, Polyak K, Firpo E, Collins S, Ohtsubo M, Massagué J (1994) Cyclins, Cdks, and cyclin kinase inhibitors. *Cold Spring Harb Symp Quant Biol* 59: 31-38

Roderick HL, Cook SJ (2008) Ca2+ signalling checkpoints in cancer: remodelling Ca2+ for cancer cell proliferation and survival. *Nat Rev Cancer* 8: 361-375

Rodrigues RR, Barry CT (2011) Gene pathway analysis of hepatocellular carcinoma genomic expression datasets. *J Surg Res* 170: e85-92

Schneider G, Oswald F, Wahl C, Greten FR, Adler G, Schmid RM (2002) Cyclosporine inhibits growth through the activating transcription factor/cAMP-responsive element-binding protein binding site in the cyclin D1 promoter. *J Biol Chem* 277: 43599-43607

Seeger C, Zoulim F, Mason W (2007) Hepadnaviridae. In *Fields Virology*, Knipe D, Howley P (eds), Vol. 2, Fifth edn, pp 2977-3030. Philadelphia: Wolters Kluwer Health, Lippincott Williams & Wilkins

Shen L, Fang J, Qiu D, Zhang T, Yang J, Chen S, Xiao S (1998) Correlation between DNA methylation and pathological changes in human hepatocellular carcinoma. *Hepatogastroenterology* 45: 1753-1759

Sherr CJ (1993) Mammalian G1 cyclins. *Cell* 73: 1059-1065

Sherr CJ (1994) G1 phase progression: cycling on cue. *Cell* 79: 551-555

Sherr CJ, Roberts JM (1995) Inhibitors of mammalian G1 cyclin-dependent kinases. *Genes Dev* 9: 1149-1163

Sherr CJ, Roberts JM (1999) CDK inhibitors: positive and negative regulators of G1-phase progression. *Genes Dev* 13: 1501-1512

Shih W-L, Kuo M-L, Chuang S-E, Cheng A-L, Doong S-L (2000) Hepatitis B virus X protein inhibits transforming growth factor-b-induced apoptosis through the activation of phosphatidylinositol 3-kinase pathway. *J Biol Chem* 275: 25858-25864

Shim YH, Park HJ, Choi MS, Kim JS, Kim H, Kim JJ, Jang JJ, Yu E (2003a) Hypermethylation of the p16 gene and lack of p16 expression in hepatoblastoma. *Mod Pathol* 16: 430-436

Shim YH, Yoon GS, Choi HJ, Chung YH, Yu E (2003b) p16 Hypermethylation in the early stage of hepatitis B virus-associated hepatocarcinogenesis. *Cancer Lett* 190: 213-219

Shintani Y, Yotsuyanagi H, Moriya K, Fujie H, Tsutsumi T, Kanegae Y, Kimura S, Saito I, Koike K (1999) Induction of apoptosis after switch-on of the hepatitis B virus X gene mediated by the Cre/loxP recombination system. *J Gen Virol* 80: 3257-3265

Shirakata Y, Koike K (2003) Hepatitis B virus X protein induces cell death by causing loss of mitochondrial membrane potential. *J Biol Chem* 278: 22071-22078

Short AD, Bian J, Ghosh TK, Waldron RT, Rybak SL, Gill DL (1993) Intracellular Ca2+ pool content is linked to control of cell growth. *Proc Natl Acad Sci U S A* 90: 4986-4990

Siddiqui A, Jameel S, Mapoles J (1987) Expression of the hepatitis B virus X gene in mammalian cells. *Proc Natl Acad Sci USA* 84: 2513-2517

Singh AK, Swarnalatha M, Kumar V (2011) c-ETS1 facilitates G1/S-phase transition by up-regulating cyclin E and CDK2 genes and cooperates with hepatitis B virus X protein for their deregulation. *J Biol Chem* 286: 21961-21970

Sitterlin D, Bergametti F, Tiollais P, Tennant BC, Transy C (2000) Correct binding of viral X protein to UVDDB-p127 cellular protein is critical for efficient infection by hepatitis B viruses. *Oncogene* 19: 4427-4431

Slagle BL, Lee TH, Medina D, Finegold MJ, Butel JS (1996) Increased sensitivity to the hepatocarcinogen diethylnitrosamine in transgenic mice carrying the hepatitis B virus X gene. *Mol Carcinog* 15: 261-269

Smyth JT, Dehaven WI, Jones BF, Mercer JC, Trebak M, Vazquez G, Putney JW (2006) Emerging perspectives in store-operated Ca2+ entry: roles of Orai, Stim and TRP. *Biochim Biophys Acta* 1763: 1147-1160

Spandau D, C. L (1988) *trans*-activation of viral enhancers by the hepatitis B virus X protein. *J Virol* 62: 427-434

Sprengel R, Kaleta EF, Will H (1988) Isolation and characterization of a hepatitis B virus endemic in herons. *J Virol* 62: 3832-3839

Su F, Schneider R (1996) Hepatitis B virus HBx protein activates transcription factor NF-kB by acting on multiple cytoplasmic inhibitors of *rel*-related proteins. *J Virol* 70: 4558-4566

Su F, Schneider R (1997) Hepatits B virus HBx protein sensitizes cells to apoptotic killing by tumor necrosis factor a. *Proc Natl Acad Sci USA* 94: 8744-8749

Su F, Theodosis C, Schneider R (2001) Role of NF-kB and myc proteins in apoptosis induced by hepatitis B virus HBx protein. *J Virol* 75: 215-225

Su Q, Schroder CH, Otto G, Bannasch P (2000) Overexpression of p53 protein is not directly related to hepatitis B x protein expression and is associated with neoplastic progression in hepatocellular carcinomas rather than hepatic preneoplasia. *Mutat Res* 462: 365-380

Swanton C, Jones N (2001) Strategies in subversion: de-regulation of the mammalian cell cycle by viral gene products. *Int J Exp Pathol* 82: 3-13

Takada S, Shirakata Y, Kaneniwa N, Koike K (1999) Association of hepatitis B virus X protein with mitochondria causes mitochondrial aggregation at the nuclear periphery, leading to cell death. *Oncogene* 18: 6965-6973

Takuwa N, Zhou W, Kumada M, Takuwa Y (1992) Ca2+/calmodulin is involved in growth factor-induced retinoblastoma gene product phosphorylation in human vascular endothelial cells. *FEBS Lett* 306: 173-175

Takuwa N, Zhou W, Kumada M, Takuwa Y (1993) Ca(2+)-dependent stimulation of retinoblastoma gene product phosphorylation and p34cdc2 kinase activation in serum-stimulated human fibroblasts. *J Biol Chem* 268: 138-145

Talavera A, Basilico C (1977) Temperature sensitive mutants of BHK cells affected in cell cycle progression. *J Cell Physiol* 92: 425-436

Tan C, Guo H, Zheng M, Chen Y, Huang W (2009) Involvement of mitochondrial permeability transition in hepatitis B virus replication. *Virus Res* 145: 307-311

Tanaka Y, Kanai F, Kawakami T, Tateishi K, Ijichi H, Kawabe T, Arakawa Y, Kawakami T, Nishimura T, Shirakata Y, Koike K, Omata M (2004) Interaction of the hepatitis B virus X protein (HBx) with heat shock protein 60 enhances HBx-mediated apoptosis. *Biochem Biophys Res Commun* 318: 461-469

Tang H, Delgermaa L, Huang F, Oishi N, Liu L, He F, Zhao L, Murakami S (2005) The transcriptional transactivation function of HBx protein is important for its augmentation role in hepatitis B virus replication. *J Virol* 79: 5548-5556

Tarn C, Bilodeau M, Hullinger R, Andrisan O (1999) Differential immediate early gene expression in conditional hepatitis B virus pX-transforming *versus* nontransforming hepatocyte cell lines. *J Biol Chem* 274: 2327-2336

Tarn C, Lee S, Hu Y, Ashendel C, Andrisani OM (2001) Hepatitis B virus X protein differentially activates RAS-RAF-MAPK and JNK pathways in X-transforming versus non-transforming AML12 hepatocytes. *J Biol Chem* 276: 34671-34680

Tarn C, Zou L, Hullinger R, Andrisani O (2002) Hepatitis B virus X protein activates the p38 mitogen-activated protein kinase pathway in dedifferentiated hepatocytes. *J Virol* 76: 9763-9772

Taub R (2004) Liver regeneration: from myth to mechanism. *Nat Rev Mol Cell Biol* 5: 836-847

Terradillos O, Billet O, Renard CA, R. L, Molina T, Briand P, Buendia M-A (1997) The hepatitis B virus X gene potentiates c-myc-induced liver oncogenesis in transgenic mice. *Oncogene* 14: 395-404

Terradillos O, de La Coste A, Pollicino T, Neuveut C, Sitterlin D, Lecoeur H, Gougeon M-L, Kahn A, Buendia M-A (2002) The hepatitis B virus X protein abrogates Bcl-2-mediated protection against Fas apoptosis in the liver. *Oncogene* 21: 377-386

Terradillos O, Pollicino T, Lecoeur H, Tripodi M, Gougeon ML, Tiollais P, Buendia MA (1998) p53-independent apoptotic effects of the hepatitis B virus HBx protein in vivo and in vitro. *Oncogene* 17: 2115-2123

Thelander L, Reichard P (1979) Reduction of ribonucleotides. *Annu Rev Biochem* 48: 133-158

Thompson MD, Monga SP (2007) WNT/beta-catenin signaling in liver health and disease. *Hepatology* 45: 1298-1305

Tomono M, Toyoshima K, Ito M, Amano H, Kiss Z (1998) Inhibitors of calcineurin block expression of cyclins A and E induced by fibroblast growth factor in Swiss 3T3 fibroblasts. *Arch Biochem Biophys* 353: 374-378

Torbenson M, Kannangai R, Abraham S, Sahin F, Choti M, Wang J (2004) Concurrent evaluation of p53, beta-catenin, and alpha-fetoprotein expression in human hepatocellular carcinoma. *Am J Clin Pathol* 122: 377-382

Tralhao J, Roudier J, Morosan S, Giannini C, Tu H, Goulenok C, Carnot F, Zavala F, Joulin V, Kremsdorf D, Brechot C (2002) Paracrine *in vivo* inhibitory effects of hepatitis B virus X protein (HBx) on liver proliferation: an alternative mechanism of HBx-related pathogenesis. *Proc Natl Acad Sci USA* 99: 6991-6996

Tsuge M, Hiraga N, Akiyama R, Tanaka S, Matsushita M, Mitsui F, Abe H, Kitamura S, Hatakeyama T, Kimura T, Miki D, Mori N, Imamura M, Takahashi S, Hayes CN, Chayama K (2010) HBx protein is indispensable for development of viraemia in human hepatocyte chimeric mice. *J Gen Virol* 91: 1854-1864

Tsuge M, Hiraga N, Takaishi H, Noguchi C, Oga H, Imamura M, Takahashi S, Iwao E, Fujimoto Y, Ochi H, Chayama K, Tateno C, Yoshizato K (2005) Infection of human hepatocyte chimeric mouse with genetically engineered hepatitis B virus. *Hepatology* 42: 1046-1054

Urban S, Hildt E, Eckerskorn C, Sirma H, Kekule A, Hofschneider PH (1997) Isolation and molecular characterization of hepatitis B virus X-protein from a baculovirus expression system. *Hepatology* 26: 1045-1053

Vermeulen K, Van Bockstaele DR, Berneman ZN (2003) The cell cycle: a review of regulation, deregulation and therapeutic targets in cancer. *Cell Prolif* 36: 131-149

Vitvitski-Trepo L, Kay A, Pichoud C, Chevallier P, de Dinechin S, Shamoon B-M, Mandart E, Trepo C, Galibert F (1990) Early and frequent detection of HBxAg and/or Anti-HBx in hepatitis B virus infection. *Hepatology* 12: 1278-1283

Walker DH, Maller JL (1991) Role for cyclin A in the dependence of mitosis on completion of DNA replication. *Nature* 354: 314-317

Wang HD, Trivedi A, Johnson DL (1998) Regulation of RNA polymerase I-dependent promoters by the hepatitis B virus X protein via activated Ras and TATA-binding protein. *Mol Cell Biol* 18: 7086-7094

Wang JH, Yun C, Kim S, Chae S, Lee YI, Kim WH, Lee JH, Kim W, Cho H (2008) Reactivation of p53 in cells expressing hepatitis B virus X-protein involves p53 phosphorylation and a reduction of Hdm2. *Cancer Sci* 99: 888-893

Wang T, Zhao R, Wu Y, Kong D, Zhang L, Wu D, Li C, Zhang C, Yu Z, Jin X (2011) Hepatitis B virus induces G1 phase arrest by regulating cell cycle genes in HepG2.2.15 cells. *Virol J* 8: 231

Wang WH, Gregori G, Hullinger RL, Andrisani OM (2004a) Sustained activation of p38 mitogen-activated protein kinase and c-Jun N-terminal kinase pathways by hepatitis B virus X protein mediates apoptosis via induction of Fas/FasL and tumor necrosis factor (TNF) receptor 1/TNF-alpha expression. *Mol Cell Biol* 24: 10352-10365

Wang X, Forrester K, Yeh H, Feitelson M, Gu J-R, Harris C (1994) Hepatitis B virus X protein inhibits p53 sequence-specific DNA binding, transcriptional activity, and association with transcription factor ERCC3. *Proc Natl Acad Sci USA* 91: 2230-2234

Wang XW, Gibson MK, Vermeulen W, Yeh H, Forrester K, Sturzbecher HW, Hoeijmakers JH, Harris CC (1995) Abrogation of p53-induced apoptosis by the hepatitis B virus X gene. *Cancer Res* 55: 6012-6016

Wang Y, Lau SH, Sham JS, Wu MC, Wang T, Guan XY (2004b) Characterization of HBV integrants in 14 hepatocellular carcinomas: association of truncated X gene and hepatocellular carcinogenesis. *Oncogene* 23: 142-148

Waris G, Huh KW, Siddiqui A (2001) Mitochondrially associated hepatitis B virus X protein constitutively activates transcription factors STAT-3 and NF-kappa B via oxidative stress. *Mol Cell Biol* 21: 7721-7730

Wei Y, Neuveut C, Tiollais P, Buendia MA (2010) Molecular biology of the hepatitis B virus and role of the X gene. *Pathol Biol (Paris)* 58: 267-272

Weil R, Sirman H, Giannini C, Kremsdorf D, Bessis C, Dargemont C, Brechot C, Israel A (1999) Direct association and nuclear import of the hepatitis B virus X protein with the NF-KB inhibitor IKBa. *Mol Cell Biol* 19: 6345-6354

Whittaker S, Marais R, Zhu AX (2010) The role of signaling pathways in the development and treatment of hepatocellular carcinoma. *Oncogene* 29: 4989-5005

WHO. (2008) Hepatitis B Fact Sheet.

Williams J, Andrisani O (1995) The hepatitis B virus X protein targets the basic region-leucine zipper domain of CREB. *Proc Natl Acad Sci USA* 92: 3819-3823

Wollersheim M, Debelka U, Hofschneider P (1988) A transactivating function encoded in the hepatitis B virus X gene is conserved in the integrated state. *Oncogene* 3: 545-552

Wong IH, Lo YM, Lai PB, Johnson PJ (2000a) Relationship of p16 methylation status and serum alpha-fetoprotein concentration in hepatocellular carcinoma patients. *Clin Chem* 46: 1420-1422

Wong IH, Lo YM, Yeo W, Lau WY, Johnson PJ (2000b) Frequent p15 promoter methylation in tumor and peripheral blood from hepatocellular carcinoma patients. *Clin Cancer Res* 6: 3516-3521

Wu BK, Li CC, Chen HJ, Chang JL, Jeng KS, Chou CK, Hsu MT, Tsai TF (2006) Blocking of G1/S transition and cell death in the regenerating liver of Hepatitis B virus X protein transgenic mice. *Biochem Biophys Res Commun* 340: 916-928

Wu J, Merlino G, Cveklova K, Mosinger B, Fausto N (1994a) Autonomous growth in serum-free medium and production of hepatocellular carcinomas by differentiated hepatocyte lines that overexpress transforming growth factor a. *Cancer Res* 54: 5964-5973

Wu J, Merlino G, Fausto N (1994b) Establishment and characterization of differentiated, nontransformed hepatocyte cell lines derived from mice transgenic for transforming growth factor a. *Proc Natl Acad Sci USA* 91: 674-678

Xu Z, Yen T, Wu L, Madden C, Tan W, Slagle B, Ou J-h (2002) Enhancement of hepatitis B virus replication by its X protein in transgenic mice. *J Virol* 76: 2579-2584

Yamashita M, Emerman M (2006) Retroviral infection of non-dividing cells: old and new perspectives. *Virology* 344: 88-93

Yang WJ, Chang CJ, Yeh SH, Lin WH, Wang SH, Tsai TF, Chen DS, Chen PJ (2009) Hepatitis B virus X protein enhances the transcriptional activity of the androgen receptor through c-Src and glycogen synthase kinase-3beta kinase pathways. *Hepatology* 49: 1515-1524

Yang Y, Ma Y, Zhen L, Chen Y, Ma W, Murakami S (1999) HBV X protein (HBX) interacts with general transcription factor TFIIB both in vitro and in vivo. *Chin Med Sci J* 14: 152-157

Yeh CT, Wong SW, Fung YK, Ou JH (1993) Cell cycle regulation of nuclear localization of hepatitis B virus core protein. *Proc Natl Acad Sci U S A* 90: 6459-6463

Yen TS (1996) Hepadnaviral X protein: review of recent progress. *J Biomed Sci* 3: 20-30

Yu DY, Moon HB, Son JK, Jeong S, Yu SL, Yoon H, Han YM, Lee CS, Park JS, Lee CH, Hyun BH, Murakami S, Lee KK (1999) Incidence of hepatocellular carcinoma in transgenic mice expressing the hepatitis B virus X-protein. *J Hepatol* 31: 123-132

Yun C, Um H-R, Jin Y, Wang J-H, Lee M-O, Park S, Lee J-H, Hyeseong C (2002) NF-kB activation by hepatitis B virus X (HBx) protein shifts the cellular fate toward survival. *Cancer Lett* 184: 97-104

Zhang JL, Zhao WG, Wu KL, Wang K, Zhang X, Gu CF, Li Y, Zhu Y, Wu JG (2005) Human hepatitis B virus X protein promotes cell proliferation and inhibits cell apoptosis through interacting with a serine protease Hepsin. *Arch Virol* 150: 721-741

Zhang X, Zhang E, Ma Z, Pei R, Jiang M, Schlaak JF, Roggendorf M, Lu M (2011) Modulation of hepatitis B virus replication and hepatocyte differentiation by MicroRNA-1. *Hepatology* 53: 1476-1485

Zhang X, Zhang H, Ye L (2006) Effects of hepatitis B virus X protein on the development of liver cancer. *J Lab Clin Med* 147: 58-66

Zhang Z, Protzer U, Hu Z, Jacob J, Liang TJ (2004) Inhibition of Cellular Proteasome Activities Enhances Hepadnavirus Replication in an HBX-Dependent Manner. *J Virol* 78: 4566-4572

Zhang Z, Torii N, Hu Z, Jacob J, Liang T (2001) X-deficient woodchuck hepatitis virus mutants behave like attenuated viruses andinduce protective immunity in vivo. *J Clin Invest* 108: 1523-1531

Zhu H, Wang Y, Chen JS, Cheng G, Xue J (2004) Transgenic mice expressing hepatitis B virus X protein are more susceptible to carcinogen induced hepatocarcinogenesis. *Exp Mol Path* 76: 44-50

Zhu R, Li BZ, Li H, Ling YQ, Hu XQ, Zhai WR, Zhu HG (2007) Association of p16INK4A hypermethylation with hepatitis B virus X protein expression in the early stage of HBV-associated hepatocarcinogenesis. *Pathol Int* 57: 328-336

Zhu YZ, Zhu R, Fan J, Pan Q, Li H, Chen Q, Zhu HG (2010) Hepatitis B virus X protein induces hypermethylation of p16(INK4A) promoter via DNA methyltransferases in the early stage of HBV-associated hepatocarcinogenesis. *J Viral Hepat* 17: 98-107

Zoratti M, Szabo I (1995) The mitochondrial permeability transition. *Biochim Biophys Acta* 1241: 139-176

Zoulim F, Saputelli J, Seeger C (1994) Woodchuck hepatitis virus X protein is required for viral infection in vivo. *J Virol* 68: 2026-2030

# 6

# Vascular Adhesion Protein-1 and Hepatocellular Cancer

Ozgur Kemik[1*], Ahu Sarbay Kemik[2] and A. Cumhur Dulger[3]
[1]*Department of General Surgery, Medical Faculty, University of Yuzuncu Yıl, Van*
[2]*Department of Biochemistry, Cerrahpasa Medical Faculty, University of Istanbul, Istanbul*
[3]*Department of Gastroenterology, Medical Faculty, University of Yuzuncu Yıl, Van*
*Turkey*

## 1. Introduction

The extravasation of leukocytes from the vasculature to the tissue space is a fundamental response of the normal immune system. A multistep model of leukocyte adhesion to vascular endothelium has been characterized, although details of the signaling differ between tissues [1-9].

Lymphocytes recirculate between blood and tissues as part of the immune surveillance process, and recent evidence suggests that specialized subsets of T cells exhibit discrete tissue-specific patterns of recirculation in vivo [2, 10].

These cells are directed to particular tissues by combinations of adhesion molecules and chemokines that control the lymphocyte recognition of and adhesion to endothelium. For example, memory T cells that recirculate to the gut lamina propria express integrin $\alpha_4\beta_7$ and bind to an endothelial ligand, namely, mucosal cell adhesion molecule-1, which is detected in gut endothelium [11]. Conversely, T cells that migrate to the skin do not express $\alpha_4\beta_7$ but do express high levels of the lymphocyte Ag, Which binds to E-selectin on dermal endothelium [12] .The liver is a major site of Ag exposure and contains large numbers of lymphocytes even under normal conditions. These lymphocytes are differentiated lymphocytes that are displaced by apoptosis [13-17]. It is thus likely that tissue-specific signals regulate lymphocyte recruitment to the liver [18].

The hepatic cells are formed into ranks by specialized endothelium that supports lymphocyte adhesion and recruitment in a low-shear environment [19]. Hepatic endothelium has a discrete phenotype compared with endothelium from other vascular beds.

Several cell adhesion molecules play an important role in this complex process and stabilize the adhesion and diapedesis of leukocytes across the endothelial barrier, similar to the manner in which human hepatic endothelium cells secrete the endothelial adhesion molecule vascular adhesion protein-1 (VAP-1)[-9].

---

[*] Corresponding Author

The VAP-1 molecule is a 170 kDa homodimeric glycoprotein that consists of two 90 kDa subunits that are held together by disulfide bonds [20]. VAP-1 has a large extracellular domain, a single-pass transmembrane domain, and a short cytoplasmic cue [21]. The molecule has ample sialic acid moieties that are required for its adhesive function, which was shown based on the inability of VAP-1 to mediate lymphocyte adhesion to desialylated vessels [20]. The leukocyte ligand for VAP-1 is presently unknown.

Serum measurements of VAP-1 are performed by enzyme-linked immunosorbent assay[22].

A possible role for VAP-1 was shown in adhesion assays. VAP-1 may have a normal physiological role in maintaining the proadhesive status of PBLs toward endothelia since its concentration in normal individuals is within the range that is used in these adhesion experiments.

Some reports have shown that significantly elevated levels of VAP-1 were found in patients with liver diseases [22, 23]. Patients had increased systemic circulation, and VAP-1 levels in these patients were higher, suggesting that VAP-1 could engender biological effects. It is interesting that patients with hepatocellular carcinoma had higher VAP-1 values than patients with inflammatory liver diseases, which agrees well with the finding of high VAP-1 expression in primary liver tumors but not in liver metastases [22-24]. Other non-hepatic inflammatory diseases were not related to increased levels of VAP-1 [23]. An increase in VAP-1 levels is specific to particular inflammatory diseases. The specificity of increased VAP-1 levels for certain liver diseases (hepatocellular carcinoma) justifies further characterization of the role of VAP-1 in the inflammatory activity of these diseases.

In conclusion, VAP-1 is present in the serum of healthy individuals at a level similar to those of most other soluble endothelial adhesion molecules [25]. The concentration of VAP-1 is higher in certain liver diseases than the levels of other known circulating endothelial adhesion molecules [23, 25].

## 2. Vascular adhesion protein-1 and hepatocellular cancer

Unmixed lymphocytes travel continuously throughout the body in search of antigens. Blood-borne lymphocytes leave the circulation by binding to the endothelium of specialized postcapillary high endothelial venules (HEVs) in lymph nodes, move through the tissue stroma, and later return to the circulation via efferent lypmhatics [26]. Elemental lymphocytes can freely circulate through both peripheral lymph nodes (PLNs) and mucosa-associated lymphatic tissues, which represent two functionally different re-circulatory systems. It has been known for some time that T cells immigrate and bind to PLN 2-5 times more frequently than B cells. On the contrary, B cells adhere 2-3 times more frequently than T cells to HEVs in mucosal lymphatic organs. When unmixed lymphocytes adhere to their related antigens, the migratory properties of the activated lymphocytes change dramatically. They no longer freely circulate through different lymphatic organs but instead selectively extravasate at sites of the original antigenic and in related lymphoid tissues [27].

Lymphocyte exchange between the circulation and tissues is essential for the appropriate function of the immune system. In the extravasation function, blood-borne cells make primary contacts with endothelial adhesion molecules, which may stimulate grappling, activation, entrenched binding, and finally transmigration [1, 27]. The grappling cells can be exposed to activating stimuli such as chemokines that can reinforce the integrin-dependent adhesion of leukocytes and migration through vessel walls using adhesion molecules from immunoglobulin and other super-families as well as local protease activity. Immune function is predicated on the continuous exchange of lymphocytes between the blood and tissue and is regulated by molecular interactions between the circulating lymphocytes and ligands on the surface of endothelial cells [28].

VAP-1 was described after monoclonal antibody (mAB) 1B2 immunoprecipitation, which gave a 170- to 180-kDa homodimeric sialoglycoprotein that was formed by two 90 kDa subunits, bound by disulfide bonds, with close sequence homology to the copper-dependent semicarbazide-sensitive amine oxidases (SSAO) [1, 20]. Both the transmembrane and soluble forms of VAP-1 exhibit monoamine oxidase activity [29]. A rabbit homolog of VAP-1 has been shown to function under in vivo conditions during the primary temporary interactions between endothelial and lymphoid cells [20]. VAP-1 has a large extracellular domain, a single-pass transmembrane domain, and a short cytoplasmic cauda [20].

Soluble adhesion molecules may have definite and adverse physiological effects. They may function as inhibitors of cell to cell adhesion by competing with their membrane-bound forms.

Serum measurements of VAP-1 were performed by enzyme-linked immunosorbent assay (ELISA). Blood was drawn into serum tubes and allowed to clot for at least 30 min, centrifuged at 3000 rpm for 10 min and kept frozen at -70°C [22]. Wells of microtiter plates were coated with 100 µl of the anti–VAP-1 mAb TK8-18 at 10 µg/ml in 0.1 M $NaHCO_3$ buffer (pH 9.6), stored at 4⁰Covernight, and then kept at 37°C for 1 h. The wells were washed 6 times with 0.1% Tween 20 in phosphate buffered saline (PBS) and then blocked by the addition of 200 µl of PBS containing 1% gelatin and 1% nonfat milk powder (blocking solution) for 45 min at room temperature to prevent nonspecific adsorption. After washing the wells 6 times with Tween/PBS, 175 µl of each serum sample was added to the wells, and the plates were left at room temperature for 1 h. The wells were then washed six times with Tween/PBS and incubated with 100 µl of the biotinylated anti–VAP-1 mAbTK8-14 or biotinylated control mAb Hermes-3 at room temperature for 1 h. After six washes with Tween/PBS, 100 µl of streptavidin–horseradish peroxidase was added to the wells, and the plates were allowed to incubate at room temperature again for 1 h. Thereafter, the plates were washed six times with Tween/PBS and finally developed with a chemoluminescence ELISA reagent (Boehringer Mannheim, Mannheim, Germany) according to the manufacturer's instructions. All serum samples were measured at 1:25 dilution. Each sample was measured in triplicate, and the anti–VAP-1 value was calculated by subtracting the mean background value of the negative control from the mean value of VAP-1 [23].

Each assay included a titration of the quantified tonsil lysate; this titration was used to generate a standard curve. To obtain a protein milieu similar to the serum samples, tonsil lysate standards were diluted in blocking solution that contained as much VAP-1–depleted human serum as the test samples contained patient serum. Calculations of the amount of sVAP-1 in the serum samples were made by comparing the specific VAP-1 values with a standard curve of titrated tonsil lysate using a linear regression analysis [23].

The adhesive function of VAP-1 is important in optimal oligosaccharide modifications since desialylated VAP-1 does not bind to lymphocytes [30]. The lymphocyte ligand of VAP-1 is unknown whereas the enzymatic reaction takes place independently within the rotund buried catalytic center of the molecule [31].

VAP-1 is postulated as a mediator of adhesion of effector lymphocytes to tumor vasculature. It is an endothelial adhesion molecule that is up-regulated at inflammation sites and mediates lymphocyte binding to inflamed endothelium [23].

Similar to the membrane-bound endothelial VAP-1 [1], circulating VAP-1 involves effusive sialic acid decorations (moieties). The finding of effusive sialic acid remnants in VAP-1 is especially noteworthy because the adhesive function of VAP-1 depends on its sialic acids [1]. VAP-1 is a deeply sialylated molecule that might be functionally active.

The probable biological effects of VAP-1 could affect the expression or function of other adhesion molecules in vivo or in vitro in primary endothelial cells and in liver endothelial cells. These effects of VAP-1 on the synthesis of other adhesion molecules such as fucosyltransferases or sulfotransferases might contribute to the significantly rising capability of VAP-1 transfectants to effect lymphocyte accession.

VAP-1 mediates the leukocyte subtype-specific recognition of HEVs under nonstatic conditions in humans, and hence, it represents a previously unknown method of achieving selectivity of the leukocyte-endothelial interactions in the multistep adhesion cascade. VAP-1 is able to mediate the adhesion of PLN and HEV. Moreover, VAP-1 extends the role of carbohydrate-dependent lymphocyte–endothelial cell interactions [20].

VAP-1 mediates HEV binding of lymphocytes but not of monocytes. Adhesion of T and B cells was independent of VAP-1. VAP-1 mediated oligosaccharide-dependent adhesion to endothelial cells under non-static harvest conditions [20], implying that it is involved in the adhesion cascade.

Hepatic endothelial cells are lined by specialized endothelium that supports lymphocyte adhesion and recruitment in an optimal low-shear environment [31]. Hepatic endothelium has a phenotype that is different from the endothelium of other vascular beds. In vivo hepatic endothelial cells express low levels of CD31 which are the most expansive entrapment receptors in other tissues [32]. Human hepatic endothelial cells secrete the endothelial adhesion molecule VAP-1 [33], which is major defective from non-inflamed vessels in extralymphoid organs [34]. The ability of VAP-1 to mediate sialic acid-dependent adhesion suggests that it could have a particular function in the liver by mediating shear-dependent adhesion in the selectins [15]. However, human liver endothelial cell behavior under conditions of shear stress is unknown.

VAP-1 on liver endothelium promotes lymphocyte adhesion under laminar shear stress but not in hepatic roaming in vivo [35]; VAP-1 is a mediator of lymphocyte transendothelial migration, but the capability of VAP-1 to promote adhesion and transendothelial migration is blocked by specific inhibitors of its enzyme activity [35]. Functional characterization of VAP-1 has not been conducted because the molecule is not expressed on the cell surface of human endothelial cell lines [22].

In some studies, rising levels of serum VAP-1 were found in patients with hepatocellular cancer [36, 37]. These results suggest that increasing levels of VAP-1 contribute to the elevated adhesion of lymphocytes to vascular endothelial cells on the periphery of primary liver tumors. This mechanism could increase the immune response at the tumor where other adhesion molecules involved in the multistep adhesion cascade are also elevated in primary liver tumors. The rise in VAP-1 expression is specific to liver tumors because other non-hepatic tumors are not associated with elevated levels of VAP-1.

VAP-1 expression occurs in the hepatic vascular bed [38, 39]. This occurrence suggests that some of the elements of the adhesion cascade in the hepatic vascular bed differ from those in post capillary venules.

VAP-1 mediated adhesion is consistent with the finding of VAP-1–dependent lymphocyte adhesion to rat peripheral lymph node endothelial cells transfected with human VAP-1 and with recent intravital studies where it has been shown to act as a brake for neutrophils in rabbit mesenteric blood vessels [39]. The precise nature of the adhesion mediated by VAP-1 was unclear, although the total number of adherent cells was reduced with the inhibition of VAP-1, suggesting that its receptor is active at different points in the adhesion cascade.

The inhibition of adhesion by blockade of VAP-1 had a marked inhibitory effect on lymphocyte transendothelial migration that was independent of its capability to assist adhesion. This effect was specific for VAP-1. It has also been proposed that VAP-1 mediates the transmigration of adherent leukocytes [28].

VAP-1 is a monoamine oxidase, and this functionality was demonstrated with soluble VAP-1 protein [40]. Recent reports suggest that the adhesive and enzymatic functions of VAP-1 are closely linked. Some specific inhibitors block the enzymatic activity of VAP-1, and the specific semicarbazide-sensitive amine oxidase inhibitor (SSAO), semicarbazide, and a broad-acting monoamine oxidase inhibitor, hydroxylamine, both decreased lymphocyte adhesion and transmigration. The enzymatic activity of VAP-1 is thought to be important in the adhesion of lymphocytes to VAP-1–transfected cells.

This effect was specific for hepatic endothelial cells that express VAP-1 since adhesion and transmigration of lymphocytes was observed. Other molecules have been shown to share adhesive and enzymatic properties, but VAP-1 is the only adhesion molecule with amino oxidase activity [23, 40]. The active site of the SSAO in VAP-1 may mediate adhesion via interactions with immobilized amine residues on the lymphocyte surfaces [40]. The fact that the inhibitors had a similar effect on transendothelial migration is the first demonstration of enzymatic regulation of this process.

The identification of VAP-1 as a new contact-initiating ligand suggests that it may be part of an optimal molecular pathway for regulating the specificity and multiplicity of the initial steps of lymphocyte–endothelial cell interactions.

VAP-1 may be a molecule that is template expressed in the liver tumor vasculature but down-regulated in some tumors during the growth of the malignancy or not up-regulated in some other tumors. Since VAP-1 clearly binds to the blood vessels of liver tumors, it is conceivable that the up-regulation of VAP-1 in liver tumors with a low level of VAP-1 expression may improve the treatment of hepatocellular carcinoma [20, 40, 41].

## 3. References

[1] Salmi M, Jalkanen JS. How do lymphocytes know where to go: current concepts and enigmas of lymphocyte homing. Adv Immunol 1997; 64: 139.
[2] Butcher EC. Leukocyteo-endothelial cell recıgnition: three steps to specificity and diversity. Cell 1991; 67: 1033.
[3] Springer TA. Traffic signals for lymphocyte recirculation and leukocyte emigration: the multistep paradigm. Cell 1994; 76: 301.
[4] Carlos TM, Harlan JM. Leukocyte-endothelial adhesion molecules. Blood 1994; 84: 2068.
[5] Osborn L. Leukocyte adhesion to endothelium in inflammation. Cell 1990; 62: 3.
[6] Picker L, Butcher EC. Physiological and molecular mechanisms of lymphocyte homing. Annu Rev Immunol 1992; 10: 561.
[7] Stoolman LM. Adhesion molecules controlling lymphocyte migration. Cell 1989; 56: 907.
[8] Shimizu Y, Newman W, Tanaka Y, Shaw S. Lymphocyte interactions with endothelial cells. Immunol Today 1992; 13: 106.
[9] Zimmerman GA, Prescott SM, McIntyre TM. Endothelial cell interactions with garnulocytes: tethering and signaling molecules. Immunol Today 1992; 13: 99.
[10] Kunkel EJ, Campbell JJ, Haraldsen G, Pan J, Boisvert J, Roberts AI, Ebert EC, Vierra MA, Goodman SB, Genovese MC. Lymphocyte CC chemokine receptor 9 and epithelial thymus-expressed chemokine expression of tissue specific chemokines as an organizing principle in regional immunity. J Exp Med 2000; 192: 761.
[11] Berlin C, Berg EL, Briskin MJ, Andrew DP, Kilshaw PJ, Holzmann B, Weismann IL, Hamman A, Butcher EC. Alpha-4 β7 integrin mediates binding to mucosal vascular addressin MAdCAM-1. Cell 1993; 74: 185.
[12] Picker LJ, Kishimoto TK, Smith CW, Warnock RA, Butcher EC. ELAM-1 is an adhesion molecule for skin-homing T cells. Nature 1991; 349: 796.
[13] Mehal ZW, Juedes AE, Crispe IN. Selective retention of activated CD8+ T cells by the normal liver. J Immunol 1999; 163: 3202.
[14] Hamann A, Klugewitz K, Austrup F, Jablonski-Westrich D. Activation induces rapid and profound alterations in the trafficking of T cells. Eur J Immunol 2000; 30: 3207.
[15] Doherty DG, Norris S, Madrigal-Estebas L, McEntee G, Traynor O, Hegarty JE, O'Farrely C. The human liver contains multiple populations of NK cells, T cells, and CD3+ CD56+ natural T cells with distinct cytotoxic activities and Th1, Th2, and Th0 cytokine secretion pattern. J Immunol 1999; 163: 2314.
[16] Lalor PF, Edwards S, McNab G, Salmi M, Jalkanen J, Adams DH. Vascular adhesion molecul-1 mediates adhesion and trans migration of lymphocytes on human hepatic endothelial cells. J Immunol 2002, 169: 983-992.
[17] Shields PL, Morland CM, Salmon M, Qin S, Hubscher SG, Adams DH, Chemokine and chemokine receptor interactions provide a mechanism for selective T cell recruitment to specific liver compartments within hepatitis C-infected liver. J Immunol 1999; 163: 6236.
[18] Salmi M, Adams DH, Jalkanen S. Lymphocyte trafficking in the intestine and liver. Am J Physiol 1998; 274: G1.
[19] Jaeschke H, Smith CW. Cell adhesion and migration. III. Leukocyte adhesion and transmigration in the liver vascularite. Am J physiol 1997; 273: G1169.

[20] Salmi M, Jalkanen S. Human vascular adhesion protein (VAP-1) is a unique sialoglycoprotein that mediates carbohydrate-dependent binding of lymphocytes to endothelial cells. J Exp Med 1996; 183: 569.
[21] Smith DJ, Salmi M, Bono P, Hellman J, Leu T, Jalkanen S. Cloning of vascular adhesion protein-1 (VAP-1) reveals a novel multifunctional adhesion molecule. J Exp Med 1998; 271: 500.
[22] Kemık O, Sumer A, Kemık A, Itık V, Dulger AC, Purisa S, Tuzun S. Human vascular adhesion protein-1: Serum levels of hepatocellular carcinoma in non-alcoholic and fatty liver diseases. World J Surg Oncol 2010; 8: 83.
[23] Kurkijarvi R, Adams DH, Leino R, Möttönen T, Jalkanen S, Salmi M. Circulation form of human vascular adhesion protein-1: Increased serum levels in inflammatory liver diseases. J Immunol 1998; 161: 1549-1557.
[24] Yoong KF, Hubscher SG, Adams DH. Vascular adhesion protein-1 and ICAM-1 support the adhesion of tumor-infiltrating lymphocytes to tumor endothelium in human hepatocellular carcinoma. J Immunol 1998; 160: 3978.
[25] Gearing AJH, Newman W. Circulating adhesion molecules in disease. Immunol Today 1993; 14: 506.
[26] Gowans JL, Knight EJ. The route re-circulation of lypmhocytes in rat. Proc R Soc Lond Ser B 1964; 159: 257-282.
[27] Butcher EJ. Lypmhocyte homing and homestosis. Science 1996; 272: 60-66.
[28] Salmi M, Jalkanen S. VAP-1: an adhesion and an enzyme. Trends Immunol 2001; 22: 211-216.
[29] Salmi M, Tohka S, Berg EL, Butcher EC, Jalkanen J. Vascular adhesion protein-1 mediates lymphocyte subtype-specific, selectin-independent recognition of vascular endothelium in human lymph nodes. J Exp Med 1997; 186: 589.
[30] Smith DJ, Salmi M, Bono P, Hellman J, Leu T, Jalkanen J. Cloning of vascular adhesion protein-1 reveals a novel multifunctional adhesion molecule. J Exp Med 1998; 188(1): 17-27.
[31] Adams DH, Hubscher N, Fisher C, Williams A, Robinson M. Expression E-selectin and E-selectin ligands in human liver inflammation. Hepatology 1996; 24: 533.
[32] Ley K, Tedder TF. Leukocyte interactions with vascular endothelium : new insights into selectin-mediated attachment and rolling. J Immunol 1995; 155: 525.
[33] McNab G, Reeves L, Salmi M, Jalkanen S, et al. Vascular adhesion protein-1 supports adhesion of T lymphocytes to hepatic endothelium : a mechanism for T cell recirculation to the liver? Gastroenterolgy 1996; 110: 522.
[34] Wong J, Johnston B, Lee D, et al. A minimal role for selectins in the recruitment of leukocytes into the inflamed liver microvasculature. J Clin Invest 1997; 99: 2782.
[35] Arvilommi AM, Salmi M, Jalkanen S. Organ-selective regulation of vascular adhesion protein-1 expression in man. Eur J Immunol 1997; 27: 1794.
[36] Salmi M, Jalkanen S. A 90kDa endothelial cell molecule mediating lymphocyte binding in humans. Science 1992; 257: 1407.
[37] Kukijarvi R, Yegutkin B, Gunson S, Jalkanen JS, Salmi M, Adams DH. Circulasting soluble vascular adhesion protein-1 accounts for the increased serum monoamine oxidase activity in chronic liver disease. Gastroenterology 2000; 119: 1096.
[38] Tohka S, Laukkanen, L, Jalkanen S, Salmi M. VAP-1 functions as a molecular brake during granulocyte rolling and mediates recruitment in vivo. FASEB J 2001; 15: 373.

[39] Ostermann G, Weber KS, Zernecke A, Schroder A, Weber C. JAM-1 is ligand of the beta-integrin LFA-1 involved in transendothelial migration of leukocytes. Nat Immunol 2002 3: 151.
[40] Jalkanen S, Salmi M. Cell surface monoamine oxidases: enzymes in search of a function. EMBO J 2001; 20: 3893.
[41] Salmi M, Kalimo K, Jalkanen S. Induction and function of vascular adhesion protein-1 at sites of inflammation. J Exp Med 1993; 178: 2255.

# 7

# Tissue Factor Pathway Inhibitor-2 Inhibits the Growth and Invasion of Hepatocellular Carcinoma Cells and is Inactivated in Human Hepatocellular Carcinoma

Yong Xu et al.*
*Pingshan People's Hospital, Shenzhen, Guangdong*
*P.R. China*

## 1. Introduction

Human tissue factor pathway inhibitor-2 (TFPI-2) is an extracellular matrix-associated Kunitz-type serine proteinase inhibitor that inhibits the plasmin- and trypsin-mediated activation of matrix metalloproteinases and inhibits tumor progression, invasion and metastasis. Previous studies have shown that TFPI-2 is downregulated in the progression of various tumors. Here we aim to investigate the expression and function of TFPI-2 in hepatocellular carcinoma (HCC). *In situ* hybridization and immunohistochemical analyses revealed that the expression of TFPI-2 in hepatocarcinoma tissues was markedly lower than that in tumor-adjacent normal hepatic tissues. Restored expression of TFPI-2 in $HepG_2$ cells inhibits cell proliferation and invasion. Taken together, our results suggest that TFPI-2 plays tumor-suppression function and its inactivation may contribute to HCC.

## 2. TFPI-2 expression in normal hepatic and hepatocarcinoma tissues

### 2.1 Tissue specimens

Human hepatocarcinoma tissues and tumor-adjacent normal hepatic tissues were obtained from HCC patients admitted to Shenzhen People's Hospital. They were stored frozen at -75°C until use.

### 2.2 In situ hybridization

Tumor specimens were fixed in formalin overnight and embedded in paraffin using standard procedures. Series sections (4um) were deparaffinized with xylene, rehydrated in a graded series of ethanol, and washed in PBS. Human TFPI-2 mRNA was detected using the

---

* Xiaolin Qin[2], Jinjing Zhou[2], Zhiguang Tu[2], Xiao Bi[3], Wuxian Li[2], Xiaoqing Fan[2] and Yi Zhang[3]
[1]*Pingshan People's Hospital, Shenzhen, Guangdong, P.R. China*
[2]*Key Laboratory of Laboratory Medical Diagnostics, Ministry of Education, Chongqing Medical University, Chongqing, P.R. China*
[3]*The Second Clinical Medical College, Jinan University, Shenzhen People's Hospital, Guangdong, P.R. China*

In Situ Hybridization Detection Kit (Boster, Wuhan, China) according to the manufacturer's instructions. Briefly, the sections were hybridized in prehybridization buffer supplemented with 0.1 ug/ml digoxigenin-labeled, 1.2-kb antisenese TFPI-2 probe overnight at 37°C and incubated with biotinylated mouse antidigoxigenin antibody (1:1000 dilution), then incubated with biotinylated peroxidase. Staining was developed with DAB. Slides were counterstained with hematoxylin, dehydrated, and mounted. The number of cells stained brown (indicating the presense of TFPI-2 mRNA) were assessed by light microscopy. The hybridization probe replaced with PBS was used as a negative control. Mature placenta tissue, known to express large amounts of TFPI-2, was used as a positive control.

### 2.3 Immunohistochemistry

Tissue sections were prepared in the same manner as above. Then the expression of TFPI-2 was determined by incubation with a mouse polyclonal antibody against human TFPI-2 (Santa Cruz, CA), horseradish peroxidase (HRP)-conjugated sheep anti-mouse lgG secondary antibodies (Chinagen, Shenzhen, China), and final detection using the non Biotin-labeled

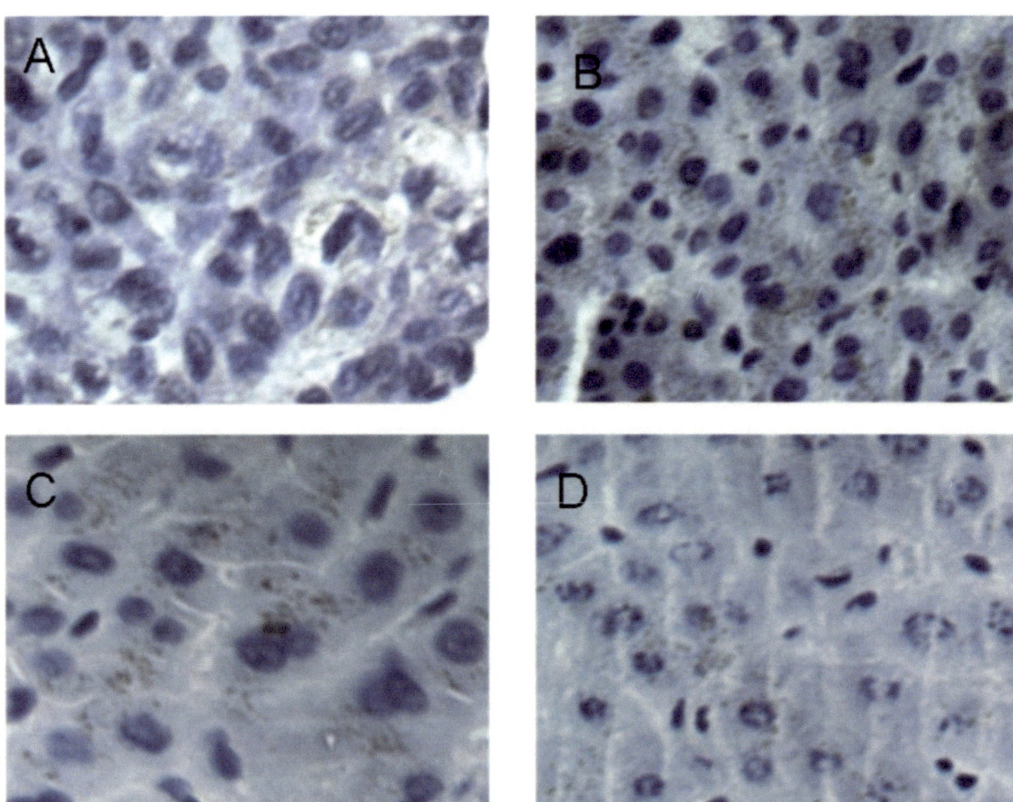


Fig. 1. TFPI-2 expression in normal hepatic and hepatocarcinoma tissues. Expression of (A) TFPI-2 mRNA in hepatocarcinoma tissue and (B) tumor-adjacent normal hepatic tissue was examined by *in situ* hybridization with a digoxigenin-labeled TFPI-2 probe. Expression of (C) TFPI-2 protein in hepatocarcinoma tissue and (D) tumor-adjacent normal hepatic tissue was examined by immunohistochemical analyses with TFPI-2 antibody. Magnification, x400.

Detection Kit (Zhongshan Goldbridge, Beijing, China) according to the manufacturer's instructions. Staining was developed with DAB, slides were counterstained with hematoxylin, dehydrated, and mounted. The primary antibody replaced with PBS was used as a negative control.Mature placenta tissue, known to express large amounts of TFPI-2,was used as a positive control.

*In situ* hybridization with TFPI-2 probe demonstrated that little or no TFPI-2 mRNA was detected in hepatocarcinoma tissue sections, while a high level of TFPI-2 mRNA was detected in tumor-adjacent normal hepatic tissue sections (Fig. 1A, B). The positive and negative controls confirmed the specifility of hybridization liquid replaced with PBS used as a negative control confirmed the absence of a specific hybridization signal (data not shown).

Further immunohistochemical analysis confirmed that TFPI-2 protein was stained strongly positive in normal hepatic tissues but was weakly stained in hepatocarcinoma tissues (Fig. 1C, D). The TFPI-2 immunostaining scores for normal hepatic tissues and hepatocarcinoma tissues were 46.60±1.80 and 22.54±1.22, respectively ($P<0.05$). Taken together, these data indicate that the expression of TFPI-2 was markedly reduced in hepatocarcinoma tissues.

## 3. TFPI-2 plasmid expression vector construct

### 3.1 TFPI-2 gene sequencing

The RNA from hepatic tissue of human fetor (Shenzhen People's Hospital) was isolated and full length TFPI-2 cDNA was amplified with RT-PCR kit (TaKaRa). The cloned gene was inserted into plasmid pcDNA2.1 (Chinagen, Shenzhen, China), and sequenced from forward and reverse direction at Shanghai Biotechnology (China), then it was inserted into eukaryotic expression vetor pcDNA3.1, a gift from Dr Tiyuan Li (Central Laboratory, Shenzhen People's Hospital) verified by enzyme digestion and sequencing.

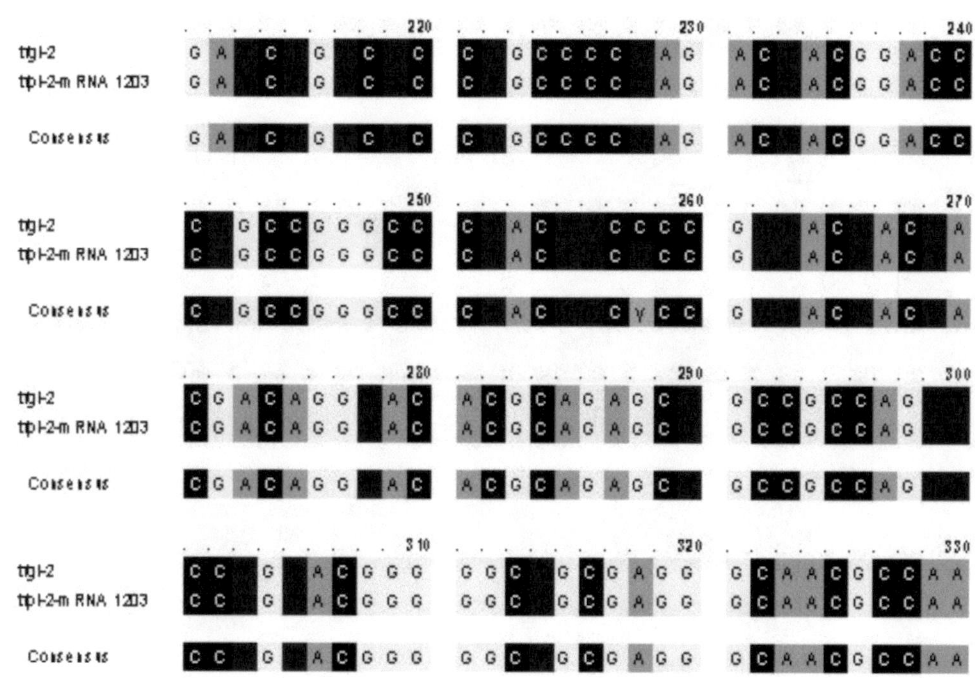

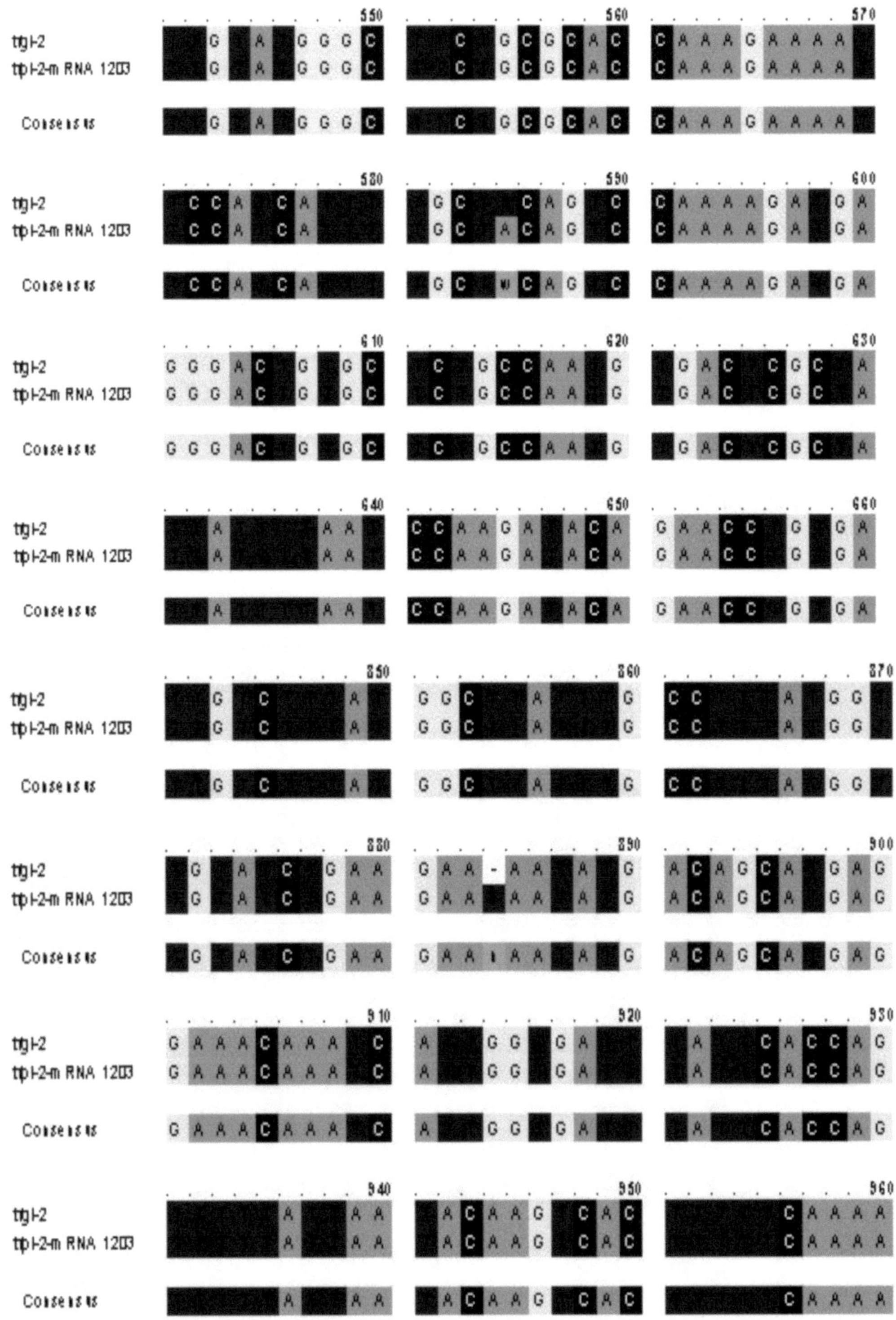

Fig. 2. Homology analysis of TFPI-2 gene

### 3.2 Plasmid construct

A 0.7-kb fragment encoding TFPI-2 cDNA was amplified from normal liver tissue with the primers 5'-GCTTTCTCGGACGCCTTGC-3' and 5'-GAATACGACCCCAAGAAATGAGTGA-3'. PCR product was purified and cloned into the BamHI and XhoI sites of the pCDNA3.1 expressing vector. The DNA sequence of the recombinant plasmid was confirmed via DNA sequencing.

The Chinese TFPI-2 gene is 1222bp. Sequencing results showed that the cloned Chinese TFPI-2 gene has three bases different (258, 585 and 884 bp) with that registered in Genbank (Fig. 2). Our sequencing results has been transmitted and accepted by Genbank, accession number is TFPI AY691946. TFPI-2 gene was inserted to eukaryotic expression vetor pcDNA3.1 successfully. The result of nucleotide sequencing confirmed that the recombinant vector pcDNA3.1-TFPI-2 was constructed accurately.

## 4. Construct $HepG_2$-TFPI-2 stable cell line

### 4.1 Cell culture and transfection

To explore the functional role of TFPI-2 in HCC, we employed $HepG_2$ cells as a model. Based on RT-PCR, we found that the expression of TFPI-2 mRNA in $HepG_2$ cells was undetected (data not shown), therefore we introduced TFPI-2 into $HepG_2$ cells by establishing $HepG_2$-TFPI-2 stable cell line.

Human hepatoma $HepG_2$ cells were obtained from Cancer Institute, Chinese Academy of Medical Sciences, and cultured in 6% $CO_2$ to 94% air and 96% humidity at 37°C in DMEM supplemented with 10% bovine calf serum (Hyclone, Logan, UT), 1.0% glutamine, 100 ug/ml strepotomycin, 100 ug/ml penicillin. The recombinant constructs or pCDNA3.1 vector was transfected into $HepG_2$ cells using Lipofectamine 2000 transfection reagent (Invitrogen) according to the manufacturer's instructions. Selection of transfected cells with 0.8 mg/ml G418 sulfate (Invitrogen) was initiated 48 h after transfection. After a 4-week selection, stable transfectants were expanded and used for the study. The $HepG_2$ cells were divided into three groups: $HepG_2$ parental cells ($HepG_2$-P), $HepG_2$ cells transfected by pCDNA3.1 vector ($HepG_2$-V) and $HepG_2$ cells transfected by TFPI-2 construct ($HepG_2$-TFPI-2).

### 4.2 RT-PCR

Total RNA was isolated from $HepG_2$ cells using TRIZOL reagent (Invitrogen) following a standard protocol. Using the 2-step RT-PCR kit (TaKaRa), cDNA was synthesized with RNA as the template. PCR amplification of human TFPI-2 and ß-actin was performed with Taq Master Mix (Promega, Madison, WI, USA) with synthesized cDNA. The primer were synthesized by Shanghai Biotechnology (China) as follows: TFPI-2 5'-ATAGGATCCACATGGACCCGCTCGC-3'
and 5'-GGCCTCGAGAAATTGCTTCTTCCGAATTTCC-3', amplicion 700 bp. ß-actin 5'-CTGGCACCACACCTTCTACAATG-3' and 5'-AATGTCACGCACGATTTCCCGC-3'. The PCR condition were: denaturing at 95°C for 30 sec, annealing at 52°C for 30 sec, and extension at 72°C for 40 sec for 32 cycles. After electrophoresis of PCR products, the data were analyzed by Image Master Tatal Laboratory ID software. The level of TFPI-2 mRNA was calculated by the ratio of density of TFPI-2 to ß-actin.

### 4.3 Western blot

$HepG_2$-P $HepG_2$-TFPI-2 and $HepG_2$-V cells were grown to 80-90% confluence in six-well plates, after which the medium was replaced with serum-free medium and incubated for 24 h. Then the cultures were washed several times with PBS and the ECM was prepared as described by Rao *et al* (15). The ECM protein were supplemented with PMSF (1 mmol/L) to inhibit the proteases. The samples was mixed with equal volume of 2×SDS sample buffer and boiled for 5 min. Equal amounts of protein were resolved on 12% sodium dodecyl sulfate (SDS)-polyacrylamid gels, and then transfected onto polyvinylidene difluoride (PVDF) membrane (Millopore). After blocking with 5% non-fat milk, the membranes were incubated, first with primary antibody at 4°C overnight and then with horseradish peroxidase (HRP)-conjugated sheep anti-mouse lgG secondary antibody. After washing, the blots were developed with a super-Enhanced Chemiluminescence Detection Kit (Applygen Technologies, Beijing, China).

By Western blot we found that a high level of TFPI-2 protein was detected in conditioned media of $HepG_2$-TFPI-2 cells but not in that of $HepG_2$-V or the $HepG_2$-P cells (Fig. 3). These results proved that we successfully introduced TFPI-2 into HepG2 cells.

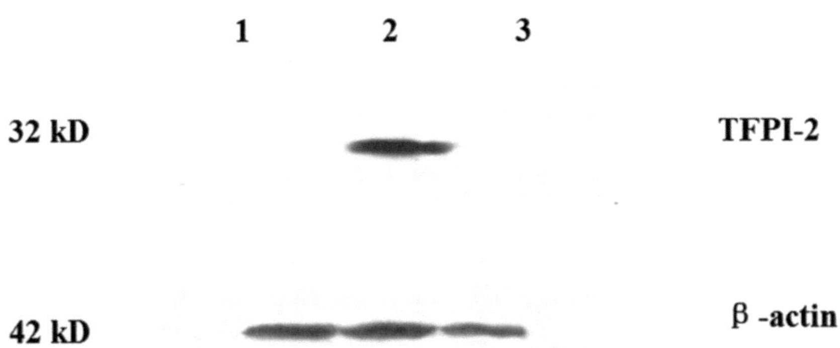


Fig. 3. Secretion of TFPI-2 in the conditioned media from $HepG_2$-TFPI-2 cells. The conditioned media were collected from lanes 1, $HepG_2$-P cells; 2, $HepG_2$-TFPI-2 cells and 3, $HepG_2$-V cells, and analyzed by Western blotting.

## 5. Cell proliferation assay

Cell proliferation was evaluated by MTT assay (sigma) according to a procedure described previously (16). In brief, every 24 h, for a total of 7 days, the cells from the three groups were harvested and 200 ul of cell suspension was added to each well in 96-well plates. A one-tenth volume of MTT solution (5 mg MTT/ml PBS) was added to each well and incubated for 2-4 h at 37°C until a purple precipitate was visible. The medium was then carefully removed, and precipitates were dissolved in 150 ul DMSO. Growth rate was plotted as the percentage of viable cells in $HepG_2$-P control (a value arbitrarily set at 100%). Each experiment was repeated at least three times with each treatment given in duplicate or triplicate. Data were presented as an average of the results from individual experiments.

We examined the effect of TFPI-2 expression on the proliferation of HepG2 cells. The viability of cells was determined by MTT assay for 7 days and cell proliferation was obviously inhibited on the fourth day in $HepG_2$-TFPI-2 cells but not in the other two groups of cells (Fig. 4). These results suggested that TFPI-2 could suppress the growth of hepatocarcinoma cells.

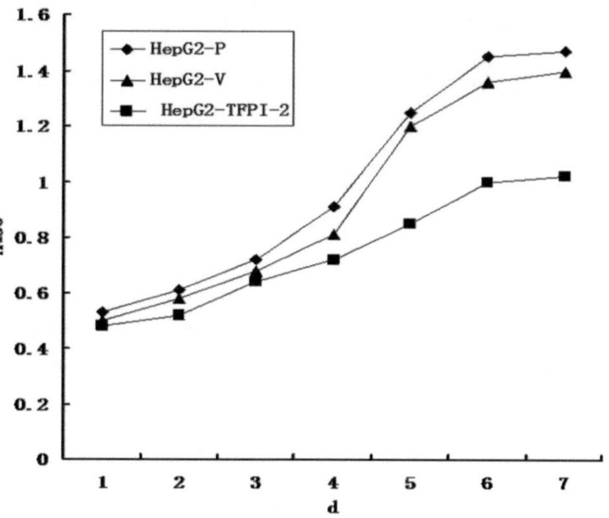


Fig. 4. The growth curve of different groups of $HepG_2$ cells ($HepG_2$-P, $HepG_2$-V and $HepG_2$-TFPI-2).

## 6. *In vitro* cell migration and invasion assay

Invasion and migration of the hepatocarcinoma cells in vitro was measured by the invasion of cells through Matrigel-coated or -uncoated transwell inserts according to a procedure described previously (17). Briefly, transwell inserts (Corning) with 8-um pore size were coated (for invasion assay) or uncoated (for migration assay) with 50 ug of Matrigel matrix (BD Biosciences). Cells suspended in serum-free DMEM medium were seeded into upper chambers (100 ul/well) at a density of 1×10^6 cells/ml (for migration assay) or 3×10^5 cells/ml (for invasion assay). The lower chambers were filled with DMEM supplemented with 10% FBS. After 24 h of incubation, cells attached to the upper side of the filter were removed, and the filters were fixed and stained with hematoxylin and eosin. At this point, there was no difference in the total number of cells (proliferation rate) among the groups in the serum-free medium. The number of cells that had migrated to the undersurface of the membrane was counted in five randomly-selected microscopic fields in each sample.

| Groups | Membranes in **matrigel invasion assay** | | | | | |
|---|---|---|---|---|---|---|
| | 1 | 2 | 3 | 4 | 5 | $\bar{x}\pm s$ |
| $HepG_2$-TFPI-2 | 45 | 53 | 39 | 48 | 41 | 49.3 ± 5.9 * |
| $HepG_2$-V | 91 | 93 | 80 | 79 | 88 | 86.2 ± 6.4 |
| $HepG_2$-P | 90 | 86 | 93 | 81 | 89 | 87.8 ± 4.5 |

| Groups | Membranes **in migration assay** | | | | | |
|---|---|---|---|---|---|---|
| | 1 | 2 | 3 | 4 | 5 | $\bar{x}\pm s$ |
| $HepG_2$-TFPI-2 | 142 | 132 | 139 | 152 | 137 | 140.4 ± 7.4 |
| $HepG_2$-V | 134 | 148 | 160 | 140 | 147 | 145.8 ± 9.8 |
| $HepG_2$-P | 150 | 166 | 159 | 142 | 147 | 152.8 ± 9.6 |

* $p< 0.05$ vs HepG2-V or HepG2-P

Table 1. In vitro invasion of different groups of HepG2 cells

We went further to examine the effect of TFPI-2 expression on the invasion of $HepG_2$ cells. Based on invasion and migration assays, we counted the cells that passed through the membranes (Table 1). The results show that the number of cells passing through the membranes was significantly lower in the $HepG_2$-TFPI-2 group than the other two groups ( $P<0.05$), indicating that TFPI-2 suppresses the invasive potential of hepatocarcinoma cells. While no significant difference in migration ability was observed in the three groups (Table 1).

## 7. Statistical analysis

All data were presented as mean±SD. Stastical analysis was performed with SPSS statistical software. The Student two-tailed *t* test was used to compare the difference between groups, $p<0.05$ was considered to be statistically significant.

TFPI-2 is a serine proteinase inhibitor which is frequently downregulated in malignant tumors (18). Previous studies have demonstrated that silencing of TFPI-2 by either histone deacetylation (19) or promoter hypermethylation contributes to its inactivation and tumor progression in several cancers including glioma (18), choricarcinoma (20), pancreatic carcinoma (17), lung carcinoma (21), breast cancer (22), melanoma (23) and hepatocarcinoma (24). In addition, the aberrant splicing form of TFPI-2 was detected during cancer progression (25), which represents an untranslated form providing another mechanism by which TFPI-2 is downregulated in tumor cells.

In this study, we investigated the expression and function of TFPI-2 in HCC. We first applied the *in situ* hybridization and immunohistochemistry methods to evaluate the expression of TFPI-2 mRNA and protein in hepatocarcinoma tissues and tumor-adjacent normal hepatic tissues. Consistent with previous studies, our results showed that TFPI-2 expression at both mRNA and protein levels was low in hepatocarcinoma tissues compared to adjacent normal hepatic tissues. These results indicated that a decreased expression of TFPI-2 is implicated in HCC.

To find the mechanism by which TFPI-2 loss contributes to HCC, we employed $HepG_2$ cells as a model. Our results demonstrate that reconstitution of TFPI-2 into $HepG_2$ cells could inhibit the proliferation and invasion of $HepG_2$ cells. Although the details for TFPI-2-mediated growth suppression are unknown, a previous study suggested that TFPI-2 induces apoptosis in glioma cells (26). Further studies are necessary to examine whether TFPI-2 promotes apoptosis of $HepG_2$ cells. In agreement with previous reports that overexpression of TFPI-2 reduced the invasion of cancer cell lines derived from melanoma (27), prostate cancer (28), choriocarcinoma (29), glioblastoma (30) or meningiomas (31), our results showed that restoration of TFPI-2 was associated with a twofold decrease in invasive ability of $HepG_2$ cells. In fact, TFPI-2 is thought to play a pivotal role in the regulation of plasmin-mediated ECM proteolysis during tumor invasion and metastasis (14). TFPI-2 inhibits the release of plasmin- or trypsin-dependent activation of pro-matrix metalloproteinase (MMP)-1 and pro-MMP-3, which leads to diminished ECM degradation and decreased invasion of HT-1080 fibrosarcoma cell lines (32, 33). In addition, TFPI-2 can inhibit MMP-2 activation in HT-1080 cells (34) and inhibit MMP-1, MMP-13, MMP-2 and MMP-9 in experimental models (35). Thus we assume that TFPI-2 inhibits HCC invasion and metastasis through modulating the activity of MMPs.

In summary, we reported that TFPI-2 expression is lost in HCC. The results of our *in vitro* studies confirm that restoration of TFPI-2 caused decreased proliferative and invasive behaviors of $HepG_2$ cells. Taken together, these data suggest that inactivation of TFPI-2 may contribute to the malignant behavior in hepatocarcinoma. Additional in vivo studies will help determine whether restoration of TFPI-2 in hepatocarcinoma cells may represent a novel therapeutic approach for HCC.

## 8. References

[1] Okuda K: Hepatocellular carcinoma: recent progress. Hepatology 15: 948-963, 1992.

[2] Enzan H, Himeno H, Iwamura S, *et al*: Alpha-smooth muscle actin-positive perisinusoidal stromal cells in human hepatocellular carcinoma. Hepatology 19: 895-903, 1994.

[3] Faouzi S, Le Bail B, Neaud V, *et al*: Myofibroblasts are responsible for collagen synthesis in the stroma of human hepatocellular carcinoma: an in vivo and in vitro study. J Hepatol 30: 275-284, 1999.

[4] Terada T, Makimoto K, Terayama N, Suzuki Y and Nakanuma Y: Alpha-smooth muscle actin-positive stromal cells in cholangiocarcinomas, hepatocellular carcinomas and metastatic liver carcinomas. J Hepatol 24: 706-712, 1996.

[5] Egeblad M and Werb Z: New functions for the matrix metalloproteinases in cancer progression. Nat Rev Cancer 2: 161-174, 2002.

[6] Stamenkovic I: Extracellular matrix remodelling: the role of matrix metalloproteinases. J Pathol 200: 448-464, 2003.

[7] Vihinen P and Kahari VM: Matrix metalloproteinases in cancer: prognostic markers and therapeutic targets. Int J Cancer 99: 157-166, 2002.

[8] Westermarck J and Kahari VM: Regulation of matrix metalloproteinase expression in tumor invasion. Faseb J 13: 781-792, 1999.

[9] Noel A, Jost M and Maquoi E: Matrix metalloproteinases at cancer tumor-host interface. Semin Cell Dev Biol 19: 52-60, 2008.

[10] Butzow R, Huhtala ML, Bohn H, Virtanen I and Seppala M: Purification and characterization of placental protein 5. Biochem Biophys Res Commun 150: 483-490, 1988.

[11] Sprecher CA, Kisiel W, Mathewes S and Foster DC: Molecular cloning, expression, and partial characterization of a second human tissue-factor-pathway inhibitor. Proc Natl Acad Sci U S A 91: 3353-3357, 1994.

[12] Miyagi Y, Yasumitsu H, Eki T, *et al*: Assignment of the human PP5/TFPI-2 gene to 7q22 by FISH and PCR-based human/rodent cell hybrid mapping panel analysis. Genomics 35: 267-268, 1996.

[13] Miyagi Y, Koshikawa N, Yasumitsu H, *et al*: cDNA cloning and mRNA expression of a serine proteinase inhibitor secreted by cancer cells: identification as placental protein 5 and tissue factor pathway inhibitor-2. J Biochem 116: 939-942, 1994.

[14] Chand HS, Du X, Ma D, *et al*: The effect of human tissue factor pathway inhibitor-2 on the growth and metastasis of fibrosarcoma tumors in athymic mice. Blood 103: 1069-1077, 2004.

[15] Rao CN, Reddy P, Liu Y, *et al*: Extracellular matrix-associated serine protease inhibitors (Mr 33,000, 31,000, and 27,000) are single-gene products with differential glycosylation: cDNA cloning of the 33-kDa inhibitor reveals its identity to tissue factor pathway inhibitor-2. Arch Biochem Biophys 335: 82-92, 1996.

[16] Tang Z, Geng G, Huang Q, *et al*: Expression of Tissue Factor Pathway Inhibitor 2 in Human Pancreatic Carcinoma and its Effect on Tumor Growth, Invasion, and Migration in vitro and in vivo. J Surg Res 2009.

[17] Sato N, Parker AR, Fukushima N, *et al*: Epigenetic inactivation of TFPI-2 as a common mechanism associated with growth and invasion of pancreatic ductal adenocarcinoma. Oncogene 24: 850-858, 2005.

[18] Konduri SD, Srivenugopal KS, Yanamandra N, *et al*: Promoter methylation and silencing of the tissue factor pathway inhibitor-2 (TFPI-2), a gene encoding an inhibitor of matrix metalloproteinases in human glioma cells. Oncogene 22: 4509-4516, 2003.

[19] Pulukuri SM, Gorantla B and Rao JS: Inhibition of histone deacetylase activity promotes invasion of human cancer cells through activation of urokinase plasminogen activator. J Biol Chem 282: 35594-35603, 2007.

[20] Hube F, Reverdiau P, Iochmann S, Rollin J, Cherpi-Antar C and Gruel Y: Transcriptional silencing of the TFPI-2 gene by promoter hypermethylation in choriocarcinoma cells. Biol Chem 384: 1029-1034, 2003.

[21] Rollin J, Iochmann S, Blechet C, *et al*: Expression and methylation status of tissue factor pathway inhibitor-2 gene in non-small-cell lung cancer. Br J Cancer 92: 775-783, 2005.

[22] Guo H, Lin Y, Zhang H, *et al*: Tissue factor pathway inhibitor-2 was repressed by CpG hypermethylation through inhibition of KLF6 binding in highly invasive breast cancer cells. BMC Mol Biol 8: 110, 2007.

[23] Nobeyama Y, Okochi-Takada E, Furuta J, *et al*: Silencing of tissue factor pathway inhibitor-2 gene in malignant melanomas. Int J Cancer 121: 301-307, 2007.

[24] Wong CM, Ng YL, Lee JM, *et al*: Tissue factor pathway inhibitor-2 as a frequently silenced tumor suppressor gene in hepatocellular carcinoma. Hepatology 45: 1129-1138, 2007.

[25] Kempaiah P, Chand HS and Kisiel W: Identification of a human TFPI-2 splice variant that is upregulated in human tumor tissues. Mol Cancer 6: 20, 2007.

[26] Tasiou A, Konduri SD, Yanamandra N, *et al*: A novel role of tissue factor pathway inhibitor-2 in apoptosis of malignant human gliomas. Int J Oncol 19: 591-597, 2001.

[27] Konduri SD, Tasiou A, Chandrasekar N, Nicolson GL and Rao JS: Role of tissue factor pathway inhibitor-2 (TFPI-2) in amelanotic melanoma (C-32) invasion. Clin Exp Metastasis 18: 303-308, 2000.

[28] Konduri SD, Tasiou A, Chandrasekar N and Rao JS: Overexpression of tissue factor pathway inhibitor-2 (TFPI-2), decreases the invasiveness of prostate cancer cells in vitro. Int J Oncol 18: 127-131, 2001.

[29] Jin M, Udagawa K, Miyagi E, *et al*: Expression of serine proteinase inhibitor PP5/TFPI-2/MSPI decreases the invasive potential of human choriocarcinoma cells in vitro and in vivo. Gynecol Oncol 83: 325-333, 2001.

[30] Yanamandra N, Kondraganti S, Gondi CS, *et al*: Recombinant adeno-associated virus (rAAV) expressing TFPI-2 inhibits invasion, angiogenesis and tumor growth in a human glioblastoma cell line. Int J Cancer 115: 998-1005, 2005.

[31] Kondraganti S, Gondi CS, Gujrati M, *et al*: Restoration of tissue factor pathway inhibitor inhibits invasion and tumor growth in vitro and in vivo in a malignant meningioma cell line. Int J Oncol 29: 25-32, 2006.

[32] Rao CN, Cook B, Liu Y, *et al*: HT-1080 fibrosarcoma cell matrix degradation and invasion are inhibited by the matrix-associated serine protease inhibitor TFPI-2/33 kDa MSPI. Int J Cancer 76: 749-756, 1998.

[33] Rao CN, Mohanam S, Puppala A and Rao JS: Regulation of ProMMP-1 and ProMMP-3 activation by tissue factor pathway inhibitor-2/matrix-associated serine protease inhibitor. Biochem Biophys Res Commun 255: 94-98, 1999.

[34] Izumi H, Takahashi C, Oh J and Noda M: Tissue factor pathway inhibitor-2 suppresses the production of active matrix metalloproteinase-2 and is down-regulated in cells harboring activated ras oncogenes. FEBS Lett 481: 31-36, 2000.

[35] Herman MP, Sukhova GK, Kisiel W, *et al*: Tissue factor pathway inhibitor-2 is a novel inhibitor of matrix metalloproteinases with implications for atherosclerosis. J Clin Invest 107: 1117-1126, 2001.

8

# Proteoglycans in Chronic Liver Disease and Hepatocellular Carcinoma: An Update

Péter Tátrai and Ilona Kovalszky
*Semmelweis University*
*Hungary*

## 1. Introduction

The last four decades witnessed a brilliant career of proteoglycans (PGs). Once regarded as mere space-fillers or passive structural components of matrices and charge-selective barriers, these fascinating molecules have been increasingly acknowledged as key players in cell-cell and cell-matrix communication, and have become recognized as modulators of most, if not all, aspects of cell behavior including survival, proliferation, and migration. Simultaneously, the range of disease processes with known involvement of PGs has steadily expanded, now covering areas as diverse as host-pathogen interactions, regulation of pathologic fibrogenesis, and tumor progression. Characteristic alterations of PGs in various human malignant tumors, including HCC, were first described more than 20 years ago (for an early review, see Tímár & Kovalszky, 1995).

PGs, glycanated proteins with extensive posttranslational modifications, consist of a protein core and one or more long, linear, sulfated polysaccharide chains, called glycosaminoglycans (GAGs). GAGs are ligated to the protein core at specific serine, threonine, or asparagine residues, although the exact signal sequences that designate the position of attachment are mostly unknown. The multifunctionality of PGs arises from their inherently complex structure: some functions are assigned to the core protein, while others are fulfilled by the GAG chains.

The synthesis of each GAG chain (recently reviewed by Ly et al., 2010) is introduced by the attachment of a short linkage region to Ser in the case of heparan sulfate (HS)/heparin and chondroitin sulfate/dermatan sulfate (CS/DS), and either Asn or Ser/Thr in the case of keratan sulfate (KS) type I and type II, respectively. During the elongation phase of GAG synthesis, acetylated hexosamine and hexuronic acid or galactose residues are added in an alternating fashion to the growing polysaccharide chain. GAGs are classified by their disaccharide composition: the dimeric building block is N-acetyl-glucosamine / glucoronic acid in HS and heparin; N-acetyl-galactosamine / glucoronic acid in CS and DS; and N-acetlyl-glucosamine / galactose in KS. Completed GAG chains then undergo various chemical modifications including *N*-deacetylation, *N*- and *O*-sulfation, and epimerization of the hexuronic acid. Heparin, for example, differs from HS in the extent of sulfation (heparin is sulfated uniformly and nearly exhaustively, whereas HS is sulfated only partially and in a patterned manner); and DS differs from CS in the degree of uronic acid epimerization (0% in CS vs. 1-100% in DS.) The extent and pattern of modifications not only vary between different GAGs and PGs, but also depend on the type and actual state of a cell, which contributes a great deal to the biological diversity of PGs. If this were still not enough of versatility, PGs may undergo further editing once they are in place: in the matrix or on the cell surface, they may be subject to the action of endoglycosidases that cleave the GAG chain, proteases that cut the protein core, and endosulfatases capable of removing sulfate groups from internal sugar residues.

Historically, PGs were sorted by the type of their GAG chain into one of the categories HSPG, CS/DSPG, or KSPG. Later, however, the discovery that several PGs carry more than one type of GAG (i.e., syndecans and betaglycan carry both HS and CS; aggrecan carries both CS and KS II) prompted a new classification based on structure and tissue localization. In this revised system, each PG belongs to one of three major families: 1) small leucine-rich proteoglycans or SLRPs; 2) modular PGs, further divided into a) hyalectans or hyaluronan-binding PGs and b) non-hyaluronan-binding PGs of the basement membrane; and 3) cell surface PGs. Nevertheless, both the old and new classifications fall short of being perfect; neither is free of overlaps, and neither can properly accommodate, for example, serglycin or endocan. In this review, we shall follow a sort of "hybrid" classification that fits best for our purposes.

A complete listing of all currently known PGs seems unnecessary here (for a comprehensive review, the Reader is referred to Esko et al., 2009); this paper is restricted in scope to PGs present in the healthy or diseased liver, and will concentrate on those involved in, or affected by, chronic liver disease and hepatocarcinogenesis. Also, with a focus on human disease, PGs reported to be present in the liver of experimental animals but not of humans will be omitted.

## 2. Proteoglycans in the liver

The healthy liver is a dominantly parenchymatous organ with relatively scarce stroma. Consequently, cell surface PGs expressed by hepatocytes are considerably more abundant than matrix PGs, either small or modular. Chronic liver diseases, on the other hand, are hallmarked by the accumulation of connective tissue, and PGs, along with other matrix constituents, become massively deposited as fibrosis progresses. Hepatocarcinogenesis is accompanied by further alterations in liver PG profile. These disease-associated changes are reflected in gene expression levels (i.e., of PG core proteins and GAG synthesis / modification enzymes), in the abundance and/or localization of PGs, and in the quantity and structure of GAGs in the tissue. Specific PGs present in the healthy or diseased liver, their pathology-related changes, as well as known or proposed functions in liver physiology or disease, are listed concisely in **Table 1** (on pages 3-4), and discussed in detail in the following sections.

### 2.1 SLRPs

The family of SLRPs, extracellular PGs characterized by relatively small (approx. 30-70 kDa) core proteins with leucine-rich repeats and conserved cysteine-containing motifs, currently counts 18 members divided into 5 classes (Schaefer & Iozzo, 2008; Schaefer & Schaefer,

| | Healthy liver | | Chronic liver disease | | | HCC | | | |
|---|---|---|---|---|---|---|---|---|---|
| | Localization | Main physiological roles | Localization | Rel. expr. | Proposed role | Localization | Rel. expr. | Proposed role | Prognostic significance |
| *SLRPs* | | | | | | | | | |
| Decorin | CV, PT CT, sin w | regulation of collagen fibrillogenesis and TGFβ signaling | fibrotic CT, sin w | ↑ | antifibrotic | stroma | ↓ | antitumor | |
| Biglycan | | regulation of TGFβ signaling; endogenous TLR ligand | fibrotic CT, sin w | ↑ | | | | | |
| *Modular HSPGs* | | | | | | | | | |
| Perlecan | all BMs, sin w, sin ECs, PT MCs, BV w | migration, proliferation, differentiation, angiogenesis | all BMs, sin w, BV w, fibrotic CT | ↑ | | vascular w | ↑ | pro-angiogenic | |
| Agrin | BD BM, PT BV w | postsynaptic differentiation, immune cell communication, cytoskeletal organization | BD BM, PT BV w | ↑ | | vascular w | ↑ | pro-angiogenic? | |
| Collagen type XVIII / endostatin | all BMs, sin w, BV w | BM organization, angiogenesis | hep, activated HSCs; all BMs, sin w↑, BV w | ↑ | | tu hep?, vascular w | ↑↓ | anti-angiogenic? | debated - high or low expr. ~ adverse progn.? |
| *Cell membrane HSPGs* | | | | | | | | | |
| Syndecan-1 | hep | Common roles of syndecans: cytoskeletal and ECM organization; cell-cell and cell-ECM interactions; co-receptor function | hep | ↑ | HBV, HCV coreceptor ??? | tu hep | ↑↓ | enhances migration; inhibits EMT | reduced expr. ~ high metastatic potential |
| Syndecan-2 | PT MCs | | | | | stromal MCs | ↑ | | |
| Syndecan-3 | PT BV ECs, HSCs | | activated HSCs, MΦs | ↑ | | BV w, ECs | | | |
| Syndecan-4 | hep | | | | | tu hep | ↑ | enhances migration | |

| | | | | | | | | | |
|---|---|---|---|---|---|---|---|---|---|
| Glypican-3 | not expressed | regulation of growth factor signaling (Wnt, Hh, IGF) | not expressed | | | tu hep | ↑ | enhances tu cell growth & migration | high expr. ~ adverse progn. |
| *Other cell membrane PGs* | | | | | | | | | |
| Betaglycan | | co-receptor for TGFβ family members | activated HSCs | ↓ | | | ↓ | tumor suppressor | high expr. ~ lower grade |
| CD44(v3) | hep (weak) | receptor for hyaluronan and other ECM components | activated progenitors | ↑ | regeneration | tu hep (cancer stem cells?) | ↑ | enhances metastasis | high expr. ~ vascular invasion |
| Neuropilin-1 | sin ECs, PT BV Ecs | axonal guidance; co-receptor for VEGFs | sin ECs; activated HSCs | ↑ | pro-fibrotic | tu BV ECs, tu hep | ↑ | pro-angiogenic? | |
| *Hyalectans* | | | | | | | | | |
| Versican | | | activated HSCs? | | | | | | |
| *Secreted PGs* | | | | | | | | | |
| Endocan | not expressed | enhances HGF signaling | not expressed | | | tu BV ECs, tu hep | ↑ | pro-angiogenic, enhances tu invasion & growth | high tu expr. & serum levels ~ adverse progn. |
| PG-100 | weakly expressed | | reactive ductules | ↑ | | | | | |

Abbreviations: BD, bile duct; BM, basement membrane; BV, blood vessel; CT, connective tissue; CV, central vein; EC, endothelial cell; EMT, epithelial-to-mesenchymal transition; HBV/HCV, hepatitis B/C virus; HSC, hepatic stellate cell; HSPG, heparan sulfate PG; MC, mesenchymal cell; MΦ, macrophage; PT, portal tract; rel. expr., expression relative to normal liver tissue; sin, sinusoid(al); SLRP, small leucine-rich PG; tu, tumor(al); w, wall

Table 1.

2010). While most SLRPs carry CS/DS or KS chains, some of them are non-classical PGs lacking GAG chains altogether, and can thus be considered as "honorary" members of the PG superfamily that have been grouped together with SLRPs on the basis of structural and functional homology. So far, only three SLRPs were found in the liver: decorin, the prototypical member of the family; biglycan; and asporin, a non-canonical, GAG-less relative of the former two. Whereas reports leave ambiguity regarding the mere presence of asporin (its mRNA was abundant in the human liver but undetectable in mice) (Lorenzo et al., 2001; Henry et al., 2001), decorin has been widely implicated in liver fibrogenesis, and may also play a role in the regulation of hepatocellular carcinoma (HCC) growth. Knowledge on biglycan in the liver is much more limited; nevertheless, mentioning will be made of it.

*Decorin*, the archetypal SLRP, is glycanated with a single CS/DS chain, and was originally described as a regulator of collagen fibrillogenesis. Later, an increasingly complex picture has emerged: decorin was found to modulate the signaling of transforming growth factor-β1 (TGF-β1), a key stimulator of fibrogenesis, and it also became evident that decorin establishes contacts with multiple receptor tyrosine kinases (RTKs) such as epidermal growth factor receptor (EGFR), insulin-like growth factor-I receptor (IGF-IR), and Met (Iozzo & Schaefer, 2010). Decorin has a broad tissue distribution, being most abundant in the skin, connective tissues, muscles, and the kidney (Kalamajski & Oldberg, 2010).

In the healthy liver, strong decorin immunoreaction is solely seen in the Glisson's capsule, with some positive labeling around central veins, and only delicate, spot-like extracellular staining in the periportal connective tissue and, occasionally, in sinusoidal walls. In the course of chronic liver injury, however, decorin accumulates in the areas of periportal and bridging fibrosis, and becomes increasingly deposited in sinusoidal walls as capillarization ensues. Co-localization studies suggest association of decorin with collagen fibers, and its interaction with TGF-β1 (Dudás et al., 2001).

Decorin can directly bind and sequester TGF-β1, or indirectly influence its effect via association with the LRP-1 receptor (Cabello-Verrugio & Brandan, 2007). While the net outcome of these interactions depends on the cell type, decorin seemed to inhibit TGF-β1-dependent fibroblast proliferation and matrix production in the context of experimental renal fibrogenesis (Isaka et al., 1996). Importantly, decorin exerted a similar inhibitory effect on a human hepatic stellate cell (HSC) line *in vitro* (Shi et al., 2006). Since activated hepatic stellate cells are the major culprits in liver fibrosis, decorin might limit worsening of the condition, and the use of decorin as a TGF-β1 blocking agent for the treatment of chronic liver disease has been repeatedly proposed (Breitkopf et al., 2005). A recent report provides indirect support to this approach, demonstrating increased susceptibility to thioacetamide-induced fibrogenesis, and impaired recovery from established fibrosis in decorin-null mice (Baghy et al., 2011). The absence of decorin, with consequently higher activity of TGF-β1, not only increased fibrogenesis but also impeded resolution of fibrosis by interfering with matrix metalloprotease action. However, the transferability of these results to human liver fibrosis is unclear. At least, massive accumulation of decorin in the course of chronic liver disease indicates that, even if interpreted as a defense mechanism, overexpression of decorin is largely inefficient in preventing fibrosis. Being itself upregulated by TGF-β1 in HSCs (Baghy et al., 2011), the deposition of decorin in the connective tissue is more likely a by-product of fibrogenesis rather than a protective reaction against it.

While little is known about the involvement of decorin in hepatic carcinogenesis, available studies unequivocally assign an antitumor role to decorin in HCC. Decorin has been reported to be downregulated in HCC tissue relative to the normal liver (Miyasaka et al., 2001; Chung et al., 2002), and it became re-expressed in the HCC cell line SMMC-7721 upon knockdown of DNA methyltransferase 1 (Fan et al., 2007), indicating active repression by the tumor cells. Moreover, decorin was found to inhibit proliferation of HuH7 cells in a concentration-dependent manner (Shangguan et al., 2009), and killed xenografted HCC cells via adenoviral gene transfer (Tralhão et al., 2003). These findings are in good agreement with the general view that decorin, via its suppressive interactions with TGF-β1 and RTKs, and upregulation of p21, attenuates cell proliferation, possibly curbs angiogenesis, and thus inhibits both primary growth and metastatic spread of tumors (Goldoni & Iozzo, 2008). However, an expected inverse correlation between decorin expression and aggressive behavior of HCC still waits to be demonstrated.

*Biglycan*, another class I member SLRP, was found to be produced by activated HSCs during rat and human fibrogenesis (Gressner et al., 1994), and it is strongly deposited in fibrotic areas along with decorin (Högemann et al., 1997). Biglycan, like decorin, is also known to interact with members of the TGFβ/BMP family (Schaefer & Iozzo, 2008); however, up to now, no mechanistic details of its contribution to liver disease have been revealed.

### 2.2 Modular and cell surface HSPGs

Just like SLRPs span multiple classes of the old PG nomenclature, HSPGs cross the borders of the new classification, with some members belonging to the non-hyaluronan-binding modular group and others to the cell surface group. However, the many common features they share owing to their HS chains speak for the conservation of the traditional HSPG category.

HSPGs are by far the most thoroughly studied representatives of the PG superfamily. This distinctive attention is all but unmerited: due to the incredibly broad spectrum of their functions, HSPGs permeate all fields of mammalian physiology (for a comprehensive review, see Bishop et al., 2007). The paradigm that GAGs can specifically bind extracellular mediators such as growth factors and cytokines, regulate their availability and activity, and assist their binding to primary receptors, has been derived from the study of HS, and knowledge on other GAGs in this respect is still lagging behind. The interaction of HS with fibroblast growth factors (FGFs) and their receptors has been characterized in greatest detail (Pellegrini, 2001), but a host of other heparin-/HS-binding growth factors and mediators have been identified (Dreyfuss et al., 2009). HS synthesis, structure, function, and modifications have been extensively reviewed elsewhere (for references, see Esko et al., 2009); hence, only a brief outline is provided here.

Following synthesis of the *N*-acetyl-glucosamine/glucuronic acid (GlcNAc/GlcUA) copolymer, the prospective heparin/HS molecule undergoes extensive modifications. GlcUA residues may be epimerized into iduronic acid (IdoUA); *N*-acetyl groups may be removed and replaced by N-sulfates; and further sulfates may be transferred to the 6-*O* and 3-*O* positions on GlcN, as well as to the 2-*O* position of IdoUA. These modifications are carried out by epimerase, *N*-deacetylase-sulfotransferases (NDSTs), and position-specific *O*-sulfotransferases (OSTs), respectively; some of these enzymes have several isoforms.

Whereas epimerized, *N*-, 2-*O*- and 6-*O*-sulfated disaccharides are predominant and uniformly distributed in heparin, HS is characterized by the alternation of unmodified (*N*-acetylated) and modified (*N*-sulfated) regions, the latter being flanked by partially modified transition zones. The rarest modification in both heparin and HS is 3-*O*-sulfation which, however, is indispensable for important biological functions such as antithrombin binding (Chen & Liu, 2005). Unlike heparin, native HS has little anticoagulant activity; on the other hand, it possesses a delicate fine structure that is pivotal in determining its specificity and affinity towards potential binding partners. Consequently, even subtle alterations in the sulfation pattern of HS may substantially affect its biological properties.

HS may be further shaped post-synthetically by the action of heparanase, a secreted endoglucuronidase capable of cleaving the polysaccharide in a limited fashion, and the SULFs, endosulfatases removing 6-*O*-sulfate groups from specific disaccharide motifs. Since these enzymes also modulate the growth factor binding properties of HS, their activities have broad implications for tumor growth, angiogenesis, and metastasis.

Of course, HSPGs possess a protein core, too, which may participate in a number of interactions. The complex modular structure of matrix HSPGs warrants their involvement in intricate protein networks within the matrix as well as between matrix and cells; thus, they often occupy a bridging position between the matrix and cell surface. Transmembrane HSPGs may similarly establish contacts with the matrix, but may also associate with other cell surface receptors or recruit cytoskeletal and signaling proteins via their cytoplasmic domain (Mythreye & Blobe, 2009).

### 2.2.1 Modular HSPGs of the basement membrane: Perlecan, agrin, and collagen type XVIII

*Perlecan.* This large HSPG, consisting of numerous modules grouped into five major domains, is secreted into the pericellular space. Perlecan, ubiquitously found in basement membranes (BMs) and other extracellular matrices, is strategically positioned to mediate signaling events related to cell migration, proliferation, and differentiation. Most of its functions are assigned to the HS chains capable of binding growth factors, but the modular protein core also participates in numerous cell-matrix and matrix-matrix interactions (Whitelock et al., 2008).

Perlecan was detected in the healthy liver in all BMs, including those of bile ducts and blood vessels; even in the poorly organized BM of sinusoids. Endothelial cells, portal mesenchymal cells, and arterial walls were also immunopositive for perlecan (Roskams et al., 1995). Accumulation of perlecan in chronic liver disease is mainly attributable to ductular reaction and sinusoidal capillarization, although perlecan appears not only in BMs but diffusely in connective tissue septa (Roskams et al., 1996; Kovalszky et al. 1998). In HCC, robust perlecan immunostaining labels the vasculature of the tumor (Roskams et al., 1998).

The role of perlecan in the pathomechanism of chronic liver diseases and HCC has not been investigated. Data on the role of perlecan in fibrogenesis are missing altogether, and inferences regarding HCC can be drawn from studies on other cancer types only. Perlecan plays a central role in both developmental and pathologic angiogenesis (Iozzo & Sanderson, 2011). Intriguingly, perlecan can either stimulate or inhibit angiogenesis by two entirely distinct mechanisms. Its stimulatory role is primarily explained by the high capacity of its

HS chains to bind vascular endothelial growth factor (VEGF) and FGF-2, two major proangiogenic factors. Deposited around tumor cells and in capillary basement membranes, perlecan is ideally situated to support neovessel growth. Perlecan is supposed to act in concert with heparanase that liberates bound growth factors from its HS chains, or alone by cross-linking VEGF receptor with integrins on the surface of endothelial cells. The antiangiogenic effect, on the other hand, is exerted by a C-terminal proteolytic fragment of perlecan, termed endorepellin. Binding of endorepellin to $\alpha_2\beta_1$-integrin, a master matrix receptor of endothelial cells, triggers disruption of the cytoskeleton and blocks endothelial migration and survival. This dual nature of perlecan notwithstanding, both experimental and clinical data indicate that the proangiogenic role dominates in human malignancies, and perlecan promotes progression of various tumor types including carcinomas of the breast, prostate, and colon, as well as metastatic melanoma (Bix & Iozzo, 2008). Although the role of perlecan in HCC progression has not yet been specifically addressed, it is tempting to speculate that it may favor neovessel growth in this hypervascular tumor type.

*Agrin.* Another large HSPG with complex domain structure, agrin shares some homology with perlecan, but possesses many unique features and is probably less ubiquitous in the body. One peculiarity of agrin is the existence of both secreted and membrane-bound isoforms. Agrin was first described as organizer of the postsynaptic receptor apparatus in neuromuscular junctions, and was subsequently shown to play a similar role in the central nervous system. It was later found in the renal glomerular basement membrane, on the surface of immune cells, and in the blood-brain barrier (Bezakova & Ruegg, 2003).

In the healthy liver, agrin is so scarce that it was understandably missed on the first survey (Gesemann et al., 1998). No sooner than its accumulation in cirrhosis and HCC raised attention could the purposeful quest find some agrin in the walls of portal blood vessels and in the BM of bile ducts (Tátrai et al., 2006). Similar to perlecan, increased deposition of agrin during chronic liver injury is associated with ductular reaction and neovessel formation in the connective tissue septa; however, in contrast with perlecan, no diffuse agrin immunostaining is seen in fibrotic areas, and agrin is virtually absent from all sinusoids, either healthy or capillarized. In HCC, agrin is deposited in a pattern similar to that of perlecan, i.e. in the wall of tumoral blood vessels. Since agrin, unlike perlecan, is missing from normal and cirrhotic sinusoids, the appearance of agrin in microvascular walls is a useful immunohistochemical marker of malignant hepatocellular transformation (Tátrai et al., 2009). To date, no mechanistic or clinical data are available on the role of agrin in HCC, or in tumor biology as a whole. With only *a priori* knowledge at hand, a proangiogenic role can be hypothesized, based on agrin's structural and functional similarities with perlecan, including the ability of its HS chains to bind growth factors and the possible interactions of its core protein with integrin receptors (Burgess et al., 2002).

*Collagen type XVIII*, a ubiquitous BM-HSPG (reviewed by Iozzo et al., 2009; Seppinen & Pihlajaniemi, 2011) combines features of collagens and modular PGs. Three variant forms of collagen type XVIII result from alternative transcription initiation sites and splicing. The shortest one is found in most vascular, muscle fiber and epithelial BMs as well as in various ocular structures, whereas the two long variants are expressed predominantly in the liver. Despite its widespread presence in vascular BMs, collagen XVIII does not seem to be essential for blood vessel development; rather, its mutations lead to malformations of the eye and the central nervous system. Main functions of collagen XVIII are linked to its role in maintaining the structural integrity of BMs, especially those in the eye, as well as to the anti-angiogenic effect of its C-terminal proteolytic fragment termed endostatin. Endostatin (O'Reilly et al., 1997), a potent endogenous inhibitor of angiogenesis, can be liberated from full-length collagen XVIII by matrix proteases, and interferes with virtually every step of the angiogenic process. It curbs proliferation and migration of endothelial cells and promotes their apoptosis; impedes the recruitment of pericytes; and reduces mobilization of endothelial progenitor cells into the circulation. The mechanism of action of endostatin is complex, involving multiple pathways such as $\alpha_5\beta_1$-integrin-, VEGFR-, and Wnt/β-catenin signaling (Seppinen & Pihlajaniemi, 2011). External administration of endostatin, either as recombinant protein or in the form of gene therapy, has been shown to suppress growth of numerous animal and xenografted human tumor types including HCC (Folkman, 2006).

As mentioned above, collagen XVIII is abundant in the healthy liver, where it is deposited both perisinusoidally and in BM zones of bile ducts, blood vessels, and peripheral nerves (Musso et al., 1998). Unlike most other extracellular matrix (ECM) proteins which are produced primarily by HSCs, collagen XVIII in the normal liver mostly originates from hepatocytes. Liver parenchymal cells produce both long variants under liver-specific transcriptional control; interestingly, variant #2 is secreted into the plasma rather than retained in the sinusoidal BM. Non-parenchymal cells such as bile duct epithelial, endothelial, and vascular smooth muscle cells express the short, ubiquitous variant (Musso et al., 2001a). Activated HSCs step on the stage in active fibrosis, and short collagen XVIII becomes a major component of remodeled BM in capillarized sinusoids; then, in quiescent cirrhosis, hepatocytes once again take over the primacy in collagen XVIII synthesis.

It seems proven that HCC cells initially maintain or even increase their expression of long collagen XVIII, and stromal cells continue to produce short collagen XVIII in HCC (Musso et al., 2001a, 2001b). Controversy exists, on the other hand, as to whether collagen XVIII levels in tumor hepatocytes increase or decrease with HCC progression. While some authors demonstrate that high tumoral expression of collagen XVIII correlates with increased VEGF activity and poor prognosis (Hu et al., 2005), others argue that, as it can be expected of an angiogenesis suppressor, collagen XVIII becomes downregulated by HCC cells in parallel with increasing tumor size, microvessel density, and clinical aggressiveness (Musso et al., 2001b). Since long collagen XVIII variants are regulated by liver-specific transcription factors, it has been suggested that their downregulation may reflect the loss of hepatocytic phenotype. It has also been proposed that decreased tumoral expression of the longest (#3) variant may favor progression by allowing higher activation of the Wnt/β-catenin pathway (Quélard et al., 2008). Variant #3 possesses a domain homologous to the Wnt-receptor frizzled which, when cleaved off proteolytically, localizes to the cell surface and blocks Wnt/β-catenin activation by sequestering Wnt3a. Thus, downregulation of variant #3 may relieve this block and allow enhanced tumor growth. Moreover, in further support of decreased tumoral expression of collagen XVIII, higher levels of endostatin were found in adjacent liver tissue relative to HCC in a tissue array-based immunohistochemical study (Yu et al., 2010).

### 2.2.2 Cell surface HSPGs: Syndecans and glypicans

*Syndecans.* All four members of this transmembrane cell surface HSPG family (reviewed by Xian et al., 2010) share highly conserved membrane-spanning domains and cytoplasmic regions, while their extracellular domains are divergent. Syndecans play prominent roles in cell-cell and cell-ECM interactions including cell adhesion, as well as in matrix organization and assembly. Via their intracellular domain they can communicate with actin-associated and signaling molecules; some of their intracellular partners are PDZ domain-containing proteins. Unlike giant multimodular HSPGs, the core protein of syndecans is rather small, ranging between 20-40 kDa. Besides HS chains, syndecan-1 and -3 may also bear CS/DS GAGs. The extracellular domain of syndecans may be cleaved off proteolytically and solubilized in a process referred to as ectodomain shedding, which is effected by matrix metalloproteinases (Couchman, 2010).

Of the four family members, syndecan-1, a ubiquitous epithelial membrane HSPG, is the most abundant in the healthy liver. Syndecan-1 is robustly expressed on hepatocytes, resulting in a primarily sinusoidal and, to a lesser extent, lateral membrane-associated immunostaining pattern. Syndecan-1 is also present on biliary epithelial cells, with basolateral accentuation, and on sinusoidal but not on portal vessel endothelial cells (Roskams et al., 1995).

Endocytic clearance of triglyceride-rich lipoprotein remnants, a major metabolic task of hepatocytes, is mediated by HS as a receptor, and syndecan-1 has been identified as the primary HSPG involved in this process (Stanford et al., 2009; Williams & Chen, 2010). Cell surface HS is also a main clue for pathogens in the recognition of their host cells and in endocytic entry (Y. Chen et al., 2008). *Plasmodium* sporozoites dock on hepatocytes using HS receptors (Pinzon-Ortiz et al., 2001); it has been suggested that blood-borne sporozoites are literally "filtered out" by liver-specific, highly sulfated HS structures (Pradel et al., 2002; Coppi et al., 2007). Furthermore, HSPGs act as receptors or co-receptors for obligate and facultative hepatotropic viruses including dengue, hepatitis B, C, and E viruses (Hilgard & Stockert, 2000; Barth et al., 2003; Schulze et al., 2007; Kalia et al., 2009). The previously established role of HS in adenoviral infection of the liver is currently a matter of debate (Di Paolo et al., 2007; Bradshaw et al., 2010; Corjon et al., 2011). Being the major liver cell membrane HSPG, syndecan-1 may plausibly turn out to be the key mediator in most hepatocyte-pathogen interactions, although at least one study has shown that syndecan-1 is dispensable for murine liver infection by *Plasmodium yoelii* (Bhanot & Nussenzweig, 2002). Theoretically, as being also expressed by hepatocytes, syndecan-4 might overtake some of the roles of syndecan-1, although it is present in minor amounts only and in a distinct, bile canalicular localization (Roskams et al., 1995).

Syndecan-2, also called fibroglycan, is a mesenchymal-type syndecan. As such, it is produced by mesenchymal cells of the portal tract, but not by quiescent HSCs (Roskams et al., 1995). Syndecan-3, despite its general reputation as a neuronal syndecan, was also detected immunohistochemically in the normal liver, where it was localized to the endothelial lining of portal blood vessels, as well as to HSCs in the sinusoids (Roskams et al., 1995).

The quantity and distribution of syndecans is affected in several ways by chronic liver disease. Regenerative hepatocytes in chronic cholestatic disease show increased syndecan-1 expression which, accompanied by a relative gain in lateral membrane localization, results in an almost honeycomb-like immunostaining pattern (Roskams et al., 1996). Similar alterations occur in cirrhosis (Tátrai et al., 2010). Additionally, reactive ductules also exhibit strong syndecan-1 immunoreaction. Syndecan-3 is intensely seen in activated HSCs and macrophages. Disturbed polarity of hepatocytes is indicated not only by a less restricted localization of syndecan-1, but also by the dispersion of granular syndecan-4 immunostaining originally concentrated around the bile canalicular pole (Roskams et al., 1996).

In most HCCs, the honeycomb pattern of syndecan-1 immunostaining is preserved, and the overall intensity is increased relative to the normal liver (Roskams et al., 1998). However, syndecan-1 may be gradually silenced in parallel with tumor progression, and reduced expression of syndecan-1 has been shown to correlate with high metastatic potential (Matsumoto et al., 1997). Downregulation of syndecan-1 during the progression of epithelial cancers is a common phenomenon which, especially when accompanied by simultaneous loss of E-cadherin, is thought to indicate epithelial-to-mesenchymal transition (Iozzo & Sanderson, 2011). Loss of tumor cell syndecan-1 expression in carcinomas, occasionally combined with aberrant stromal expression of the same protein, is typically considered as a predictor of poor prognosis (for references, see Máthé et al., 2006). Stromal syndecan-1 in HCC has not been reported, but abnormal cytoplasmic, or even nuclear, staining in tumor cells was observed. Unlike syndecan-1, syndecan-2 in HCC appears on stromal mesenchymal cells, and syndecan-3 in vessel walls and on endothelial cells. Syndecan-4 is strikingly enhanced in HCC, with some tumor cells showing intense and diffuse cytoplasmic immunostaining.

The functions of syndecans in chronic liver disease and HCC are largely unknown. Upregulation and increased shedding of syndecan-1 is characteristic of wound healing (Manon-Jensen et al., 2010), and fibrosis is a process analogous to wound healing in many aspects. Indeed, the amount of syndecan-1 ectodomains shed into the serum has been reported to reflect the severity of fibrosis (Zvibel at al., 2009). Additionally, it can be speculated that enhanced and broadened expression of syndecan-1 on the surface of hepatocytes may facilitate entry of hepatitis viruses, and thus create a positive feedback loop that may contribute to the perpetuation of infection in the fibrotic/cirrhotic liver (András Kiss, personal communication).

The role of syndecan-1 in tumorigenesis and tumor progression is contradictory, and varies with tumor stage and type: it is downregulated in some carcinomas (e.g., certain breast cancers) but overexpressed by other tumors (e.g., pancreatic cancers, myelomas) (Manon-Jensen et al., 2010). Based on an *in vitro* study performed with multiple HCC cell lines, it has been proposed that syndecan-1 and -4 may assist in the binding of the chemokine CCL5/RANTES, and thus promote migration and invasion of tumor cells (Charni et al., 2009).

*Glypicans.* The glypican family (reviewed by Filmus et al., 2008) consists of six glycosyl-phosphatidylinositol-anchored HSPGs with relatively small (555-580 amino acid) core proteins, and HS chains located close to the cell surface. Glypicans may also shed from the cell surface (and hence appear in the serum), and may undergo proteolytic cleavage. The main function of glypicans lies in regulating the signaling of Wnts, Hedgehogs (Hh's), FGFs, and bone morphogenetic proteins (BMPs). Research has mostly been focused on glypican-3, luckily for us, since this is the only member of the family with true relevance to the liver. Glypican-3 exerts opposite effects on Wnt and Hh pathways: it facilitates binding of Wnts to frizzled and increases signaling, whereas it competes with patched for Hh binding, and directs Hh toward endocytic breakdown, leaving smoothened and its signal cascade inactive (Filmus et al., 2008).

In the liver, glypican-3 behaves as an oncofetal antigen: it is expressed in the fetal but not in the adult liver, and becomes re-expressed in hepatocytes upon malignant transformation only. Quite intriguingly, although glypican-3 appears to be a negative regulator of growth during development and regeneration of the liver (Liu et al., 2009, 2010), and its forced expression suppresses hepatocyte proliferation in mice (Lin et al., 2011), glypican-3 is nearly uniformly overexpressed in human liver cancers, and glypican-3-positive HCCs have significantly worse prognosis when compared to the relatively few glypican-3-negative cases (Shirakawa et al., 2009). In fact, glypican-3 has recently emerged as one of the most promising immunocytochemical, immunohistochemical and serum markers of HCC. Glypican-3, in combination with other markers, has been shown to facilitate detection of early HCC both in biopsies and from the serum (Roskams & Kojiro, 2010; Malaguarnera et al., 2010).

Glypican-3 is thought to promote HCC progression through multiple mechanisms. Overexpression of glypican-3 in HCC was not only found to correlate with enhanced nuclear localization of β-catenin (indicating its role as a stimulator of Wnt signaling), but also with increased expression of matrix metalloproteinases, members of the FGF signaling pathway, and SULF2 (Akutsu et al., 2010). Oncogenic potential of GPC-3 may be related to its ability to stimulate IGF-II / IGF-1R interaction, too (Cheng et al., 2008). Activation of all the above-mentioned molecules and pathways had been observed previously in HCC, and hypotheses can now be formulated as to whether and how they are mechanistically related to the upregulation of glypican-3. Yet it is difficult to foresee at the moment how the supposed anti-proliferative and pro-oncogenic effects of glypican-3 can be consolidated into a single self-consistent theory. Also, while some important details of the transcriptional regulation of glypican-3 have been elucidated (Morford et al., 2007), the basis for its re-activation in HCC remains to be investigated.

### 2.2.3 Enzymes involved in HS synthesis and modification

As chronic liver diseases and HCC bring about profound alterations in HSPG synthesis, it is logical to expect accompanying changes in the levels and/or activities of enzymes involved in HS synthesis and modification. Moreover, it has been demonstrated that besides a rise in its quantity, the fine structure (and, consequently, the biological activity) of HS also becomes altered in HCC (Dudás et al., 2000). So far, however, very little attention has been directed toward the expression and activity of NDSTs and OSTs (the enzymes transferring sulfates on the nascent HS chain) in the healthy and diseased liver. The role of heparanase and SULFs in HCC progression has apparently attracted more interest.

*NDSTs and OSTs.* NDSTs substitute the acetyl group with sulfate on glucosamine, while OSTs place sulfates on selected disaccharide units at the 6-*O*- and 3-*O*-positions of glucosamine, as well as at the 2-*O*-position of the uronic acid. *N*-sulfation, uronic acid epimerization, and *O*-sulfation are not independent steps; rather, they follow a hierarchy suggested by the above order (Murphy et al., 2004). Both NDST isoforms NDST-1 and -2 have been reported to be present and enzymatically active in the healthy liver, although NDST-2 does not seem to contribute to HS sulfation (Ledin et al., 2006). Out of the many 2-, 3- and 6-OSTs, only a few isoforms have been detected in the normal liver (Shworak et al., 1999). The relative neglect of these enzymes in research is probably unjust, as they make key contributions to the synthesis of functional liver HS. Specifically, *N*- and 2-*O*-sulfated (and probably also 6-*O*-sulfated) HS is necessary for remnant lipoprotein uptake (Stanford et al., 2010; K. Chen et al., 2010), and various highly sulfated HS motifs are required for the interaction of parenchymal cells with pathogens such as *Plasmodium* sporozoites or hepatitis B and C viruses (Barth et al., 2006; Coppi et al., 2007; Schulze et al., 2007). Suppressed NDST expression in diabetes has been suggested to impair lipoprotein uptake and thus worsen dyslipidemia (Williams et al., 2005).

Both NDST isoforms, as well as 3-OST-1 and 6-OST-1 have been found to be overexpressed in fibrotic liver diseases and HCC. The enzymes 2-OST-1 and 3-OST-3B, on the other hand, were highly expressed in the normal liver but not significantly upregulated in disease (Tátrai et al., 2010). Although the clinicopathologic significance of these alterations are unknown, it can be speculated that overexpression of 3-OST-1, the 3-OST isoform most potent in the synthesis of anticoagulant HS (Girardin et al., 2005), coupled with release of liver HS into the bloodstream by heparanase, may contribute to the coagulopathy observed in some cirrhotic patients. Altered HS structure created by hyperactive 3-OSTs may also influence signaling pathways involved in oncogenesis.

*Heparanase* (reviewed by Levy-Adam et al., 2010) is an endo-β-D-glucuronidase capable of cleaving HS chains in a limited fashion. Fragmentation of HS by heparanase (HPSE) breaks the integrity of the ECM and BMs, and mobilizes bound growth factors. Such remodeling of the ECM is generally thought to promote multiple steps of tumor progression including angiogenesis, invasion, and metastasis. Hence, it is not surprising that high expression of HPSE is an unfavorable prognostic factor in most tumor types (Barash et al, 2010). In fact, the mechanism of action of HPSE in tumors is much more complex and goes beyond growth factor mobilization. E.g., increased HPSE activity enhances syndecan-1 shedding, either directly or via induction of MMP-9; moreover, it influences clustering, PKCα-mediated signaling, and internalization of syndecan-1 (Yang et al., 2007; Fux et al., 2009). HPSE also stimulates the production of hepatocyte growth factor (HGF) in an enzymatic activity-independent fashion. Shed syndecan-1 may form active complexes with HGF, and further potentiate tumor growth (Ramani et al., 2011). Additional non-enzymatic effects of HPSE include enhanced Erk phosphorylation, as well as activation of the AKT and EGFR pathways (Fux et al., 2009).

HPSE is detected in the developing liver, but not in the healthy adult organ. It becomes induced, however, during liver regeneration (Goldshmidt et al., 2004), and elevated HPSE mRNA levels were measured in fibrogenic liver diseases (Tátrai et al., 2010), although other studies have found no difference in the amount of HPSE protein between normal liver tissue and cirrhosis (Xiao et al., 2003; G. Chen et al., 2008). Despite its overall pro-oncogenic profile, literature data are equivocal on the role of HPSE in HCC progression (for a recent review, see Dong & Wu, 2010). The majority of papers report on the elevation of HPSE mRNA and/or protein in HCC relative to both adjacent non-tumorous and normal liver tissue, and most investigations have found significant positive correlation between tumoral HPSE levels, HCC progression, and adverse prognosis. In some studies, however, the levels of HPSE mRNA were found to be decreased in HCC when compared to adjacent non-cancerous tissue (Ikeguchi et al., 2002, 2003), and mean HPSE mRNA expression was shown to be elevated in HCC relative to the healthy liver but lower than in fibrogenic diseases (Tátrai et al., 2010). In explanation of a supposed tumor-inhibitory effect it has been proposed that, as opposed to the stimulatory effect of moderate HPSE activity, excessive HS fragmentation by HPSE may be detrimental to FGF-2 signaling and may therefore lead to increased apoptosis rates (Ikeguchi et al., 2003; Dong & Wu, 2010).

*SULFs* (reviewed by Bret et al., 2011) are secreted endosulfatases that remove specific 6-*O*-sulfates from HS. Both SULF1 and SULF2 have broad tissue distribution in the healthy human organism (Morimoto-Tomita et al., 2002). Although they catalyze the same reaction and possess similar substrate specificities, the two enzymes appear to exert distinct effects. In mice, Sulf2 can complement the lack of Sulf1 during embryonic development, whereas Sulf2-knockout animals are born with severe central nervous system defects and die by day 14 postnatally (Kalus et al., 2009). Such differences in regulation and mechanism of action may explain the surprising observation that SULF1 and SULF2 act oppositely in the process of tumorigenesis: unlike SULF1 that is generally regarded as a tumor suppressor, SULF2 is a pro-oncogenic endosulfatase overexpressed in several tumor types including HCC (Bret et al., 2011).

In the healthy liver, SULF1 mRNA is expressed at low levels; SULF2 mRNA is approx. 10 times more abundant. On the other hand, while average SULF2 mRNA levels are only slightly increased during chronic liver disease and HCC, SULF1 mRNA is robustly overexpressed in both conditions (Tátrai et al., 2010). Nevertheless, SULF1 has been proven to behave as a suppressor of HCC growth both *in vitro* and *in vivo*. By desulfating HS, it inhibits the co-receptor function of HSPGs in multiple heparin-binding growth factor – tyrosine kinase receptor pathways, and forced overexpression of SULF1 in HCC cell lines results in delayed xenograft growth (Lai et al., 2008a). While SULF1 is downregulated in 30% of resected HCCs only, it was found to be silenced in 82% of established HCC cell lines (Lai et al., 2008b). This discrepancy between primary tumors and cell lines can possibly be explained by selection bias associated with *in vitro* culturing.

SULF2, as a contrast, was found to be upregulated in 8/11 (72%) HCC cell lines and approx. 60% of primary tumors, and patients with the highest SULF2 expression had significantly worse prognosis (Lai et al., 2008c). SULF2 enhances FGF-2 signaling, thereby promoting tumor cell growth and migration. Moreover, SULF2 upregulates both glypican-3 and Wnt3a expression of cancer cells, and facilitates release of Wnt3a from glypican-3 by desulfating its HS chains; the outcome is boosted Wnt/β-catenin signaling (Lai et al., 2010).

### 2.3 Other transmembrane PGs

Membrane-spanning PGs other than syndecans include betaglycan, melanoma chondroitin sulfate proteoglycan (also known as CSPG4), neuropilin-1, and the variant forms of CD44 (Couchman, 2010). Similar to syndecans, these transmembrane PGs may also interact with a plethora of extracellular partners; further, although their short intracytoplasmic domains lack intrinsic enzymatic activity, they may recruit cytoskeleton-associated and signaling molecules, often via their PDZ binding site. Since CSPG4, despite its discovery in several human tissues and cancer types after melanoma, has not been identified in the liver, it is omitted from our discussion.

*Betaglycan*, also referred to as type III TGFβ receptor, can be substituted with either HS or CS/DS (Couchman, 2010). As its alternate name indicates, betaglycan acts as a co-receptor for members of the TGFβ family. Like neuropilin-1 (see below), betaglycan also has a close relative, endoglin, which shares sequence homology, some details of domain structure, and related functions with betaglycan, but lacks attached GAG (Bernabeu et al., 2009). Betaglycan seems to be implicated in epithelial-to-mesenchymal transition (EMT), and betaglycan-null mouse embryos die *in utero* due to multiple malformations involving the heart and the liver (Stenvers et al., 2003). Paradoxically, while betaglycan is required to sustain TGFβ signaling in embryonic cells undergoing EMT, it is silenced by most neoplastic cells embarking on the same process (Bernabeu et al., 2009). On the whole, betaglycan is considered as a suppressor of cancer progression that inhibits tumor cell migration, proliferation, invasion, and tumor angiogenesis; accordingly, it becomes downregulated in many human malignancies (Gatza et al., 2010).

Although betaglycan expression of the healthy human liver tissue has not been investigated, it was shown to be expressed by cultured human and rat HSCs and myofibroblasts, and its mRNA levels decreased during transition from HSC to myofibroblast (Weiner et al., 1996; Meurer et al., 2005). In line with its accepted role as a tumor suppressor, expression of betaglycan mRNA was found to be reduced in 7/10 HCCs relative to the corresponding normal liver tissues, and its levels were inversely correlated with tumor grade (Bae et al., 2009).

*CD44*, a ubiquitous cell surface receptor of hyaluronan and other ECM components, is expressed in numerous variant forms (reviewed by Sackstein, 2011). Part of its diversity stems from a strikingly complex genomic structure: the human CD44 gene, besides 10 'standard' exons, contains 9 functional 'variant' exons that can be alternatively spliced. Additionally, CD44 may undergo extensive posttranslational modifications, comprising the attachment of CS/DS, KS, and - in the presence of the v3 exon - also HS chains (van der Voort et al., 1999; Sackstein, 2011). The smallest form of CD44, termed CD44s, lacks all variant exons, and it is primarily expressed on cells of hematopoietic origin, including stem and progenitor cells, and mature but naïve lymphocytes. The larger, GAG-bearing variants (CD44v forms) appear on normal and cancerous epithelia, as well as on activated and malignantly transformed hematopoietic cells (Sackstein, 2011). A role for CD44 in tumor progression has long been suggested (Naor et al., 1997). More recently, standard and variant CD44 forms have been recognized as cancer stem cell markers (Keysar & Jimeno, 2010), and CD44 is among the genes that identify liver cancer stem cells (Liu et al., 2011).

In the normal liver, only few hepatocytes were observed to exhibit weak membrane expression of CD44 (Endo & Terada, 2000). Elevated CD44 mRNA levels were measured in chronic liver diseases where the liver progenitor cell population is activated. High CD44 mRNA expression was restricted to progenitor cells and reactive ductules, indicating that CD44 is a 'stemness' marker not only for cancer stem cells, but for non-malignant liver progenitors, too (Spee et al., 2010).

Standard and variant forms of CD44 were upregulated in approx. half of HCCs investigated. High expression of CD44 on tumor cells was found to be associated with vascular invasion, and correlated with poorer disease outcome (Mathew et al., 1996; Endo & Terada, 2000). In an *in vitro* study, v3-containing, HS-decorated CD44 variants, but not the forms lacking the v3 exon, have been demonstrated to confer metastatic phenotype to an otherwise non-metastatic HCC cell line, SKHep1 (Barbour et al., 2003). Therefore, high expression of CD44, and of CD44v3 in particular, might be positively correlated with a dominance of 'stem-like' character and aggressive behavior of HCC cells.

*Neuropilin-1* (NRP1) is a single-span transmembrane PG glycosylated with HS or CS/DS (Couchman, 2010). Just like its non-PG relative neuropilin-2, NRP1 has first been described as a co-receptor for class 3 semaphorins, soluble signal molecules implicated in axonal guidance and vascular patterning (Adams & Eichmann, 2010). Later, neuropilins have also been identified as accessory receptors of VEGFs. NRP1 affects VEGFR signaling in a way that enhances migration and survival of endothelial cells, modulates vascular permeability, and stimulates angiogenesis (Koch et al., 2011).

During development, NRP1 is broadly expressed in the vasculature, preferentially in arteries (Koch et al., 2011). In the adult liver, NRP1 immunostaining positively labels both sinusoidal and portal vessel endothelial cells, but not the hepatocytes (Bergé et al., 2011). When sinusoidal endothelium is subjected to increased shear stress, either *in vitro* or during liver regeneration following partial hepatectomy, NRP1 becomes upregulated in concert with other proangiogenic factors such as VEGF and angiopoetin-1 (Kraizer et al., 2001; Braet et al., 2004). NRP1 is also induced in HSCs upon activation, and has been shown to promote progression of fibrosis by stimulating platelet-derived growth factor- (PDGF-) dependent chemotaxis and TGFβ-mediated matrix deposition of myofibroblasts (Cao et al., 2010).

In HCC, NRP1 expression is seen not only in endothelial cells of tumoral vessels, but - in approx. 50% of cases, and with variable intensity - in tumor hepatocytes, too. The significance of tumor cell NRP1 is unclear, but blocking NRP1-VEGF interaction was shown to inhibit vascular remodeling and growth of primary murine HCC (Bergé et al., 2011).

### 2.4 Hyalectans

Hyalectans are hyaluronan- and lectin-binding PGs of the ECM. They all share a tridomain structure, with the central domain carrying the majority of GAG chains (the number of which varies from 3 in brevican up to 100 in aggrecan), and the N- and C-terminal domains making contact with hyaluronan and lectins, respectively (Schaefer & Schaefer, 2010). Strategically positioned around hyaluronan, a principal ECM component, hyalectans regulate matrix assembly, and mediate a plethora of cell-ECM interactions. The group currently counts four members: versican, aggrecan, neurocan, and brevican.

Although the CS/DSPG versican is expressed throughout the body, is known to regulate a multitude of cellular processes, and has been reported to contribute to the progression of several tumor types (Ricciardelli et al., 2009; Theocharis et al., 2010), no specific investigations have been targeted to versican in the liver, except for a single study where versican was detected in activated rat HSCs (Szende et al., 1992). With respect to the liver, even less is known about aggrecan, a CS/KSPG primarily found in cartilage and brain, and the CSPGs brevican and neurocan which have never been observed outside of the central nervous system (Theocharis et al., 2010).

### 2.5 Secreted PGs: Endocan and PG-100

Secreted PGs are 'odd one outs' in the new classification of PGs, being neither anchored to the cell surface nor immobilized in the ECM. *Endocan* (Béchard et al., 2001), or endothelial cell-specific molecule-1 (ESM-1), is a soluble PG by default which is secreted by endothelial cells directly into the bloodstream. Production of endocan by endothelial cells is boosted by both inflammatory and pro-angiogenic mediators; endocan, in turn, enhances HGF signaling. Endocan has been shown to be overexpressed in several human tumor types, and elevated serum levels in late-stage cancer patients is regarded as an adverse prognostic factor (Abid et al., 2006; Sarrazin et al., 2006).

| | Proposed effect | Therapeutic action | Reference | Level of evidence |
|---|---|---|---|---|
| Decorin | antifibrotic | The protein inhibits matrix production of activated HSCs | Shi et al., 2006 | in vitro |
| | antitumor | The protein inhibits proliferation of HuH7 cells | Shangguan et al., 2009 | in vitro |
| | antitumor | Adenovirus-mediated gene transfer exhibits oncolytic activity on xenografted HCC | Tralhão et al., 2003 | in vivo |
| Collagen type XVIII / endostatin | antitumor | Adenovirus-mediated delivery of endostatin inhibits HCC xenograft growth | Li et al., 2004 | in vivo |
| | antitumor | Adeno-associated virus-mediated delivery of endostatin reduces growth and vascularization of HCC xenograft | Liu et al., 2005 | in vivo |
| | antitumor | Forced expression of endostatin in xenografted HCC cells potentiates the action of doxorubicin | Liu et al., 2007 | in vivo |
| Syndecan-1 and -4 | antitumor | Knockdown reduces CCL5/RANTES-dependent migration of HCC cells | Charni et al., 2009 | in vitro |
| Glypican-3 | antitumor | Humanized antibodies to GPC3 evoke NK-mediated ADCC of HCC cells (phase I clinical trial recruiting) | Ishiguro et al., 2008 | in vivo |
| | antitumor | A GPC3-derived peptide vaccine sensitizes CTLs against HCC cells | Yoshikawa et al., 2011 | phase I clinical trial |
| SULF1 | antitumor | Forced expression inhibits HCC xenograft growth and potentiates the effect of HDAC inhibitors | Lai et al., 2006 | in vivo |
| Neuropilin-1 | antifibrotic | Knockout or silencing decreases motility of activated HSCs | Cao et al., 2010 | in vitro / in vivo |
| | antitumor | Blocking inhibits growth and vascular remodeling of primary murine HCC | Bergé et al., 2011 | in vivo |
| Endocan | antitumor | Silencing inhibits growth and migration of HCC cells | Kang et al., 2011 | in vitro |

Table 2. Proteoglycans in future therapies of chronic liver disease

Endocan is differentially expressed in the endothelium of HCC blood vessels, being absent from the sinusoids of both peritumoral non-malignant and healthy liver tissue; thus, immunohistochemistry for endocan helps visualize HCC vasculature (Huang et al., 2009). Endocan-positive microvessel density (MVD), unlike CD34-positive MVD, was shown to be predictive of poor survival, and high expression of endocan by tumoral endothelial cells correlated with the angiogenic and invasive potential of the tumor (Huang et al., 2009; L. Y. Chen et al., 2010). In a recent study, endocan production by tumoral hepatocytes has also been reported, and silencing of endocan has been shown to inhibit tumor cell growth and migration *in vitro* (Kang et al., 2011).

*PG-100* is the PG form of macrophage colony-stimulating factor and, as such, is a 'part-time' PG that may exist in a GAG-less or CS/DS-substituted form, the latter exhibiting less than 1% of cytokine activity compared with the non-PG variant (Schwarz et al., 1990; Partenheimer et al. 1995). PG-100 was first discovered in the conditioned medium of osteosarcoma cells, and later found to be produced by other cell types including endothelia (Nelimarkka et al., 1997). PG-100 was only faintly immunostained in the normal liver, whereas in active fibrosis it was strongly visualized in bile duct epithelia, and thus proposed as a marker of ductular reaction (Högemann et al., 1997). The significance of this elevated expression remains to be clarified.

## 3. Outlook: PGs in future therapies of chronic liver disease and HCC

PGs are emerging therapeutic targets in inflammatory, fibrogenic and malignant diseases. As a summary to this review, in **Table 2** we have collected some (however, by no means all) current attempts to exploit the multiple actions of PGs for countering the progression of chronic liver disease and HCC. Such experiments may involve delivery of PGs with supposed therapeutic effect, inhibition of those known to promote the pathologic process, modulation of HS structure, or application of HS-mimicking molecules. Some PGs expressed in the liver may be well-studied therapeutic targets in other organs or tumor types (e.g. perlecan, heparanase), yet have not been included in the list because their therapeutic potential has not been addressed specifically in the context of liver disease. The level of evidence (*in vitro, in vivo*) is also indicated in the table.

Therapeutic approaches targeting glypican-3 have reached closest to human application; some phase I clinical trials have been completed or are underway. Several other PGs show remarkable promise, but these apparently have a longer way ahead.

## 4. Acknowledgement

Publication of this article was supported by the grants Nos. 67925 and 100904 from the Hungarian Scientific Research Fund (OTKA).

## 5. References

Abid, M. R., Yi, X., Yano, K., Shih, S. C. & Aird, W. C. (2006). Vascular endocan is preferentially expressed in tumor endothelium. *Microvascular Research*, Vol.72, No.3, (November 2006), pp. 136-145, ISSN 0026-2862

Adams, R. H. & Eichmann, A. (2010). Axon guidance molecules in vascular patterning. *Cold Spring Harbor Perspectives in Biology*, Vol.2, No.5, (May 2010), a001875, ISSN 1943-0264

Akutsu, N., Yamamoto, H., Sasaki, S., Taniguchi, H., Arimura, Y., Imai, K. & Shinomura, Y. (2010). Association of glypican-3 expression with growth signaling molecules in hepatocellular carcinoma. *World Journal of Gastroenterology*, Vol.16, No.28, (July 2010), pp. 3521-3528, ISSN 1007-9327

Bae, H. J., Eun, J. W., Noh, J. H., Kim, J. K., Jung, K. H., Xie, H. J., Park, W. S., Lee, J. Y. & Nam, S. W. (2009). Down-regulation of transforming growth factor beta receptor type III in hepatocellular carcinoma is not directly associated with genetic alterations or loss of heterozygosity. *Oncology Reports*, Vol.22, No.3, (September 2009), pp. 475-480, ISSN 1021-335X

Baghy, K., Dezso, K., Laszlo, V., Fullar, A., Peterfia, B., Paku, S., Nagy, P., Schaff, Z., Iozzo, R. V. & Kovalszky, I. (2011). Ablation of the decorin gene enhances experimental hepatic fibrosis and impairs hepatic healing in mice. *Laboratory Investigation*, Vol.91, No.3, (March 2011), pp. 439-451, ISSN 1530-0307

Barash, U., Cohen-Kaplan, V., Dowek, I., Sanderson, R. D., Ilan, N. & Vlodavsky, I. (2010). Proteoglycans in health and disease: new concepts for heparanase function in tumor progression and metastasis. *FEBS Journal*, Vol.277, No.19, (October 2010), pp. 3890-3903, ISSN 1742-4658

Barbour, A. P., Reeder, J. A., Walsh, M. D., Fawcett, J., Antalis, T. M. & Gotley, D. C. (2003). Expression of the CD44v2-10 isoform confers a metastatic phenotype: importance of the heparan sulfate attachment site CD44v3. *Cancer Research*, Vol.63, No.4, (February 2003), pp. 887-892, ISSN 0008-5472

Barth, H., Schafer, C., Adah, M. I., Zhang, F., Linhardt, R. J., Toyoda, H., Kinoshita-Toyoda, A., Toida, T., Van Kuppevelt, T. H., Depla, E, Von Weizsacker, F., Blum, H.E. & Baumert, T. F. (2003) Cellular binding of hepatitis C virus envelope glycoprotein E2 requires cell surface heparan sulfate. *The Journal of Biological Chemistry*, Vol.278, No.42, (October 2003), pp. 41003-41012, ISSN 0021-9258

Barth, H., Schnober, E. K., Zhang, F., Linhardt, R. J., Depla, E., Boson, B., Cosset, F. L., Patel, A. H., Blum, H. E. & Baumert, T. F. (2006). Viral and cellular determinants of the hepatitis C virus envelope-heparan sulfate interaction. *Journal of Virology*, Vol.80, No.21, (November 2006), pp. 10579-10590, ISSN 0022-538X

Bechard, D., Gentina, T., Delehedde, M., Scherpereel, A., Lyon, M., Aumercier, M., Vazeux, R., Richet, C., Degand, P., Jude, B., Janin, A., Fernig, D. G., Tonnel, A. B. & Lassalle, P. (2001). Endocan is a novel chondroitin sulfate/dermatan sulfate proteoglycan that promotes hepatocyte growth factor/scatter factor mitogenic activity. *The Journal of Biological Chemistry*, Vol.276, No.51, (December 2001), pp. 48341-48349, ISSN 0021-9258

Berge, M., Allanic, D., Bonnin, P., de Montrion, C., Richard, J., Suc, M., Boivin, J. F., Contreres, J. O., Lockhart, B. P., Pocard, M., Levy, B. I., Tucker, G. C., Tobelem, G. & Merkulova-Rainon, T. (2011). Neuropilin-1 is upregulated in hepatocellular carcinoma and contributes to tumour growth and vascular remodelling. *Journal of Hepatology*, (February 2011), doi:10.1016/j.jhep.2011.01.033, ISSN 0168-8278

Bernabeu, C., Lopez-Novoa, J. M. & Quintanilla, M. (2009). The emerging role of TGF-beta superfamily coreceptors in cancer. *Biochimica et Biophysica Acta*, Vol.1792, No.10, (October 2009), pp. 954-973, ISSN 0006-3002

Bezakova, G. & Ruegg, M. A. (2003). New insights into the roles of agrin. *Nature Reviews Molecular Cell Biology*, Vol.4, No.4, (April 2003), pp. 295-308, ISSN 1471-0072

Bhanot, P. & Nussenzweig, V. (2002). Plasmodium yoelii sporozoites infect Syndecan-1 deficient mice. *Molecular and Biochemical Parasitology*, Vol.123, No.2, (August 2002), pp. 143-144, ISSN 0166-6851

Bishop, J. R., Schuksz, M. & Esko, J. D. (2007). Heparan sulphate proteoglycans fine-tune mammalian physiology. *Nature*, Vol.446, No.7139, (April 2007), pp. 1030-1037, ISSN 1476-4687

Bix, G. & Iozzo, R. V. (2008). Novel interactions of perlecan: unraveling perlecan's role in angiogenesis. *Microscopy Research and Technique*, Vol.71, No.5, (May 2008), pp. 339-348, ISSN 1059-910X

Bradshaw, A. C., Parker, A. L., Duffy, M. R., Coughlan, L., van Rooijen, N., Kahari, V. M., Nicklin, S. A. & Baker, A. H. (2010). Requirements for receptor engagement during infection by adenovirus complexed with blood coagulation factor X. *PLoS Pathogens*, Vol.6, No.10, (2010), pii: e1001142. ISSN 1553-7374

Braet, F., Shleper, M., Paizi, M., Brodsky, S., Kopeiko, N., Resnick, N. & Spira, G. (2004). Liver sinusoidal endothelial cell modulation upon resection and shear stress in vitro. *Comparative Hepatology*, Vol.3, No.1, (September 2004), p. 7, ISSN 1476-5926

Breitkopf, K., Haas, S., Wiercinska, E., Singer, M. V. & Dooley, S. (2005). Anti-TGF-beta strategies for the treatment of chronic liver disease. *Alcoholism, Clinical and Experimental Research*, Vol.29, No.11 Suppl, (November 2005), pp. 121S-131S, ISSN 0145-6008

Bret, C., Moreaux, J., Schved, J. F., Hose, D. & Klein, B. (2011). SULFs in human neoplasia: implication as progression and prognosis factors. *Journal of Translational Medicine*, Vol.9, (2011), p. 72, ISSN 1479-5876

Burgess, R. W., Dickman, D. K., Nunez, L., Glass, D. J. & Sanes, J. R. (2002). Mapping sites responsible for interactions of agrin with neurons. *Journal of Neurochemistry*, Vol.83, No.2, (October 2002), pp. 271-284, ISSN 0022-3042

Cabello-Verrugio, C. & Brandan, E. (2007). A novel modulatory mechanism of transforming growth factor-beta signaling through decorin and LRP-1. *The Journal of Biological Chemistry*, Vol.282, No.26, (June 2007), pp. 18842-18850, ISSN 0021-9258

Cao, S., Yaqoob, U., Das, A., Shergill, U., Jagavelu, K., Huebert, R. C., Routray, C., Abdelmoneim, S., Vasdev, M., Leof, E., Charlton, M., Watts, R. J., Mukhopadhyay, D. & Shah, V. H. (2010). Neuropilin-1 promotes cirrhosis of the rodent and human liver by enhancing PDGF/TGF-beta signaling in hepatic stellate cells. *Journal of Clinical Investigation*, Vol.120, No.7, (July 2010), pp. 2379-2394, ISSN 1558-8238

Charni, F., Friand, V., Haddad, O., Hlawaty, H., Martin, L., Vassy, R., Oudar, O., Gattegno, L., Charnaux, N. & Sutton, A. (2009). Syndecan-1 and syndecan-4 are involved in RANTES/CCL5-induced migration and invasion of human hepatoma cells. *Biochimica et Biophysica Acta*, Vol.1790, No.10, (October 2009), pp. 1314-1326, ISSN 0006-3002

Chen, G., Dang, Y. W., Luo, D. Z., Feng, Z. B. & Tang, X. L. (2008). Expression of heparanase in hepatocellular carcinoma has prognostic significance: a tissue microarray study. *Oncology Research*, Vol.17, No.4, (2008), pp. 183-189, ISSN 0965-0407

Chen, J. & Liu, J. (2005). Characterization of the structure of antithrombin-binding heparan sulfate generated by heparan sulfate 3-O-sulfotransferase 5. *Biochimica et Biophysica Acta*, Vol.1725, No.2, (September 2005), pp. 190-200, ISSN 0006-3002

Chen, K., Liu, M. L., Schaffer, L., Li, M., Boden, G., Wu, X. & Williams, K. J. (2010). Type 2 diabetes in mice induces hepatic overexpression of sulfatase 2, a novel factor that suppresses uptake of remnant lipoproteins. *Hepatology*, Vol.52, No.6, (December 2010), pp. 1957-1967, ISSN 1527-3350

Chen, L. Y., Liu, X., Wang, S. L. & Qin, C. Y. (2010). Over-expression of the Endocan gene in endothelial cells from hepatocellular carcinoma is associated with angiogenesis and tumour invasion. *The Journal of International Medical Research*, Vol.38, No.2, (March-April 2010), pp. 498-510, ISSN 0300-0605

Chen, Y., Gotte, M., Liu, J. & Park, P. W. (2008). Microbial subversion of heparan sulfate proteoglycans. *Molecules and Cells*, Vol.26, No.5, (November 2008), pp. 415-426, ISSN 1016-8478

Cheng, W., Tseng, C. J., Lin, T. T., Cheng, I., Pan, H. W., Hsu, H. C. & Lee, Y. M. (2008). Glypican-3-mediated oncogenesis involves the Insulin-like growth factor-signaling pathway. *Carcinogenesis*, Vol.29, No.7, (July 2008), pp. 1319-1326, ISSN 1460-2180

Chung, E. J., Sung, Y. K., Farooq, M., Kim, Y., Im, S., Tak, W. Y., Hwang, Y. J., Kim, Y. I., Han, H. S., Kim, J. C. & Kim, M. K. (2002). Gene expression profile analysis in human hepatocellular carcinoma by cDNA microarray. *Molecules and Cells*, Vol.14, No.3, (December 2002), pp. 382-387, ISSN 1016-8478

Coppi, A., Tewari, R., Bishop, J. R., Bennett, B. L., Lawrence, R., Esko, J. D., Billker, O. & Sinnis, P. (2007). Heparan sulfate proteoglycans provide a signal to Plasmodium sporozoites to stop migrating and productively invade host cells. *Cell Host & Microbe*, Vol.2, No.5, (November 2007), pp. 316-327, ISSN 1934-6069

Corjon, S., Gonzalez, G., Henning, P., Grichine, A., Lindholm, L., Boulanger, P., Fender, P. & Hong, S. S. (2011). Cell entry and trafficking of human adenovirus bound to blood factor X is determined by the fiber serotype and not hexon:heparan sulfate interaction. *PLoS One*, Vol.6, No.5, (2011), e18205, ISSN 1932-6203

Couchman, J. R. (2010). Transmembrane signaling proteoglycans. *Annual Review of Cell and Developmental Biology*, Vol.26, (November 2010), pp. 89-114, ISSN 1530-8995

Di Paolo, N. C., Kalyuzhniy, O. & Shayakhmetov, D. M. (2007). Fiber shaft-chimeric adenovirus vectors lacking the KKTK motif efficiently infect liver cells in vivo. *Journal of Virology*, Vol.81, No.22, (November 2007), pp. 12249-12259, ISSN 0022-538X

Dong, S. & Wu, X. Z. (2010). Heparanase and hepatocellular carcinoma: promoter or inhibitor? *World Journal of Gastroenterology*, Vol.16, No.3, (January 2010), pp. 306-311, ISSN 1007-9327

Dreyfuss, J. L., Regatieri, C. V., Jarrouge, T. R., Cavalheiro, R. P., Sampaio, L. O. & Nader, H. B. (2009). Heparan sulfate proteoglycans: structure, protein interactions and cell signaling. *Anais da Academia Brasileira de Ciências*, Vol.81, No.3, (September 2009), pp. 409-429, ISSN 1678-2690

Dudas, J., Kovalszky, I., Gallai, M., Nagy, J. O., Schaff, Z., Knittel, T., Mehde, M., Neubauer, K., Szalay, F. & Ramadori, G. (2001). Expression of decorin, transforming growth factor-beta 1, tissue inhibitor metalloproteinase 1 and 2, and type IV collagenases in chronic hepatitis. *American Journal of Clinical Pathology*, Vol.115, No.5, (May 2001), pp. 725-735, ISSN 0002-9173

Dudas, J., Ramadori, G., Knittel, T., Neubauer, K., Raddatz, D., Egedy, K. & Kovalszky, I. (2000). Effect of heparin and liver heparan sulphate on interaction of HepG2-derived transcription factors and their cis-acting elements: altered potential of hepatocellular carcinoma heparan sulphate. *The Biochemical Journal*, Vol.350 Pt 1, (August 2000), pp. 245-251, ISSN 0264-6021

Endo, K. & Terada, T. (2000). Protein expression of CD44 (standard and variant isoforms) in hepatocellular carcinoma: relationships with tumor grade, clinicopathologic parameters, p53 expression, and patient survival. *Journal of Hepatology*, Vol.32, No.1, (January 2000), pp. 78-84, ISSN 0168-8278

Esko, J. D., Kimata, K. & Lindahl, U. (2009). Proteoglycans and Sulfated Glycosaminoglycans. In: *Essentials of Glycobiology. 2nd edition,* Varki, A., Cummings, R. D., Esko, J. D., Freeze, H. H., Stanley, P., Bertozzi, C. R., Hart, G. W., Etzler, M. E. (Ed.), Chapter 16, Cold Spring Harbor Laboratory Press, ISBN 978-0879697709, Cold Spring Harbor (NY), USA

Fan, H., Zhao, Z., Quan, Y., Xu, J., Zhang, J. & Xie, W. (2007). DNA methyltransferase 1 knockdown induces silenced CDH1 gene reexpression by demethylation of methylated CpG in hepatocellular carcinoma cell line SMMC-7721. *European Journal of Gastroenterology and Hepatology*, Vol.19, No.11, (November 2007), pp. 952-961, ISSN 0954-691X

Filmus, J., Capurro, M. & Rast, J. (2008). Glypicans. *Genome Biology*, Vol.9, No.5, (2008), p. 224, ISSN 1465-6914

Folkman, J. (2006). Antiangiogenesis in cancer therapy--endostatin and its mechanisms of action. *Experimental Cell Research*, Vol.312, No.5, (March 2006), pp. 594-607, ISSN 0014-4827

Fux, L., Ilan, N., Sanderson, R. D. & Vlodavsky, I. (2009). Heparanase: busy at the cell surface. *Trends in Biochemical Sciences*, Vol.34, No.10, (October 2009), pp. 511-519, ISSN 0968-0004

Gatza, C. E., Oh, S. Y. & Blobe, G. C. (2010). Roles for the type III TGF-beta receptor in human cancer. *Cellular Signaling*, Vol.22, No.8, (August 2010), pp. 1163-1174, ISSN 1873-3913

Gesemann, M., Brancaccio, A., Schumacher, B. & Ruegg, M. A. (1998). Agrin is a high-affinity binding protein of dystroglycan in non-muscle tissue. *The Journal of Biological Chemistry*, Vol.273, No.1, (January 1998), pp. 600-605, ISSN 0021-9258

Girardin, E. P., Hajmohammadi, S., Birmele, B., Helisch, A., Shworak, N. W. & de Agostini, A. I. (2005). Synthesis of anticoagulantly active heparan sulfate proteoglycans by glomerular epithelial cells involves multiple 3-O-sulfotransferase isoforms and a limiting precursor pool. *The Journal of Biological Chemistry*, Vol.280, No.45, (November 2005), pp. 38059-38070, ISSN 0021-9258

Goldoni, S. & Iozzo, R. V. (2008). Tumor microenvironment: Modulation by decorin and related molecules harboring leucine-rich tandem motifs. *International Journal of Cancer*, Vol.123, No.11, (December 2008), pp. 2473-2479, ISSN 1097-0215

Goldshmidt, O., Yeikilis, R., Mawasi, N., Paizi, M., Gan, N., Ilan, N., Pappo, O., Vlodavsky, I. & Spira, G. (2004). Heparanase expression during normal liver development and following partial hepatectomy. *The Journal of Pathology*, Vol.203, No.1, (May 2004), pp. 594-602, ISSN 0022-3417

Gressner, A. M., Krull, N. & Bachem, M. G. (1994). Regulation of proteoglycan expression in fibrotic liver and cultured fat-storing cells. *Pathology, Research and Practice*, Vol.190, No.9-10, (October 1994), pp. 864-882, ISSN 0344-0338

Henry, S.P., Takanosu, M., Boyd, T.C., Mayne, P.M., Eberspaecher, H., Zhou,W., de Crombrugghe, B., Hook, M. & Mayne, R. Expression pattern and gene characterization of asporin. A newly discovered member of the leucine-rich repeat protein family. *The Journal of Biological Chemistry*, Vol.276, No.15 (April 2001), pp. 12212-12221, ISSN 1083-351X

Hilgard, P. & Stockert, R. (2000). Heparan sulfate proteoglycans initiate dengue virus infection of hepatocytes. *Hepatology*, Vol.32, No.5, (November 2000), pp. 1069-1077, ISSN 0270-9139

Hogemann, B., Edel, G., Schwarz, K., Krech, R. & Kresse, H. (1997). Expression of biglycan, decorin and proteoglycan-100/CSF-1 in normal and fibrotic human liver. *Pathology, Research and Practice*, Vol.193, No.11-12, (1997), pp. 747-751, ISSN 0344-0338

Hu, T. H., Huang, C. C., Wu, C. L., Lin, P. R., Liu, S. Y., Lin, J. W., Chuang, J. H. & Tai, M. H. (2005). Increased endostatin/collagen XVIII expression correlates with elevated VEGF level and poor prognosis in hepatocellular carcinoma. *Modern Pathology*, Vol.18, No.5, (May 2005), pp. 663-672, ISSN 0893-3952

Huang, G. W., Tao, Y. M. & Ding, X. (2009). Endocan expression correlated with poor survival in human hepatocellular carcinoma. *Digestive Diseases and Sciences*, Vol.54, No.2, (February 2009), pp. 389-394, ISSN 1573-2568

Ikeguchi, M., Hirooka, Y. & Kaibara, N. (2003). Heparanase gene expression and its correlation with spontaneous apoptosis in hepatocytes of cirrhotic liver and carcinoma. *European Journal of Cancer*, Vol.39, No.1, (January 2003), pp. 86-90, ISSN 0959-8049

Ikeguchi, M., Ueta, T., Yamane, Y., Hirooka, Y. & Kaibara, N. (2002). Quantitative analysis of heparanase messenger RNA expression in hepatocellular carcinoma. *Journal of Surgical Oncology*, Vol.81, No.3, (November 2002), pp. 148-154; disscusion 154, ISSN 0022-4790

Iozzo, R. V. & Sanderson, R. D. (2011). Proteoglycans in cancer biology, tumour microenvironment and angiogenesis. *Journal of Cellular and Molecular Medicine*, Vol.15, No.5, (May 2011), pp. 1013-1031, ISSN 1582-4934

Iozzo, R. V. & Schaefer, L. (2010). Proteoglycans in health and disease: novel regulatory signaling mechanisms evoked by the small leucine-rich proteoglycans. *FEBS Journal*, Vol.277, No.19, (October 2010), pp. 3864-3875, ISSN 1742-4658

Iozzo, R. V., Zoeller, J. J. & Nystrom, A. (2009). Basement membrane proteoglycans: modulators Par Excellence of cancer growth and angiogenesis. *Molecules and Cells*, Vol.27, No.5, (May 2009), pp. 503-513, ISSN 0219-1032

Isaka, Y., Brees, D. K., Ikegaya, K., Kaneda, Y., Imai, E., Noble, N. A. & Border, W. A. (1996). Gene therapy by skeletal muscle expression of decorin prevents fibrotic disease in rat kidney. *Nature Medicine*, Vol.2, No.4, (April 1996), pp. 418-423, ISSN 1078-8956

Ishiguro, T., Sugimoto, M., Kinoshita, Y., Miyazaki, Y., Nakano, K., Tsunoda, H., Sugo, I., Ohizumi, I., Aburatani, H., Hamakubo, T., Kodama, T., Tsuchiya, M. & Yamada-Okabe, H. (2008). Anti-glypican 3 antibody as a potential antitumor agent for human liver cancer. *Cancer Research*, Vol.68, No.23, (December 2008), pp. 9832-9838, ISSN 1538-7445

Kalamajski, S. & Oldberg, A. (2010). The role of small leucine-rich proteoglycans in collagen fibrillogenesis. *Matrix Biology*, Vol.29, No.4, (May 2010), pp. 248-253, ISSN 1569-1802

Kalia, M., Chandra, V., Rahman, S. A., Sehgal, D. & Jameel, S. (2009). Heparan sulfate proteoglycans are required for cellular binding of the hepatitis E virus ORF2 capsid protein and for viral infection. *Journal of Virology*, Vol.83, No.24, (December 2009), pp. 12714-12724, ISSN 1098-5514

Kalus, I., Salmen, B., Viebahn, C., von Figura, K., Schmitz, D., D'Hooge, R. & Dierks, T. (2009). Differential involvement of the extracellular 6-O-endosulfatases Sulf1 and Sulf2 in brain development and neuronal and behavioural plasticity. *Journal of Cellular and Molecular Medicine*, Vol.13, No.11-12, (November-December 2009), pp. 4505-4521, ISSN 1582-4934

Kang, Y. H., Ji, N. Y., Lee, C. I., Lee, H. G., Kim, J. W., Yeom, Y. I., Kim, D. G., Yoon, S. K., Park, P. J. & Song, E. Y. (2011). ESM-1 silencing decreased cell survival, migration, and invasion and modulated cell cycle progression in hepatocellular carcinoma. *Amino Acids*, Vol.40, No.3, (March 2011), pp. 1003-1013, ISSN 1438-2199

Keysar, S. B. & Jimeno, A. (2010). More than markers: biological significance of cancer stem cell-defining molecules. *Molecular Cancer Therapeutics*, Vol.9, No.9, (September 2010), pp. 2450-2457, ISSN 1538-8514

Koch, S., Tugues, S., Li, X., Gualandi, L. & Claesson-Welsh, L. (2011). Signal transduction by vascular endothelial growth factor receptors. *The Biochemical Journal*, Vol.437, No.2, (July 2011), pp. 169-183, ISSN 1470-8728

Kovalszky, I., Nagy, P., Szende, B., Lapis, K., Szalay, F., Jeney, A. & Schaff, Z. (1998). Experimental and human liver fibrogenesis. *Scandinavian Journal of Gastroenterology Supplement*, Vol.228, (1998), pp. 51-55, ISSN 0085-5928

Kraizer, Y., Mawasi, N., Seagal, J., Paizi, M., Assy, N. & Spira, G. (2001). Vascular endothelial growth factor and angiopoietin in liver regeneration. *Biochemical and Biophysical Research Communications*, Vol.287, No.1, (September 2001), pp. 209-215, ISSN 0006-291X

Lai, J. P., Oseini, A. M., Moser, C. D., Yu, C., Elsawa, S. F., Hu, C., Nakamura, I., Han, T., Aderca, I., Isomoto, H., Garrity-Park, M. M., Shire, A. M., Li, J., Sanderson, S. O., Adjei, A. A., Fernandez-Zapico, M. E. & Roberts, L. R. (2010). The oncogenic effect of sulfatase 2 in human hepatocellular carcinoma is mediated in part by glypican 3-dependent Wnt activation. *Hepatology*, Vol.52, No.5, (November 2010), pp. 1680-1689, ISSN 1527-3350

Lai, J. P., Sandhu, D. S., Shire, A. M. & Roberts, L. R. (2008a). The tumor suppressor function of human sulfatase 1 (SULF1) in carcinogenesis. *Journal of Gastrointestinal Cancer*, Vol.39, No.1-4, (2008), pp. 149-158, ISSN 1941-6628

Lai, J. P., Thompson, J. R., Sandhu, D. S. & Roberts, L. R. (2008b). Heparin-degrading sulfatases in hepatocellular carcinoma: roles in pathogenesis and therapy targets. *Future Oncology*, Vol.4, No.6, (December 2008), pp. 803-814, ISSN 1744-8301

Lai, J. P., Sandhu, D. S., Yu, C., Han, T., Moser, C. D., Jackson, K. K., Guerrero, R. B., Aderca, I., Isomoto, H., Garrity-Park, M. M., Zou, H., Shire, A. M., Nagorney, D. M., Sanderson, S. O., Adjei, A. A., Lee, J. S., Thorgeirsson, S. S. & Roberts, L. R. (2008c). Sulfatase 2 up-regulates glypican 3, promotes fibroblast growth factor signaling, and decreases survival in hepatocellular carcinoma. *Hepatology*, Vol.47, No.4, (April 2008), pp. 1211-1222, ISSN 1527-3350

Lai, J. P., Yu, C., Moser, C. D., Aderca, I., Han, T., Garvey, T. D., Murphy, L. M., Garrity-Park, M. M., Shridhar, V., Adjei, A. A. & Roberts, L. R. (2006). SULF1 inhibits tumor growth and potentiates the effects of histone deacetylase inhibitors in hepatocellular carcinoma. *Gastroenterology*, Vol.130, No.7, (June 2006), pp. 2130-2144, ISSN 0016-5085

Ledin, J., Ringvall, M., Thuveson, M., Eriksson, I., Wilen, M., Kusche-Gullberg, M., Forsberg, E. & Kjellen, L. (2006). Enzymatically active N-deacetylase/N-sulfotransferase-2 is present in liver but does not contribute to heparan sulfate N-sulfation. *The Journal of*

*Biological Chemistry*, Vol.281, No.47, (November 2006), pp. 35727-35734, ISSN 0021-9258

Levy-Adam, F., Ilan, N. & Vlodavsky, I. (2010). Tumorigenic and adhesive properties of heparanase. *Seminars in Cancer Biology*, Vol.20, No.3, (June 2010), pp. 153-160, ISSN 1096-3650

Li, L., Huang, J. L., Liu, Q. C., Wu, P. H., Liu, R. Y., Zeng, Y. X. & Huang, W. L. (2004). Endostatin gene therapy for liver cancer by a recombinant adenovirus delivery. *World Journal of Gastroenterol*, Vol.10, No.13, (July 2004), pp. 1867-1871, ISSN 1007-9327

Lin, C. W., Mars, W. M., Paranjpe, S., Donthamsetty, S., Bhave, V. S., Kang, L. I., Orr, A., Bowen, W. C., Bell, A. W. & Michalopoulos, G. K. (2011). Hepatocyte proliferation and hepatomegaly induced by phenobarbital and 1,4-bis [2-(3,5-dichloropyridyloxy)] benzene is suppressed in hepatocyte-targeted glypican 3 transgenic mice. *Hepatology*, Vol.54, No.2, (August 2011), pp. 620-630, ISSN 1527-3350

Liu, B., Bell, A. W., Paranjpe, S., Bowen, W. C., Khillan, J. S., Luo, J. H., Mars, W. M. & Michalopoulos, G. K. (2010). Suppression of liver regeneration and hepatocyte proliferation in hepatocyte-targeted glypican 3 transgenic mice. *Hepatology*, Vol.52, No.3, (September 2010), pp. 1060-1067, ISSN 1527-3350

Liu, B., Paranjpe, S., Bowen, W. C., Bell, A. W., Luo, J. H., Yu, Y. P., Mars, W. M. & Michalopoulos, G. K. (2009). Investigation of the role of glypican 3 in liver regeneration and hepatocyte proliferation. *American Journal of Pathology*, Vol.175, No.2, (August 2009), pp. 717-724, ISSN 1525-2191

Liu, F., Tan, G., Li, J., Dong, X., Krissansen, G. W. & Sun, X. (2007). Gene transfer of endostatin enhances the efficacy of doxorubicin to suppress human hepatocellular carcinomas in mice. *Cancer Science*, Vol.98, No.9, (September 2007), pp. 1381-1387, ISSN 1347-9032

Liu, H., Peng, C. H., Liu, Y. B., Wu, Y. L., Zhao, Z. M., Wang, Y. & Han, B. S. (2005). Inhibitory effect of adeno-associated virus-mediated gene transfer of human endostatin on hepatocellular carcinoma. *World Journal of Gastroenterology*, Vol.11, No.22, (June 2005), pp. 3331-3334, ISSN 1007-9327

Liu, L. L., Fu, D., Ma, Y. & Shen, X. Z. (2011). The Power and the Promise of Liver Cancer Stem Cell Markers. *Stem Cells and Development*, (August 2011), ISSN 1557-8534

Lorenzo, P., Aspberg, A., Onnerfjord, P., Bayliss, M.T., Neame, P.J. & Heinegard, D. (2001). Identification and characterization of asporin. A novel member of the leucine-rich repeat protein family closely related to decorin and biglycan. *The Journal of Biological Chemistry*, Vol.276, No.15 (April 2001), pp. 12201-12211, ISSN 1083-351X

Ly, M., Laremore, T.N. & Linhardt, R.J. (2010). Proteoglycomics: recent progress and future challenges. *OMICS: a Journal of Integrative Biology*, Vol.14, No.4, (August 2010), pp. 389-399, ISSN 1557-8100

Malaguarnera, G., Giordano, M., Paladina, I., Berretta, M., Cappellani, A. & Malaguarnera, M. (2010). Serum markers of hepatocellular carcinoma. *Digestive Diseases and Sciences*, Vol.55, No.10, (October 2010), pp. 2744-2755, ISSN 1573-2568

Manon-Jensen, T., Itoh, Y. & Couchman, J. R. (2010). Proteoglycans in health and disease: the multiple roles of syndecan shedding. *FEBS Journal*, Vol.277, No.19, (October 2010), pp. 3876-3889, ISSN 1742-4658

Mathe, M., Suba, Z., Nemeth, Z., Tatrai, P., Fule, T., Borgulya, G., Barabas, J. & Kovalszky, I. (2006). Stromal syndecan-1 expression is an adverse prognostic factor in oral carcinomas. *Oral Oncology*, Vol.42, No.5, (May 2006), pp. 493-500, ISSN 1368-8375

Mathew, J., Hines, J. E., Obafunwa, J. O., Burr, A. W., Toole, K. & Burt, A. D. (1996). CD44 is expressed in hepatocellular carcinomas showing vascular invasion. *Journal of Pathology*, Vol.179, No.1, (May 1996), pp. 74-79, ISSN 0022-3417

Matsumoto, A., Ono, M., Fujimoto, Y., Gallo, R. L., Bernfield, M. & Kohgo, Y. (1997). Reduced expression of syndecan-1 in human hepatocellular carcinoma with high metastatic potential. *International Journal of Cancer*, Vol.74, No.5, (October 1997), pp. 482-491, ISSN 0020-7136

Meurer, S. K., Tihaa, L., Lahme, B., Gressner, A. M. & Weiskirchen, R. (2005). Identification of endoglin in rat hepatic stellate cells: new insights into transforming growth factor beta receptor signaling. *The Journal of Biological Chemistry*, Vol.280, No.4, (January 2005), pp. 3078-3087, ISSN 0021-9258

Miyasaka, Y., Enomoto, N., Nagayama, K., Izumi, N., Marumo, F., Watanabe, M. & Sato, C. (2001). Analysis of differentially expressed genes in human hepatocellular carcinoma using suppression subtractive hybridization. *British Journal of Cancer*, Vol.85, No.2, (July 2001), pp. 228-234, ISSN 0007-0920

Morford, L. A., Davis, C., Jin, L., Dobierzewska, A., Peterson, M. L. & Spear, B. T. (2007). The oncofetal gene glypican 3 is regulated in the postnatal liver by zinc fingers and homeoboxes 2 and in the regenerating liver by alpha-fetoprotein regulator 2. *Hepatology*, Vol.46, No.5, (November 2007), pp. 1541-1547, ISSN 1527-3350

Morimoto-Tomita, M., Uchimura, K., Werb, Z., Hemmerich, S. & Rosen, S. D. (2002). Cloning and characterization of two extracellular heparin-degrading endosulfatases in mice and humans. *The Journal of Biological Chemistry*, Vol.277, No.51, (December 2002), pp. 49175-49185, ISSN 0021-9258

Murphy, K. J., Merry, C. L., Lyon, M., Thompson, J. E., Roberts, I. S. & Gallagher, J. T. (2004). A new model for the domain structure of heparan sulfate based on the novel specificity of K5 lyase. *The Journal of Biological Chemistry*, Vol.279, No.26, (June 2004), pp. 27239-27245, ISSN 0021-9258

Musso, O., Rehn, M., Saarela, J., Theret, N., Lietard, J., Hintikka, Lotrian, D., Campion, J. P., Pihlajaniemi, T. & Clement, B. (1998). Collagen XVIII is localized in sinusoids and basement membrane zones and expressed by hepatocytes and activated stellate cells in fibrotic human liver. *Hepatology*, Vol.28, No.1, (July 1998), pp. 98-107, ISSN 0270-9139

Musso, O., Theret, N., Heljasvaara, R., Rehn, M., Turlin, B., Campion, J. P., Pihlajaniemi, T. & Clement, B. (2001a). Tumor hepatocytes and basement membrane-Producing cells specifically express two different forms of the endostatin precursor, collagen XVIII, in human liver cancers. *Hepatology*, Vol.33, No.4, (April 2001), pp. 868-876, ISSN 0270-9139

Musso, O., Rehn, M., Theret, N., Turlin, B., Bioulac-Sage, P., Lotrian, D., Campion, J. P., Pihlajaniemi, T. & Clement, B. (2001b). Tumor progression is associated with a significant decrease in the expression of the endostatin precursor collagen XVIII in human hepatocellular carcinomas. *Cancer Research*, Vol.61, No.1, (January 2001), pp. 45-49, ISSN 0008-5472

Mythreye, K. & Blobe, G. C. (2009). Proteoglycan signaling co-receptors: roles in cell adhesion, migration and invasion. *Cellular Signaling*, Vol.21, No.11, (November 2009), pp. 1548-1558, ISSN 1873-3913

Naor, D., Sionov, R. V. & Ish-Shalom, D. (1997). CD44: structure, function, and association with the malignant process. *Advances in Cancer Research*, Vol.71, (1997), pp. 241-319, ISSN 0065-230X

Nelimarkka, L., Kainulainen, V., Schonherr, E., Moisander, S., Jortikka, M., Lammi, M., Elenius, K., Jalkanen, M. & Jarvelainen, H. (1997). Expression of small extracellular chondroitin/dermatan sulfate proteoglycans is differentially regulated in human endothelial cells. *The Journal of Biological Chemistry*, Vol.272, No.19, (May 1997), pp. 12730-12737, ISSN 0021-9258

O'Reilly, M. S., Boehm, T., Shing, Y., Fukai, N., Vasios, G., Lane, W. S., Flynn, E., Birkhead, J. R., Olsen, B. R. & Folkman, J. (1997). Endostatin: an endogenous inhibitor of angiogenesis and tumor growth. *Cell*, Vol.88, No.2, (January 1997), pp. 277-285, ISSN 0092-8674

Partenheimer, A., Schwarz, K., Wrocklage, C., Kolsch, E. & Kresse, H. (1995). Proteoglycan form of colony-stimulating factor-1 (proteoglycan-100). Stimulation of activity by glycosaminoglycan removal and proteolytic processing. *Journal of Immunology*, Vol.155, No.12, (December 1995), pp. 5557-5565, ISSN 0022-1767

Pellegrini, L. (2001). Role of heparan sulfate in fibroblast growth factor signalling: a structural view. *Current Opinion in Structural Biology*, Vol.11, No.5, (October 2001), pp. 629-634, ISSN 0959-440X

Pinzon-Ortiz, C., Friedman, J., Esko, J. & Sinnis, P. (2001). The binding of the circumsporozoite protein to cell surface heparan sulfate proteoglycans is required for plasmodium sporozoite attachment to target cells. *The Journal of Biological Chemistry*, Vol.276, No.29, (July 2001), pp. 26784-26791, ISSN 0021-9258

Pradel, G., Garapaty, S. & Frevert, U. (2002). Proteoglycans mediate malaria sporozoite targeting to the liver. *Molecular Microbiology*, Vol.45, No.3, (August 2002), pp. 637-651, ISSN 0950-382X

Quelard, D., Lavergne, E., Hendaoui, I., Elamaa, H., Tiirola, U., Heljasvaara, R., Pihlajaniemi, T., Clement, B. & Musso, O. (2008). A cryptic frizzled module in cell surface collagen 18 inhibits Wnt/beta-catenin signaling. *PLoS One*, Vol.3, No.4, (2008), e1878, ISSN 1932-6203

Ramani, V. C., Yang, Y., Ren, Y., Nan, L. & Sanderson, R. D. (2011). Heparanase plays a dual role in driving hepatocyte growth factor (HGF) signaling by enhancing HGF expression and activity. *The Journal of Biological Chemistry*, Vol.286, No.8, (February 2011), pp. 6490-6499, ISSN 1083-351X

Ricciardelli, C., Sakko, A. J., Ween, M. P., Russell, D. L. & Horsfall, D. J. (2009). The biological role and regulation of versican levels in cancer. *Cancer Metastasis Reviews*, Vol.28, No.1-2, (June 2009), pp. 233-245, ISSN 1573-7233

Roskams, T., De Vos, R., David, G., Van Damme, B. & Desmet, V. (1998). Heparan sulphate proteoglycan expression in human primary liver tumours. *Journal of Pathology*, Vol.185, No.3, (July 1998), pp. 290-297, ISSN 0022-3417

Roskams, T. & Kojiro, M. (2010). Pathology of early hepatocellular carcinoma: conventional and molecular diagnosis. *Seminars in Liver Disease*, Vol.30, No.1, (February 2010), pp. 17-25, ISSN 1098-8971

Roskams, T., Moshage, H., De Vos, R., Guido, D., Yap, P. & Desmet, V. (1995). Heparan sulfate proteoglycan expression in normal human liver. *Hepatology*, Vol.21, No.4, (April 1995), pp. 950-958, ISSN 0270-9139

Roskams, T., Rosenbaum, J., De Vos, R., David, G. & Desmet, V. (1996). Heparan sulfate proteoglycan expression in chronic cholestatic human liver diseases. *Hepatology*, Vol.24, No.3, (September 1996), pp. 524-532, ISSN 0270-9139

Sackstein, R. (2011). The biology of CD44 and HCELL in hematopoiesis: the 'step 2-bypass pathway' and other emerging perspectives. *Current Opinion in Hematology*, Vol.18, No.4, (July 2011), pp. 239-248, ISSN 1531-7048

Sarrazin, S., Adam, E., Lyon, M., Depontieu, F., Motte, V., Landolfi, C., Lortat-Jacob, H., Bechard, D., Lassalle, P. & Delehedde, M. (2006). Endocan or endothelial cell specific molecule-1 (ESM-1): a potential novel endothelial cell marker and a new target for cancer therapy. *Biochimica et Biophysica Acta*, Vol.1765, No.1, (January 2006), pp. 25-37, ISSN 0006-3002

Schaefer, L. & Iozzo, R.V. (2008). Biological functions of the small leucine-rich proteoglycans: from genetics to signal transduction. *The Journal of Biological Chemistry*, Vol.283, No.31 (August 2008), pp. 21305-21309, ISSN 1083-351X

Schaefer, L. & Schaefer, R.M. (2010). Proteoglycans: from structural compounds to signaling molecules. *Cell and Tissue Research*, Vol.339, No.1 (January 2010), pp. 237-246, ISSN 1432-0878

Schulze, A., Gripon, P. & Urban, S. (2007). Hepatitis B virus infection initiates with a large surface protein-dependent binding to heparan sulfate proteoglycans. *Hepatology*, Vol.46, No.6, (December 2007), pp. 1759-1768, ISSN 1527-3350

Schwarz, K., Breuer, B. & Kresse, H. (1990). Biosynthesis and properties of a further member of the small chondroitin/dermatan sulfate proteoglycan family. *The Journal of Biological Chemistry*, Vol.265, No.35, (December 1990), pp. 22023-22028, ISSN 0021-9258

Seppinen, L. & Pihlajaniemi, T. (2011). The multiple functions of collagen XVIII in development and disease. *Matrix Biology*, Vol.30, No.2, (March 2011), pp. 83-92, ISSN 1569-1802

Shangguan, J. Y., Dou, K. F., Li, X., Hu, X. J., Zhang, F. Q., Yong, Z. S. & Ti, Z. Y. (2009). [Effects and mechanism of decorin on the proliferation of HuH7 hepatoma carcinoma cells in vitro]. *Xi Bao Yu Fen Zi Mian Yi Xue Za Zhi*, Vol.25, No.9, (September 2009), pp. 780-782, ISSN 1007-8738

Shi, Y. F., Zhang, Q., Cheung, P. Y., Shi, L., Fong, C. C., Zhang, Y., Tzang, C. H., Chan, B. P., Fong, W. F., Chun, J., Kung, H. F. & Yang, M. (2006). Effects of rhDecorin on TGF-beta1 induced human hepatic stellate cells LX-2 activation. *Biochimica et Biophysica Acta*, Vol.1760, No.11, (November 2006), pp. 1587-1595, ISSN 0006-3002

Shirakawa, H., Suzuki, H., Shimomura, M., Kojima, M., Gotohda, N., Takahashi, S., Nakagohri, T., Konishi, M., Kobayashi, N., Kinoshita, T. & Nakatsura, T. (2009). Glypican-3 expression is correlated with poor prognosis in hepatocellular carcinoma. *Cancer Science*, Vol.100, No.8, (August 2009), pp. 1403-1407, ISSN 1349-7006

Shworak, N. W., Liu, J., Petros, L. M., Zhang, L., Kobayashi, M., Copeland, N. G., Jenkins, N. A. & Rosenberg, R. D. (1999). Multiple isoforms of heparan sulfate D-glucosaminyl 3-O-sulfotransferase. Isolation, characterization, and expression of human cdnas and identification of distinct genomic loci. *The Journal of Biological Chemistry*, Vol.274, No.8, (February 1999), pp. 5170-5184, ISSN 0021-9258

Spee, B., Carpino, G., Schotanus, B. A., Katoonizadeh, A., Vander Borght, S., Gaudio, E. & Roskams, T. (2010). Characterisation of the liver progenitor cell niche in liver diseases: potential involvement of Wnt and Notch signalling. *Gut*, Vol.59, No.2, (February 2010), pp. 247-257, ISSN 1468-3288

Stanford, K. I., Bishop, J. R., Foley, E. M., Gonzales, J. C., Niesman, I. R., Witztum, J. L. & Esko, J. D. (2009). Syndecan-1 is the primary heparan sulfate proteoglycan mediating hepatic clearance of triglyceride-rich lipoproteins in mice. *Journal of Clinical Investigation*, Vol.119, No.11, (November 2009), pp. 3236-3245, ISSN 1558-8238

Stanford, K. I., Wang, L., Castagnola, J., Song, D., Bishop, J. R., Brown, J. R., Lawrence, R., Bai, X., Habuchi, H., Tanaka, M., Cardoso, W. V., Kimata, K. & Esko, J. D. (2010). Heparan sulfate 2-O-sulfotransferase is required for triglyceride-rich lipoprotein clearance. *The Journal of Biological Chemistry*, Vol.285, No.1, (January 2010), pp. 286-294, ISSN 1083-351X

Stenvers, K. L., Tursky, M. L., Harder, K. W., Kountouri, N., Amatayakul-Chantler, S., Grail, D., Small, C., Weinberg, R. A., Sizeland, A. M. & Zhu, H. J. (2003). Heart and liver defects and reduced transforming growth factor beta2 sensitivity in transforming growth factor beta type III receptor-deficient embryos. *Molecular and Cellular Biology*, Vol.23, No.12, (June 2003), pp. 4371-4385, ISSN 0270-7306

Szende, B., Lapis, K., Kovalszky, I. & Timar, F. (1992). Role of the modified (glycosaminoglycan producing) perisinusoidal fibroblasts in the CCl4-induced fibrosis of the rat liver. *In Vivo*, Vol.6, No.4, (July-August 1992), pp. 355-361, ISSN 0258-851X

Tatrai, P., Dudas, J., Batmunkh, E., Mathe, M., Zalatnai, A., Schaff, Z., Ramadori, G. & Kovalszky, I. (2006). Agrin, a novel basement membrane component in human and rat liver, accumulates in cirrhosis and hepatocellular carcinoma. *Laboratory Investigation*, Vol.86, No.11, (November 2006), pp. 1149-1160, ISSN 0023-6837

Tatrai, P., Egedi, K., Somoracz, A., van Kuppevelt, T. H., Ten Dam, G., Lyon, M., Deakin, J. A., Kiss, A., Schaff, Z. & Kovalszky, I. (2010). Quantitative and qualitative alterations of heparan sulfate in fibrogenic liver diseases and hepatocellular cancer. *Journal of Histochemistry and Cytochemistry*, Vol.58, No.5, (May 2010), pp. 429-441, ISSN 1551-5044

Tatrai, P., Somoracz, A., Batmunkh, E., Schirmacher, P., Kiss, A., Schaff, Z., Nagy, P. & Kovalszky, I. (2009). Agrin and CD34 immunohistochemistry for the discrimination of benign versus malignant hepatocellular lesions. *American Journal of Surgical Pathology*, Vol.33, No.6, (June 2009), pp. 874-885, ISSN 1532-0979

Theocharis, A. D., Skandalis, S. S., Tzanakakis, G. N. & Karamanos, N. K. (2010). Proteoglycans in health and disease: novel roles for proteoglycans in malignancy and their pharmacological targeting. *FEBS Journal*, Vol.277, No.19, (October 2010), pp. 3904-3923, ISSN 1742-4658

Timar, J. & Kovalszky, I. (1995). Differential expression of proteoglycans on the surface of malignant cells and in the tumor stroma, In: *Tumor Matrix Biology*, Ádány, R. (Ed.), pp.23-53, CRC Press, ISBN 0-8493-4882-X, Boca Raton, Florida, USA.

Tralhao, J. G., Schaefer, L., Micegova, M., Evaristo, C., Schonherr, E., Kayal, S., Veiga-Fernandes, H., Danel, C., Iozzo, R. V., Kresse, H. & Lemarchand, P. (2003). In vivo selective and distant killing of cancer cells using adenovirus-mediated decorin gene transfer. *FASEB Journal*, Vol.17, No.3, (March 2003), pp. 464-466, ISSN 1530-6860

van der Voort, R., Taher, T. E., Wielenga, V. J., Spaargaren, M., Prevo, R., Smit, L., David, G., Hartmann, G., Gherardi, E. & Pals, S. T. (1999). Heparan sulfate-modified CD44 promotes hepatocyte growth factor/scatter factor-induced signal transduction through the receptor tyrosine kinase c-Met. *The Journal of Biological Chemistry*, Vol.274, No.10, (March 1999), pp. 6499-6506, ISSN 0021-9258

Weiner, O. H., Zoremba, M. & Gressner, A. M. (1996). Gene expression of syndecans and betaglycan in isolated rat liver cells. *Cell and Tissue Research*, Vol.285, No.1, (July 1996), pp. 11-16, ISSN 0302-766X

Whitelock, J. M., Melrose, J. & Iozzo, R. V. (2008). Diverse cell signaling events modulated by perlecan. *Biochemistry*, Vol.47, No.43, (October 2008), pp. 11174-11183, ISSN 1520-4995

Williams, K. J. & Chen, K. (2010). Recent insights into factors affecting remnant lipoprotein uptake. *Current Opinion in Lipidology*, Vol.21, No.3, (June 2010), pp. 218-228, ISSN 1473-6535

Williams, K. J., Liu, M. L., Zhu, Y., Xu, X., Davidson, W. R., McCue, P. & Sharma, K. (2005). Loss of heparan N-sulfotransferase in diabetic liver: role of angiotensin II. *Diabetes*, Vol.54, No.4, (April 2005), pp. 1116-1122, ISSN 0012-1797

Xian, X., Gopal, S. & Couchman, J. R. (2010). Syndecans as receptors and organizers of the extracellular matrix. *Cell and Tissue Research*, Vol.339, No.1, (January 2010), pp. 31-46, ISSN 1432-0878

Xiao, Y., Kleeff, J., Shi, X., Buchler, M. W. & Friess, H. (2003). Heparanase expression in hepatocellular carcinoma and the cirrhotic liver. *Hepatology Research*, Vol.26, No.3, (July 2003), pp. 192-198, ISSN 1386-6346

Yang, Y., Macleod, V., Miao, H. Q., Theus, A., Zhan, F., Shaughnessy, J. D., Jr., Sawyer, J., Li, J. P., Zcharia, E., Vlodavsky, I. & Sanderson, R. D. (2007). Heparanase enhances syndecan-1 shedding: a novel mechanism for stimulation of tumor growth and metastasis. *The Journal of Biological Chemistry*, Vol.282, No.18, (May 2007), pp. 13326-13333, ISSN 0021-9258

Yoshikawa, T., Nakatsugawa, M., Suzuki, S., Shirakawa, H., Nobuoka, D., Sakemura, N., Motomura, Y., Tanaka, Y., Hayashi, S. & Nakatsura, T. (2011). HLA-A2-restricted glypican-3 peptide-specific CTL clones induced by peptide vaccine show high avidity and antigen-specific killing activity against tumor cells. *Cancer Science*, Vol.102, No.5, (May 2011), pp. 918-925, ISSN 1349-7006

Yu, D. C., Chen, J., Sun, X. T., Zhuang, L. Y., Jiang, C. P. & Ding, Y. T. (2010). Mechanism of endothelial progenitor cell recruitment into neo-vessels in adjacent non-tumor tissues in hepatocellular carcinoma. *BMC Cancer*, Vol.10, (2010), p. 435, ISSN 1471-2407

Zvibel, I., Halfon, P., Fishman, S., Penaranda, G., Leshno, M., Or, A. B., Halpern, Z. & Oren, R. (2009). Syndecan 1 (CD138) serum levels: a novel biomarker in predicting liver fibrosis stage in patients with hepatitis C. *Liver International*, Vol.29, No.2, (February 2009), pp. 208-212, ISSN 1478-3231

# 9

# Chemically Induced Hepatocellular Carcinoma and Stages of Development with Biochemical and Genetic Modulation: A Special Reference to Insulin-Like-Growth Factor II and Raf Gene Signaling

Biswajit Mukherjee*, Miltu Kumar Ghosh and Chowdhury Mobaswar Hossain
*Department of Pharmaceutical Technology, Jadavpur University, Kolkata India*

## 1. Introduction

### 1.1 Liver and its physiology

The liver, the largest organ in the body, predominantly functions as a biochemical laboratory where metabolism takes place. It has both endocrine and exocrine functions; and is also involved in numerous metabolic activities and acting as a storage depot. Once the nutritional substances and other chemicals such as drugs, carcinogens etc. reach in liver, they are metabolized by hepatic enzymes. The organ is located on the right side of the abdomen just beneath the diaphragm in human. Liver is a solid organ consisting of several lobes. Each lobe is constituted with numerous lobules which are in general hexagonal in shape (Figure 1). The center of each lobule is occupied by the central vein and the periphery of the lobule is delineated by a close arrangement of hepatic artery, portal vein, and bile duct; called "portal triads". The portal triads appear at the vertices of the hexagonal lobules. The vessels generated from the portal triads ramify and distribute along the sides of the lobule, and open into the sinusoids which have thin epithelial lining, a discontinuous layer of fenestrated endothelial cells. The liver has different types of cells. Oval cells are generally found near the portal triad. This rare cell-type has been claimed as hepatic stem cells by some researchers (Zamule et al., 2011). However, the major cell-type in liver is the polygonal hepatic parenchymal cells (hepatocytes). Hepatic lobules are made up of more than 80% hepatocytes which have an average size of 25 μ and occupy 70-90% of liver mass, depending on the species. They have clear cell membrane; sometimes with two nuclei. They have large deposits of glycogen, often with lipid droplets and basophilic materials. They also contain other cellular organelles such as mitochondria, rough endoplasmic reticulum (granular) and smooth endoplasmic reticulum (agranular), golgi apparatus, and lysosomes. The hepatocytes are arranged in stacks of anastomosing plates, separated by an anastomosing

* Corresponding Author

system of sinusoids. One or two cells thick hepatocytes appear radiating from central vein towards the periphery. They metabolize and excrete into sinusoids or bile canaliculi. They can undergo cell division to produce more hepatocytes. Other than the endothelial cells, the liver sinusoids contain phagocytic cells derived from monocytes, known as Kupffer cells. These macrophages phagocytize particulates and cell debris. Another hepatic cell-type is known as the ito cell. These are adipose or stellate cells.

Liver undertakes several important functions in our body. It

- produces bile which contains bile salts (sodium glycocholate, sodium taurocholate). The bile salts emulsify fats and oils and thus help in the digestion of them.
- involves in carbohydrate and fat metabolism, hemoglobin metabolism and lipid synthesis.
- stores many chemicals such as glycogens, vitamins, minerals and several metabolites.
- involves in detoxification and removal of many toxic chemicals, including drugs, carcinogens, and various toxins through bile from the body.
- converts circulating ammonia into urea by urea cycle (Ornithine cycle) and thereby reduces ammonia level in blood.
- produces serum proteins such as albumin, clotting factors.

### 1.2 Hepatic regenerative capability

Under normal condition in an adult, liver maintains its size. However, liver has the regenerative capacity. Under various stress conditions, liver-size may increase. Numerical

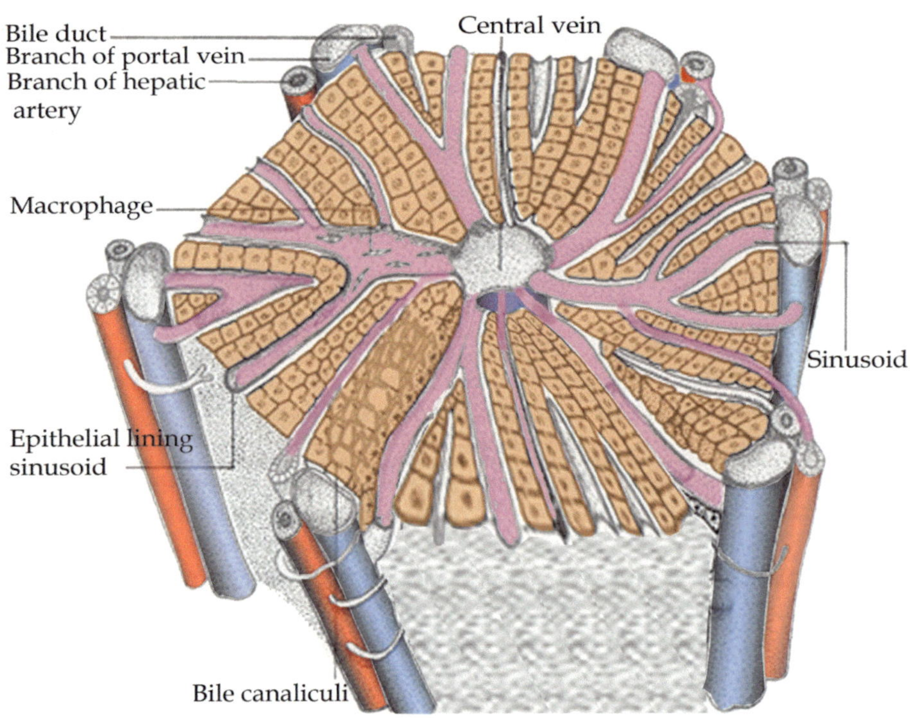


Fig. 1. Histological structure of a liver lobule

increase in hepatic cells by rapid cell division (hyperplasia) or increase in cell-size (hypertrophy) primarily causes enlargement of the tissue (Michalopoulos & DeFrances, 1997). Exposure to high levels of chemical toxicants causes increase in liver-size about 2-3 times of its normal size to combat the enhanced metabolic pressure exerted by chemical exposure (Michalopoulos & DeFrances, 1997). By regeneration process liver replaces the necrotic/ dead cells or the cells damaged due to toxicity. During hepatic continual regeneration process, the increased collagen synthesis and deposition result in fibrosis. This alongwith further continual hepatic cell damage due to various stress conditions cause liver cirrhosis (Lv et al., 2006). In cirrhosis, liver morphology alters. Scarring and nodularity appear. Normal hepatic function suffers and hepatic homeostasis decreases.

### 1.3 Liver cancer and its types

Cancer is the uncontrolled proliferation of cells that is caused by the multi-genetic defects. When the phenomenon occurs in liver cells, this is called hepatic cancer or liver cancer. The cancerous process begins in a few cells and the cells become immortal. They invade adjacent cells, intrude other nearby tissues (sometimes tissues at a distance) and metastasize. Uncontrolled proliferation of the cells causes solid mass formation in liver, resulting hepatic tumor. The predominant risk factors and etiological agents responsible for hepatocellular carcinoma in humans have been identified as chronic infection with hepatitis B virus or hepatitis C virus, exposure to aflatoxin B1 or other chemical carcinogens, and alcoholic cirrhosis and cirrhosis associated with genetic liver diseases.

#### 1.3.1 Primary liver cancer

Primary liver cancer means that the cancerous process occurs and develops primarily in liver and does not start from the spread of cancerous cells located outside the liver. It is the most common type of hepatic cancer. There may be several causes of primary liver cancer. Chronic viral infections such as hepatitis B or C, some toxins, chemical induced hepatic damage, radiation-induced hepatic damage, and chronic liver diseases such as cirrhosis can cause primary liver cancer. Primary liver cancer has different types, too.

##### 1.3.1.1 Hepatocellular carcinoma (also called hepatoma)

Hepatocellular carcinoma is the incidence of primary liver cancer in liver parenchyma cells or hepatocytes. People suffering from liver chronic diseases such as cirrhosis of liver are more prone to hepatocellular carcinoma. This is common to adult patients. However, in children and teenagers, similar pattern of the disease is called hepatoblastoma.

##### 1.3.1.2 Cholangiocarcinoma

When primary liver cancer occurs in bile ducts it is called cholangiocarcinoma.

##### 1.3.1.3 Angiosarcoma and hemangiosarcoma

These are fast growing rare type liver cancers.

##### 1.3.1.4 Angiosarcoma

This rare form of rapidly growing fatal tumor develops in the endothelial cells of blood vessel of the liver.

#### 1.3.1.5 Hemangiosarcoma

This is also developed from the lining of blood vessel, however, with relatively a slow speed. Blood-filled channels and spaces can be delineated under microscope. This is highly invasive type of cancer. It is commonly found in children. In patients suffering from hemangiosarcoma, the rapture of tumor leads to bleeding to death.

### 1.3.2 Secondary liver cancer

Malignant cells migrated from any tissues other than liver may invade hepatic tissue and develop neoplastic tumor in liver. This is described as secondary liver cancer. Spread of cancerous cells from outside the liver to the liver through blood flow or through the lymphatic system, the anchorage of the cells in liver, angiogenesis (formation of new blood vessels for supply of food and oxygen for new cells), and cellular proliferation leading to solid growth of mass are the possible sequences of secondary liver cancer. It is also called as metastatic cancer.

### 1.3.3 Experimental liver cancer in animals

Cancer in general is a multistage complex process by which uncontrolled proliferation of cells occurs. To understand the underlying mechanism in the process of development of the disease and its progress, it is important to develop the strategy to combat the dreadful disease. The need for the development of various in vivo cancer models has been in demand. Experimental liver cancer in animals is thus developed for studying the progress of the disease scientifically minutely in vivo and to develop therapeutic and other combating strategies to fight against it. There are various in vivo animal models already available for the purpose. Generally, virus-induced, radiation-induced, neoplastic cell-transplanted and chemical-induced liver cancer animal models have been widely studied.

## 2. Hepatocarcinogenesis

Hepatocarcinogenesis is the development of liver cancer due to the exposure of carcinogen (a chemical that produces cancer). Many hepatocarcinogens such as aflatoxins, acetylaminofluorene, diethylnitrosamine have been successfully used to develop hepatocarcinogenesis in animals. Experimentally, hepatocarcinogenesis is developed using different carcinogens and also in different animal species. Several genetic and epigenetic changes such as chromosomal deletions, rearrangements, aneuploidy, gene amplification, and mutations, formation of DNA adducts, DNA strand-break, modulation of DNA methylation, and modulation of cell signaling pathways, due to direct or indirect effect of carcinogen exposure lead to neoplastic transformation of hepatocytes in experimental animals. Hepatocarcinogenesis is a multistage complex process, which is preceded by early appearance of morphologically and genetically altered hepatic focal lesions, also known as preneoplastic lesions. Initially monoclonal populations of hepatocytes evolve primarily due to carcinogenic insult. These aberrant monoclonal populations of regenerative hepatocytes (focal lesions) develop hyperplastic nodules to dysplastic nodules, leading to hepatocellular carcinoma.

## 3. Hepatocellular carcinoma

The most common primary malignant tumor of liver is hepatocellular carcinoma. This primary liver cancer is also called hepatoma. As described above, liver has different types of cells such as hepatocytes, billiary cells, blood cells, Kupffer cells, ito cells, perisinusoidal cells etc. However, about more than 80% of liver tissue consists of hepatocytes. The majority of primary liver cancer (>90%) arises from hepatocytes and is called hepatocellular carcinoma. During hepatocarcinogenesis, initial carcinogen insult results in initiated cells from normal liver parenchyma cells or hepatocytes by genetic alteration following an interaction generally with DNA. Subsequent tumor promotion by chronic exposure of carcinogen or a tumor promoter such as phenobarbital develop clonally selected expansions of initiated cell populations called hepatic altered foci by fixing the mutations for further genetic changes. Additional accumulations of genetic changes within these foci produce hyperplastic nodules that ultimately lead to the development of hepatocellular carcinoma.

### 3.1 Stages of hepatocellular carcinoma

Transformation of the initiated hepatocytes into hepatocellular carcinoma is a multistage complex process. Based on the various morphological (such as appearance, size, shape, growth) and biochemical (such as variation in staining patterns, and altered enzyme expression patterns) changes of these hepatocytes, leading to hepatocellular carcinoma, various stages of development of the disease, namely *initiation*, *promotion* and *progression,* have been described to understand the progress of the disease in a more defined way and to develop better therapeutic strategies.

#### 3.1.1 Initiation

Exposure of genotoxic agents such as aflatoxins, 2-acetylaminofluorene, diethylnitrosamine, ionizing radiation etc. alters DNA sequence, causing mutations in the hepatocytes that

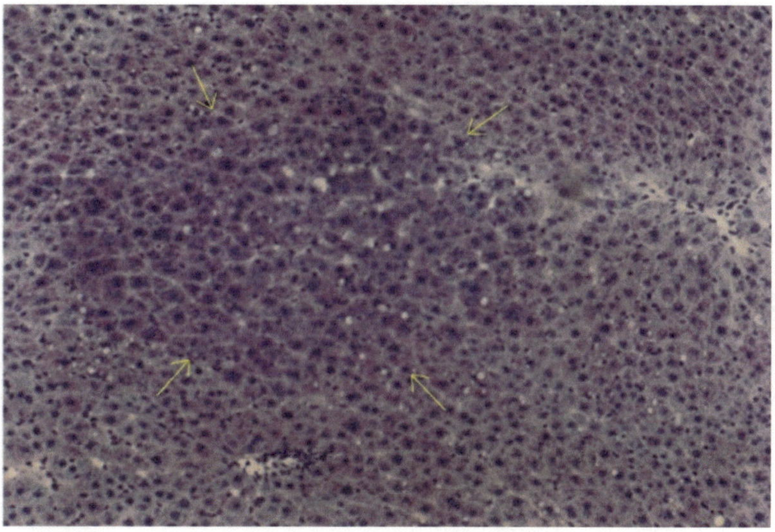

Fig. 2. Glycogen-stored early preneoplastic focal lesion (shown by yellow arrows) in rat hepatic tissue with Periodic Acid Schiff reaction. (Mukherjee et al. 2005)

develop potential to begin the transformation of normal cells to cancer cells. The mutations generally activate proto-oncogenes and/or inactivate tumor suppressor genes to develop hepatocellular carcinoma in the carcinogenic mechanism. The chemicals that cause the process (initiation) are called "initiators". Initiation is an irreversible process for a small population of cells. It occurs with a single/ brief exposure to a carcinogen. Electrophilic moieties generated by genotoxic agents generally bind with DNA to form DNA adduct, hamper cellular DNA repair mechanism, and develop permanent DNA lesions. Thus, the normal cell becomes an initiated cell. The initiated cells can develop focal lesions (Figure 2), one or more of which can act as sites of origin for the subsequent development of malignant neoplasia (Farber & Sarma 1987).

### 3.1.2 Promotion

Initiated hepatocytes are unable to grow autonomously (Farber & Sarma 1987), although they gain the potential to favor proliferation by possessing alterations in gene and protein expressions. Upon exposure to an environment where initiated cells are at greater risk, further genetic alterations begin, causing some reversible changes in the initiated cell populations. Repeated or long-term exposure to a promoting agent (phenobarbital, dietary fat, ethanol, estrogens, chronic exposure of carcinogens) or by some processes (e.g., partial hepatectomy), or by physiological condition (e.g., the neonatal liver) or diseased liver (virus infected or cirrhotic liver), the initiated cells induce focal proliferations. It begins with a selective, clonal amplification of the initiated cells into focal proliferations.

### 3.1.3 Progression

One or more focal lesions from the promotion phase further proceed for more genetic and enzymatic alterations in the constituted hepatocytes, forming enzyme-altered foci. Such a lesion may form from a single lesion or by merging several lesions and may be large enough to form a macroscopic structure (hepatic nodule) (Figure 3) in the liver. They sometimes

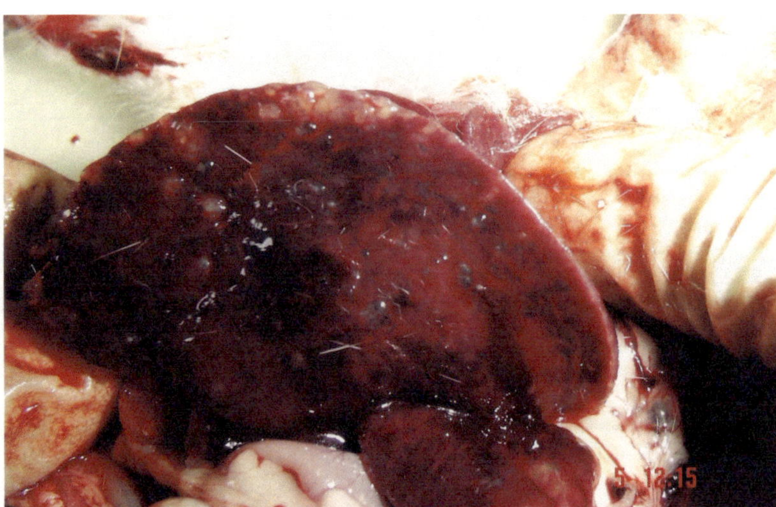


Fig. 3. An external morphology of liver tumor of a carcinogen-control rat showing multiple grayish-white and greenish-white hyperplastic nodules on the liver surface. (Das et al. 2010)

look grey or whitish gray or greenish (because of the presence of bile in them). Eventually by a slow process through lots of biochemical and genetic alterations those hepatic altered foci or hepatic nodules develop increasingly malignant cellular characteristics and are transformed into neoplasia without any further external stimulus or intervention (Farber & Sarma 1987).

## 4. Sequential changes in hepatocellular lineages leading to hepatocellular carcinoma

Etiology of hepatocellular carcinoma has probably been studied and analyzed in the best defined manner. Various groups of scientists have studied minutely and described the process of development of hepatocellular carcinoma during hepatocarcinogenesis. Other than initiation, promotion and progression models, Bannasch and his coworkers (Bannasch, 1995) have established and described the involvement of defined cellular lineages in the process of development of liver cancer. Predominant sequential cellular changes during the development of hepatocellular carcinoma commence with glycogenotic clear and acidophilic (due to proliferation of smooth endoplasmic reticulum) cell focal lesions and progress through intermediate phenotype of mixed cell population to glycogen poor basophilic (ribosome rich) cell phenotypes (Figure 4). The group has described few other cellular lineages. In the tigroid basophilic lineage, initially the cells have abundant highly ordered stacks of the rough endoplasmic reticulum and thereby they have uniqueness. The scientist group further reported that the lineage is common to the animals treated with a low dose treatment of hepatocarcinogen (Gournay et al., 2002). Another type of cellular lineage has been found to involve in the development of hepatocellular carcinoma. Rats when treated with non-genotoxic peroxisome proliferators or woodchucks chronically infected with woodchuck hepatitis virus showed foci with glycogen-poor cytoplasm containing abundantly granular acidophilic (mitochondria and peroxisome proliferators) and basophilic (ribosome) components (Bannasch et al., 1998). They named it amphiphilic cell lineage.

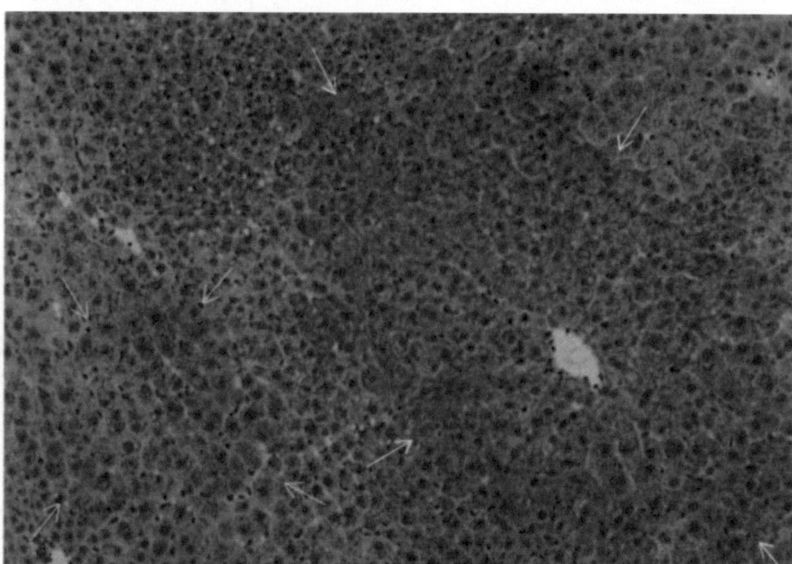

Fig. 4. Mixed cell focal lesion (shown by green arrows) and basophilic lesion (shown by blue arrows) in diethylnitrosamine-treated rat liver. (Mukherjee et al. 2007)

## 5. Biochemical modulation in hepatocellular carcinoma

As discussed above, from the beginning of initiation process to the development of neoplasm, various biochemical and genetic changes occur in the affected cells. Some of these changes are well-distinguishable and vary along with the stages of development during various cancer processes including hepatocarcinogenesis. They have been described as preneoplastic or neoplastic markers, depending on the developmental stages (Pérez-Carreón et al., 2006). Liver is the largest organ in our body and it takes major role in metabolism. It has several enzymes which take part in metabolism and detoxification of various chemicals, including drugs. Most of these enzymes were discovered during investigation of drug metabolism in liver and thus they are called hepatic drug metabolizing enzymes. In liver, glutathione and related enzymes such as glutathione peroxidase, glutathione reductase, superoxide dismutase, catalase and many other hepatic drug metabolizing enzymes and isoenzymes, such as glutathione-S-transferases (GSHT), UDP-glucuronyl transferases (UDPGT), cytochrome-c-reductase, cytochrome P-450 content and cytochrome $b_5$, have been identified as possible markers of preneoplastic and neoplastic hepatocytes (Mukherjee et al., 2005; Sarkar et al., 1994). They are categorized as Phase I and Phase II drug metabolizing enzymes/ isoenzymes. Variation in different such enzyme and isoenzyme levels, enzyme expression patterns assessed by histochemistry, lipid peroxidation profile, oxidative stress markers etc., during hepatocarcinogenesis, has been studied and reviewed by several workers (Sarkar et al., 1994,). Conjugation of toxic metabolites with cellular macromolecules such as proteins and nucleic acids, may lead to several health problems including cancer. The enzymes (glutathione S-transferases, arylhydrocarbon hydroxylases, UDP-glucuronic trasferases, cytochrome monooxygenases etc.) and isoenzymes (cytochrome $b_5$, cytochrome C etc.) are mostly involved in the detoxification process in liver. In Phase I hepatic metabolic reaction, oxygenation and hydroxylation reactions and in Phase II metabolic reaction in liver, glucuronidation and transferase reactions are very predominant. Glucuronic acid is transferred from uridine diphosphate glucuronic acid to a drug or phase I metabolite by the enzyme UDPGT (Vessey, 1996). Thus inefficient phase II processes cause increased deposition of phase I toxic metabolites. Another very important class of transferase enzymes is GSHT. They take enormous role in phase II detoxification process in liver. They detoxify electrophilic groups and thus inactivate even the function of carcinogens or mutagens. Satoh and Hatayama (Satoh & Hatayama, 2002) reported that specific different forms of GSHT are expressed during initiation, promotion and neoplastic cell populations. In the different developmental stages of hepatocellular carcinoma, glutathione peroxidase and reduced triphosphopyridine nucleotide (TPNH)-cytochrome-c-reductase activities, cytochrome $b_5$ and P-450 contents, glutathione content and superoxide dismutase and catalase activities were found to vary. Activities of these enzymes or their levels in hepatocellular carcinoma were always lower than those in initiation and promotion stages (Vessey, 1996). These reports suggest that the effects of Phase I hepatic drug metabolism is dwindled in hepatocellular carcinoma. The importance of glucose-6-phosphatase (G6P) in preneoplastic and neoplastic liver cannot be ruled out. The enzyme catalyzes in the final biochemical reactions of both gluconeogenesis and glycogenolysis (Nordlie & Sukalski, 1986; Shieh et al., 2003). This enzyme has an important role in blood glucose homeostasis (Nordlie & Sukalski, 1986). Histochemical demonstrations of G6P exhibited less pronounced activity in some cancer lesions and enhanced activity in the others. G6P-negative hepatocellular carcinoma (Figure 5) was also found to be basophilic (Mukherjee et al., 2007; Hwang et al., 2004).

Reports suggest that mutation in the G6P gene, G727T, leads to hepatocellular carcinoma (Nordlie & Sukalski, 1986).

Upon exposure of carcinogens, mutagens or other xenobiotics, reactive oxygen species are generated in the cells. Intracellular reactive oxygen species produce different types of DNA

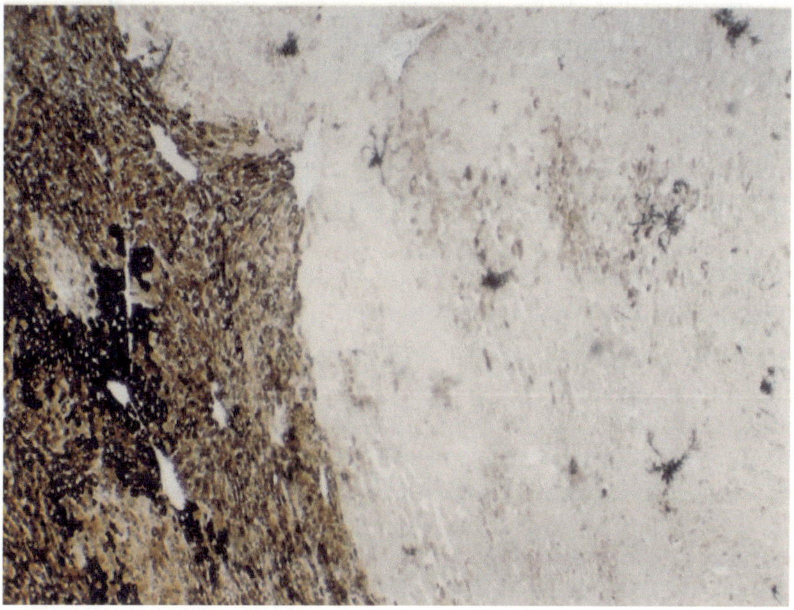

A

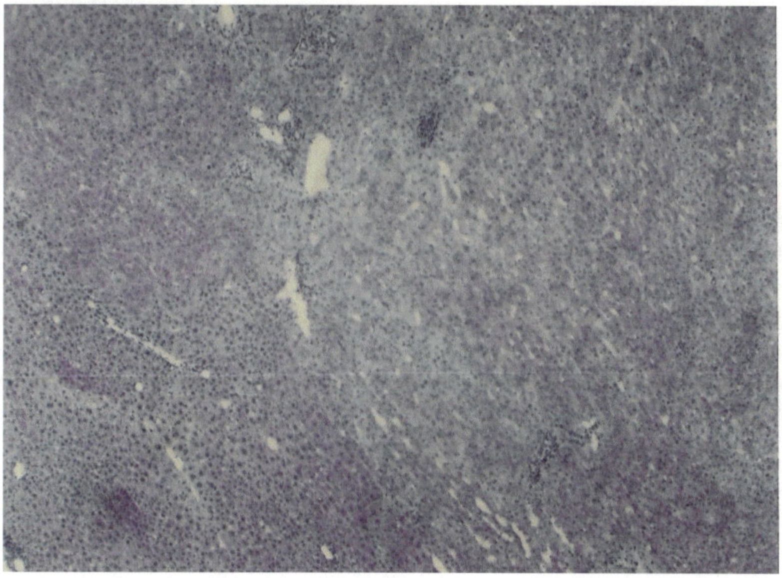

B

Fig. 5. No predominant glucose-6-phosphatase expression in tumor area (A) of a basophilic tumor (B). (Mukherjee at al. 2007)

damage, including chromosomal aberrations, sister chromatid exchanges, and mutations (Dahm, 1996), leading to the initiation and/ or promotion and/ or progression of the cancerous process. Oxidative stress resulting from the imbalance of free radicals and the cellular antioxidant defense enzyme systems is reported to induce damage to cellular membranes and nuclear DNA, which results in lipid peroxidation and oxidative DNA damage, respectively (Dahm, 1996). Oxidation of the C8 of guanine which gives rise to the formation of modified base 8-hydroxy-2'-deoxyguanosine (8-OHdG) is one of the most abundant types of oxidative DNA damage (Kasai & Nishimura, 1986). It is therefore considered as a sensitive biomarker for cancer development and an important molecular epidemiological assessment of cancer risk due to oxidative stress (Romano et al., 2000). The lipid peroxidation, another important chemical reaction owing to the oxidative stress during hepatocarcinogenesis, is known to influence tumor growth (Gelderblom,2001).

## 6. Signaling of hepatocellular carcinoma: A special reference to the genes, Insulin-like-growth factor II (IGF II) and c-raf.1

Accumulation of mutations in a variety of genes transforms phenotypes of cancer cells. Mutations are found in several important genes, including p73, p53, rb, APC, DLC-1(deleted in liver cancer), p16, PTEN, IGF-2, BRCA2, SOCS-1, Smad2 and Smad4, ß-catenin, c-myc, and cyclinD1, in hepatocellular carcinoma (Farber & Sarma, 1987). These gene products normally modulate biochemical pathways that regulate cell death and cell proliferation. Deregulation of signaling pathways during the development of hepatocellular carcinoma affects normal cellular processes such as cell cycle and apoptosis. Many growth factors such as insulin-like growth factor I and II (IGF I/II) have ubiquitous role in the development of the disease. Raf/MEK/ ERK/MAP (Mitogen Activated Protein) kinase pathway, Akt pathway, Wnt pathway and Ink4A pathway are some of the predominant pathways involved in the neoplastic conversion of normal cells. However, here our focus is to establish the role of IGF II and c-raf.1 in Raf/MEK/ ERK/MAP kinase pathway during the development of hepatocellular carcinoma in hepatocarcinogenesis.

### 6.1 Insulin-like growth factor II (IGF II)

Insulin-like growth factor II (IGF II), a mitogenic polypeptide, has been widely implicated in the pathogenesis of neoplasm of different tissues including the liver of rats and men (Li et al., 1998; Mukherjee et al., 2005). This growth factor is found to express in neonatal life (in the first few days after birth) and then during neoplasia in rodents and men (Li et al., 1998; Mukherjee et al., 2007). IGF II in signaling for cancer cell proliferation is mediated through the Raf growth factor (Das et al., 2010). IGF II activates c-raf through signaling proteins such as Grb2 and Ras. Thus, the pathological implication of the overexpression of these two genes during the development of hepatocellular carcinoma cannot be ignored.

The correlation between IGF II expression and cancer development has been reported in a number of works (Mukherjee et al., 2005, 2007; Li et al., 1998). In a majority of liver carcinoma, IGF-II mRNA expression was reactivated and high levels of IGF-II expression were detected. We also investigated to understand the stage(s) at which IGF II gene activates during carcinogenesis. In our study, IGF II overexpression was observed in the early hepatic altered lesions (Figure 6A, B, C, D) and in hepatocellular carcinoma (Figure 7) (Mukherjee et

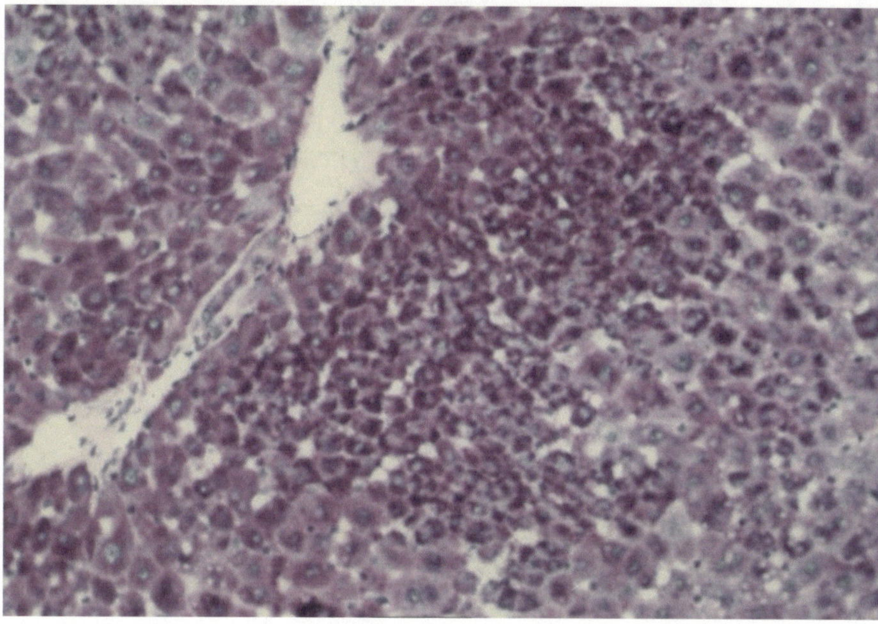

Fig. 6. A. Hepatic section of an experimental animal showing glycogen-stored early preneoplastic focal lesion with Periodic Acid Schiff reaction. (Mukherjee et al. 2007)

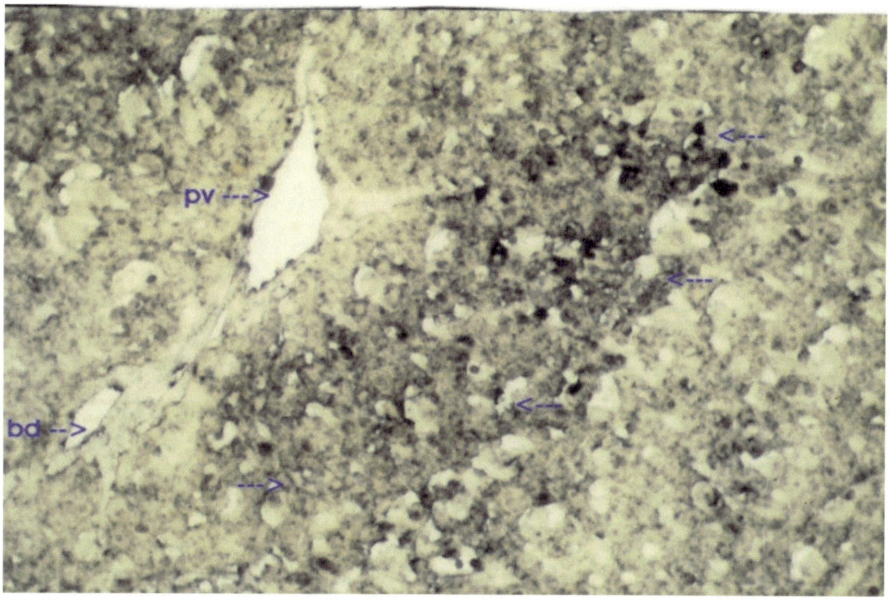


Fig. 6. B. IGF II mRNA-expressed glycogen storage early preneoplastic lesion detected with Digoxigenin-labeled antisense IGF II mRNA by *in situ* hybridization from the consecutive section. pv – portal vein. bd – bile duct. (Mukherjee et al. 2005)

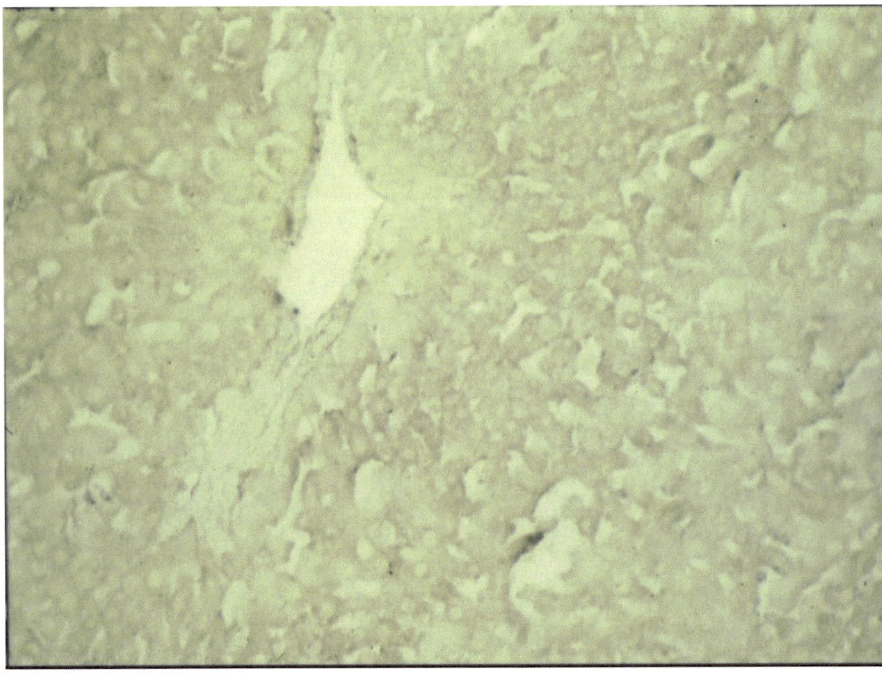

Fig. 6. C. Consecutive hepatic section after Digoxigenin-labeled sense IGF II mRNA treatment during *in situ* hybridization method. (Mukherjee et al. 2007)

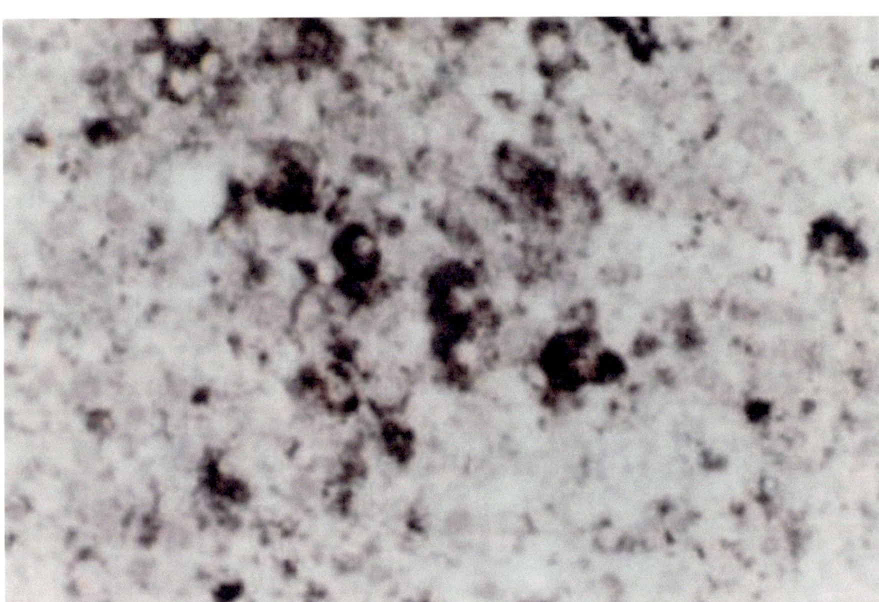

Fig. 6. D. IGF II-expressed one of the early preneoplastic lesions in an animal of initiation group. (Mukherjee et al.2005)

al., 2005). IGF II gene expressed in the sequence of events leading from glycogen-rich-acidophilic lesions to glycogen poor basophilic lesions through intermediate type lesions to hepatocellular carcinoma with an expression pattern of "high-low-high" in terms of degree of expression. More precisely, IGF II overexpression was found to be predominant in hepatocellular carcinoma and partially in early preneoplastic lesions. Thus, the gene has an essential role at the initiation stage of carcinogenesis (first few weeks) and during hepatocellular carcinoma development.

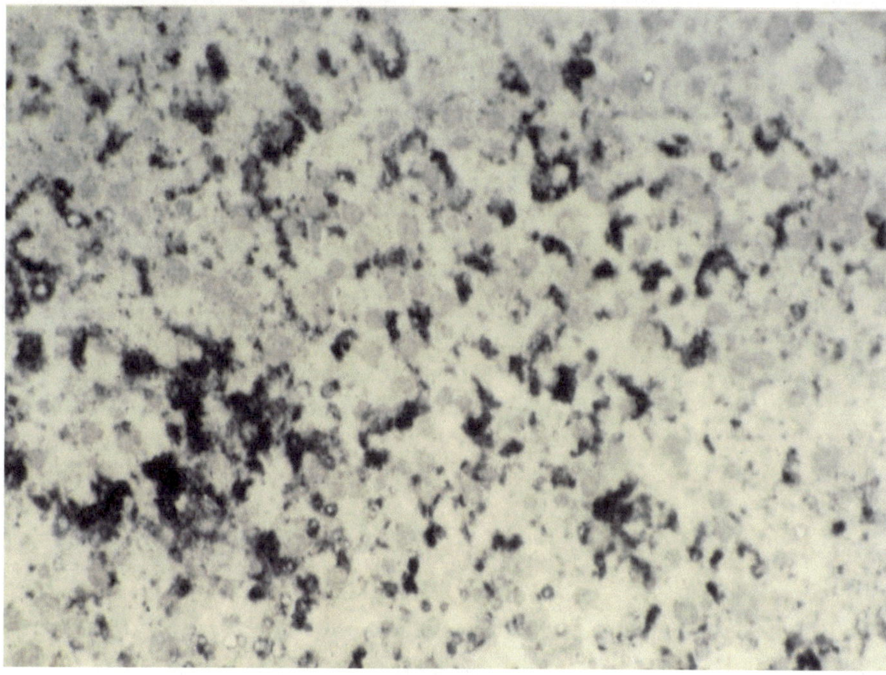

Fig. 7. IGF II mRNA expression in hepatocytes in tumor area (hepatocellular carcinoma) in experimental animals. (Mukherjee et al. 2005)

### 6.2 The Ras/raf/MEK/ ERK/MAP kinase pathway

The MAP kinase pathway has probably undergone the most extensive characterization in the process of development of hepatocellular carcinoma. Binding of a growth factor to a tyrosine kinase receptor causes receptor phosphorylation, leading to the formation of a molecular complex with an adaptor protein growth factor receptor bound-2 (Grb2), Grb-2 associated binder 1 and signal relay protein SH-2 domain-containing tyrosine phosphatase-2. This is then localized in the plasma membrane. Other protein such as an exchange factor, Son-of-sevenless (SOS) joins. This complex activates ras while exchange GDP to GTP in the ras/raf/MEK/ERK/MAP kinase pathway. Ras/raf/MEK/ ERK/MAP kinase pathway is known to involve in cell proliferation, dedifferentiation, angiogenesis and cell survival process (Rapp, 1991). Activation of the components of this pathway has been reported to contribute to tumorigenesis, including liver cancer. The GTPase (Guanine neucleotides triphosphate)-Ras and the serine/threonine kinase raf (signaling regulators) regulate the signaling process immediately by activating raf which then phosphorylates the mitogen/extracellular protein kinase kinases, MEK-1 and MEK-2. MEK proteins then phosphorylate the downstream extracellular signal-regulated kinase (ERK) signaling molecules, ERK-1 and ERK-2. GTPase-Ras is a switch protein which alternates between an active on state with a bound GTP and an inactive off state with a bound GDP (Polakis & McCormick, 1992). Activation of ERK-1 and ERK-2 regulates many target proteins and gene regulation proteins in cytoplasm and nucleus. Ras protein of this pathway is found to involve other signaling pathways such as phosphoinositol-3-kinase/Akt pathway, Phospholipase C/protein kinase C pathway and Ral guanine nucleotide dissociation stimulator pathway.

The c-raf.1 is a direct downstream effector of ras. The signaling molecule c-raf.1 is one of the three highly conserved members (raf A, raf B and c-raf.1) of the raf gene family, which code for serine threonine-specific protein kinases in ras-mediated signal transduction pathway (Daum et al., 1994; Rapp, 1991; Sebolt-Leopold, 2000). The c-raf.1 has a crucial role in diverse signal transduction pathways (Rapp, 1991). The c-raf.1 protein kinase has oncogenic potential and is found to be up-regulated in tumors (Störm SM et al. 1993; Stanton VP Jr et al. 1987) and highly expressed in hepatocellular carcinoma too (Rapp,1991; Störm et al., 1993). An excessive activation of the MAPK pathway was observed in hepatocellular carcinoma (Rapp,1991). This findings and another findings that shows overexpression of c-raf in hepatocellular carcinoma in all the 30 different tissue specimens as tested by Hwang et al. (Hwang et al., 2004) thus suggest the predominant role of the raf protein as well as ras/raf/MEK/ERK/MAP kinase pathway in hepatocellular carcinoma. In a phase-wise study (initiation/ promotion/ hepatocellular carcinoma) in rat hepatocarcinogenesis model (Mukherjee et al., 2007), we

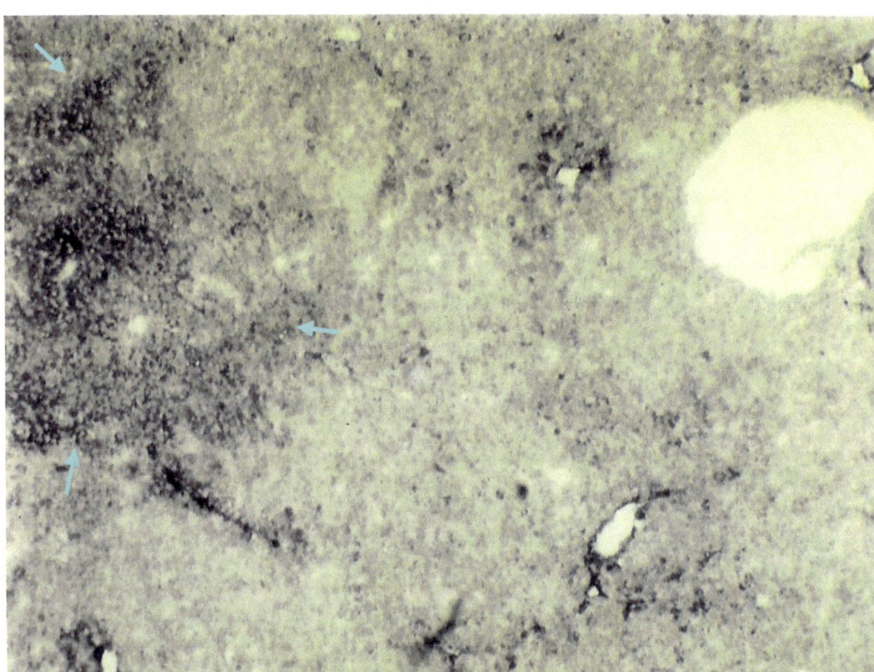

Fig. 8. A predominant raf-expressed late basophilic lesion (shown by arrows) in animal of cancer control group. (Das et al. 2009)

wanted to investigate the stage(s) at which c-raf.1 overexpression occurs. Our findings (as studied by in-situ hybridization) suggest that overexpression of the gene (Figure 8) occurs at the late stage basophilic focal lesions and in hepatocellular carcinoma. Further, c-raf.1 mediated activation of ras/raf/MEK/ERK/MAP kinase pathway may be a late stage phenomenon during the development of hepatocellular carcinoma and the activation may be either through c-raf.1 oncogenic mutation or by constitutive c-raf.1 activation by other deregulated proteins such as growth factors during hepatocarcinogenesis. Thus, constitutive activation of this pathway at one or more steps, particularly at ras or raf, can lead to a malignant state. However, no predominant difference is noticed between constitutive activation of Raf and Ras (Zang et al., 2002).

## 7. Conclusion

Unlike IGF II, c-raf.1 overexpression was observed in the late basophilic lesions associated with hepatocellular carcinoma. Thus, IGF II may have a role in activation of c-raf.1 signaling in the late stage of development of cancer. The role of raf.1 protein in IGF-induced signaling has been reported (Evert et al., 2004). But, when does it happen during the process of development of hepatocellular carcinoma? The c-raf.1 gene overexpression was predominantly found in hepatocellular carcinoma and late basophilic foci. Thus, the overexpression of c-raf.1 has been considered as a late-stage phenomenon during hepatocarcinogenesis (Bannasch, 2010). However, overexpression of c-raf.1 in very early lesion was also reported (He & Gascon- Barre, 1997). In our study, the dissection of animals after 7-8 weeks of carcinogenic insult did not show any raf.1-expressed lesions. Further, it was reported that c-raf.1 expressed in the basophilic tumors (Hwang et al., 2004). IGF II gene overexpression was noticed in the preneoplastic lesions and in hepatocellular carcinoma. On the other hand, overexpression of c-raf.1 gene was seen in the basophilic lesions associated with hepatocellular carcinoma as well as in tumor. While correlating the expression patterns of IGF II and c-raf.1, it suggests that IGF II-induced cellular signaling may be mediated through and/or affected by c-raf.1 in hepatocellular carcinoma and in the late stage of development of cancer. Thus, IGF II mediated c-raf.1 activation may drive late preneoplastic lesions towards neoplasia.

## 8. Acknowledgement

The work has been carried out, using the fund from Indian Council of Medical Research (ICMR), grant no. 58/7/2009-BMS

## 9. References

Bannasch, P. (1995). Sequential cellular and molecular changes during hepatocarcinogenesis. *Verh Dtsch Ges Patho*,79, pp.(72-83), ISSN: 0070-4113.

Bannasch, P. (2010). Hepatocellular glycogenosis and hepatic neoplasms.*Toxicol Pathol.* 38, 6, pp. (1000-1002), ISSN: 1533-1601.

Bannasch,P., D'Intron,A., Leonetti, P., Metzgen, C., Klimek,F., Mayer,D. (1998). Early aberrations of energy metaboloisim in carcinogenesis. In: *Cell growth and oncogenesis*. (eds. Bannasch,P., Kanduc,D., Papa,S., Tager,JM., ) Birkhauser Verlasi, Basel, Boston, Berlin), pp. (191-212). ISBN: 3-7643-5727-4.

Dahm, LJ.,Jones,DP.(1996). Mechanisms of chemically induced liver disease. In: Zakin D, Boyer TD, eds. Hepatology: a textbook of liver disease, 3rd ed. Philadelphia: WB Saunders: pp.(875–890), ISBN:7216-8821 -7.

Das,T., F,Patra., Mukherjee, B. (2010). Effect of antisense oligomer in controlling c-raf.1 overexpression during diethylnitrosamine-induced hepatocarcinogenesis in rat. *Cancer Chemother Pharmacol*, (May, 2010) 65, pp.(309–318), ISSN: 0344-5704.

Daum, G., Eisenmann-Tappe, I., Fries, HW., Troppmair, J., Rapp, U.R. (1994). The ins and outs of Raf kinases. *Trends Biochem. Sci*, 19,11, pp(474-480), ISSN: 0968-0004.

Evert, M., Sun, J., Pichler, S., Slavova, N., Schneider-Stock, R., Dombrowski, F. (2004). Insulin receptor, insulin receptor substrate-1, raf-1, and mek-1 during hormonal hepatocarcinogenesis by intrahepatic pancreatic islet transplantation in diabetic rats. *Cancer Res*, 64, pp.(8093-8100) ISSN: 0008-5472.

Farber, E., and Sarma, DSR. (1987). Biology of disease. hepatocaronogenesis, a dynamic cellular perspective.*Lab. Invest*, 56, pp. (4 -22), ISSN: 0023-6837.

Gelderblom,W.C.A.,Abel,S., Smuts,CM.,Marnewick,J., Marasas, W.F.O., Lemmer, ER., Ramljak, D. (2001). Fumonisin-induced hepatocarcinogenesis: mechanisms related to cancer initiation and promotion. *Environmental Health Perspectives Supplements*,109, 2, (May 2001),pp.( 291-300), ISSN:10780475.

Gournay,J., Auvigne, I., Pichard,V., Ligeza,C., Bralet MP, Ferry, N.(2002). In vivo cell lineage analysis during chemical hepatocarcinogenesis in rats using retroviral-mediated gene transfer: evidence for dedifferentiation of mature hepatocytes. *Lab Invest*, 82, 6, (Jun, 2002), pp. (781-788), ISSN: 0023-6837.

He, RK., Gascon-Barre, M. (1997). Influence of the vitamin D status on the early hepatic response to carcinogen exposure in rats. *J Pharmacol Exp Ther,* 281,1, (April,1997), pp.(464–469), ISSN: 0022-3565.

Hwang, Y., Choi, J., Kim, S. (2004). Over-expression of c-raf-1 protooncogene in liver cirrhosis and hepatocellular carcinoma. *Hepatology* Res. 29, 2,(June,2004), pp (113–121), ISSN: 1527-3350.

Kasai,H.,Nishimura,S.(1986). Hydroxylation of guanine in nucleosides and DNA at C-8 position by heated glucose and oxygen radical-forming agents. *Environ. Health Perpect*, 67, pp. (111–116), ISSN: 0091-6765.

Li, SL., Xu, ZDX., Kimura, G., Sun, Y., Kawachi, MH., Wilson, TG., Wilczynk, S., Yamaguchi, YE.. (1998). Expression of insulin like growth factor (IGF)-II in human prostate, breast, bladder and paraganglioma tumors. *Cell Tissue Res*, 291,3, pp(469-479), ISSN: 0302-766X.

Lv, P., Luo, HS., Zhou, XP., Paul, SC., Xiao, YJ, Si, XM.,Liu, SQ. (2006).Thalidomide prevents rat liver cirrhosis via inhibition of oxidative stress. *J. Pathology – Research and Practice*, 202,11, pp. (777–788), ISSN: 0344-0338.

Michalopoulos, GK., DeFrances, MC. (1997). Liver regeneration. *Science*, 276, 5309, (Apr 4, 1997), pp. (60-66), ISSN: 0036-8075.

Mukherjee,B., Das,T., Datta, S. (2007). Changes in the antioxidant defense and hepatic drug metabolizing enzyme and isoenzyme levels, 8-hydroxydeoxyguanosine formation and expressions of c-raf.1 and insulin-like growth factor II genes during the stages of development of hepatocellular carcinoma in rats. *European Journal of Cancer Prevention*, 16, 4, (August, 2007), pp. (363–371), ISSN: 0959-8278.

Mukherjee,B.,Ghosh,S.,Das,T.,Doloi, M. (2005). Characterization of insulin-like growth factor II (IGF II) mRNA positive hepatic altered foci and IGF II expression in hepatocellular carcinoma during diethylnitrosamine-induced hepatocarcinogenesis in rats. *J Carcinogenesis*, 4,1, pp(1-14), ISSN: 0974-6773.

Nordlie,RC., Singh,J., Sukalski,KA.(1986). N-acetylglucosamine-insensitive glucose phosphorylation in isolated hepatocytes from rats fasted for 48 h. *Biochim Biophys Acta*,889,2,(Nov 28,1986),pp(179-82), ISSN: 0006-3002.

Pérez-Carreón,JI.,López-García,C., Fattel-Fazenda,S.,Arce-Popoca,E., Alemán-Lazarini,L., Hernández-García,S.,Le Berre, V., Sokol,S., Francois, JM.,Villa-Treviño,S. (2006). Gene expression profile related to the progression of preneoplastic nodules toward hepatocellular carcinoma in rats. *Neoplasia*, 8,5,( May,2006),pp. 373–383, ISSN: 1476-5586.

Polakis, P., McCormick, F. (1992). Interactions between p21ras proteins and their GTPase activating proteins. *Cancer Surv*, 12,pp.(25-42), ISSN: 0261-242.

Rapp, UR. (1991). Role of Raf-1 serine/threonine protein kinase in growth factor signal transduction. *Oncogene*, 6,4,pp.(495–500), ISSN: 0950-9232.

Romano,G.,Sgambato, A., Mancini, R., Capellui,G., Giovagnoli, MR., Flaminii, G. (2000). 8-Hydroxy-2'-deoxyguanosine in cervical cells: correlation with grade of dysplasia and human papillomavirus infection. *Carcinogenesis*, 21, pp.(1143-1147), ISSN: 0143-3334.

Sarkar, A., Mukherjee, B., Chatterjee, M., (1994). Inhibition of β-carotene on 2- acetyl amino fluorine-induced hepatocarcinogenesis in rats; reflection in hepatic drug metabolism. *Carcinogenesis*, 15,5,pp.(1055–1060), ISSN: 0143-3334.

Satoh,K.,Hatayama,I.(2002).Anomalous elevation of glutathione S-transferase P- form (GST-P) in the elementary process of epigenetic initiation of chemical hepatocarcinogenesis in rats. *Carcinogenesis*, 23,7, pp(1193-1198), ISSN: 0143-3334.

Sebolt-Leopold, J. (2000). Development of anticancer drugs targeting the MAP kinase pathway. *Oncogene*, 19,56,(27 December 2000), pp.(6594–6599), ISSN: 0950-9232.

Shieh, JJ., Pan, CJ., Mansfield, BC., Chou, JY. (2003). A glucose-6-phosphate hydrolase, widely expressed outside the liver, can explain age-dependent resolution of hypoglycemia in glycogen storage disease type. *J Biol Chem*, 278,47, (November, 2003), pp. (47098–47103),ISSN: 1083-351X.

Stanton, VP. Jr., Cooper GM. (1987). Activation of human raf transforming genes by deletion of normal amino-terminal coding sequences. *Mol. Cell. Biol*, 7, 3, pp(1171-1179), ISSN: 0270-7306.

Störm, SM., Rapp, UR. (1993). Oncogene activation: c-raf-1 gene mutations in experimental and naturally occurring tumors. *Toxicol Lett*, 94, 1, (January, 2010),pp.(201–210), ISSN: 1653-9168.

Vessey, DA. (1996). Metabolism of xenobiotics by the human liver. In: Zakin D, Boyer TD, eds. Hepatology: a textbook of liver disease, 3rd ed. Philadelphia: WB Saunders, pp.(257–305), ISBN:7216-8821 -7.

Zamule,SM.,Coslo,DM.,Chen,F.,Omiecinski,CJ.(2011). Differentiation of human embryonic stem cells along a hepatic lineage. *Chemico-Biological Interactions* 190, 1, (March, 2011) pp.(62–72), ISSN: 0009-2797.

Zang, M., Hayne, C., and Luo, Z. (2002). Interaction between active Pak1 and Raf-1 is necessary for phosphorylation and activation of Raf-1. *J. Biol. Chem*, 277, pp. (4395-4405), ISSN: 1083-351X.

# 10

# Hepatocellular Carcinoma: Insights from the Centrosome Abnormalities

Ying Chen[1] and Qingzhong Kong[2]
[1]*School of Life Science and Technology, Henan Institute of Science and Technology, Xinxiang City, Henan Province*
[2]*Shandong Lanjin Pharmaceuticals Co., LTD, Jinan Hi-tech Zone, Jinan City, Shandong Province*
*China*

## 1. Introduction

Hepatocellular carcinoma (HCC) ranks the third in cancer-related death in the world. In Africa and Asia, the incidence of HCC, and death rate in particular, is even higher than other types of cancer. Chronic inflammation, mainly caused by viruses such as hepatitis B virus (HBV) and hepatitis C virus (HCV), has long been regarded as the major player in HCC development. However, increasing genes and/or tremendous epigenetic factors, and interactions thereof, have appeared to be involed in HCC development (Beasley & Lin, 1978; Arbuthnot & Kew, 2001). Although great efforts have been made in the past, early diagnosis and effective treatment to the patients in the late stage are still difficult. Centrosome amplification, a distinct feature in most cancer cells, has been widely studied recently in leukemia and increasing types of solid tumors. In HCC, however, there are few studies reported. What roles may centrosome play in hepatocellular carcinoma? What insights may it shine in guiding cancer therapies? And so on. We, in this chapter, would like to discuss the relations between centrosome and HCC development, through which, hopefully, novel therapeutic approaches are developed based on targeting the centrosome as a whole instead of just some proteins on it.

## 2. Centrosome in cancer

Centrosomes are tiny complex organelles, near the nucleus of an interphase cell, serving as microtubule organizing center (MTOC) involved in fundamental cellular activities such as cell polarity, cellular adhension, mobility, signal and molecule transport. These cellular processes are inseparable with important cellular events, such as cell cycle, DNA synthesis, DNA repair, apoptosis regulation, signal transduction, and carcinogenesis (Whitehead & Salisbury, 1999; Rieder et al., 2001; Palazzo et al., 2000). When cell enters into M phase, two newly duplicated centrosomes move to the opposing sites and form the poles of the mitosis spindle. Mitosis spindle play key roles in maintaining genetic stability, with the roles of centrosome in carcinogenesis having long been noticed by Theodor Boveri (Boveri T, 1914). Recently the centrosome was even described as a core part of "cell brain" (Kong et al., 2002).

### 2.1 The roles of centrioles in centrosome duplication

The important roles that centrosome plays in carcinogenesis should be understood together with the understanding of the centrioles embedded in the centrosome. Normal structure and/or function of centrosome requires the exactly controlled centrioles cycle. In fact, in most cells the reproductive capacity of centrosome does depend on its centriole contents, and centrosome would not duplicate if centrosome lacks centrioles. Therefore, strictly controlled mechanisms to regulate the centriole duplication in one cell cycle, appear to particularly important, as abnormality of centrioles may promote genetic instability, centrosome mis-segregation and/or apoptosis (Schatten et al., 2000).

As known, centrioles embedded in a cloud of electron-dense materials called pericentriolar material (PCM), which is responsible for formation of centrosome leading to bipolar mitosis, which, in turn, results in genetic stabilities. In cell cycle, centrosome cycle can be divided into centriole disorientation and disengagement, centriole duplication, centrosome maturation, centrosome separation, and procentriole assembly (Azimzadeh & Bornens, 2007). In G1 phase, the orthogonal arrangement of the two centrioles is lost and the distance between the two centrioles increased. Then, the amorphous central tube forms perpendicular to mother centriole, subsequently, nine individual microtubules around it assemble to procentriole. S and G2 phase trigger the newly generated daughter centrioles elongation until they reach to the same size of their mothers. Once cells enter into M phase, the two parental centrioles disconnect fully and finally lose their orthogonal relationship. In the end, PCM separates to give rise to each own cloud of PCM.

However, these two centrioles are not identical in cell since centriole only originated from a pre-existing one called the mother centriole. The new one, being about 80% of the length of the mother centriole, is called the daughter centriole (Azimzadeh & Bornens, 2007). Only mother centriole has external appendages functioning as docking site for microtubules and mediating centriole attachment to plasma membrane. PCM also plays important roles in directing microtubule nucleation by minus ends at proteinaceous complexes around mother centriole. Therefore, the mother centriole may be a major player in "licensing" event to ensure that one cell contains only one newly duplicated centriole in rigorous centriole duplication cycle. Support of this idea came from the finding that once daughter centriole formed from mother centriole, the centriole duplication process would have been inhibited, even though the cell was in a permissive condition (Tsou & Stearns, 2006a). In other words, the centriole duplication was determined by the mother centriole. Does this mean that in M phase, the separated duplication centriole each can be as a template to give rise to a new centriole? The prevailing view is that cytoplasm symaptic with mother centriole controls the centriole duplication. In S phase, even if the newly synthesized centriole has been ablated by laser, centriole duplication cycle cannot restart (Balczon et al., 1995; Loncarek et al., 2008). It is noteworthy that in S phase arrested CHO, HeLa and U2OS cells, mother centriole generates more than one daughter centriole, indicating mother centriole must have a mechanism to count the number of newly formed centriole (Loncarek et al., 2008; Jones & Winey, 2006; Tsou & Stearns, 2006b). Once this mechanism attenuated, the number of daughter centriole is out of the control of mother one. Today, we know that some mother centrole proteins may be the major players in this process, such as PLK4, SAS-6, and pericentrin. Support of this further came from the experiment that HIV-16 E7 oncoprotein can induce multiple daughter centriole at single mother centriole by cyclin E/CDK2 and

PLK4 over-expression both in normal primary cells and in tumor cell lines (Kleylein-Sohn et al., 2007; Duensing et al., 2007; Strnad et al., 2007). These findings may help to explain why supernumerary centrosomes are found in most cancer cells. However, there may be other ways to form newly synthesized centriole. De novo assembly of centriole has been found in the centriole that lacks of oocyte in most species (Manandhar et al., 2005; Riparbelli & Callaini, 2003; Szollosi & Ozil, 1991). *De novo* centriole assembly can be activated only in somatic cells with the centrioles removed either by microsurgery or by laser ablation in spite of the cell is transformed or not (Khodjakov et al., 2002; La Terra et al., 2005). Under this circumstance, the *de novo* assembled centriole is usually supernumerary, displacement, and malformed. In addition, the minimal pericentriolar material, lower microtubule nucleation capacity, and disjoin centriole pairs are the common features. Obviously, *de novo* assembly centriole is deleterious consequences in somatic cells, so *de novo* assembly pathway always inhibited by canonical centriole duplication cycle as a well-defined cloud of PCM (Young et al., 2000). Thus the elegant centriole duplication mechanism ensures that only one centrosome is in interphase cells unless two in M phase.

### 2.2 Centrosome abnormalities in cancer

Given that centrosome abnormalities, including increased number and centrosome structural abnormalities, is a hallmark in most, if not all, cancer cells, some questions remain to be elucidated: why supernumerary centrosomes are common features in cancer cell; how do they arise; and are they the causes or consequences of tumorigenesis (Lingle et al., 1998; Pihan et al., 1998). Recent studies showed that centrosome abnormalities in cancers can originate either by centrosome overduplication or by *de novo* synthesis of centrosomes (Duensing, 2005). Several centriole maturity markers, including ODF2/cenexin, ε-tubulin, ninein, ninein-like protein, adenomatous polyposis coli, EB1, centriolin, and Cep170, which only located in the mother centriole, can be used to distinguish the centriole duplication either from centrosome supernumerary or vice versa (Huber et al., 2008; Chang et al., 2003; Ibi et al., 2011; Louie et al., 2004; Hinchcliffe, 2003; Guarguaglini et al., 2005). No matter what is causal factor in inducing centosome overduplication, the extra centrosome can form multipolar mitosis, which leads to unequal chromosomes separation, therefore, promoting tumorigenesis. In addition, only centrosome amplification has been recently shown to initiate tumorigenesis in flies (Basto et al., 2008). Although the relation between centrosome abnormalities and chromosome instability (CIN) has long been regarded as a hen-and-egg problem, increasing studies intent to support the findings that extra centrosomes are major players in directly inducing chromosome missegregation, which, in turn, facilitates the evolution of more malignant phenotypes (Ganem et al., 2009).

As known that centrosome supernumerary and CIN are deleterious to cancer cells, the question is then how cancer cells survive. If the number of tumor cell having abnormal centrosome is less, the negative effects on the cell fates can be neglected. However, if most of the tumor cells have extra centrosomes, then there must be some mechanism to limit the detrimental consequences of supernumerary centrosome and CIN. Based on the findings that not all of extra centrosomes are activated to form MTOC and the normal cells harboring extra centrosome can survive, to date, bipolar spindle has been regarded as the major mechanism to prevent multipolar mitosis in supernumerary centrosomal tumor cells (Godinho et al., 2009). In principle, bipolar division is an effective way to eliminate extra centrosome. In fact, several research groups have found that some cell lines, which contain extra centrosomes, undergo bipolar divisions by clustering extra centrosomes. Interestingly, this phenomenon has been observed in some non-transformed cells that harbor extra centrosomes. Why is the centrosome clustering such a so popular event in supernumerary centrosome cells? It is highly possible that bipolar mitoses may be the best way to reduce the selective pressure. Although the exact mechanisms through which centrosome clustering is coordinated are not fully elucidate, recent studies have indicated that SAC, some MT motor proteins, such as Ncd/HEST, a kinesin family, and dynein, may be major players (Godinho et al., 2009).

Centrosome amplification has long been regarded as a distinct feature in most cancer cells. Abnormal centrosome biology, either centrosome amplification or structural abnormalities, frequently occur in most types of tumors including testicular germ cell, liposarcoma, adrenocortical, bronchial, bladder, cerebral primitive neuroectodermal, cervical, prostate, breast, squamous cell carcinomas of the head and neck, myeloma, and T-cell leukemia (Pihan et al., 1998; Duensing, 2005; Kramer et al., 2005; Nigg, 2002; Nigg, 2007; Giehl et al., 2005). Recent proteomic studies showed that abnormal centrosome may be the consequences of centrosome protein dysregulation. Up to now, More than 500 proteins have been identified and localized in centrosome, suggesting that centrosome may function as a central docking platform, where regulatory complexes converge and cross-talk by signaling pathway through microtubule network (Andersen et al., 2003). These centrosome localized proteins are generally divided into two classes: 1) structure proteins, including alpha tubulin, beta tubulin, gamma-tubulin, gamma-tubulin complex components 1-6, centrin 2 and 3, AKAP450, pericentrin/kendrin, ninein, pericentriolar material 1 (PCM1), ch-TOG protein, C-Nap1, Cep250, Cep2, centriole-associated protein CEP110, Cep1, centriolin, centrosomal P4.1 associated protein (CPAP), CLIP-associating proteins CLASP1 and CLASP 2, ODF2, cenexin, Lis1, Nudel, EB1, centractin, myomegalin; 2) temporary proteins, including oncogenes, tumor suppressor genes, ubiquitination and degradation related proteins, DNA damage checkpoint proteins, cell cycle regulated proteins, such as Survivin, Ras, Rad6, HER2/neu, p53, Rb, p21, APC, Gadd4, including APC/C, brca1, Cdc20, Cdh1, ATM, ATR, BRCA1, Chk1, including cyclin B1, Cdks, Chks, Plks, aurora kinases, and Neks. Over-expression of these centrosome proteins, mainly temporary proteins, has been demonstrated to induce tumor-like features. Since more and more known and yet-to-be known key proteins are found to be docked to centrosome, regarding centrosome together with centrioles and microtubules as the center of cell or called cell brain appears to be reasonable.

### 2.3 Roles of the centrosome in HBV virus infection

About 15% of all human cancers were caused by tumor viruses, mainly including human T-cell leukemia virus (HTLV-I), HBV, HCV, human papillomavirus (HPV), Epstein–Barr virus (EBV), Kaposi's sarcoma herpesvirus (KSHV) (Parkin, 2006). Whether virus need to entry into the cell or out from the cell, the cytoplasm is a very viscous milieu to preclude efficient directional movements by free diffusion (Suzuki & Craigie, 2007). What can they do to cope with this problem? Intracellular viral pathogens has evolved numerous mechanisms to hijack the host for their own profit during their life cycles. As centrosome is a perinuclear organelle and functions as an MTOC, which, in turn, is responsible for MT assembly and mediates MT-dependent trafficking due to MTs minus ends anchoring to the PCM and the plus ends extending towards the cell periphery, it is reasonable to believe that centrosome is the most appropriate candidate (Afonso et al., 2007). In fact, centrosome, particularly the pericentriole may act as progeny virus assembly site because of the high local concentration of chaperons, and play as a transfer station controlling virus cytoplasm - nuclear transport through MTs (Brown et al., 1996a, 1996b). The evidence stems from that microtubule depolymerizing agents can affect the ability of incoming viruses to reach to their replication site and viral protein assembly. This is why viruses such as HBV and HCV exploit the host cell's centrosomal capabilities and recruit centrosomal material for their own survival within host cells (Scaplehorn & Way, 2004; Coppens et al., 2006).

As for HCC, more than 85% of the cases are attributed to HBV infections (World Health Organization Scientific Group on Prevention and Control of Hepatocellular Carcinoma, 1983; Goncalves et al., 1998; Brechot et al., 2000). HBV is a DNA virus, which can lead to centrosome abnormalities, either supernumerary or dysfunction. Among HBV virus encoded proteins, only X proteins (HBx) is an oncoprotein associated with dysregulated cell division and cell death mainly caused by centrosome abnormal. Among HBx binding partners, HBXIP, a centrosome associated protein in mitotic cells, controls the virus cellular movement by binding to the motor protein, dynein (Chisari & Ferrari, 1995). HBXIP is a cytosolic survivin adaptor belonging to BIR-family chromosome passenger protein involved in cell apoptosis and division controlling. In Reed group, it is reported that HBXIP functions as a regulator in prometaphase and at telophase through centrosome duplication and cytokinesis pathway (Fujii et al., 2006). In HBV virus infected cells, the functions of cellular HBXIP may be dysregulated by HBx oncoprotein, which promote amplification of centrosomes, multipolar mitotic spindle formation, and CIN, and eventually creating tumorigenesis. Over-expression of HBXIP can trigger formation of extra centrosomes, which results in tripolar and multipolar spindles formation in premetaphase, whereas down-regulation of HBXIP may lead to monopolar spindle formation, regardless of p53 status. This may partly explain the contradictory findings that the centrosome abnormalities were caused by p53 and vice versa. Interestingly, pericentrin , the primary signal, transports signal to HBx and HBXIP to regulate centrosome functions (Wen et al., 2008). These findings explain why pericentriole is an assembly site for most virus infection and centrosome is a major hijacking target in virus entry and out process. Besides, 20 kDa centrin 2 has been found only in the cell expressiong HBx. Chromosome region maintenance 1 (CRM1), which is a transport receptor that mediates nuclear export of proteins, was found to mediates HBx nuclear export through Crm1/Ran GTPase-mediated pathway (Rousselet, 2009). Once exported from the nuclear by Crm1, HBx can be transported to pericentriole to assembly and budding sites. And pericentrin, main component of pericentriole, identified as five novel nuclear export signals (NESs) could bind to Crm1 (Forgues et al., 2003). Any disruption of specific nuclear cytoplasm transport pathways is crucial for the productive life cycle of some viruses. Clearly, centrosome and associated MTs plays pivotal roles in virus life cycle (Greber & Way, 2006).

### 2.3.1 The roles of centrosome-associated proteins in HBV induced HCC

More recently, a growing list of centrosome located proteins associated with carcinogenesis have been identified, such as PLK4, Aurora-A/STK 15/ BTAK, p53, NF-κB, and so on. In normal cells, the balance of apoptosis and proliferation must maintain at a stable level, whereas viruses usually hamper the host apoptosis to facilitate virus reproduction. The proteins involved in this process include p53, NF-κB, MAPK (Pang et al., 2006). HBx may influence apoptosis by interacting with the NF-κB signaling cascade or p53 (Wang et al., 1995; Becker et al., 1998; Livezey et al., 2002), whereas stimulate cell proliferation through the activation of cyclin-dependent kinase activities (Bouchard et al., 2001). p53, the tumor suppressor and key surveillance factor, has recently been detected to be mutated in HCC. In HCC, HBx inactivates p53 and p53-mediated activation of p21 (Ogden et al., 2000; Park et al., 2009), which, in turn, do not act as the "stop signal" for cell division. On the other hand, inactivated p53 no longer binds DNA in an effective way and acts as the negative signal for cell division, inducing an uncontrolled cell cycle-specific manner, which, in turn, leads to multiple copies of centrosome duplication in cell cycle. p53 mutation accompanied with centrosome aberration can induce genetic instability and this defective surveillance checkpoint mechanism ensures cancer cell reentering the cell cycle, thereby leading to series of catastrophic cascade, such as uncontrolled cell growth, pro-oncogenes activation, and tumors formation. NF-κB, the oncogene, promotes cell division, which can be augmented by mutant p53 through activation IKKα and IKKβ and enhancing NF-κB activity, therefore promoting cancer cell utilization of aerobic glycolysis preferentially for energy provision. Studies found in HBx expression cells, NF-κB was highly up-regulated and accompanied with extending life span, which indicated that cells enhance endogenous NF-κB transcriptional activity, harboring p53 mutations through a selective survival advantage in inflammatory microenvironments, and that p53 mutations may promote cancer under conditions of chronic inflammation (Park et al., 2006). More recently, the studies showed that HBx, but not export-defective mutant, can bind to and sequester Crm1 in the cytoplasm, thereby altering Crm1/Ran GTPase-dependent nuclear export of the NF-κB/IκBα complex (Forgues et al., 2003). In addition, all these findings suggested that HBx may act as several centrosome associated proteins to regulate cell apoptosis and proliferation benefitting for virus reproduction.

In addition, several centrosome associated kinases have been shown to induce chromosomal instability, leading to aneuploidy and cell transformation, such as Aurora-A, PLK4. Frequently occurred over-expression and amplification of Aurora-A, which can promote tumor formation and progression by causing unbalanced chromosomal segregation and centrosome aberrations in human cancer, lately have been detected in HCC (Benten et al., 2009). Centrosomal proteins such as Aurora-A and p53 may regulate each other in carcinogenesis. p53 protein could suppress the Aurora-A induced centrosome amplification and cellular transformation in a trans-activation-independent manner in HCC. Aurora-A over-expression was found to be correlated with p53 mutation, and tumors with both Aurora-A over-expression and p53 mutation usually have worse prognosis than that with p53 mutation alone (Jeng et al., 2004). This indicates that both of p53 and Aurora-A contribute to tumor progression and poor prognosis. Similar results have been found in PLK abnormal expression cells. Polo-like kinases (Plks), potential regulators of M phase, functions in mitotic entry, spindle pole activities and cytokinesis, which are broadly conserved despite physical and molecular differences in these processes in disparate organisms (de Carcer et al., 2011). PLK1-4 proteins are aberrantly regulated and possess different roles in human HCC, with PLK1 acting as an oncogene and PLK2-4 being presumably tumor suppressor genes. Plk4, major risk factor for primary liver cancer, localizes to centrioles throughout the cell cycle and is essential for centriole duplication (Pellegrino et al, 2010). In Plk4 down expression HCC cells, cell cycle progression was impaired with delay in M phase completion by dysregulation of cyclins D1, E, and B1, and of cdk1, whereas multipolar spindle formation was increased 6-fold and p53 activation and p21 expression were suppressed (Pellegrino et al., 2010; Ward et al, 2011).

### 2.3.2 The roles of centrosome in signaling pathway in HBV-induced HCC

Network of signaling pathway provides a robust mechanism for cells to respond to various biological stimuli. Although little is known about the roles of centrosome in signal transduction, a growing body of evidence has demonstrated that many signaling proteins localize at centrosome, being the targets of HBx. For example, protein kinase C (PKC) and its major substrate MARCKS (myristoylated alanine-rich C-kinase substrate), exerting multiple roles, such as controlling microtubule organization, spindle function, and cytokinesis, were found to colocalize to pericentrin and gamma-tubulin within MTOCs (Kim et al., 2008; Michaut et al., 2005). HBx activates PKC, which is transient and differs from activation of PKC by the ras oncogene product or phorbol ester in that it does not lead to rapid down-regulation of the enzyme subsequent to the activation. Previous studies have implicated protein kinase C (PKC) as upstream regulators of the MAPK. Interestingly, both of PKC and MAPK are required for phosphorylation of HBx, which, in turn, alters its subcellular localization and dysregulation of cell cycle progression, leading to hepatocarcinogenesis in HBV-infected cells. Besides, phosphoinositide 3-kinase (PI3K), a family of enzymes linked to extraordinarily diverse group of cellular functions, are involved in cancer (Lee et al., 2001; Yun et al., 2004, Wang et al., 2011). In HBV-infected cells, PI3K/Akt pathway can be activated through Akt phosphorylation by HBXIP, which also induce up-regulate cyclin D and down-regulate p21 and p53 expression, promoting cell proliferation (Wang, et al., 2011).

Cell adhesion to the extracellular matrix (ECM) is an important process that controls cell morphology, migration, proliferation, and so on. Integrin bridges cell and ECM, enduring pulling forces to promote cell migration. Otherwise, cell attachment to ECM is a basic requirement to build a multicellular organism, during this process integrin transmits surrounding signals into cytoplasm. The cytoplasmic domain of β1 integrin acts as a proximal receptor kinase to phosphorylate downstream targets regulating integrin-mediated signal transduction. If β1 integrin cytoplasmic domain mutation occurs, it will inhibit MT nucleation from the centrosomes and also disrupts cytokinesis, most likely due to spindle defects such as multipolar spindles (Reverte et al., 2006). In addition, cell migration also requires the orientation of the spindle during asymmetric cell division. Integrin linked kinase (ILK), a serine/threonine protein kinase, has also been shown to localize to the centrosome and to play a role in spindle assembly (Fielding et al., 2008). Interestingly, ILK signaling effectors such as Akt, GSK3 and β-catenin have also been found at the centrosome and mitotic spindles, indicating that centrosome associated proteins play important roles in spindle assembly. Recent evidence suggests that β-catenin involves in two signaling transduction pathways, cell-adhesion signaling and Wnt signaling pathway in which process β-catenin–T-cell factor (TCF) complex transcriptionally regulates gene expression

(Nelson & Nusse, 2004). No matter which way β-catenin involves, the intracellular β-catenin level is critical to its functions, therefore, HBx can regulate β-catenin, which plays an important role in various aspects of liver biology including cancer development, either by GSK-3, which directly suppress its activation via Src, or indirectly inhibit its activation by ERK signaling, or by p53, in which process HBx stabilize p53 expression leading to β-catenin degeneration (Hsieh et al., 2011; Wu et al., 2008; Jung et al., 2007). Importantly, β-catenin, a component of centrosome, interacts with centrosomal proteins to regulate mitotic centrosome separation (Bahmanyar, 2010) by forming a complex with the centrosomal proteins Nek2, C-Nap1 and Rootletin (Bahmanyar et al., 2008; Hadjihannas et al., 2010). Depletion of β-catenin in asynchronous cells results in monopolar spindles with unseparated centrosomes (Bahmanyar et al., 2008), whereas expression of mutation β-catenin causes increased centriole splitting in G1-S (Bahmanyar et al., 2008; Hadjihannas et al., 2010). These findings suggest that cell adhesion is a major target for HBx both on cell migration and on signaling transduction.

## 3. Centrosome abnormalities in the development of drug resistance

As signaling center, centrosome plays important roles in the development of drug resistance. Many centrosome-associated proteins are involved in chemo-resistance process, such as Her-2/neu, bcl-2, c-myc, ras, c-jun, MDM2, p210 BCR-abl, or mutant p53. In fact, abnormal centrosome itself may lead to formation of poly- or monopolarity spindle resulting in chromatin mis-segregation, which further result in or accelerate inactivation of tumor suppressor genes and/or activation of tumor genes, thereby leading to the development of chemoresistance. Support of this idea comes from the recent finding that p53 status determines tumor response to anti-angiogenic therapy and heat shock proteins (HSPs) varies with tumor progressions (Chen & Kong, 2009; Ciocca & Calderwood, 2005).

### 3.1 Centrosome clustering pathway as a target in cancer therapy

Centrosome clustering pathway is indispensable in cells with supernumerary centrosomes ensuring the success of cell division. Interference in this process could be lethal to tumor cells containing extra centrosomes (Kwon et al., 2008). Therefore, proper interference centrosome clustering pathway may raise the possibility of developing a new therapeutic strategy. HSET, the human homologue of the KAR3 family of minus end-directed kinesin-like motors, may be one of the most appropriate such candidates, as HSET depletion destroys centrosome clustering pathway and induces multipolar divisions and hence abnormal chromosome segregation or aneuploidy. Besides, HEST is essential only for clustering extra centrosomes in cancer cell but not in normal cells, by bundling the minus end of MT in acentrosomal spindles (Mountain et al., 1999). These results indicate that inhibition of HSET can selectively kill cells with extra centrosomes without affecting the viability of cells that contain normal centrosome numbers. In addition, HEST has been found to be involved in cell-cell adhesion by influencing the cells shape, then inducing low integrin -1 expression, and eventually resulting in tumor environment changes (Amendola et al., 2001). Taken together, HSET inhibitor may have a relative low toxicity compared with other mitosis-blocking agents involving centrosme, including checkpoint with forkhead and ring finger domains (CHFR), Aurora A, B, and C, Polo-like kinases (Plk1-4), and Nek kinases (NIMA1-11).

### 3.2 Targeting the centrosome as a whole in HCC therapy

As stated above, most of the key proteins are associated with cancer development. Selective inhibitors of these proteins such as p53, kinase C (PKC), proteasome, Aurora, NEDD1, and centrosome-associated regulators, therefore, have recently been tried in drug development (Graff et al., 2005; Montagut et al., 2005; Godl et al., 2005; Warner et al., 2006; Wang et la., 2009; Tillement et al., 2009). Since most of the key cellular proteins are localized to the centrosome, and centrosome abnormalities has long been found to be one of the most common features in a variety of human cancers and to be one of the earliest events in cancer development, as compared to p53 mutation and telomerase up-regulation that have been long regarded as the major factors contributing to the development of carcinogenesis. Centrosome is naturally becoming a candidate target in cancer therapy. In addition, chromosome instability (CIN) may be the fundamental cause in the development of drug resistance, and centrosome together with centrioles abnormalities are closely associated CIN, the whole complex consisting of the centrosome and centrioles may be a most promising candidate in cancer therapy.

Since increasing key proteins are found to be localized on centrosome and/or centrioles. And each protein exerts its yet unknown functions alone or through centrosome and/or centrioles. Selective targeting centrosome as a whole like mentioned previously (Kong, 2003a, 2003b, 2003c) or through combination of chemotherapeutic drugs that work through different mechanisms is expected to be reasonable and promising. Kong proposed that centrosome can be crystallized with tetrazolium salts (Kong et al., 2002). Although there is no further evidence to affirm whether it works or not in clinic, it seems to be reasonable that the crystallized centrosome may not function as the centre of the cell to mediate important cellular events. In other words, all key enzymes located in the centrosome will not function normally, and the cellular structures that are rich in the enzymes will be functionally and structurally frozen or restrained (Kong et al., 2002; Chen & Kong, 2006). Therefore, selective targeting centrosome as a whole unlike traditional approaches aiming at single protein or pathway is worthy of trying.

## 4. Conclusion

Centrosome works as an integrated complex in regulating important cellular events. Disrupting centrosome structurally and functionally may trigger malignant transformation. Although the roles of centrosome in carcinogenesis have been elucidated in some types of cancer, the roles of the centrosome in HCC development, particularly in cancer therapy, are largely uncovered. As discussed above, centrosome serves as a platform for HBV virus infection through centrosome-associated proteins, then transforming cell to immortalization. It is reasonable to believe that the drugs targeting centrosome-associated proteins should be developed to stop cancer cells proliferation and exert their efficacy when combined with conventional therapeutic agents. However, centrosome is an open prison, where proteins can bind and release in a precisely time-dependent manner in different cell cycle. Selective targeting centrosome as a whole, instead of a single protein or pathway, is, therefore, particularly worthy of trying.

## 5. References


Afonso, P.V.; Zamborlini, A.; Saib, A. & Mahieux, R. (2007). Centrosome and retroviruses: The dangerous liaisons. *Retrovirol* 4, 27.

Amendola, R.; Martinez, R.; Negroni, A.; Venturelli, D.; Tanno, B.; Calabretta, B. & Raschlla, G. (2001). DR-nm23 expression affects neuroblastoma cell differentiation, integrin expression, and adhesion characteristics. *Med Pediatr Oncol* 36, 93-96.

Andersen, J.S.; Wilkinson, C.J.; Mayor, T.; Mortensen, P.; Nigg, E.A. & Mann, M. (2003). Proteomic characterization of the human centrosome by protein correlation profiling. *Nature* 426, 570-574.

Arbuthnot, P. & Kew, M. (2001). Hepatitis B virus and hepatocellular carcinoma. *Int J Exp Pathol* 82, 77-100.

Azimzadeh, J. & Bornens, M. (2007). Structure and duplication of the centrosome. *J Cell Sci* 120, 2139-2142.

Bahmanyar, S.; Kaplan, D.D.; Deluca, J.G.; Giddings, T.H.Jr.; O'Toole, E.T.; Winey, M.; Salmon, E.D.; Casey, P.J.; Nelson, W.J. & Barth, A.I. (2008). beta-Catenin is a Nek2 substrate involved in centrosome separation. *Genes Dev* 22(1), 91-105.

Bahmanyar, S.; Guiney, E.L.; Hatch, E.M.; Nelson, W.J. & Barth, A.I. (2010). Formation of extra centrosomal structures is dependent on beta-catenin. *J Cell Sci* 123(Pt18), 3125-3135.

Balczon, R.; Bao, L.; Zimmer, WE.; Brown, K.; Zinkowski, R.P. & Brinkley, B.R. (1995). Dissociation of centrosome replication events from cycles of DNA synthesis and mitotic division in hydroxyurea-arrested Chinese hamster ovary cells. *J Cell Biol* 130, 105-115.

Basto, R.; Brunk, K.; Vinadogrova, T.; Peel, N.; Franz, A.; Khodjakov, A. & Raff, J.W. (2008). Centrosome amplification can initiate tumorigenesis in flies. *Cell* 133(6), 1032-1042.

Beasley, R.P. & Lin C.C. (1978). Hepatoma risk among HbsAg carriers. *Am J Epid* 108, 247.

Becker, S.A.; Lee, T.H.; Butel, J.S. & Slagle, B.L. (1998). Hepatitis B virus X protein interferes with cellular DNA repair. *J Virol* 72, 266-272.

Benten, D.; Keller, G.; Quaas, A.; Schrader, J.; Gontarewicz, A.; Balabanov, S.; Braig, M.; Wege, H.; Moll, J.; Lohse, A.W. & Brummendorf, T.H. (2009). Aurora kinase inhibitor PHA-739358 suppresses growth of hepatocellular carcinoma in vitro and in a xenograft mouse model. *Neoplasia* 11(9), 934-944.

Bouchard, M.; Giannakopoulos, S.; Wang, E.H.; Tanese, N. & Schneider, R.J. (2001). Hepatitis B virus HBx protein activation of Cyclin A–Cyclin-Dependent Kinase 2 complexes and G1 transit via a Src kinase pathway. *J Virol* 75(9), 4247-4257.

Boveri T. (1914). *Zur Frage der Entstehung Maligner Tumoren.* Jena: Fischer Verlag. 1929 English translation by M Boveri reprinted as '*The Origin of Malignant Tumors*' Baltimore: Williams and Wilkins Co.

Brechot, C.; Gozuacik, D.; Murakami, Y. & Paterlini-Brechot, P. (2000). Molecular basis for the development of hepatitis B virus (HBV)-related heaptocellular carcinoma (HCC). *Semin Cancer Biol* 10, 211-231.

Brown, C.R.; Doxsey, S.J.; Hong-Brown, L.Q.; Martin, R.L. & Welch, W.J. (1996a). Molecular chaperones and the centrosome. A role for TCP-1 in microtubule nucleation. *J Biol Chem* 271(2), 824-832.

Brown, C.R.; Hong-Brown, L.Q.; Doxsey, S.J. & Welch, W.J. (1996b). Molecular chaperones and the centrosome. A role for HSP 73 in centrosomal repair following heat shock treatment. *J Biol Chem* 271(2), 833-840.

Chang, P.; Thomas, H.; Giddings, Jr.; Winey, M. & Stearn, T. (2003). ε-Tubulin is required for centriole duplication and microtubule organization. *Nature Cell Bio* 5, 71-76.

Chen, Y. & Kong, Q. (2006). Cell brain: insight into hepatocarcinogenesis. *Med Hypotheses* 67, 44-52.

Chen, Y. & Kong, Q. (2009). Evaluation of centrosome abnormalities and p53 inactivation in chemical induced hepatocellular carcinoma. *Neoplasma* 56(2), 169-76.

Chisari, F.V. & Ferrari, C. (1995). Hepatitis B virus immunopathogenesis. *Annu Rev Immunol* 13, 29-60.

Ciocca, D.R. & Calderwood, S.K. (2005). Heat shock proteins in cancer: diagnostic, prognostic, predictive, and treatment implications. *Cell Stress Chaperones* 10(2), 86-103.

Coppens, I.; Dunn, J.D.; Romano, J.D.; Pypaert, M.; Zhang, H. & Boothroyd, J.C. (2006). *Toxoplasma gondii* sequesters lysosomes from mammalian hosts in the vacuolar space. *Cell* 125, 261-274.

de Carcer, G.; Manning, G. & Malumbres, M. (2011). From Plk1 to Plk5: functional evolution of Polo-like kinases. *Cell Cycle* 10(14), in print.

Duensing, S. (2005). A tentative classification of centrosome abnormalities in cancer. *Cell Biol Int* 29, 352-359.

Duensing, A.; Liu, Y.; Perdreau, S.A.; Kleylein-Sohn, J.; Nigg, E.A. & Duensing, S. (2007). Centriole overduplication through the concurrent formation of multiple daughter centrioles at single maternal templates. *Oncogene* 26, 6280-6288.

Fielding, A.B.; Dobreva, I.; McDonald, P.C.; Foster, L.J. & Dedhar, S. (2008). Integrin-linked kinase localizes to the centrosome and regulates mitotic spindle organization. *J Cell Biol* 180 (4), 681-689.

Forgues, M.; Difilippantonio, M.J.; Linke, S.P.; Ried ,T.; Nagashima, K.; Feden, J.; Valerie, K.; Fukasawa, K. & Wang, X.W. (2003). Involvement of Crm1 in hepatitis B virus X protein-induced aberrant centriole replication and abnormal mitotic spindles. *Mol Cell Biol* 23(15), 5282-5292.

Fujii, R.; Zhu, C.; Wen, Y.; Marusawa, H.; Bailly-Maitre, B.; Matsuzawa, S.; Zhang, H.; Kim, Y.; Bennett, C.F.; Jiang, W. & Reed, J.C. (2006). HBXIP, cellular target of hepatitis B virus oncoprotein, is a regulator of centrosome dynamics and cytokinesis. *Cancer Res* 66(18), 9099-9107.

Ganem, N.J.; Godinho, S.A. & Pellman, D. (2009). A mechanism linking extra centrosomes to chromosomal instability. *Nature* 460(7252), 278-282.

Giehl, M.; Fabarius, A.; Frank, O.; Hochhaus, A.; Hafner, M.; Hehlmann, R. & Seifarth, W. (2005). Centrosome aberrations in chronic myeloid leukemia correlate with stage of disease and chromosomal instability. *Leukemia* 19, 1192-1197.

Godinho, S.A.; Kwon, M. & Pellman, D. (2009). Centrosomes and cancer: how cancer cells divide with too many centrosomes. *Cancer Metastasis Rev* 28, 85-98.

Godl, K.; Gruss, O.J.; Eickhoff, J.; Wissing, J.; Blencke, S.; Weber, M.; Deqen, H.; Brehmer, D.; Orfi, L.; Horvath, Z.; Keri, G.; Muller, S.; Cotton, M.; Ullrich, A. & Daub, H. (2005). Proteomic characterization of the angiogenesis inhibitor SU6668 reveals multiple impacts on cellular kinase signaling. *Cancer Res* 65(15), 6919-26.

Goncalves, C.S.; Pereira, F.E. & Zago, M. (1988). Hepatocellular carcinoma. *Arq Gastroenterol* 25, 207-217.

Graff, J.R.; McNulty, A.M.; Hanna, K.R.; Konicek, B.W.; Lynch, R.L.; Bailey, S.N.; Banks, C.; Capen, A.; Goode, R.; Lewis, J.E.; Sams, L.; Huss, K.L.; Campbell, R.M.; Iversen, P.W.; Neubauer, B.L.; Brown, T.J.; Musib, L.; Geeqanaqe, S. & Thornton, D. (2005). The protein kinase Cβ-selective inhibitor, enzastaurin (LY317615.HCl), suppresses signaling through the AKT pathway, induces apoptosis, and suppresses growth of human colon cancer and glioblastoma xenografts. *Cancer Res* 65(16), 7462-7469.

Greber, U.F. & Way, M. (2006). A Superhighway to Virus Infection. *Cell* 124, 741-754.

Guarguaglini, G.; Duncan, P.I.; Stierhof, Y.D.; Holmstrom, T.; Duensing, S. & Nigg, E.A. (2005). The forkhead-associated domain protein Cep170 interacts with Polo-like Kinase 1 and serves as a marker for mature centrioles. *Mol Biol Cell* 16(3), 1095-1107.

Hadjihannas, M.V.; Bruckner, M. & Behrens, J. (2010). conductin/axin2 and Wnt signaling regulates centrosome cohesion. *EMBO Rep* 11(4), 317-324.

Hinchcliffe, E.H. (2003). Cell cycle: seeking permission from the mother centriole. *Curr Biol* 13, R646-648.

Hsieh, A.; Kim, H.S.; Lim, S.O.; Yu, D.Y. & Jung, G. (2011). Hepatitis B viral X protein interacts with tumor suppressor adenomatous polyposis coli to activate Wnt/β-catenin signaling. *Cancer Lett* 300(2), 162-172.

Huber, D.; Geisler, S.; Monecke, S. & Hoyer-Fender, S. (2008). Molecular dissection of ODF2/Cenexin revealed a short stretch of amino acids necessary for targeting to the centrosome and the primary cilium. *Eur J Cell Biol* 87(3), 137-146.

Ibi, M.; Zou, P.; Inoko, A.; Shiromizu, T.; Matsuyama, M.; Hayashi, Y.; Enomoto, M.; Mori, D.; Hirotsune, S.; Kiyono, T.; Tsukita, S.; Goto, H. & Inagaki, M. (2011). Trichoplein controls microtubule anchoring at the centrosome by binding to Odf2 and ninein. *J Cell Sci* 124(Pt 6), 857-864.

Jeng, Y.M.; Peng, S.Y.; Lin, C.Y. & Hsu, H.C. (2004). Overexpression and amplification of Aurora-A in hepatocellular carcinoma. *Clin Cancer Res* 10(6), 2065-2071.

Jones, M.H. & Winey, M. (2006). Centrosome duplication: is asymmetry the clue? *Cur Biol* 16, R808-810.

Jung, J.K.; Kwun, H.J.; Lee, J.O.; Arora, P. & Jang, K.L. (2007). Hepatitis B viral X protein differentially affects the ubiquitin-mediated proteasomal degradation of beta-catenin depending on the status of cellular p53. *J Gen Virol* 88(Pt8), 2144-2154.

Khodjakov, A.; Rieder, C.L.; Sluder, G.; Cassels, G.; Sibon, O. & Wang, C.L. (2002). *De novo* formation of centrosomes in vertebrate cells arrested during S phase. *J Cell Biol* 158, 1171-1181.

Kleylein-Sohn, J.; Westendorf, J.; Le Clech, M.; Habedanck, R.; Stierhof, Y.D. & Nigg, E.A.(2007). Plk4-induced centriole biogenesis in human cells. *Dev Cell* 13, 190-202.

Kim, J.; Choi, Y.L.; Vallentin, A.; Hunrichs, B.S.; Hellerstein, M.K.; Peehl, D.M. & Mochy-Rosen, D. (2008). Centrosomal PKCbetaII and pericentrin are critical for human prostate cancer growth and angiogenesis. *Cancer Res* 68(16), 6831-6839.

Kong, Q.; Sun, J. & Kong, L.D. (2002). Cell brain crystallization for cancer therapy. *Med Hypotheses* 59(4), 367-372.

Kong, Q. (2003a). Cell brain: a new focus in the postgenomic era. *Med Hypotheses* 61(1), 114-119.

Kong, Q. (2003b). Cell brain abnormalities in cancer development. *Med Hypotheses* 61(1), 120-125.

Kong, Q. (2003c). The centrosome-centered cell brain in apoptosis. *Med Hypotheses* 61(1), 126-132.

Kramer, A.; Neben, K. & Ho, A.D. (2005). Centrosome aberrations in hematological malignancies. *Cell Biol Int* 29, 375-383.

Kwon, M.; Godinho, S.A.; Chandhok, N.S.; Ganem, N.J.; Azioune, A.; Thery, M. & Pellman, D. (2008). Mechanisms to suppress multipolar divisions in cancer cells with extra centrosomes. *Genes Dev* 22, 2189-2203.

La Terra, S.; English, C.N.; Hergert, P.; McEwen, B.F.; Sluder, G. & Khodjakov, A. (2005). The *de novo* centriole assembly pathway in HeLa cells: cell cycle progression and centriole assembly/maturation. *J Cell Biol* 168, 713-722.

Lee, Y.I.; Kim, S.O.; Kwon, H.J.; Park, J.G.; Sohn, M.J. & Jeong, S.S. (2001). Phosphorylation of purified recombinant hepatitis B virus-X protein by notogen-activated protein kinase and protein kinase C in vitro. *J Virol Methods* 95(1-2), 1-10.

Lingle, W.L.; Lutz, W.H.; Ingle, J.N.; Maihle, N.J. & Salisbury, J.L. (1998). Centrosome hypertrophy in human breasttumors: implications for genomic stability and cell polarity. *Proc Natl Acad USA* 95(6), 2950-2955.

Livezey, K.W.; Negorev, D. & Simon, D. (2002). Increased chromosomal alterations and micronuclei formation in human hepatoma HepG2 cells transfected with the hepatitis B virus HBX gene. *Mutat Res* 505, 63-74.

Loncarek, J.; Hergert, P.; Magidson, V. & Khodjakov, A. (2008). Control of daughter centriole formation by the pericentriolar material. *Nat Cell Biol* 10, 322-328.

Louie, R.K.; Bahmanyar, S.; Siemers, K.A.; Votin, V.; Chang, P.; Stearns, T.; Nelson, W.J. & Barth, A.I. (2004). Adenomatous polyposis coli and EB1 localize in close proximity of the mother centriole and EB1 is a functional component of centrosomes. *J Cell Sci* 117(Pt 7), 1117-1128.

Manandhar, G.; Schatten, H. & Sutovsky, P. (2005). Centrosome reduction during gametogenesis and its significance. *Biol Reprod* 72, 2-13.

Michaut, M.A.; Williams, C.J. & Schultz, R.M. (2005). Phosphorylated MARCKS: a novel centrosome component that also defines a peripheral subdomain of the cortical actin cap in mouse eggs. *Dev Biol* 280(1), 26-37.

Montagut, C.; Rovira, A.; Mellado, B.; Gascon, P.; Ross, J.S. & Albanell, J. (2005). Preclinical and clinical development of the proteasome inhibitor bortezomib in cancer treatment. *Drugs Today* 41 (5), 299-315.

Mountain, V.; Simerly, C.; Howard, L.; Ando, A.; Schatten, G. & Compton, D.A. (1999). The kinesin-related protein, HSET, opposes the activity of Eg5 and cross-links microtubules in the mammalian mitotic spindle. *J Cell Biol* 147, 351-366.

Nelson, W.J. & Nusse, R. (2004). Convergence of Wnt, beta-catenin, and cadherin pathways. *Science* 303(5663), 1483-1487.

Nigg, E.A. (2002). Centrosome aberrations: cause or consequence of cancer progression? *Nat Rev Cancer* 2(11), 815-825.

Nigg, E.A. (2007). Centrosome duplication: of rules and licenses. *Trends Cell Biol* 17(5), 215-221.

Ogden, S.K.; Lee, K.C. & Barton, M.C. (2000). Hepatitis B Viral Transactivator HBx Alleviates p53-mediated Repression of a-Fetoprotein Gene Expression. *J Biol Chem* 275, 27806-27814.

Palazzo, R.E.; Vogel, J.M.; Schnackenberg, B.J.; Hull, D.R. & Wu, X. (2000). Centrosome maturation. *Curr Top Dev Biol* 49, 449-470.

Pang, R.; Tse, E. & Poon, R.T. (2006). Molecular pathways in hepatocellular carcinoma. *Cancer Lett* 240, 157-169.

Park, S.G.; Chung, C.; Kang, H.; Kin, J.Y. & Jung, G. (2006). Up-regulation of cyclin D1 by HBx is mediated by NF-kappaB2/BCL3 complex through kappaB site of cyclin D1 promoter. *J Biol Chem* 281(42), 31770-31777.

Park, S.G.; Min, J.Y.; Chung, C.; Hsieh, A. & Jung, G. (2009). Tumor suppressor protein p53 induces degradation of the oncogenic protein HBx. *Cancer Lett* 282(2), 229-237.

Parkin, D.M. (2006). The global health burden of infection-associated cancers in the year 2002. *Int J Cancer* 118, 3030-3044.

Pellegrino, R.; Calvisi, D.F.; Ladu, S.; Ehemann, V.; Staniscia, T.; Ecert, M.; Dombrowski, F.; Schirmacher, P. & Longerich, T. (2010). Oncogenic and tumor suppressive roles of polo-like kinases in human hepatocellular carcinoma. *Hepatol* 51(3), 857-868.

Pihan, G.A.; Purohit, A.; Wallace, J.; Knecht, H.; Woda, B.; Quesenberry, P. & Doxsey, S.J. (1998). Centrosome defects and genetic instability in malignant tumors. *Cancer Res* 58, 3974-3985.

Reverte, C.G.; Benware, A.; Jones, C.W. & LaFlamme, S.E. (2006). Perturbing integrin function inhibits microtubule growth from centrosomes, spindle assembly, and cytokinesis. *J Cell Biol* 174(4), 491-497.

Rieder, C.L.; Faruki, S. & Khodjakov, A. (2001). The centrosome in vertebrates: more than a microtubule-organizing center. *Trends Cell Biol* 11(10), 413-419.

Riparbelli, M.G. & Callaini, G. (2003). Drosophila parthenogenesis: a model for de novo centrosome assembly. *Dev Biol* 260, 298-313.

Rousselet, A. (2009). Inhibiting Crm1 causes the formation of excess acentriolar spindle poles containing NuMA and B23, but does not affect centrosome numbers. *Biol Cell* 101, 679-693.

Scaplehorn, N. & Way, M. (2004). Manipulation of centrosomes and the microtubule cytoskeleton during infectionbyintracellular pathogens, In: *Wiley-VCA Verlag GmbH & CoKGaG*, 371-400.

Schatten, H.; Wiedemeier, A.M.; Taylor, M.; Lubahn, D.B; Greenberg, N.M.; Besch-Williford, C.; Rosenfeld, C.S.; Day, J.K. & Ripple, M. (2000). Centrosome-centriole abnormalities are markers for abnormal cell divisions and cancer in the transgenic adenocarcinoma mouse prostate (TRAMP) model. *Biol Cell* 92(5), 331-340.

Strnad, P.; Leidel, S.; Vinogradova, T.; Euteneuer, U.; Khodjakov, A. & Gonczy, P. (2007). Regulated HsSAS-6 levels ensure formation of a single procentriole per centriole during the centrosome duplication cycle. *Dev Cell* 13, 203-213.

Suzuki, Y. & Craigie, R. (2007). The road to chromatin - nuclear entry of retroviruses. *Nat Rev Microbiol* 5(3), 187-196.

Szollosi, D. & Ozil, J.P. (1991). *De novo* formation of centrioles in parthenogenetically activated, diploidized rabbit embryos. *Biol Cell* 72, 61-66.

Tillement, V.; Haren, L.; Roullet, N.; Etievant, C. & Merdes, A. (2009). The centrosome protein NEDD1 as a potential pharmacological target to induce cell cycle arrest. *Mol Cancer* 8: 10.

Tsou, M.B. & Stearns, T. (2006a). Mechanism limiting centrosome duplication to once per cell cycle. *Nature* 442, 947-951.

Tsou, M.F. & Stearns, T. (2006b). Controlling centrosome number: licenses and blocks. *Cur Opin Cell Biol* 18, 74-78.

Wang, F.Z.; Fei, H.R.; Lian, L.H; Wang, J.M. & Qiu, Y.Y. (2011). Hepatitis B x-interacting protein induces HepG2 cell proliferation through activation of the phosphatidylinositol 3-kinase/Akt pathway. *Exp Biol Med* 236(1), 62-69.

Wang, X.W.; Gibson, M.K.; Vermeulen, W.; Yeh, H.; Forrester, K.; Sturzbecher, H.W.; Hoeijmakers, J.H. & Harris, C.C. (1995). Abrogation of p53-induced apoptosis by the hepatitis B virus X gene. *Cancer Res* 55, 6012-6016.

Wang, Y.; Ji, P.; Liu, J.; Broaddus, R.R.; Xue, F. & Zhang, W. (2009). Centrosome-associated regulators of the G(2)/M checkpoint as targets for cancer therapy. *Mol Cancer* 8: 8.

Ward, A.; Morettin, A.; Shum, D. & Hudson, J.W. (2011). Aberrant methylation of *Polo-like kinase* CpG islands in *Plk4* heterozygous mice. *BMC Cancer* 11, 71.

Warner, S.L.; Gray, P.J. & Von Hoff, D.D. (2006). Tubulin-associated drug targets: Aurora kinases, polo-like kinases, and others. *Semin Oncol* 33(4): 436-48.

Wen, Y.; Golubkov, V.S.; Strongin, A.Y.; Jiang, W. & Reed, J.C. (2008). Interaction of hepatitis B viral 0ncoprotein with cellular target HBXIP dysregulates centrosome dynamics and mitotic spindle formation. *J Biol Chem* 283, 2793-2803.

Whitehead, C.M. & Salisbury, J.L. (1999). Regulation and regulatory activities of centrosome. *J Cell Biochem* 32-33(Suppl), 192-199.

World Health Organization Scientific Group on Prevention and Control of Hepatocellular Carcinoma. (1983). Prevention of primary liver cancer: Report on a meeting of a WHO scientific group. *Lancet* 1, 463-465.

Wu, C.C.; Hsu, S.L. & Hwang, G.Y. (2008). HBx inhibits the growth of CCL13-HBX-stable cells via the GSK-3beta/beta-catenin cascade. *Kuo CY Intervirol* 51(2), 130-136.

Young, A.; Dictenberg, J.B.; Purohit, A.; Tuft, R. & Doxsey, S.J. (2000). Cytoplasmic dynein-mediated assembly of pericentrin and γ-tubulin onto centrosomes. *Mol Biol Cell* 11, 2047-2056.

Yun, C.; Cho, H.; Kim, S.J.; Lee, J.H.; Park, S.Y.; Chan, G.K. & Cho, H. (2004). Mitotic aberration coupled with centrosome amplification is induced by hepatitis B virus X oncoprotein via the Ras-mitogen-activated protein/extracellular signal-regulated kinase-mitogen-activated protein pathway. *Mol Cancer Res* 2(3), 159-169.

# 11

# Cytoplasmic Connexin32 and Self-Renewal of Cancer Stem Cells: Implication in Metastasis

Yasufumi Omori[1], Yohei Kawasaki[1,2], Qingchang Li[1,3], Toshiaki Yoshioka[1], Yohei Yamamoto[1] and Katsuhiko Enomoto[1]
[1]*Department of Molecular and Tumour Pathology, Akita University Graduate School of Medicine*
[2]*Department of Otorhinolaryngology, Akita University Graduate School of Medicine*
[3]*Department of Pathology, College of Basic Medical Sciences, China Medical University*
[1,2]*Japan*
[3]*China*

## 1. Introduction

Gap junction is a unique intercellular channel which connects directly the cytoplasm of two neighbouring cells, and allows small ($M_r$ < 1000) water-soluble molecules to travel between the cells throughout a tissue, thus serving as a tool of cell-cell communication (Goodenough et al., 1996). In general, gap junction plays crucial roles in tissue and cellular homeostasis and has long been known to suppress carcinogenesis in many tissues (Crespin et al., 2009; Leithe et al., 2006). In the liver, one of the organs where gap junctions are well developed, down-regulation of gap junction between hepatocytes is one of hallmarks for hepatocarcinogenesis (V.A. Krutovskikh et al., 1991). Gap junction is completely disrupted in not only hepatocellular carcinoma but also even precancerous lesions such as GST-P foci (Fitzgerald et al., 1989). A gap junction channel is composed of two hemichannels, which dock with each other to make a complete channel. Hemichannels are provided by each of two neighbouring cells and are called "connexons." The connexon is a hexamer of connexin protein, which forms connexin family consisting of more than 20 members in mammals (Beyer & Berthoud, 2009; Sohl & Willecke, 2003). Among them, connexin26 and connexin32 proteins are co-expressed in the hepatocyte (Nicholson et al., 1987; Vinken et al., 2008). During hepatocarcinogenesis, expression of connexin26 protein is abolished. On the other hand, connexin32 protein is reduced in expression but remains expressed not in plasma membrane but in cytoplasm, resulting in total loss of functional gap junction from both hepatocellular carcinoma and its precancerous lesions. More interestingly, the amount of connexin32 protein in cytoplasm often increases in the correspondence with tumour progression and/or the grade of malignancy (Fig. 1) (V. Krutovskikh et al., 1994). Therefore, although connexin32 protein localised in cytoplasm is non-functional as a gap junction component, it may contribute to tumour progression such as invasion and metastasis.

It has long been believed that the tumour is composed of monoclonal cells and thus is a homogenous cell population. According to this idea, every tumour cell should have the ability to develop a new tumour elsewhere and possible heterogeneity should be made only

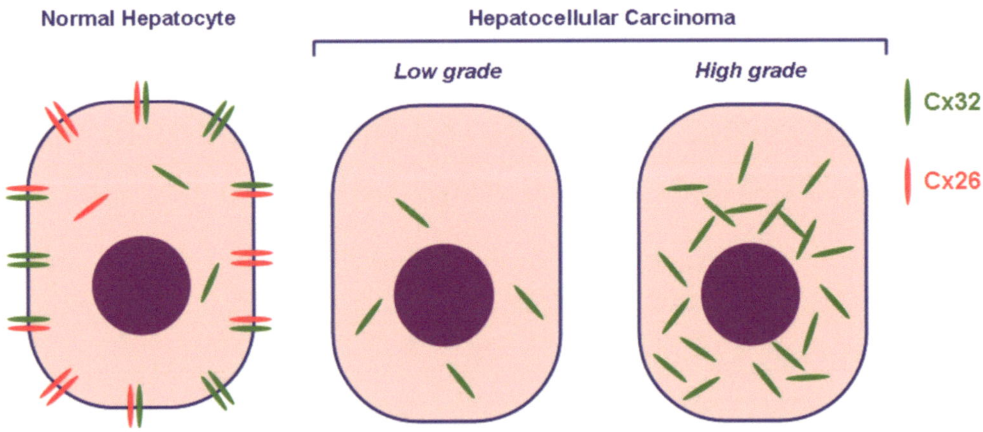


Fig. 1. Expression patterns and subcellular localisation of connexin26 and connexin32 proteins in HCC.

by spontaneous mutations during tumour development and progression. On the other hand, recent intensive studies have revealed that there is cellular hierarchy in a tumour tissue, ranging from stem-like cells to mature tumour cells (Jordan et al., 2006). This latter idea indicates that the tumour is *per se* a heterogeneous cell population and that only stem-like cells within a tumour tissue have the ability to reconstitute a daughter tumour identical to its mother tumour consisting of heterogeneous cells. These two theories are not necessarily contradictory to each other. Since a certain mutation acquired in a single normal cell is the very first event of carcinogenesis, tumour cells in the same tumour are reasonably monoclonal. It is also true that accumulation of different mutations in individual tumour cells creates heterogeneity in a tumour tissue. The concept on cellular hierarchy in tumour tissues is not brand-new but was already proposed long time ago, *i.e.*, in the first half of the 20th century (Fialkow et al., 1967; Furth & Kahn, 1937), and has recently been revisited by many scientists with the help of various cutting-edge methods. Today, the stem-like cell is called "cancer stem cell (CSC)" or "tumour-initiating cell (TIC)," depending on individual preferences. Hereafter, CSC is applied for stem-like cell in this chapter. Usually, a tumour tissue contains only a very small number of CSCs and resultantly, almost all cells constituting a tumour mass are non-CSCs. While CSCs isolated from a tumour can develop a tumour when xenografted into immunodeficient animals such as SCID mice, non-CSCs cannot. Therefore practically, CSCs are considered to be a subpopulation having tumorigenicity. Since no absolute marker for CSC has so far been known in any kind of cancers, CSCs are indistinguishable from non-CSCs. All we can do is just to enrich CSCs from the bulk of a tumour by using various markers and a cell sorting system (Klonisch et al., 2008). For example, since CSCs of glioblastoma are contained exclusively in the CD133-positive fraction, we can enrich them by isolating the CD133-positive fraction (Singh et al., 2003, 2004). However, since a few non-CSCs are also CD133-positive, no means to purify glioblastoma CSCs have become available yet.

CSCs of hepatocellular carcinoma (HCC) have also been investigated in many laboratories, some of which have succeeded in identifying the CSCs in surgical specimen (Ma et al., 2007;

Yang et al., 2008a, 2008b; Yin et al., 2007). Surprisingly, presence of CSCs was confirmed in not only HCC *in vivo* but also HCC-derived cell lines, including human HuH7 cells (Chiba et al., 2006). This finding indicates that there is cellular hierarchy even in immortalised cell lines and that cell lines are not always homogenous cell populations. Thus, employing HuH7 cells, we have investigated roles of cytoplasmic connexin32 protein in metastasis especially in terms of CSC population control.

## 2. Cytoplasmic connexin32-mediated control of CSC population and its pro-metastatic roles in HuH7 cells

### 2.1 Cytoplasmic localisation of connexin protein in cancer

It is universally accepted that connexin protein is a component of gap junction and thus localised in plasma membrane, where gap junction channels form large clusters called gap junction plaques (Yeager, 2009). When tissue sections are subjected to immunohistochemical staining, these gap junction plaques make impressive punctate signals in a cell-cell contact area (Momiyama et al., 2003). On the other hand, when connexin protein is retained in cytoplasm, their specific signals are often vague and ignored as a kind of background noises (Omori & Yamasaki, 1998). Finally, a certain number of surgical specimens where no gap junction plaques are formed are likely to be categorised as negative for connexin protein regardless of whether or not it is expressed in cytoplasm.

| Histotype of tumour | Connexin | Reference |
|---|---|---|
| Hepatocellular carcinoma, moderately and poorly differentiated | Cx32 and Cx43 | V. Krutovskikh et al. (1994)<br>Oyamada et al. (1990) |
| Adenocarcinoma of the prostate, poorly differentiated | Cx32 and Cx43 | Mehta et al. (1999) |
| Invasive ductal carcinoma (NOS[1]) of the breast, grade II and III | Cx26 | Jamieson et al. (1998) |
| Lymph node metastases of breast cancer | Cx26 and Cx43 | Kanczuga-Koda et al. (2006) |
| Oesophageal squamous cell carcinoma, poor prognostic group | Cx26 | Inose et al. (2009) |

[1]Not otherwise specified

Table 1. Cytoplasmic connexin proteins in human cancers

It is well known that gap junctional communication is severely impaired or abolished in almost all tumours during and after the early stage of carcinogenesis (Mesnil et al., 2005). Although downregulation of gap junctional communication results from a decrease in the expression level of connexin mRNA and/or protein in many cases (Leithe et al., 2006), accumulating evidences from careful studies have indicated, as shown in Table 1, that cytoplasmic localisation of connexin protein, probably due to a defect of membrane trafficking, is not rare, and that it is likely one of the mechanisms for the downregulation of gap junctional communication. We estimate that such cytoplasmic localisation of connexin could have been observed in human tumours much more frequently than reported. Connexin protein in cytoplasm is non-functional as a gap junction. Does such cytoplasmic connexin play any roles instead of gap junction? Several reports have described suggestive observations on cytoplasmic connexin and tumour progression (Table 1).

V. Krutovskikh et al. (1994) examined 20 surgical samples of human hepatocellular carcinoma for the expression pattern of connexin32 protein and found that poorly differentiated HCC exhibited stronger signals of connexin32 protein in cytoplasm than well differentiated HCC. Mehta et al. (1999) immunostained 20 primary and 20 metastatic lesions of human prostate cancer along with normal counterparts to detect connexin32 and connexin43 proteins. While both connexin32 and connexin43 proteins gave punctate signals in cell-cell contact areas of acinar epithelial cells in both normal and well differentiated adenocarcinoma tissues, both of the connexin proteins were localised in cytoplasm without forming gap junction plaques in poorly differentiated and undifferentiated carcinoma tissues. Jamieson et al. (1998) examined the immunohistochemical expression of connexin26 and connexin43 proteins in 27 cases of invasive ductal carcinoma (not otherwise specified) as well as normal and benign tumour tissues of the human breast and revealed that connexin26 protein was expressed in cytoplasm in a great majority of the examined cancer samples with grade II or III malignancy while no connexin26 protein was detected in either normal or benign tumour samples. More interestingly, Kanczuga-Koda et al. (2006) clearly showed that the cytoplasmic expression of both connexin26 and connexin43 proteins was much more frequent in tumours that metastasised to lymph nodes than in the primary lesions of human breast cancers. Most recently, Inose et al. (2009) examined 123 cases of oesophageal squamous cell carcinoma in expression and subcellular localisation of connexin26 protein. While no expression of connexin26 protein was detected anywhere in normal counterparts, connexin26 protein was expressed in 60 cases (49%) and was localised in not plasma membrane but cytoplasm in these cases. Furthermore, they found the direct correlation between connexin26 expression and the frequency of lymph node metastases, suggesting that cytoplasmic expression of connexin26 protein should be related to cancer progression and poor prognosis rather than carcinogenesis.

Therefore, while disruption of gap junction is a common early event during carcinogenesis, cytoplasmic accumulation of connexin protein seems to accelerate progression of the developed tumours.

### 2.2 Accumulation of cytoplasmic connexin32 and enhancement of self-renewal of CSCs in HuH7 HCC cells

As mentioned above, connexin32 protein translocates from plasma membrane to cytoplasm during hepatocarcinogenesis and its expression level correlates with the grade of malignancy and with the extent of progression in developed HCCs. Since the essential element in a cancer tissue is the CSCs but not matured tumour cells, connexin32 protein in cytoplasm may control progression of HCCs by modulating CSC population. Furthermore, the presence of CSCs in human HuH7 cells had already been proven. We, thus, analysed alteration of CSC population by cytoplasmic connexin32 protein in HuH7 cells (Kawasaki et al., 2011).

### 2.2.1 Overexpression of connexin32 protein and its subcellular localisation in HCC-derived cells

Disruption of gap junction in association with translocation of connexin32 protein from plasma membrane to cytoplasm is a common feature of HCCs (V. Krutovskikh et al., 1994; V.A. Krutovskikh et al., 1995). Consistently, we confirmed that this aberrant expression pattern of connexin32 protein was conserved in liver cancer-derived cell lines such as HuH7 (Nakabayashi et al., 1982), Li-7 (Hirohashi et al., 1979), and HepG2 (Aden et al., 1979) cells, the first two of which are derived from HCC and the third one is from hepatoblastoma. These cells are deficient in sorting of connexin32 protein into plasma membrane as is HCC. To examine the effects of cytoplasmic connein32 protein on CSC population, we established a Tet-off-based inducible expression system (Gossen & Bujard, 1992) of connexin32 in HuH7 and Li-7 cells (Li et al., 2007). In this system, expression of exogenous connexin32 mRNA can be blocked by doxycycline. To the contrary, withdrawal of doxycycline from the culture medium induces overexpression of connexin32 mRNA and protein. As shown in Fig. 2, all the clones examined exhibited a significant induction. Especially, the clone 15-1 of HuH7 Tet-off Cx32 cells expressed a 4-time-larger amount of connexin32 protein in the doxycycline-free medium than in the doxycycline-supplemented one.

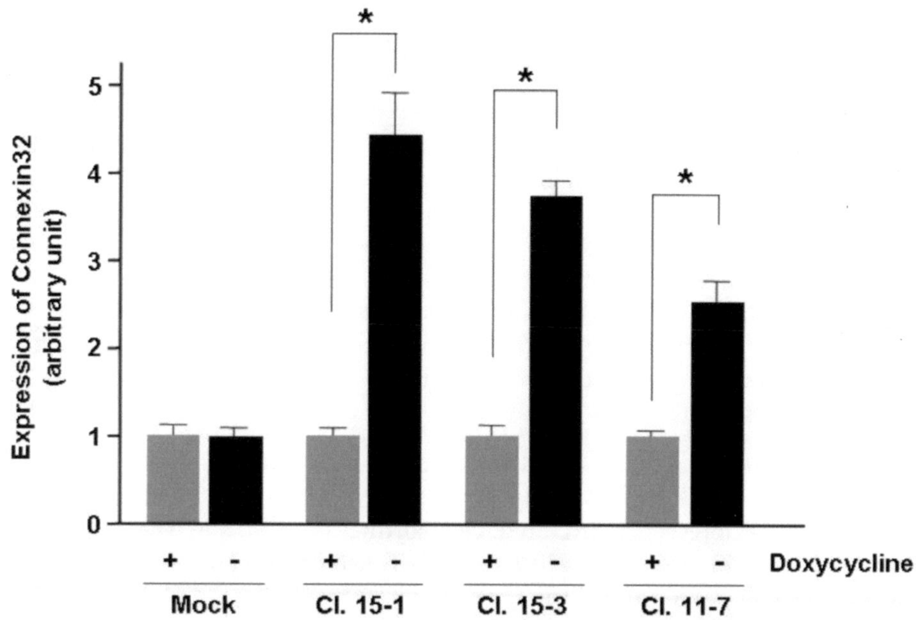


Fig. 2. Expression level of connexin32 protein in HuH7 Tet-off Cx32 and mock cells in the presence or absence of doxycycline. Densitometric analysis of immunoblottings for connexin32 protein. *$p < 0.01$ (n = 3)

Since either HuH7 or Li-7 cell line has no mutation within the coding region of GJB1 (human connexin32 gene), the exogenous connexin32 protein is identical to the endogenous one and both proteins should behave in the same manner. As expected, connexin32 protein overexpressed in HuH7 cells was co-localised with Golgi-58K protein, as revealed by immunofluorescence, in the doxycycline-deprived condition (Fig. 3), indicating that connexin32 protein was localised in Golgi apparatuses in HuH7 cells instead of plasma membrane.

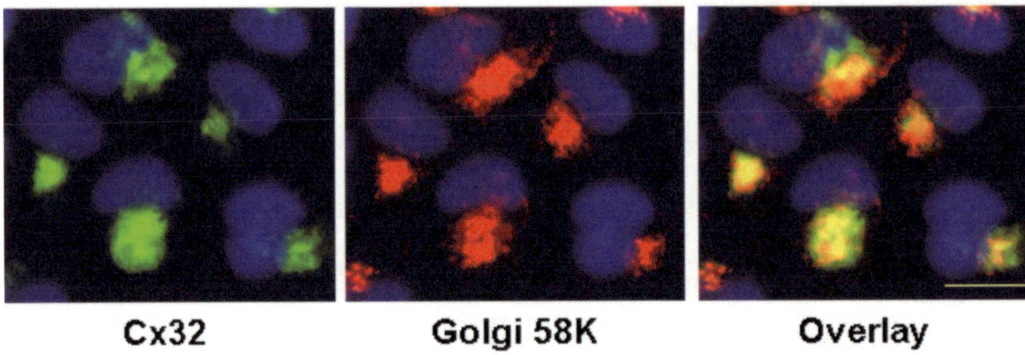


Fig. 3. Indirect immunofluorescence of connexin32 protein (left) and Golgi 58K protein (middle) in HuH7 Tet-off Cx32 cells in the absence of doxycycline. Nuclei were stained with diamidine phenylindole dihydrochloride. Note that signals of both connexin32 and Golgi 58K proteins are co-localised (right). Scale bar, 20 μm.

#### 2.2.2 CSCs of HuH7 cells are contained exclusively in the side population

Various CSC markers have been proposed in many cancers (Hill & Perris, 2007; Klonisch et al., 2008). Among them, we chose "side population" because Chiba et al. (2006) had already proven that CSCs of HuH7 cells are efficiently enriched in the side population with little contamination of non-CSCs. Besides side population, we tried another marker CD133, which had also been reported to be expressed in CSCs of HuH7 cells (Ma et al., 2007; Suetsugu et al., 2006). However, CD133-positive cells accounted for ~60% of the whole population in HuH7 cells (Kawasaki et al., 2011; Ma et al., 2007, 2008). Although the CD133-positive fraction may contain the whole CSC population, the major part of CD133-positive fraction should consist of non-CSCs. So the efficiency of CD133-driven enrichment of CSCs is quite low.

"Side population" is defined as a small subset of cells presenting a highly active efflux of Hoechst 33342 dye. As illustrated in Fig. 4, the side population is thus resistant to the dye and detected by fluorescence-activated cell sorting (FACS). On the other hand, the fraction which is stained with Hoechst 33342 is called "the main population." It is well known that the side population is the fraction into which stem cells in normal tissues are efficiently enriched (Falciatori et al., 2004; Goodell et al., 1996; Shimano et al., 2003). As is the case not only with normal tissues, a number of recent studies on various, otherwise not all, malignant tumours have revealed that the cells from the side population but not from the main population display a series of phenotypes signifying CSC (Grichnik et al., 2006; Hirschmann-Jax et al., 2004; Kondo et al., 2004; Moserle et al., 2008; Szotek et al., 2006; Wang et al., 2007).

To confirm that CSCs of our HuH7 Tet-off Cx32 cells are contained exclusively in the side population, we xenografted the side population and the main population subcutaneously into a flank of SCID mice after cell sorting and examined tumorigenicity of the grafts (Table 2). While 1 x $10^5$ cells from the side population developed a tumour at each of six mice examined, 1 x $10^5$ cells from the main population could form no palpable tumours in any mice, indicating that the CSC population resides only in the side population in our HuH7 Tet-off Cx32 and mock cells as well as in parental HuH7 cells. The side population-derived tumours are histologically identical to tumours raised from unsorted HuH7 Tet-off Cx32 cells.

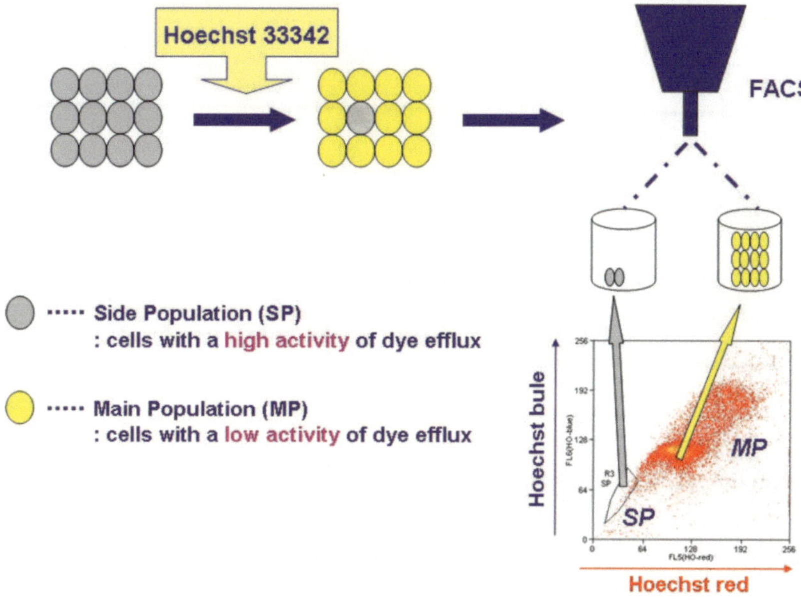


Fig. 4. Schematic diagram on side and main populations.

| | HuH7 Tet-off Cx32 | | | | | | HuH7 Tet-off Mock | | | | | |
|---|---|---|---|---|---|---|---|---|---|---|---|---|
| | SP | | MP | | US | | SP | | MP | | US | |
| Doxycycline | + | - | + | - | + | - | + | - | + | - | + | - |
| No. of mice bearing tumour | 6 | 6 | 0 | 0 | 2 | 3 | 6 | 6 | 0 | 0 | 3 | 3 |

SP: side population; MP: main population; US: unsorted
Six mice per each group were xenografted with 1 x $10^5$ cells from each fraction.

Table 2. Tumorigenicity of xenografts subcutaneously implanted into SCID mice

### 2.2.3 Overexpression of cytoplasmic connexin32 protein expands the side population

Considering the side population to be a CSC marker of HuH7 cells, we analysed the effects of cytoplasmic connexin32 protein on the CSC population by measuring the size of side population with FACS. In an experiment (Fig. 5), when HuH7 Tet-off Cx32 cells were cultured continuously for 10 days in the presence of 4 μg/ml of doxycycline, the verapamil-sensitive side population accounted for 0.27% of the whole population. In contrast, the side population in the cells cultured in a doxycycline-free medium expanded to up to 7.44% of the whole population. Fig. 5 shows that, in HuH7 Tet-off Cx32 cells, the proportion of the side population to the whole population is approximately 25 times higher in a doxycycline-free medium than in a doxycycline-supplemented one. Such a doxycycline-dependent alteration of the size of side population is not observed in HuH7 Tet-off mock cells. Therefore, it is concluded that the cell population expressing a higher level of cytoplasmic connexin32 protein contains a larger side population (Kawasaki et al., 2011).

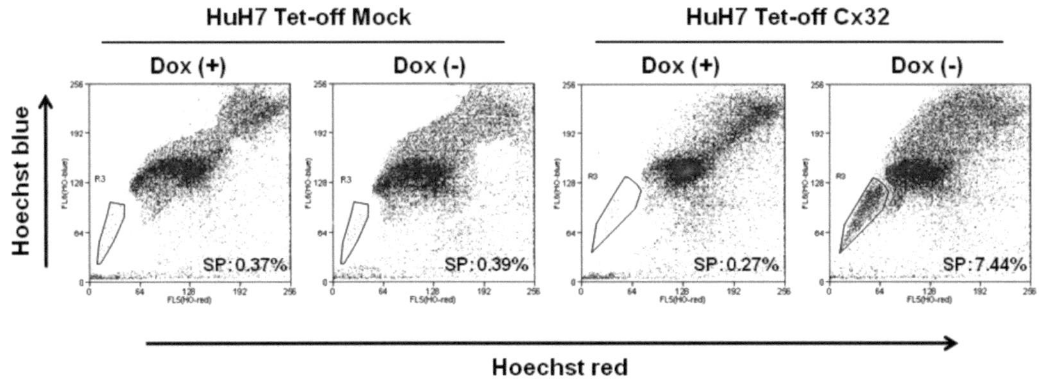


Dox: doxycycline; SP: side population

Fig. 5. FACS analysis of the side population in HuH7 Tet-off Cx32 and mock cells.

### 2.2.4 Overexpression of cytoplasmic connexin32 protein enhances self-renewal of CSCs

Similarly to stem cells in normal tissues, as far as maintained in monolayer culture with a serum-supplemented growth medium, CSCs are obliged to produce non-CSCs, which eventually predominate over CSCs. To avoid maturation of CSCs, they must be cultured in a serum-free medium on a non-attachment dish or in a serum-free semi-solid medium. In this condition, they proliferate as sphere-like cellular aggregates and sustain their undifferentiated state without maturing to non-CSCs, resulting in a pure culture of CSCs (Hermann et al., 2007; Kondo, 2007; Tirino et al., 2008). To define the roles of cytoplasmic connexin32 protein in self-renewal of CSCs, we isolated both the side population and main population separately by FACS and incubated each of them in a serum-free semi-solid medium with or without doxycycline for 20 days. As shown in Fig. 6, the main population had almost no capacity for sphere formation, whereas the side population exhibited an efficient ability to develop numerous large spheres, confirming that the side population of our HuH7 Tet-off Cx32 and the mock cells represented CSCs. As expected, spheres derived from the side population of HuH7 Tet-off Cx32 cells were increased in both number and size in a doxycycline-free medium compared with in a doxycycline-supplemented one (Fig. 6). On the other hand, the side population of HuH7 Tet-off mock cells showed similar capacities for sphere formation regardless of the presence or absence of doxycycline. These results clearly indicate that cytoplasmic accumulation of connexin32 protein enhances self-renewal of CSCs in HuH7 cells (Kawasaki et al., 2011).

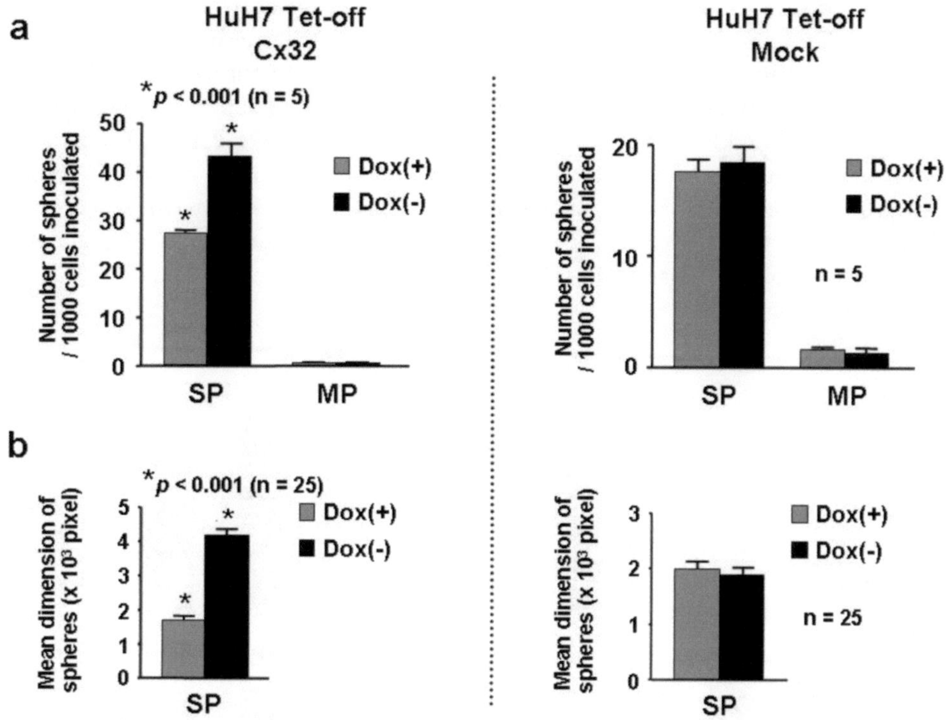


Fig. 6. CSC sphere formation assay in serum-free semisolid medium. The number (a) and the size (b) of developed CSC spheres are presented. SP: side population; MP: main population; Dox: doxycycline

### 2.3 Cytoplasmic connexin32-mediated induction of metastasis in HuH7 cells

As mentioned earlier, accumulation of different connexin proteins in cytoplasm has often been observed in cancers with high grade malignancy and/or in those of advanced stage (Table 1). Also in HCC, the expression level of cytoplasmic connexin32 protein is elevated as the differentiation state becomes poorer, strongly suggesting that accumulation of connexin32 protein in cytoplasm should contribute to progression of the developed HCC. We, thus, examined the effects of overexpression of cytoplasmic connexin32 protein on migration *in vitro* and metastasis *in vivo* (Li et al., 2007).

#### 2.3.1 Overexpression of cytoplasmic connexin32 protein enhances motility of HuH7 cells

Upregulation of cell motility is one of the most important steps during tumour metastasis (Thiery, 2002). We examined the effect of the overexpressed cytoplasmic connexin32 on cell motility by performing a serum-stimulated transwell migration assay (Li et al., 2007). Motility of all the examined clones of HuH7 Tet-off Cx32 cells was significantly upregulated in a doxycycline-free medium compared with in a doxycycline-supplemented one, while doxycycline did not affect motility of HuH7 Tet-off mock cells (Fig. 7). Much interestingly, the Cx32-transfected HeLa cell clone which exhibited a high level of gap junctional communication had a much lower motility than mock-transfected HeLa cells. Therefore, it is suggested that connexin32-mediated gap junctional communication should downregulate cell motility, which, to the contrary, cytoplasmic connexin32 protein upregulates. We further investigated whether overexpression of cytoplasmic connexin32 could affect invasiveness of HuH7 Tet-off Cx32 cells by evaluating the ability of HuH7 Tet-off Cx32 cells and mock cells to invade the basement membrane matrix in the presence or absence of doxycycline. When HuH7 Tet-off Cx32 cells were induced to overexpress cytoplasmic connexin32 protein in a doxycycline-free medium, they exhibited a significantly high level of invasiveness (Li et al., 2007).

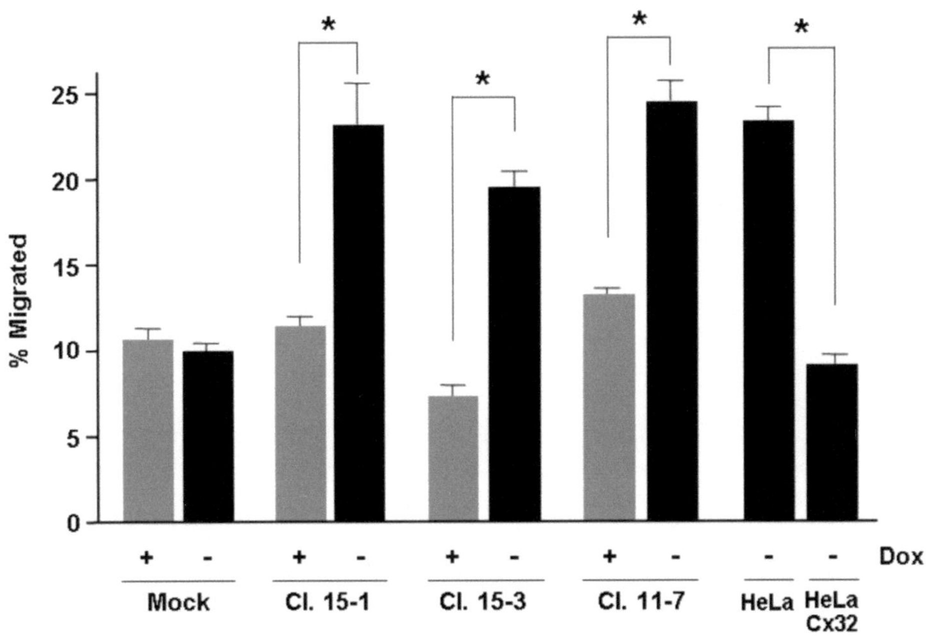


Dox: doxycycline. $^{*}p < 0.01$ (n = 6)

Fig. 7. Transwell migration assay. Three clones of HuH7 Tet-off Cx32 cells and their mock cells as well as HeLa and Cx32-transfected HeLa cells were examined on the motility.

### 2.3.2 Overexpression of cytoplasmic connexin32 protein induces a metastatic ability in non-metastatic HuH7 cells

We examined how HuH7 Tet-off Cx32 cells overexpressing cytoplasmic connexin32 protein behaved *in vivo* when they were grafted into the liver of immunodeficient SCID mice (Li et al., 2007). Each mouse was given 2 x $10^6$ cells of HuH7 Tet-off Cx32 cells along with mock cells into a subserosal area of the liver and was autopsied 8 weeks after the implantation to observe tumour development and metastases (Fig. 8). For administration of doxycycline, drink water was supplemented with 2 mg/ml doxycycline throughout the experiment period.

As summarised in Table 3, five out of six mice developed tumours at the implanted sites in each of the doxycycline (+) and the doxycycline (-) groups. The tumour sizes were not distinct between the doxycycline (+) and the doxycycline (-) groups. On the other hand, macroscopic metastatic lesions were found in all of the five tumour-bearing mice in the doxycycline (-) group but in none of the mice in the doxycycline (+) group (Table 3). This clearly indicates that the overexpressed cytoplasmic connexin32 protein can give the metastatic ability to HuH7 Tet-off Cx32 cells. Micrometastases and portal vein tumour thrombi were also frequently observed in livers of the doxycycline (-) group given HuH7 Tet-off Cx32 cells.

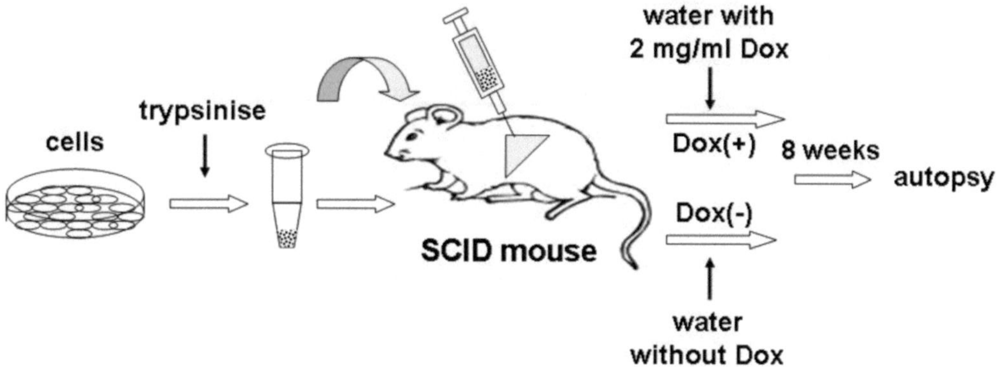


Dox: doxycycline

Fig. 8. Schematic illustration for orthotopic xenograft.

| Implanted cells | Doxycycline | No. of mice examined | No. of mice bearing tumour | No. of mice with metastases |
|---|---|---|---|---|
| HuH7 Tet-off Cx32 | + | 6 | 5 | 0 |
| | - | 6 | 5 | 5 |
| HuH7 Tet-off mock | + | 4 | 4 | 0 |
| | - | 4 | 4 | 0 |

[1]Li et al., 2007

Table 3. Tumorigenicity and metastasis of orthotopic xenografts in the liver of SCID mice[1]

Taken together, accumulation of connexin32 protein in cytoplasm should be a pro-metastatic event during progression of HCC.

## 3. Conclusive remarks

In this chapter, we reviewed the literatures describing cytoplasmic connexin proteins in different cancers including HCC and presented our previous studies demonstrating that accumulation of cytoplasmic conneixin32 protein enhanced self-renewal of CSCs in HCC-derived cells and resulted in induction of metastasis. What is the impact of the number of CSCs upon metastasis?

In our studies, we hypothesised that expansion of the CSC population should mediate the pro-metastatic function of cytoplasmic connexin32 protein. It is incontestable that cell motility and invasiveness are essential factors for metastasis. What these two factors modulate most directly is the length of the latent period between development of a primary tumour and that of its first metastatic focus. On the other hand, the number of CSCs in a tumour should be related closely to the number of metastatic lesions that develop because CSCs are so-called functional seeds that are tumorigenic at a destination site of cell migration while non-CSCs are sterile (Fig. 9) (Jordan et al., 2006). Each metastatic lesion arises from a single CSC but not from non-CSCs. A recent report clearly demonstrated that tumour cells began to circulate in peripheral blood even at the early phase of cancer development, when no risk for metastasis was clinically estimated (Hüsemann et al., 2008; Riethdorf et al., 2008). Taken together, the proportion of CSCs to the whole population in a tumour should be more relevant to the extent of metastasis than the bulk of tumour cells in migration. So it is quite reasonable that cytoplasmic connexin32 protein should enhance the metastatic potential of HCC by expanding its CSC population.

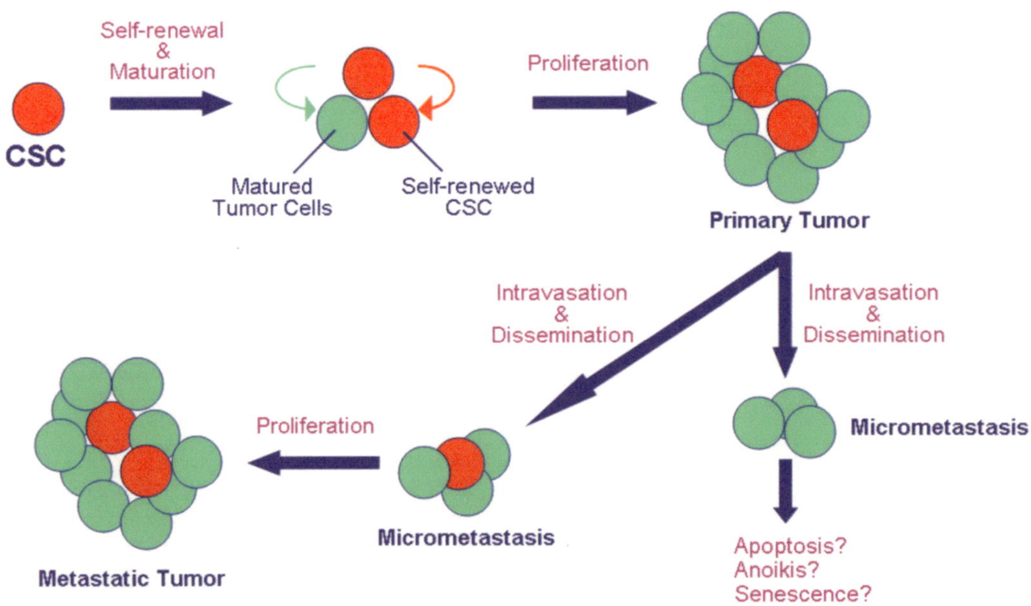


Fig. 9. Each metastatic tumour should be originated from a single cancer stem cell.

For the past five decades, connexin-mediated gap junctional communication has been believed to be one of mechanisms for tumour suppression. This was actually the case. Gap junctional communication efficiently suppressed tumour development in many organs as revealed by both *in vitro* and *in vivo* experiments. Today, connexin proteins are, however, beyond gap junction (Goodenough & Paul, 2003)! A great variety of structures, functions, and behaviours of connexin proteins are known, *i.e.*, hemichannel (Jiang & Gu, 2005), mitochondrial connexin (Boengler et al., 2005), oncogenic connexin (Banerjee et al., 2010; Boengler et al., 2005; Ito et al., 2000), cytoplasmic connexin (Omori et al., 2007), fragmented connexin, and then, gap junction. Therefore, the functions of connexin proteins in cancers are not always suppressive to either cell proliferation or tumour progression (Naus & Laird, 2010). Complex and diverse functions of connexin proteins still remain to be elucidated in this new era. In other words, we will acquire, in near future, novel important knowledge that is presently masked by connexin.

## 4. Acknowledgment

The authors are very grateful to Ms. Reiko Ito and Ms. Yuko Doi for their technical assistance, and to Ms. Eriko Kumagai for her secretarial work. This work was supported in part by a Grant-in-Aid for Scientific Research from the Ministry of Education, Culture, Sports, Science and Technology of Japan (to Y. Omori, Grant No. 21590427). Q. Li was recipient of Japanese Government (MEXT) Scholarship (#022101).

## 5. References

Aden, D.P., Fogel, A., Plotkin, S., Damjanov, I., & Knowles, B.B. (1979). Controlled synthesis of HBsAg in a differentiated human liver carcinoma-derived cell line. *Nature*, Vol.282, pp. 615-616, ISSN 0028-0836

Banerjee, D., Gakhar, G., Madgwick, D., Hurt, A., Takemoto, D., & Nguyen, T.A. (2010). A novel role of gap junction connexin46 protein to protect breast tumors from hypoxia. *International Journal of Cancer*, Vol.127, pp. 839-848, ISSN 0020-7136

Beyer, E.C., & Berthoud, V.M. (2009). The family of connexin genes, IN: *Connexins*, Harris, A.L. & Locke, D., pp. 3-26, Humana Press, ISBN 978-1-934115-46-6, New York

Boengler, K., Dodoni, G., Rodriguez-Sinovas, A., Cabestrero, A., Ruiz-Meana, M., Gres, P., Konietzka, I., Lopez-Iglesias, C., Garcia-Dorado, D., Di Lisa, F., Heusch, G., & Schulz, R. (2005). Connexin 43 in cardiomyocyte mitochondria and its increase by ischemic preconditioning. *Cardiovascular Research*, Vol.67, pp. 234-244, ISSN 0008-6363

Chiba, T., Kita, K., Zheng, Y.W., Yokosuka, O., Saisho, H., Iwama, A., Nakauchi, H., & Taniguchi, H. (2006). Side population purified from hepatocellular carcinoma cells harbors cancer stem cell-like properties. *Hepatology*, Vol.44, pp. 240-251, ISSN 0270-9139

Crespin, S., Defamie, N., Cronier, L., & Mesnil, M. (2009). Connexins and carcinogenesis, IN: *Connexins*, Harris, A.L. & Locke, D., pp. 529-542, Humana Press, ISBN 978-1-934115-46-6, New York

Falciatori, I., Borsellino, G., Haliassos, N., Boitani, C., Corallini, S., Battistini, L., Bernardi, G., Stefanini, M., & Vicini, E. (2004). Identification and enrichment of spermatogonial stem cells displaying side-population phenotype in immature mouse testis. *FASEB Journal*, Vol.18, pp. 376-378, ISSN 0892-6638

Fialkow, P.J., Gartler, S.M., & Yoshida, A. (1967). Clonal origin of chronic myelocytic leukemia in man. *Proceedings of the National Academy of Sciences of the United States of America*, Vol.58, pp. 1468-1471, ISSN 0027-8424

Fitzgerald, D.J., Mesnil, M., Oyamada, M., Tsuda, H., Ito, N., & Yamasaki, H. (1989). Changes in gap junction protein (connexin 32) gene expression during rat liver carcinogenesis. *Journal of Cellular Biochemistry*, Vol.41, pp. 97-102, ISSN 0730-2312

Furth, J., & Kahn, M.C. (1937). The transmission of leukemia of mice with a single cell. *American Journal of Cancer*, Vol.31, pp. 276-282, ISSN 0099-7013

Goodell, M.A., Brose, K., Paradis, G., Conner, A.S., & Mulligan, R.C. (1996). Isolation and functional properties of murine hematopoietic stem cells that are replicating in vivo. *Journal of Experimental Medicine*, Vol.183, pp. 1797-1806, ISSN 0022-1007

Goodenough, D.A., Goliger, J.A., & Paul, D.L. (1996). Connexins, connexons, and intercellular communication. *Annual Review of Biochemistry*, Vol.65, pp. 475-502, ISSN 0066-4154

Goodenough, D.A., & Paul, D.L. (2003). Beyond the gap: functions of unpaired connexon channels. *Nature Reviews. Molecular Cell Biology*, Vol.4, pp. 285-294, ISSN 1471-0072

Gossen, M., & Bujard, H. (1992). Tight control of gene expression in mammalian cells by tetracycline-responsive promoters. *Proceedings of the National Academy of Sciences of the United States of America*, Vol.89, pp. 5547-5551, ISSN 0027-8424

Grichnik, J.M., Burch, J.A., Schulteis, R.D., Shan, S., Liu, J., Darrow, T.L., Vervaert, C.E., & Seigler, H.F. (2006). Melanoma, a tumor based on a mutant stem cell? *Journal of Investigative Dermatology*, Vol.126, pp. 142-153, ISSN 0022-202X

Hüsemann, Y., Geigl, J.B., Schubert, F., Musiani, P., Meyer, M., Burghart, E., Forni, G., Eils, R., Fehm, T., Riethmuller, G., & Klein, C.A. (2008). Systemic spread is an early step in breast cancer. *Cancer Cell*, Vol.13, pp. 58-68, ISSN 1535-6108

Hermann, P.C., Huber, S.L., Herrler, T., Aicher, A., Ellwart, J.W., Guba, M., Bruns, C.J., & Heeschen, C. (2007). Distinct populations of cancer stem cells determine tumor growth and metastatic activity in human pancreatic cancer. *Cell Stem Cell*, Vol.1, pp. 313-323, ISSN 1934-5909

Hill, R.P., & Perris, R. (2007). "Destemming" cancer stem cells. *Journal of National Cancer Institute*, Vol.99, pp. 1435-1440, ISSN 0027-8874

Hirohashi, S., Shimosato, Y., Kameya, T., Koide, T., Mukojima, T., Taguchi, Y., & Kageyama, K. (1979). Production of alpha-fetoprotein and normal serum proteins by xenotransplanted human hepatomas in relation to their growth and morphology. *Cancer Research*, Vol.39, pp. 1819-1828, ISSN 0008-5472

Hirschmann-Jax, C., Foster, A.E., Wulf, G.G., Nuchtern, J.G., Jax, T.W., Gobel, U., Goodell, M.A., & Brenner, M.K. (2004). A distinct "side population" of cells with high drug efflux capacity in human tumor cells. *Proceedings of the National Academy of Sciences of the United States of America*, Vol.101, pp. 14228-14233, ISSN 0027-8424

Inose, T., Kato, H., Kimura, H., Faried, A., Tanaka, N., Sakai, M., Sano, A., Sohda, M., Nakajima, M., Fukai, Y., Miyazaki, T., Masuda, N., Fukuchi, M., & Kuwano, H. (2009). Correlation between connexin 26 expression and poor prognosis of esophageal squamous cell carcinoma. *Annals of Surgical Oncology*, Vol.16, pp. 1704-1710, ISSN 1068-9265

Ito, A., Katoh, F., Kataoka, T.R., Okada, M., Tsubota, N., Asada, H., Yoshikawa, K., Maeda, S., Kitamura, Y., Yamasaki, H., & Nojima, H. (2000). A role for heterologous gap junctions between melanoma and endothelial cells in metastasis. *Journal of Clinical Investigation*, Vol.105, pp. 1189-1197, ISSN 0021-9738

Jamieson, S., Going, J.J., D'Arcy, R., & George, W.D. (1998). Expression of gap junction proteins connexin 26 and connexin 43 in normal human breast and in breast tumours. *Journal of Pathology*, Vol.184, pp. 37-43, ISSN 0022-4782

Jiang, J.X., & Gu, S. (2005). Gap junction- and hemichannel-independent actions of connexins. *Biochimica et Biophysica Acta*, Vol.1711, pp. 208-214, ISSN 0006-3002

Jordan, C.T., Guzman, M.L., & Noble, M. (2006). Cancer stem cells. *New England Journal of Medicine*, Vol.355, pp. 1253-1261, ISSN 0028-4793

Kanczuga-Koda, L., Sulkowski, S., Lenczewski, A., Koda, M., Wincewicz, A., Baltaziak, M., & Sulkowska, M. (2006). Increased expression of connexins 26 and 43 in lymph node metastases of breast cancer. *Journal of Clinical Pathology*, Vol.59, pp. 429-433, ISSN 0021-9746

Kawasaki, Y., Omori, Y., Li, Q., Nishikawa, Y., Yoshioka, T., Yoshida, M., Ishikawa, K., & Enomoto, K. (2011). Cytoplasmic accumulation of connexin32 expands cancer stem cell population in human HuH7 hepatoma cells by enhancing its self-renewal. *International Journal of Cancer*, Vol.128, pp. 51-62, ISSN 0020-7136

Klonisch, T., Wiechec, E., Hombach-Klonisch, S., Ande, S.R., Wesselborg, S., Schulze-Osthoff, K., & Los, M. (2008). Cancer stem cell markers in common cancers - therapeutic implications. *Trends in Molecular Medicine*, Vol.14, pp. 450-460, ISSN 1471-4914

Kondo, T., Setoguchi, T., & Taga, T. (2004). Persistence of a small subpopulation of cancer stem-like cells in the C6 glioma cell line. *Proceedings of the National Academy of Sciences of the United States of America*, Vol.101, pp. 781-786, ISSN 0027-8424

Kondo, T. (2007). Stem cell-like cancer cells in cancer cell lines. *Cancer Biomarkers*, Vol.3, pp. 245-250, ISSN 1574-0153

Krutovskikh, V., Mazzoleni, G., Mironov, N., Omori, Y., Aguelon, A.M., Mesnil, M., Berger, F., Partensky, C., & Yamasaki, H. (1994). Altered homologous and heterologous gap-junctional intercellular communication in primary human liver tumors associated with aberrant protein localization but not gene mutation of connexin 32. *International Journal of Cancer*, Vol.56, pp. 87-94, ISSN 0020-7136

Krutovskikh, V.A., Oyamada, M., & Yamasaki, H. (1991). Sequential changes of gap-junctional intercellular communications during multistage rat liver carcinogenesis: direct measurement of communication in vivo. *Carcinogenesis*, Vol.12, pp. 1701-1706, ISSN 0143-3334

Krutovskikh, V.A., Mesnil, M., Mazzoleni, G., & Yamasaki, H. (1995). Inhibition of rat liver gap junction intercellular communication by tumor-promoting agents in vivo. Association with aberrant localization of connexin proteins. *Laboratory Investigation*, Vol.72, pp. 571-577, ISSN 0023-6837

Leithe, E., Sirnes, S., Omori, Y., & Rivedal, E. (2006). Downregulation of gap junctions in cancer cells. *Critical Reviews in Oncogenesis*, Vol.12, pp. 225-256, ISSN 0893-9675

Li, Q., Omori, Y., Nishikawa, Y., Yoshioka, T., Yamamoto, Y., & Enomoto, K. (2007). Cytoplasmic accumulation of connexin32 protein enhances motility and metastatic ability of human hepatoma cells in vitro and in vivo. *International Journal of Cancer*, Vol.121, pp. 536-546, ISSN 0020-7136

Ma, S., Chan, K.W., Hu, L., Lee, T.K., Wo, J.Y., Ng, I.O., Zheng, B.J., & Guan, X.Y. (2007). Identification and characterization of tumorigenic liver cancer stem/progenitor cells. *Gastroenterology*, Vol.132, pp. 2542-2556, ISSN 0016-5085

Ma, S., Lee, T.K., Zheng, B.J., Chan, K.W., & Guan, X.Y. (2008). CD133+ HCC cancer stem cells confer chemoresistance by preferential expression of the Akt/PKB survival pathway. *Oncogene*, Vol.27, pp. 1749-1758, ISSN 0950-9232

Mehta, P.P., Perez-Stable, C., Nadji, M., Mian, M., Asotra, K., & Roos, B.A. (1999). Suppression of human prostate cancer cell growth by forced expression of connexin genes. *Developmental Genetics*, Vol.24, pp. 91-110, ISSN 0192-253X

Mesnil, M., Crespin, S., Avanzo, J.L., & Zaidan-Dagli, M.L. (2005). Defective gap junctional intercellular communication in the carcinogenic process. *Biochimica et Biophysica Acta*, Vol.1719, pp. 125-145, ISSN 0006-3002

Momiyama, M., Omori, Y., Ishizaki, Y., Nishikawa, Y., Tokairin, T., Ogawa, J., & Enomoto, K. (2003). Connexin26-mediated gap junctional communication reverses the malignant phenotype of MCF-7 breast cancer cells. *Cancer Science*, Vol.94, pp. 501-507, ISSN 1347-9032

Moserle, L., Indraccolo, S., Ghisi, M., Frasson, C., Fortunato, E., Canevari, S., Miotti, S., Tosello, V., Zamarchi, R., Corradin, A., Minuzzo, S., Rossi, E., Basso, G., & Amadori, A. (2008). The side population of ovarian cancer cells is a primary target of IFN-alpha antitumor effects. *Cancer Research*, Vol.68, pp. 5658-5668, ISSN 0008-5472

Nakabayashi, H., Taketa, K., Miyano, K., Yamane, T., & Sato, J. (1982). Growth of human hepatoma cell lines with differentiated functions in chemically defined medium. *Cancer Research*, Vol.42, pp. 3858-3863, ISSN 0008-5472

Naus, C.C., & Laird, D.W. (2010). Implications and challenges of connexin connections to cancer. *Nature Reviews. Cancer*, Vol.10, pp. 435-441, ISSN 1474-175X

Nicholson, B., Dermietzel, R., Teplow, D., Traub, O., Willecke, K., & Revel, J.P. (1987). Two homologous protein components of hepatic gap junctions. *Nature*, Vol.329, pp. 732-734, ISSN 0028-0836

Omori, Y., & Yamasaki, H. (1998). Mutated connexin43 proteins inhibit rat glioma cell growth suppression mediated by wild-type connexin43 in a dominant-negative manner. *International Journal of Cancer*, Vol.78, pp. 446-453, ISSN 0020-7136

Omori, Y., Li, Q., Nishikawa, Y., Yoshioka, T., Yoshida, M., Nishimura, T., & Enomoto, K. (2007). Pathological significance of intracytoplasmic connexin proteins: Implication in tumor progression. *Journal of Membrane Biology*, Vol.218, pp. 73-77, ISSN 0022-2631

Oyamada, M., Krutovskikh, V.A., Mesnil, M., Partensky, C., Berger, F., & Yamasaki, H. (1990). Aberrant expression of gap junction gene in primary human hepatocellular carcinomas: increased expression of cardiac-type gap junction gene connexin 43. *Molecular Carcinogenesis*, Vol.3, pp. 273-278, ISSN 0899-1987

Riethdorf, S., Wikman, H., & Pantel, K. (2008). Review: Biological relevance of disseminated tumor cells in cancer patients. *International Journal of Cancer*, Vol.123, pp. 1991-2006, ISSN 0020-7136

Shimano, K., Satake, M., Okaya, A., Kitanaka, J., Kitanaka, N., Takemura, M., Sakagami, M., Terada, N., & Tsujimura, T. (2003). Hepatic oval cells have the side population phenotype defined by expression of ATP-binding cassette transporter ABCG2/BCRP1. *American Journal of Pathology*, Vol.163, pp. 3-9, ISSN 0002-9440

Singh, S.K., Clarke, I.D., Terasaki, M., Bonn, V.E., Hawkins, C., Squire, J., & Dirks, P.B. (2003). Identification of a cancer stem cell in human brain tumors. *Cancer Research*, Vol.63, pp. 5821-5828, ISSN 0008-5472

Singh, S.K., Hawkins, C., Clarke, I.D., Squire, J.A., Bayani, J., Hide, T., Henkelman, R.M., Cusimano, M.D., & Dirks, P.B. (2004). Identification of human brain tumour initiating cells. *Nature*, Vol.432, pp. 396-401, ISSN 0028-0836

Sohl, G., & Willecke, K. (2003). An update on connexin genes and their nomenclature in mouse and man. *Cell Communication and Adhesion*, Vol.10, pp. 173-180, ISSN 1541-9061

Suetsugu, A., Nagaki, M., Aoki, H., Motohashi, T., Kunisada, T., & Moriwaki, H. (2006). Characterization of CD133+ hepatocellular carcinoma cells as cancer stem/progenitor cells. *Biochemical and Biophysical Research Communications*, Vol.351, pp. 820-824, ISSN 0006-291X

Szotek, P.P., Pieretti-Vanmarcke, R., Masiakos, P.T., Dinulescu, D.M., Connolly, D., Foster, R., Dombkowski, D., Preffer, F., Maclaughlin, D.T., & Donahoe, P.K. (2006). Ovarian cancer side population defines cells with stem cell-like characteristics and Mullerian Inhibiting Substance responsiveness. *Proceedings of the National Academy of Sciences of the United States of America*, Vol.103, pp. 11154-11159, ISSN 0027-8424

Thiery, J.P. (2002). Epithelial-mesenchymal transitions in tumour progression. *Nature Reviews. Cancer*, Vol.2, pp. 442-454, ISSN 1474-175X

Tirino, V., Desiderio, V., d'Aquino, R., De Francesco, F., Pirozzi, G., Graziano, A., Galderisi, U., Cavaliere, C., De Rosa, A., Papaccio, G., & Giordano, A. (2008). Detection and characterization of CD133+ cancer stem cells in human solid tumours. *PLoS One*, Vol.3, pp. e3469, ISSN 1932-6203

Vinken, M., Henkens, T., De Rop, E., Fraczek, J., Vanhaecke, T., & Rogiers, V. (2008). Biology and pathobiology of gap junctional channels in hepatocytes. *Hepatology*, Vol.47, pp. 1077-1088, ISSN 0270-9139

Wang, J., Guo, L.P., Chen, L.Z., Zeng, Y.X., & Lu, S.H. (2007). Identification of cancer stem cell-like side population cells in human nasopharyngeal carcinoma cell line. *Cancer Research*, Vol.67, pp. 3716-3724, ISSN 0008-5472

Yang, Z.F., Ho, D.W., Ng, M.N., Lau, C.K., Yu, W.C., Ngai, P., Chu, P.W., Lam, C.T., Poon, R.T., & Fan, S.T. (2008a). Significance of CD90+ cancer stem cells in human liver cancer. *Cancer Cell*, Vol.13, pp. 153-166, ISSN 1535-6108

Yang, Z.F., Ngai, P., Ho, D.W., Yu, W.C., Ng, M.N., Lau, C.K., Li, M.L., Tam, K.H., Lam, C.T., Poon, R.T., & Fan, S.T. (2008b). Identification of local and circulating cancer stem cells in human liver cancer. *Hepatology*, Vol.47, pp. 919-928, ISSN 0270-9139

Yeager, M. (2009). Gap junction channel structure, IN: *Connexins*, Harris, A.L. & Locke, D., pp. 27-75, Humana Press, ISBN 978-1-934115-46-6, New York

Yin, S., Li, J., Hu, C., Chen, X., Yao, M., Yan, M., Jiang, G., Ge, C., Xie, H., Wan, D., Yang, S., Zheng, S., & Gu, J. (2007). CD133 positive hepatocellular carcinoma cells possess high capacity for tumorigenicity. *International Journal of Cancer*, Vol.120, pp. 1444-1450, ISSN 0020-7136

# 12

# The Involvement of the ERK-Hypoxia-Angiogenesis Signaling Axis and HIF-1 in Hepatocellular Carcinoma

Ilias Mylonis and George Simos
*Laboratory of Biochemistry, School of Medicine, University of Thessaly & Institute of Biomedical Research and Technology (BIOMED), Centre for Research and Technology – Thessaly (CE.RE.TE.TH)*
*Greece*

## 1. Introduction

Hepatocellular carcinoma (HCC) is the most common primary liver cancer and is associated with high resistance to drugs and high mortality. There are multiple factors that influence its molecular pathogenesis but two well established characteristics of malignant transformation in HCC are its hypervascular nature and the upregulation of the Raf/MEK/ERK signaling cascade. MAPK pathway activation can be triggered by important risk factors of hepatocarcinogenesis such as HBV or HCV infection. Furtermore, its deregulation is well documented in human HCC patients and is associated with poor prognosis (Bruix & Llovet, 2009). Constitutive stimulation of both ERK isoforms has been frequently observed in both HCC samples and hepatocarcinoma-derived cell lines and plays a prominent role in the proliferation, invasion and metastasis of HCC cells (Min et al., 2010). These processes are also associated with neoangiogenesis and aberrant vessel formation, which in turn depend on the development of hypoxic regions and VEGF overexpression frequently observed in tumor samples (Rosmorduc & Housset, 2010). The master regulators of the cellular response to oxygen deprivation are the hypoxia inducible transcription factors (HIFs). Their activation results in expression of many genes that contribute to survival and proliferation of malignant cells and, more importantly, resistance to conventional treatments and poor patient outcome (Poon, E. et al., 2009). Interestingly, hypoxia has been observed to lead to ERK activation, which can further stimulate HIF transcriptional activity. This can result in increased expression of HIF target genes that include pro-angiogenic factors and other proteins that facilitate adaptation of tumor cells to their environment (Dimova et al., 2009). In this chapter, we will discuss the cross-talk between these pathways, their contribution to HCC development and progression and their potential as targets of combined therapeutic approaches.

## 2. Hepatocellular carcinoma

Hepatocellular Carcinoma (HCC) is the fifth most common and third in lethality cancer. It is characterized by intrinsic drug-metabolizing activity that confers resistance to chemotherapeutic treatment. Mortality is associated with metastasis, recurrence and new tumor development and diagnosis is usually made at intermediate or late stage so that only ~ 20% of cases can undergo surgery that includes resection, ablation or transplantation. Unfortunately, due to the genomic heterogeneity of HCC tumors, the exact molecular pathogenetic and oncogenic alterations that lead to HCC initiation and progression are not completely understood and require further investigation. However, there are several risk factors and pathways known to be associated with the occurrence and development of this type of cancer (Villanueva et al., 2010).

Probably the most important predisposing factor for the development of HCC is liver cirrhosis that usually results from viral infection (HBV or HCV), alcohol abuse or contamination with Aflatoxin B1. Other contributing factors include inflammation and non-alcoholic fatty liver disease (NAFLD). All of these factors can lead to HCC development by triggering cellular events such as proto-oncogene activation, ROS generation and genetic alterations or instability (Frau et al., 2010). Genetic studies of human HCCs resulted in the identification of gene mutations and expression profile alterations. The identified deregulated genes can be associated with important signaling pathways and shed more light in the molecular events that contribute to HCC pathogenesis. According to these analyses, there are three subgroups of human HCC cancers, genetic profile of which corresponds to the deregulation of specific signaling events (Hoshida et al., 2010). One of them is characterized by over-expression of growth factors (EGF, IGF II and HGF being the most prominent) and induction of major signaling pathways such as PI3K/AKT/mTOR and RAS/RAF/MAPK, which affect cell proliferation and survival and, moreover, contribute to the aggressive phenotype of the disease. In another subgroup, the affected genes are related to cell differentiation and liver development. These genes are found downstream of the WNT or the highly similar Hedgehog pathway and their involvement in human hepatocarcinogenesis is still under investigation. Whereas, in the third less-defined group, the early stages of the disease are linked to inflammation-related pathways, with interleukin-6 being a major signaling molecule (Villanueva et al., 2010; Zender et al., 2010). However, all these signaling pathways do not function independently in the context of HCC tumors but they cooperate and influence one another contributing to the progression of the disease.

From these and other studies it has been made clear that ERK pathway activation and neo-angiogenesis are two characteristics of HCCs that greatly facilitate malignant transformation, as they are involved in tumor development, growth and metastasis. Another aspect of HCC, common to many solid tumors, is the creation of hypoxic areas as a result of increased metabolic rate, irregular angiogenesis and tissue inflammation (Rosmorduc & Housset, 2010). The central regulatory elements of cell response to oxygen deprivation are the hypoxia inducible transcription factors (HIFs). After their activation, HIFs induce the expression of their targets, which in their turn facilitate adaption of the cells to the hypoxic environment of the tumor and contribute to survival, proliferation and aggressiveness of cancer cells.

## 3. ERK pathway and HCC

Extracellular-signal regulated kinases 1 and 2 (ERK 1/2 or else p44/42 MAPK) are serine/threonine protein kinases both homologous and highly similar in their regulatory mechanisms and functions. They are expressed in all cell types and they integrate extracellular signals such as growth factors and cytokines into cellular responses that promote gene expression, proliferation, survival and migration. ERK activation relies on the binding of ligands to cell membrane receptors and the subsequent activation of the RAS/RAF/MEK signaling cascade resulting in the phosphorylation and activation of ERK1/2 (Pearson et al., 2001). It is well documented that sustained ERK activity is important for the development of many types of tumors including hepatocellular carcinoma. As it has been already mentioned, there is activation of Ras pathway and significant increase of phosphorylated ERK levels in all HCC-derived cell lines. However, Ras mutations that could account for sustained pathway activation are rare in human HCCs (Min et al., 2010). One explanation for constistutive ERK activation in HCCs can be that HBV or HCV viral infection interferes and activates the ERK signaling cascade facilitating thus hepatocarcinogenesis (Chin et al., 2007; Zhao et al., 2005). Another reason may lie with the fact that there is global suppression of negative regulators that control the ERK signaling cascade in HCC cell lines. It has been shown that Ras inhibitors are inactivated in HCC-derived cell lines probably as a result of deregulated methylation and genomic instability (Calvisi et al., 2006). Furthermore, the Raf kinase inhibitor protein (RKIP) has been observed to be downregulated in HCC cells (Lee, H.C. et al., 2006). Significant decrease has also been detected in the phosphatase DUSP1, which restrains ERK activity by dephosphorylation, as a result of ubiquitin-mediated proteolysis triggered by sustained ERK activation in HCC (Calvisi et al., 2008).

The constitutive activation of ERK signaling is essential for cell survival, proliferation and invasion of human HCC cells since Ras pathway inhibition results in growth suppression and cell death. Moreover, siRNA-mediated silencing of ERK2 or elimination of ERK1/2 phosphorylation by silencing of MEK1 resulted in inhibition of cell proliferation and tumor growth suppression in xenograft animal models (Bessard et al., 2008; Gailhouste et al., 2010). Activation of the Raf/MEK/ERK pathway in human HCC biopsy samples can be used as a biomarker of the disease because nuclear phosphorylated ERK levels are higher in tumor samples (Abou-Alfa et al., 2006). Finally, ERK pathway activation is associated with poor patient outcome whereas, inversely, elevated expression levels of pathway inhibitors such as DUSP1 are observed in tumor samples of patients with longer survival time (Calvisi et al., 2008).

The importance of the ERK pathway for HCC occurrence and progression made it an important candidate for targeted therapeutic approaches as shown in case of sorafenib. Sorafenib, a multikinase inhibitor, impedes cell proliferation by targeting the Raf/MEK/ERK signaling cascade at the level of Raf kinase (for which it was originally developed) and also exhibits antiangiogenic properties by targeting the tyrosine kinase activities of the vascular endothelial growth factor receptor-2/-3 (VEGFR-2/-3) and the platelet derived growth factor receptor beta (PDGFR-β) (Liu, L. et al., 2006; Wilhelm et al., 2004). Sorafenib has been recently approved as the first effective systemic drug for treating advanced HCC showing a significant (almost 3 months) increase in patient survival. Also, due to its tolerability in single agent trials, it has been evaluated in combination with other anticancer therapies, including cytotoxic chemotherapy and anti-angiogenic therapy (Llovet et al., 2008). The effectiveness of sorafenib in clinical evaluation highlights the potential of targeting the ERK pathway in the treatment of HCC. Recent experimental studies have shown that treatment with MEK inhibitors (AZD6244, PD0325901) inhibited cancer cell proliferation and tumor growth in human HCC cell lines and HCC xenografts in animal models (Hennig et al., 2010; Huynh et al., 2007). Moreover, when AZD6244 was tested in combination with sorafenib, it enhanced the anti-tumor activity of sorafenib, suggesting the potential value of ERK pathway inhibition in combinational therapeutic approaches (Huynh et al., 2010).

## 4. Angiogenesis and HCC

HCC progression requires the development and maintenance of adequate blood supply. This requires vascular endothelial cell proliferation and migration in order to establish a new vascular network. The transformation from a poorly vascular nodule to the hypervascular malignant phenotype of the disease has become a hallmark for diagnosis, treatment and possible future therapeutic approaches (Fernandez et al., 2009). Formation of new vessels with abnormal architecture is linked to fibrinogenesis and cirrhosis, processes that cause extensive cell damage and can lead to malignancy (Rosmorduc & Housset, 2010). The ability to form new vessels is critical not only for the emergence of HCC but also for the growth of metastatic nests and the transition from early to advanced stages of the disease. Indeed, impairing the blood supply that feeds the tumor with transarterial chemoembolization is an effective treatment for patients with advanced HCC and improves their survival (Llovet & Bruix, 2003).

Neoangiogenesis in HCC is a process stimulated by hypoxia, growth factors, oncogenes and nutrient concentration followed by the release of pro-angiogenic growth factors and activation of endothelial cells. The most prominent pro-angiogenic signal, as revealed in a number of studies, is vascular endothelial growth factor (VEGF) (Fernandez et al., 2009; Rosmorduc & Housset, 2010). Its expression can be induced as a result of hypoxia, oncogenic signaling and viral infection, involving MAPK pathway activation and transcriptional regulation by AP1 and HIF-1α (Hassan et al., 2009). Its significant role in HCC is shown by the fact that cells isolated from human tumors are able to produce VEGF by themselves. Hypoxia further enhances VEGF expression both by regulation at the transcriptional level and by stabilization of VEGF mRNA (von Marschall et al., 2001). Moreover, VEGF and its receptors (VEGFR-1 and VEGFR-2) are found over-expressed in patients' samples and their increased levels have been associated with the aggressive phenotype of the disease (Imura et al., 2004). In line with this observation, increased concentration of VEGF in serum samples is directly connected to poor patient outcome after resection or ablation (Poon, R.T. et al., 2004; Poon, R.T. et al., 2007).

Other factors that promote tumor angiogenesis in HCC are FGFs (Fibroblast growth factors), angiopoietins (Ang-2) and platelet-derived growth factor (PDGF). There is evidence that bFGF over-expression is involved in vascular endothelial cell proliferation during tumor angiogenesis in human HCC (Imura et al., 2004). Furthermore, Ang-2 levels as well as its activity through the Tie-2 receptor are increased in human samples and have been correlated with neovascularization and microvessel density (MVD) (Mitsuhashi et al., 2003). Finally, animal studies have shown that the involvement of PDGF-C in HCC development is linked to its role in the initiation of fibrosis (Campbell et al., 2005). Interestingly, it appears that all these factors team up with the VEGF signaling cascade in order to provoke normal or aberrant vessel formation in HCCs.

Since vascular formation is very important for tumor progression and transition to malignancy, it represents an intriguing therapeutic target for the treatment of HCC. At present, there are several drugs undergone investigation in experimental models or humans and some of them are already in use in various types of cancer. Most of the tested inhibitors target selectively the VEGF pathway and induce arrest of endothelial cell proliferation, regression of the existing vessels or suppress the mobilization of endothelial progenitor cells from bone marrow. These agents range from monoclonal antibodies (mAb) targeting VEGF-A, like bevacizumab (Avastin), to small molecules that inhibit autophosphorylation of VEGF receptors like sorafenib (Nexavar), the single agent that was approved for the treatment of advanced hepatocellular carcinoma in 2007 (Fernandez et al., 2009).

## 5. Hypoxia and HCC

As many other solid tumors, HCC is characterized by the development of hypoxia. Even in normal liver, emergence of hypoxic conditions can result from its division into areas with different capabilities of oxygen delivery (i.e., 60 to 65 mmHg in the portal area to 30 to 35 mmHg in the perivenous area) and increased cellular metabolic activity, which leads to high oxygen consumption (Rosmorduc & Housset, 2010). Apart from that, the response to trauma or inflammation can cause aberrant vessel formation, irregular blood flow and, finally, poor oxygenation of the cells. Cells respond to oxygen deprivation by activating a number of genes that allow them to adapt and survive. More importantly, hepatocellular carcinoma cells not only survive but also show significant stimulation of their proliferation under hypoxia as opposed to other cancer cell lines (Gwak et al., 2005).

Hypoxia promotes tumor progression through several mechanisms. Under hypoxic conditions, cells shift their metabolism from oxidative phosphorylation to anaerobic glycolysis by the induction of genes that encode glucose transporters, glycolytic enzymes and proteins that remove glycolysis by-products (e.g. lactic acid) from cancer cells. As mentioned above, HCC tumors exhibit epigenetic alterations and signaling pathways activation that stimulate proliferation. These may be supported by tumor hypoxia, which affects the methylation status of HCC cells and, more importantly, activates the ERK pathway (Liu, Q. et al., 2011; Minet et al., 2000). Another very important contribution of hypoxia to HCC development is the stimulation of angiogenesis. Two of the central pro-angiogenic factors in HCC, namely VEGF and angiopoietin 2, are induced in hypoxic conditions and promote the abnormal vessel formation and branching observed in these tumors. Key mediators of these responses and central components of hypoxia signaling within the cell are the hypoxia inducible factors (HIFs).

HIFs are heterodimeric transcriptional complexes that respond to changes of cellular oxygen concentration and activate the expression of hypoxia target genes. These genes encode for proteins involved in processes critical for oncogenesis such as survival, proliferation, invasion and metastasis. Active HIF heterodimers are composed of the constitutively expressed HIF-β subunit (or ARNT; Aryl hydrocarbon Receptor Nuclear Translocator) and the regulated HIF-α subunit, which is over-expressed in many tumors and causes HIF activation and increased transcription of its targets (Semenza, 2010). HCC is not an exception and expression levels of HIF-1α are increased in all stages of the disease and correlate to its progress.

There is plenty of evidence linking HIF-1α to both early and late HCC stages. The genetic instability observed during the premalignant state of HCC can be caused by viral infection. HCV core protein induces HIF-1α and HIF-dependent transcriptional activation of the VEGF gene in HCC-derived cells (Hassan et al., 2009). Liver angiogenesis has been indeed observed in biopsy samples of HCV patients and is possibly an essential step for HCV-related oncogenesis. HIF-1α mRNA and protein levels are also increased in premalignant dysplastic nodules, as observed in both human and animal samples, and cause up-regulation of a number of genes that promote angiogenesis (VEGF), glucose transport (GLUT1) and PI3K/AKT pathway activation (growth factor IGF-II and hepatocyte growth factor receptor c-Met) (Nakamura et al., 2007). Interestingly, it has also been shown that HIF-1α expression at this stage is hypoxia-independent and its levels rise as the disease progresses (Tanaka et al., 2006). These findings indicate the important role of this transcription factor in abnormal gene expression that occurs during early HCC development.

As already mentioned, hypervascularity is a prominent feature of progression to HCC malignancy and HIF-1α over-expression is also directly associated with VEGF expression, microvessel density (MVD) and microvenous invasion in human HCC samples (Huang et al., 2005). Deregulation of the HIF pathway, which comes as a result of HIF-1α over-expression, is often associated with resistance to radiotherapy and chemotherapy, which renders hypoxic tumors highly aggressive and metastatic (Poon, E. et al., 2009). This is also true for primary HCC, in which HIF-1α expression is associated with poor response to radiotherapy, metastasis and low survival rates (Xiang et al., 2011). Therefore, understanding HIF-α regulation may provide valuable information in order to target the HIF pathway as a means for combinational therapeutic strategies against HCC.

## 6. HIF-α structure and regulation

Three HIF-α isoforms have been so far identified: HIF-1α, HIF-2α and HIF-3α. HIF-1α and -2α have similar structure and are rapidly induced in response to hypoxia. The third family member is not well understood. It exists in several splice variants, one of which acts as a dominant negative regulator of HIF-dependent gene expression as it binds to the HIF-1α subunit to form a nonfunctional complex. Whereas HIF-1α shows broad tissue distribution, HIF-2α is cell-type specific and was shown to have distinct biological roles. However, HIF-1 and HIF-2 can regulate both overlapping and distinct target genes (Poon, E. et al., 2009). More specifically, liver cells express both isoforms, albeit, with different kinetic profiles: HIF-1α responds quickly but returns to basal levels early. In contrast, HIF-2α expression is delayed but prolonged, suggesting a coordinated response of the two subunits to hypoxia (Wiesener et al., 2003).

Both HIF-1α and HIF-2α contain basic helix loop helix (bHLH) and PER-ARNT-SIM (PAS) domains in their $NH_2$-terminal regions that mediate heterodimerization and binding to specific DNA regulatory sequences called hypoxia response elements (HREs) (Fig. 1). The PAS domain contains two conserved repeats termed PAS-A and PAS-B. In their C-terminal regions, both contain transactivation domains (TAD) that mediate the transcription of their targets. Oxygen sensitivity and regulation relies in a structural feature called oxygen depended degradation (ODD) domain that lies inside the central region of HIF-α (Semenza, 2003).

In terms of its oxygen-dependent or -independent regulation, HIF-1α is more extensively investigated. HIF-2α, on the other hand, is regulated in a similar fashion by oxygen but many elements of its oxygen-independent regulation still remain unclear. Under normal oxygen conditions, HIF-1α is constantly produced and destroyed in a process that involves von Hippel-Lindau (VHL)-mediated polyubiquitination and subsequent proteasomal degradation (Schofield & Ratcliffe, 2005). Interaction of HIF-1α with VHL, a tumor suppressor protein and a subunit of an E3 ubiquitin ligase complex, requires the hydroxylation of two proline residues within the ODD domain of HIF-1α. This hydroxylation is mediated by three conserved prolyl hydroxylases (termed PHDs or HPHs), the activity of which depends on the availability of oxygen, iron and 2-oxoglutarate (Semenza, 2001). When oxygen becomes sparse, hydroxylation is impaired, HIF-1α is stabilized and is imported into the nucleus, where it dimerizes with ARNT and activates the expression of its target genes. However, oxygen dependent-regulation does not only rely on HIF-1α destruction alone but also on the control of its activity. Another oxygen-sensitive hydroxylase called FIH (Factor Inhibiting HIF-1) modifies HIF-1α in one asparagine residue situated inside its C-terminal TAD region (Asn803) and interferes with the association of HIF-1α with the transcriptional co-activator CBP/p300 (Lancaster et al., 2004a).

Apart from oxygen tension, HIF-1α expression and activity are additionally stimulated by oxygen-independent mechanisms that respond to oncogenic activation, growth factors, cytokines and variations of the cellular environment (e.g. pH). There are multiple levels at which cells can control HIF-1α activity, ranging from transcriptional and translational regulation to post-translational modifications. Its transcriptional activation responds to inflammatory stimuli as IKKβ activation causes increased HIF-1α gene expression in a NF-κB-dependent fashion in the liver of hypoxic mice (Rius et al., 2008). The signal transducer and activator of transcription 3 (Stat3) is also involved in the regulation of HIF-1α mRNA synthesis (Niu et al., 2008) and mediates the transcriptional suppression of HIF-1α by the eIF2α kinase PKR (Papadakis et al., 2010). Activation of the phosphatidylinositol 3-kinase/AKT pathway leads to elevated translation of HIF-1α mRNA and increased HIF-1α protein levels (Bardos & Ashcroft, 2005). Post-translationally, HIF-1α is regulated either through its association with other proteins or its modification by number of different enzymes. Protein interactions like binding to the molecular chaperone HSP90 can increase HIF-1α stability by inhibiting VHL-independent degradation (Isaacs et al., 2002; Katschinski et al., 2004). On the other hand, the protein RACK1 competes with HSP90 for binding to the HIF-1α N-terminal PAS-A domain. The RACK1-HIF-1α interaction, which is stabilized by the protein SSAT1 and inhibited by Sept9-v1, promotes increased ubiquitination and degradation of HIF-1α irrespective of oxygen levels (Amir et al., 2009; Baek et al., 2007; Liu, Y.V. et al., 2007). MgcRacGAP (male germ cell RacGTPase Activating Protein), identified using the yeast two-hybrid system, is another protein that interacts with and inhibits HIF-1α. MgcRacGAP over-expression inhibits HIF-1α transcriptional activity, without lowering HIF-1α protein levels or altering its subcellular localization (Lyberopoulou et al., 2007).

Apart from hydroxylation, other posttranslational modifications of HIF-1α include SUMOylation, acetylation, S-nitrosylation and phosphorylation by a number of different kinases. HIF-1α can be SUMOylated but the role of this modification remains controversial; certain reports claim that SUMO conjugate stabilizes HIF-1α while others suggest that deSUMOylation of HIF-1α is necessary for its stability and activity (Bae et al., 2004; Berta et al., 2007; Carbia-Nagashima et al., 2007; Cheng et al., 2007). In contrast, acetylation of HIF-1α by the acetyltransferase ARD1 has a negative impact by facilitating its interaction with VHL (Jeong et al., 2002), although its effect on HIF-1α stability has also been later disputed (Wei & Yu, 2007). Nitrogen oxide (NO) can interfere with PHD function as well as cause HIF-1α S-nitrosylation, which can stabilize HIF-1α in tumor-associated macrophages (Li et al., 2007; Wei & Yu, 2007).

Direct HIF-1α phosphorylation can be an efficient way to rapidly and reversibly regulate HIF-1 activity in response to different stimuli. HIF-1α phosphorylations can be activating, such as the one at $Thr^{796}$ in the C-TAD domain of HIF-1α that impairs his interaction with FIH-1 (Lancaster et al., 2004b). On the contrary, phosphorylation by glycogen synthase kinase 3 (GSK3) at three residues ($Ser^{551}/Thr^{555}/Ser^{589}$) within the HIF-1α N-TAD drives HIF-1α to VHL-independent proteasomal degradation and down-regulates its activity (Flugel et al., 2007). We have recently described HIF-1α phosphorylation by casein kinse 1 (CK1) which also negatively affects HIF-1 activity (Kalousi et al., 2010). CK1δ targets $Ser^{247}$ in the PAS-B domain of HIF-1α and does not affect its stability or localization but interferes with the ability of HIF-1α to form an active complex with ARNT under hypoxia. Over-expression of CK1δ inhibited, whereas, inhibition or silencing of CK1δ stimulated the activity of HIF-1 in several different cell lines, including hepatoma-derived cancer cells. Furthermore, inhibition of CK1 activity in HCC- cells (Huh7) resulted in significantly higher proliferation rates under hypoxia, highlighting the importance of HIF-1 activity for hypoxic adaptation and suggesting an anti-proliferative role for CK1δ (Kalousi et al., 2010). Others, recent but less characterized modifications of HIF-1α include phosphorylation of $Ser^{696}$ by ATM kinase and $Ser^{576}/Ser^{657}$ by Plk3, both of which activate HIF-1α by stabilizing its protein levels (Cam et al., 2010; Xu et al., 2010). Finally, the longer known, best studied and probably most relevant to HCC direct phosphorylation of HIF-1α is the one mediated by ERK (p44/42 MAPK), which will discussed extensively in the next section.

Transcriptional activity of HIF-1α ultimately depends on its nuclear accumulation. In order to enter the nucleus HIF-1α uses more than one import pathways. The first one involves the presence of a classical bipartite-type nuclear localization signal (NLS) in the C-terminal part of HIF-1α and interaction with importin α to mediate its translocation to the nucleus (Depping et al., 2008; Kallio et al., 1998; Luo & Shibuya, 2001). Moreover, recent work from our lab has shown that HIF-1α active transport through the nuclear pore complex can be mediated by multiple import receptors that, apart from importin α family members, also include importins 4 and 7 (Chachami et al., 2009) . Interaction with importins 4 and 7 involves the $NH_2$-terminal part of HIF-1α (amino acids 1-251), which also contains the bHLH and PAS-A domains, but the exact nature of the NLS that mediates their association is still unclear. The operation of more than one different pathways may ensure the fast and efficient translocation of HIF-1α inside the nucleus as part of an effective cellular response to hypoxic stimuli (Fig. 1). However, the time that HIF-1α spends inside the nucleus and, ultimately, its activity depends also on its nuclear export rate, which is mediated by the major mammalian exportin CRM1 and regulated by the Raf/MEK/ERK pathway (see below).

## 7. ERK pathway and HIF-1α

The MAPK pathway is one of the two best known major signal transduction pathways regulating HIF-1α activity (the other is PI3K/AKT). Apart from being induced by growth factors, cytokines and oncogenes, the MAPK pathway is also activated by hypoxia in several different cell lines including hepatoma HepG2 cells (Liu, C. et al., 2005; Minet et al., 2000; Mottet et al., 2002) and was suggested to affect both HIF-1α mRNA translation and HIF-1 transcriptional activity (Fukuda et al., 2002; Richard et al., 1999). This was shown by the use of MEK1 inhibitor PD98059 which decreased HIF-1-dependent gene expression in a number of cell lines including the hepatoma-derived Hep3B (Minet et al., 2000; Salceda et al., 1997). Also, studies from our own and other groups using Gal4-HIF-1α fusion proteins have shown that the ERK pathway is involved in hypoxia-dependent HIF-1α transactivation domain function in different cell lines (Lee, E. et al., 2002; Mylonis et al., 2006). Finally, HIF-1α can be directly phosphorylated by ERK (p44/p42 MAPK) both in vitro and in vivo but is not a direct target of the other MAPK family members (p38 or c-JNK) (Dimova et al., 2009).

Although there had been efforts to identify the exact HIF-1α sites phosphorylated by ERK, these remained unknown until quite recently. The issue was clarified by our recent work using in vitro phosphorylation assays, mass spectrometry and site directed mutagenesis, which led to the indentification of two conserved serine residues ($Ser^{641}$ and $Ser^{643}$) as the major ERK phosphorylation sites on HIF-1α (Mylonis et al., 2006). Furthermore, inhibition of HIF-1α phosphorylation by mutagenesis of the ERK target sites (conversion of both $Ser^{641}/Ser^{643}$ into Ala) or treatment with the ERK pathway inhibitor PD98059 impaired nuclear accumulation of HIF-1α and, consequently, decreased its transcriptional activity. However, when cells expressing the phosphorylation-deficient mutant of HIF-1α were treated with Leptomycin B (a specific inhibitor of CRM1-dependent nuclear export) nuclear localization of the mutant HIF-1α was restored and its activity was partially recovered, suggesting that lack of ERK-depended phosphorylation reduces nuclear concentration of HIF-1α by excessive nuclear export into the cytoplasm (Mylonis et al., 2006).

These first results indicated that the mechanism by which ERK phosphorylation regulates HIF-1α activity lies downstream of its synthesis and stabilization steps and involves regulated nucleocytoplasmic shuttling. However, this kind of regulation requires that HIF-1α possesses a nuclear export signal (NES) in addition to its NLS. We were, indeed, able to show the presence of such a signal in the form of an atypical hydrophobic NES ($^{632}$M**E**D**IKILI**$^{639}$), situated in close proximity to the serine residues 641/643 modified by ERK (Mylonis et al., 2008). This NES interacts strongly with CRM1 but only when ERK-dependent phosphorylation of HIF-1α is impaired. These data also support the idea that regulation of HIF-1α nuclear shuttling is the major - if not exclusive - mechanism through which ERK-mediated phosphorylation controls HIF-1 activity since phospho-mimetic mutation of $Ser^{641}$ into Glu or mutation of the NES renders the mutant form of HIF-1α largely resistant to MAPK-pathway inhibition. Furthermore, the NES mutation "suppressed" the $Ser^{641}/Ser^{643}$→Ala double mutation and HIF-1α lacking both NES and ERK-sites regained wild-type properties in terms of localization and activity (Mylonis et al., 2008). Taken together, our data, which were also confirmed in a hepatoma-derived cell line (Huh7), support the following model, also shown in Fig. 1. After stabilization, HIF-1α interacts with multiple nuclear import receptors (importins α/β, 4 and 7) and is transported into the nucleus through the nuclear pore compexes (NPCs). Once in the nucleoplasm and with the HIF-1α NES exposed, there are two possible scenarios. If the MAPK/ERK pathway is inactive, as in a quiescent cell, CRM1 will bind to the NES and return HIF-1α to the cytoplasm, keeping, thus, its nuclear concentration and subsequent activity low. However, if ERK is active (in response to hypoxia or other oncogenic stimuli), it will phosphorylate HIF-1α and mask its NES, thereby trapping HIF-1α inside the nucleus, promoting its accumulation and maximizing its activity. Subsequent interaction with ARNT will form an active HIF-1 heterodimer, which can bind to DNA and stimulate transcription. This model does not exclude the possibility that ERK-mediated phosphorylation has additional, albeit minor, effects on HIF-1α regulation such as promoting interaction of phosphorylated HIF-1α with another nuclear factor or stimulating the activity of HIF-1α partners such as CBP/p300 (Sang et al., 2003).

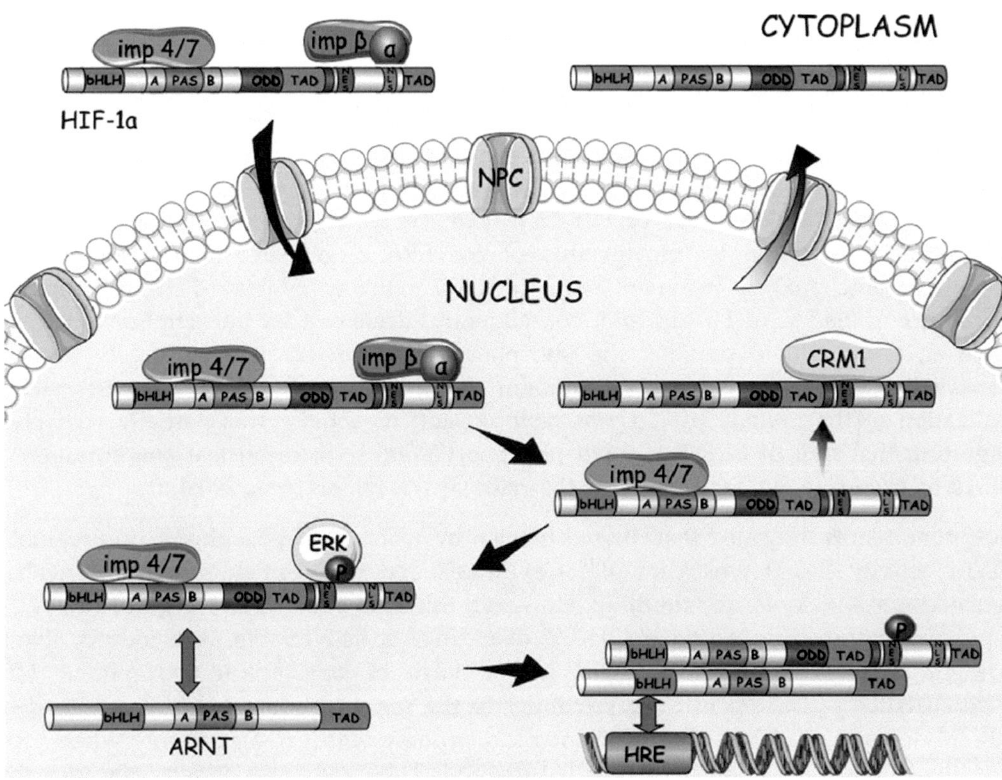


Fig. 1. HIF-1α regulation by ERK-mediated phosphorylation.

This schematic model shows how nucleocytoplasmic shuttling and activity of HIF-1α is controlled by ERK. HIF-1α is transported into the nucleus by nuclear import receptors (importins α/β, 4 and 7) but also contains an NES. In the absence of modification by ERK, binding of CRM1 to the NES returns HIF-1α to the cytoplasm and limits its activity by shortening its intranuclear resident time. When ERK phosphorylates HIF-1α, the NES is masked, interaction with CRM1 is inhibited and HIF-1α is allowed to accumulate inside the nucleus and attain maximal activity by forming an active HIF-1 heterodimer with ARNT and binding to DNA to stimulate transcription (see text for relevant references).

The link between ERK and HIF-1 appears not to be unidirectional. Many reports have shown that hypoxia induces the expression of several members of the DUSP (dual specificity phosphatase also called MAPK phosphatase, MKP) family, which inactivate the MAPKs, including ERK, by dephosphorylation (Bermudez et al., 2011; Bernaudin et al., 2002; Laderoute et al., 1999; Liu, C. et al., 2005; Seta et al., 2001). Expression of DUSP1 in HepG2 cells may be the reason for the loss of ERK activation after prolonged exposure to hypoxia (Liu, C. et al., 2005), suggesting that hypoxia-inducible DUSPs may play a critical role in the spatio-temporal regulation of MAPK signaling. Furthermore, HIF-1 is itself required for the induction of DUSP6 (Bermudez et al., 2011), suggesting the operation of the negative feedback loop shown in Fig. 2. Since excessive and prolonged activation of ERK or HIF-1 may lead to apoptosis (Cagnol et al., 2006; Carmeliet et al., 1998), this negative feedback may act to limit ERK and, consequently, HIF-1α activity to a threshold compatible with cell survival and proliferation under hypoxia. On the other hand, HIF-1 has been recently shown to inhibit DUSP2 transcription causing DUSP2 suppression and prolonged phosphorylation of ERK, which increased chemoresistance and malignancy in human cancer cells under hypoxia (Lin et al., 2011). This suggests the additional operation of a feed-forward (or positive feedback) loop (also shown in Fig. 2) that can explain the down-regulation of DUSP2 and parallel elevation of ERK and HIF-1 activity in hypoxic cancer cells. It is, however, ambiguous the fact that hypoxic DUSP2 suppression was not observed in hepatoma cell lines and clinical samples of cancerous liver had similar levels of DUSP2 mRNA as those derived from normal tissue (Lin et al., 2011) suggesting limited and tissue-specific relevance of this mechanism.

This tight connection between ERK activity and HIF-1α can be targeted for controlling HIF-1 activity (Fig. 2). Indeed, nuclear accumulation and activity of HIF-1α was impaired when cancer cells were treated with natural occurring compounds such as flavonoids that inhibit the MAPK pathway and ERK-dependent HIF-1α phosphorylation (Triantafyllou et al., 2008). Moreover, the transient expression of a 43 amino acid HIF-1α peptide that contains the ERK modification sites and can be itself an ERK substrate (termed MTD: MAPK target domain) caused nuclear exclusion and loss of activity of endogenous HIF-1α (Mylonis et al., 2008). Finally, we have recently shown that the flavonoid kaempferol could act as a potent inhibitor of hepatoma cancer (Huh7) cell viability by inhibiting ERK activation and causing cytoplasmic mislocalization and inactivation of HIF-1α (Mylonis et al., 2010). Kaempferol could play a dual role in impairing cancer cell growth. It exhibited a mild effect on Huh7 cell survival under normal oxygen concentration, most likely due to inhibition of the MAPK pathway, which is critical for cell proliferation. However, kaempferol exerted a much stronger negative effect under hypoxia, apparently by additionally blocking HIF-1 activity required for cell viability at 0.1 - 1% $O_2$, conditions that are physiologically more relevant to those inside a tumor growing in vivo. This provided proof-of-principle for the potential use of kaempferol or other HIF-1α phosphorylation inhibitors as anti-HCC agents, since they could selectively target cancer cells normally exposed to hypoxia. The potential of kaempferol to inhibit both ERK and HIF-1 was at low μM concentration ($IC_{50}$ close to 5 μM), which falls within the plasma flavonoid concentration range achievable by dietary intake alone (Gates et al., 2007; Manach et al., 2005). As a naturally occurring dietary substance without known side effects, kaempferol could be a good candidate for further evaluation, as chemopreventive or therapeutic compound, in controlled prospective studies of HCC patients along or in combination with other established conservative and interventional therapies.

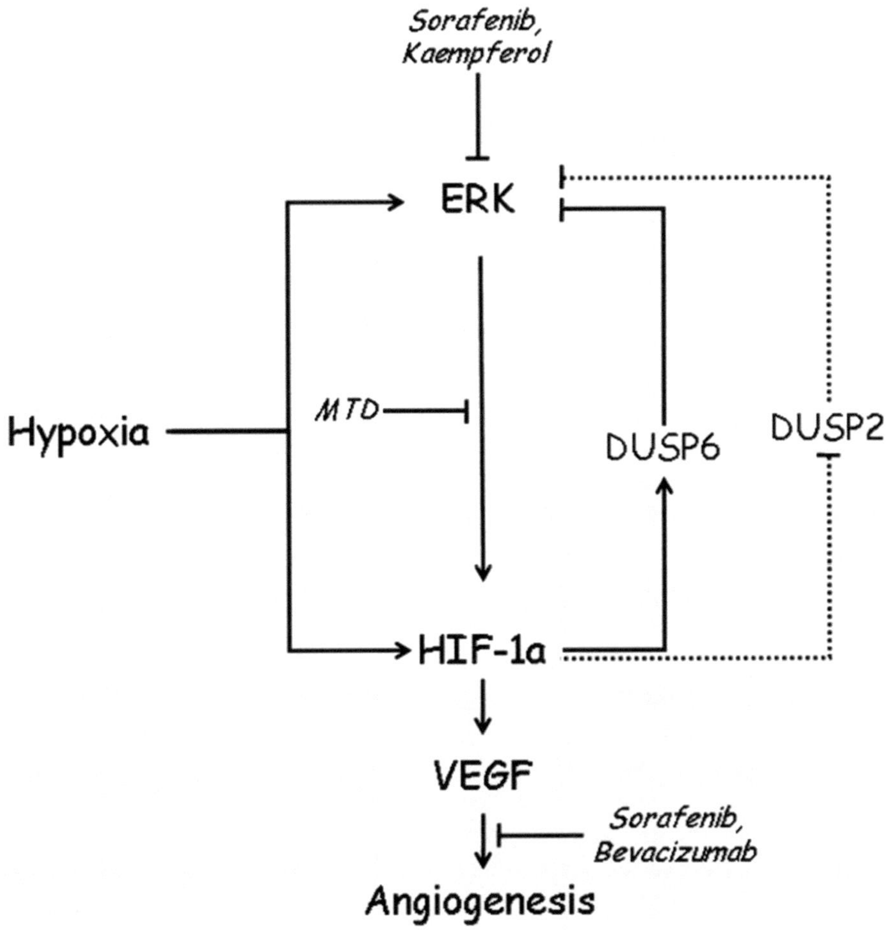


Fig. 2. The hypoxia-ERK-HIF-angiogenesis axis, feedback regulations and possible sites of targeted intervention.

HIF-1α, induced by hypoxia and activated by ERK-mediated phosphorylation, stimulates the production of VEGF that promotes angiogenesis. Induction of DUSP6 (and possibly other DUSPs, not shown) by HIF-1 deactivates ERK as a negative feedback mechanism, while suppression of DUSP2 can be part of an opposing feed-forward mechanism (not occurring in liver cells). This circuitry can be interrupted by agents that inhibit ERK activation (such as sorafenib and kaempferol), block HIF-1α phosphorylation (such as MTD) or impair VEGF function (such as sorafenib and bevacizumab). For further details and relevant reference see text.

## 8. Targeting the HIF pathway in HCC

Induction of the HIF- pathway may not come as a result of the cancer alone, but it can also be attributed to conventional HCC treatment such as chemoembolization which has been widely used in unresectable cases of hepatocellular carcinoma (Llovet & Bruix, 2003). However, restriction of the blood flow in the treated tissue generates hypoxic conditions and activation of the HIF pathway, which may lead to a phenotypic change that renders cancer cells more invasive and metastatic, with subsequent failure of treatment as shown in animal primary liver cancers (Patsenker et al., 2009). Therefore, suppression of HIF-1 activity can be especially beneficial when combined with conventional treatments or future therapeutic agents that target other pathways related to HCC. This is already evident in experimental models, in which inhibition of HIF-1α expression enhanced the efficacy of doxorubicin in suppressing HCC cell growth through stimulation of apoptosis and down-regulation of VEGF (Liu, F. et al., 2008).

Cell based methods have been used to screen for HIF-1 inhibitors and many small molecules have been identified that impair cancer cell growth by reducing HIF-1α protein levels - through blocking its expression or enhancing its degradation - or by impairing its transcriptional activity (Semenza, 2010; Wilson & Hay, 2011). Another novel method to identify HIF-1 inhibitors is screening, recognition and isolation of new bioactive compounds from natural sources with molecularly imprinted polymers (MIPs), which have been developed using as templates known compounds that interfere with HIF-1 activity (Lakka et al., 2011). Of course, the potential application of these agents in cancer therapy relies on the outcome of clinical trials. However, the search for HIF-1 inhibitors revealed that several already tested and established anti-cancer drugs such as topotecan, a topoisomerase inhibitor, geldanamycin, an HSP90 inhibitor, and trichostatin A, a histone deacetylase inhibitor, can also block HIF-1 activity (Ibrahim et al., 2005; Poon, E. et al., 2009; Rapisarda et al., 2004). Given the ERK-HIF connection, extensively discussed above, another way to suppress HIF-1 would be to inhibit the Raf/MEK/ERK signaling pathway. The approval of sorafenib, a Raf inhibitor and anti-angiogenic agent, as single agent against HCC probably demonstrates this principle. Although, the effect of sorafenib on HIF-1 activity has not been directly studied in HCC, sorafenib has been shown to interfere with the HIF pathway in models of melanoma and neuroblastoma (Kumar et al., 2007; Nilsson et al., 2010). It is possible that combination of sorafenib with other agents that also target ERK (such as kaempferol or other naturally occurring substances with similar properties), HIF-1α (such as MTD) or VEGF (such as bevacizumab or inhibitors of the VEGF receptor) could be more efficient in treating HCC and preventing acquirement of resistance (Fig. 2).

## 9. Conclusion

Aberrant angiogenenesis, MAPK pathway activation and hypoxia contribute to the aggressiveness of hepatocellular carcinoma. This property is further enhanced by the fact that these processes positively influence one another in a way that adds up to the severity of the disease. Furthermore, they all involve as key component HIF-1α (Fig. 2), so its targeting provides an attractive strategy to treat hypoxic and highly angiogenic tumours like HCC. Combination of HIF-1α inhibitors with existing treatments or new targeted therapies like sorafenib may prove to be beneficial for the treatment of the disease.

## 10. Acknowledgements

The authors acknowledge financial support in the context of the project 09SYN-12-682, which is implemented under the auspices of NSRF and the National Range Action "COOPERATION" and co-funded by the Greek Government and the European Union -

European Regional Development Fund. The authors also wish to thank Prof. G. Dalekos, Dept. of Medicine, for helpful discussions and comments on the manuscript.

## 11. References

Abou-Alfa, G. K.; Schwartz, L.; Ricci, S.; Amadori, D.; Santoro, A.; Figer, A.; De Greve, J.; Douillard, J. Y.; Lathia, C.; Schwartz, B.; Taylor, I.; Moscovici, M. & Saltz, L. B. (2006). Phase II study of sorafenib in patients with advanced hepatocellular carcinoma. *Journal of Clinical Oncology,* Vol.24, No. 26, (Sep 10 2006), pp. 4293-4300, ISSN 1527-7755

Amir, S.; Wang, R.; Simons, J. W. & Mabjeesh, N. J. (2009). SEPT9_v1 up-regulates hypoxia-inducible factor 1 by preventing its RACK1-mediated degradation. *Journal of Biological Chemistry,* Vol.284, No. 17, (Apr 24 2009), pp. 11142-11151, ISSN 0021-9258

Bae, S. H.; Jeong, J. W.; Park, J. A.; Kim, S. H.; Bae, M. K.; Choi, S. J. & Kim, K. W. (2004). Sumoylation increases HIF-1alpha stability and its transcriptional activity. *Biochemical and Biophysical Research Communications,* Vol.324, No. 1, (Nov 5 2004), pp. 394-400, ISSN 0006-291x

Baek, J. H.; Liu, Y. V.; McDonald, K. R.; Wesley, J. B.; Zhang, H. & Semenza, G. L. (2007). Spermidine/spermine N(1)-acetyltransferase-1 binds to hypoxia-inducible factor-1alpha (HIF-1alpha) and RACK1 and promotes ubiquitination and degradation of HIF-1alpha. *Journal of Biological Chemistry,* Vol.282, No. 46, (Nov 16 2007), pp. 33358-33366, ISSN 0021-9258

Bardos, J. I. & Ashcroft, M. (2005). Negative and positive regulation of HIF-1: a complex network. *Biochimica et Biophysica Acta,* Vol.1755, No. 2, (Jul 25 2005), pp. 107-120, ISSN 0006-3002

Bermudez, O.; Jouandin, P.; Rottier, J.; Bourcier, C.; Pages, G. & Gimond, C. (2011). Post-transcriptional regulation of the DUSP6/MKP-3 phosphatase by MEK/ERK signaling and hypoxia. *Journal of Cellular Physiology,* Vol.226, No. 1, (Jan 2011), pp. 276-284, ISSN 1097-4652

Bernaudin, M.; Nedelec, A. S.; Divoux, D.; MacKenzie, E. T.; Petit, E. & Schumann-Bard, P. (2002). Normobaric hypoxia induces tolerance to focal permanent cerebral ischemia in association with an increased expression of hypoxia-inducible factor-1 and its target genes, erythropoietin and VEGF, in the adult mouse brain. *Journal of Cerebral Blood Flow and Metabolism,* Vol.22, No. 4, (Apr 2002), pp. 393-403, ISSN 0271-678X

Berta, M. A.; Mazure, N.; Hattab, M.; Pouyssegur, J. & Brahimi-Horn, M. C. (2007). SUMOylation of hypoxia-inducible factor-1alpha reduces its transcriptional activity. *Biochemical and Biophysical Research Communications,* Vol.360, No. 3, (Aug 31 2007), pp. 646-652, ISSN 0006-291X

Bessard, A.; Fremin, C.; Ezan, F.; Fautrel, A.; Gailhouste, L. & Baffet, G. (2008). RNAi-mediated ERK2 knockdown inhibits growth of tumor cells in vitro and in vivo. *Oncogene,* Vol.27, No. 40, (Sep 11 2008), pp. 5315-5325, ISSN 1476-5594

Bruix, J. & Llovet, J. M. (2009). Major achievements in hepatocellular carcinoma. *Lancet,* Vol.373, No. 9664, (Feb 21 2009), pp. 614-616, ISSN 1474-547X

Cagnol, S.; Van Obberghen-Schilling, E. & Chambard, J. C. (2006). Prolonged activation of ERK1,2 induces FADD-independent caspase 8 activation and cell death. *Apoptosis,* Vol.11, No. 3, (Mar 2006), pp. 337-346, ISSN 1360-8185

Calvisi, D. F.; Ladu, S.; Gorden, A.; Farina, M.; Conner, E. A.; Lee, J. S.; Factor, V. M. & Thorgeirsson, S. S. (2006). Ubiquitous activation of Ras and Jak/Stat pathways in human HCC. *Gastroenterology,* Vol.130, No. 4, (Apr 2006), pp. 1117-1128, ISSN 0016-5085

Calvisi, D. F.; Pinna, F.; Meloni, F.; Ladu, S.; Pellegrino, R.; Sini, M.; Daino, L.; Simile, M. M.; De Miglio, M. R.; Virdis, P.; Frau, M.; Tomasi, M. L.; Seddaiu, M. A.; Muroni, M. R.; Feo, F. & Pascale, R. M. (2008). Dual-specificity phosphatase 1 ubiquitination in extracellular signal-regulated kinase-mediated control of growth in human hepatocellular carcinoma. *Cancer Research,* Vol.68, No. 11, (Jun 1 2008), pp. 4192-4200, ISSN 1538-7445

Cam, H.; Easton, J. B.; High, A. & Houghton, P. J. (2010). mTORC1 signaling under hypoxic conditions is controlled by ATM-dependent phosphorylation of HIF-1alpha. *Molecular Cell,* Vol.40, No. 4, (Nov 24 2010), pp. 509-520, ISSN 1097-4164

Campbell, J. S.; Hughes, S. D.; Gilbertson, D. G.; Palmer, T. E.; Holdren, M. S.; Haran, A. C.; Odell, M. M.; Bauer, R. L.; Ren, H. P.; Haugen, H. S.; Yeh, M. M. & Fausto, N. (2005). Platelet-derived growth factor C induces liver fibrosis, steatosis, and hepatocellular carcinoma. *Proceedings of the National Academy of Sciences of the USA,* Vol.102, No. 9, (Mar 1 2005), pp. 3389-3394, ISSN 0027-8424

Carbia-Nagashima, A.; Gerez, J.; Perez-Castro, C.; Paez-Pereda, M.; Silberstein, S.; Stalla, G. K.; Holsboer, F. & Arzt, E. (2007). RSUME, a small RWD-containing protein, enhances SUMO conjugation and stabilizes HIF-1alpha during hypoxia. *Cell,* Vol.131, No. 2, (Oct 19 2007), pp. 309-323, ISSN 0092-8674

Carmeliet, P.; Dor, Y.; Herbert, J. M.; Fukumura, D.; Brusselmans, K.; Dewerchin, M.; Neeman, M.; Bono, F.; Abramovitch, R.; Maxwell, P.; Koch, C. J.; Ratcliffe, P.; Moons, L.; Jain, R. K.; Collen, D. & Keshert, E. (1998). Role of HIF-1alpha in hypoxia-mediated apoptosis, cell proliferation and tumour angiogenesis. *Nature,* Vol.394, No. 6692, (Jul 30 1998), pp. 485-490, ISSN 0028-0836

Chachami, G.; Paraskeva, E.; Mingot, J. M.; Braliou, G. G.; Gorlich, D. & Simos, G. (2009). Transport of hypoxia-inducible factor HIF-1alpha into the nucleus involves importins 4 and 7. *Biochemical and Biophysical Research Communications,* Vol.390, No. 2, (Dec 11 2009), pp. 235-240, ISSN 1090-2104

Cheng, J.; Kang, X.; Zhang, S. & Yeh, E. T. (2007). SUMO-specific protease 1 is essential for stabilization of HIF1alpha during hypoxia. *Cell,* Vol.131, No. 3, (Nov 2 2007), pp. 584-595, ISSN 0092-8674

Chin, R.; Earnest-Silveira, L.; Koeberlein, B.; Franz, S.; Zentgraf, H.; Dong, X.; Gowans, E.; Bock, C. T. & Torresi, J. (2007). Modulation of MAPK pathways and cell cycle by replicating hepatitis B virus: factors contributing to hepatocarcinogenesis. *Journal of Hepatology,* Vol.47, No. 3, (Sep 2007), pp. 325-337, ISSN 0168-8278

Depping, R.; Steinhoff, A.; Schindler, S. G.; Friedrich, B.; Fagerlund, R.; Metzen, E.; Hartmann, E. & Kohler, M. (2008). Nuclear translocation of hypoxia-inducible factors (HIFs): involvement of the classical importin alpha/beta pathway. *Biochimica et Biophysica Acta,* Vol.1783, No. 3, (Mar 2008), pp. 394-404, ISSN 0006-3002

Dimova, E. Y.; Michiels, C. & Kietzmann, T. (2009). Kinases as upstream regulators of the HIF system: their emerging potential as anti-cancer drug targets. *Current Pharmaceutical Design,* Vol.15, No. 33, 2009), pp. 3867-3877, ISSN 1873-4286

Fernandez, M.; Semela, D.; Bruix, J.; Colle, I.; Pinzani, M. & Bosch, J. (2009). Angiogenesis in liver disease. *Journal of Hepatology,* Vol.50, No. 3, (Mar 2009), pp. 604-620, ISSN 0168-8278

Flugel, D.; Gorlach, A.; Michiels, C. & Kietzmann, T. (2007). Glycogen synthase kinase 3 phosphorylates hypoxia-inducible factor 1alpha and mediates its destabilization in a VHL-independent manner. *Molecular and Cellular Biology,* Vol.27, No. 9, (May 2007), pp. 3253-3265, ISSN 0270-7306

Frau, M.; Biasi, F.; Feo, F. & Pascale, R. M. (2010). Prognostic markers and putative therapeutic targets for hepatocellular carcinoma. *Molecular Aspects of Medicine,* Vol.31, No. 2, (Apr 2010), pp. 179-193, ISSN 1872-9452

Fukuda, R.; Hirota, K.; Fan, F.; Jung, Y. D.; Ellis, L. M. & Semenza, G. L. (2002). Insulin-like Growth Factor 1 Induces Hypoxia-inducible Factor 1-mediated Vascular Endothelial Growth Factor Expression, Which is Dependent on MAP Kinase and Phosphatidylinositol 3-Kinase Signaling in Colon Cancer Cells. *Journal of Biological Chemistry,* Vol.277, No. 41, (Oct 11 2002), pp. 38205-38211, ISSN 0021-9258

Gailhouste, L.; Ezan, F.; Bessard, A.; Fremin, C.; Rageul, J.; Langouet, S. & Baffet, G. (2010). RNAi-mediated MEK1 knock-down prevents ERK1/2 activation and abolishes human hepatocarcinoma growth in vitro and in vivo. *International Journal of Cancer,* Vol.126, No. 6, (Mar 15 2010), pp. 1367-1377, ISSN 1097-0215

Gates, M. A.; Tworoger, S. S.; Hecht, J. L.; De Vivo, I.; Rosner, B. & Hankinson, S. E. (2007). A prospective study of dietary flavonoid intake and incidence of epithelial ovarian cancer. *International Journal of Cancer,* Vol.121, No. 10, (Nov 15 2007), pp. 2225-2232, ISSN 1097-0215

Gwak, G. Y.; Yoon, J. H.; Kim, K. M.; Lee, H. S.; Chung, J. W. & Gores, G. J. (2005). Hypoxia stimulates proliferation of human hepatoma cells through the induction of hexokinase II expression. *Journal of Hepatology,* Vol.42, No. 3, (Mar 2005), pp. 358-364, ISSN 0168-8278

Hassan, M.; Selimovic, D.; Ghozlan, H. & Abdel-kader, O. (2009). Hepatitis C virus core protein triggers hepatic angiogenesis by a mechanism including multiple pathways. *Hepatology,* Vol.49, No. 5, (May 2009), pp. 1469-1482, ISSN 1527-3350

Hennig, M.; Yip-Schneider, M. T.; Wentz, S.; Wu, H.; Hekmatyar, S. K.; Klein, P.; Bansal, N. & Schmidt, C. M. (2010). Targeting mitogen-activated protein kinase kinase with the inhibitor PD0325901 decreases hepatocellular carcinoma growth in vitro and in mouse model systems. *Hepatology,* Vol.51, No. 4, (Apr 2010), pp. 1218-1225, ISSN 1527-3350

Hoshida, Y.; Toffanin, S.; Lachenmayer, A.; Villanueva, A.; Minguez, B. & Llovet, J. M. (2010). Molecular classification and novel targets in hepatocellular carcinoma: recent advancements. *Seminars in Liver Disease,* Vol.30, No. 1, (Feb 2010), pp. 35-51, ISSN 1098-8971

Huang, G. W.; Yang, L. Y. & Lu, W. Q. (2005). Expression of hypoxia-inducible factor 1alpha and vascular endothelial growth factor in hepatocellular carcinoma: Impact on neovascularization and survival. *World Journal of Gastroenterology,* Vol.11, No. 11, (Mar 21 2005), pp. 1705-1708, 1007-9327 (Print) ISSN 1007-9327

Huynh, H.; Ngo, V. C.; Koong, H. N.; Poon, D.; Choo, S. P.; Toh, H. C.; Thng, C. H.; Chow, P.; Ong, H. S.; Chung, A.; Goh, B. C.; Smith, P. D. & Soo, K. C. (2010). AZD6244 enhances the anti-tumor activity of sorafenib in ectopic and orthotopic models of human hepatocellular carcinoma (HCC). *Journal of Hepatology,* Vol.52, No. 1, (Jan 2010), pp. 79-87, ISSN 0168-8278

Huynh, H.; Soo, K. C.; Chow, P. K. & Tran, E. (2007). Targeted inhibition of the extracellular signal-regulated kinase kinase pathway with AZD6244 (ARRY-142886) in the treatment of hepatocellular carcinoma. *Molecular Cancer Therapeutics,* Vol.6, No. 1, (Jan 2007), pp. 138-146, ISSN 1535-7163

Ibrahim, N. O.; Hahn, T.; Franke, C.; Stiehl, D. P.; Wirthner, R.; Wenger, R. H. & Katschinski, D. M. (2005). Induction of the hypoxia-inducible factor system by low levels of heat shock protein 90 inhibitors. *Cancer Research,* Vol.65, No. 23, (Dec 1 2005), pp. 11094-11100, ISSN 0008-5472

Imura, S.; Miyake, H.; Izumi, K.; Tashiro, S. & Uehara, H. (2004). Correlation of vascular endothelial cell proliferation with microvessel density and expression of vascular endothelial growth factor and basic fibroblast growth factor in hepatocellular carcinoma. *Journal of Medical Investigation,* Vol.51, No. 3-4, (Aug 2004), pp. 202-209, ISSN 1343-1420

Isaacs, J. S.; Jung, Y. J.; Mimnaugh, E. G.; Martinez, A.; Cuttitta, F. & Neckers, L. M. (2002). Hsp90 regulates a von Hippel Lindau-independent hypoxia-inducible factor-1 alpha-degradative pathway. *Journal of Biological Chemistry,* Vol.277, No. 33, (Aug 16 2002), pp. 29936-29944, ISSN 0021-9258

Jeong, J. W.; Bae, M. K.; Ahn, M. Y.; Kim, S. H.; Sohn, T. K.; Bae, M. H.; Yoo, M. A.; Song, E. J.; Lee, K. J. & Kim, K. W. (2002). Regulation and destabilization of HIF-1alpha by ARD1-mediated acetylation. *Cell,* Vol.111, No. 5, (Nov 27 2002), pp. 709-720, ISSN 0092-8674

Kallio, P. J.; Okamoto, K.; O'Brien, S.; Carrero, P.; Makino, Y.; Tanaka, H. & Poellinger, L. (1998). Signal transduction in hypoxic cells: inducible nuclear translocation and recruitment of the CBP/p300 coactivator by the hypoxia-inducible factor-1alpha. *EMBO Journal,* Vol.17, No. 22, (Nov 16 1998), pp. 6573-6586, ISSN 0261-4189

Kalousi, A.; Mylonis, I.; Politou, A. S.; Chachami, G.; Paraskeva, E. & Simos, G. (2010). Casein kinase 1 regulates human hypoxia inducible factor HIF-1. *Journal of Cell Science,* Vol.123, No.17, (Sep 1 2010), pp. 2976-2986, ISSN 1477-9137

Katschinski, D. M.; Le, L.; Schindler, S. G.; Thomas, T.; Voss, A. K. & Wenger, R. H. (2004). Interaction of the PAS B domain with HSP90 accelerates hypoxia-inducible factor-1alpha stabilization. *Cellular Physiology and Biochemistry,* Vol.14, No. 4-6, 2004), pp. 351-360, ISSN 1015-8987

Kumar, S. M.; Yu, H.; Edwards, R.; Chen, L.; Kazianis, S.; Brafford, P.; Acs, G.; Herlyn, M. & Xu, X. (2007). Mutant V600E BRAF increases hypoxia inducible factor-1alpha expression in melanoma. *Cancer Research,* Vol.67, No. 7, (Apr 1 2007), pp. 3177-3184, ISSN 0008-5472

Laderoute, K. R.; Mendonca, H. L.; Calaoagan, J. M.; Knapp, A. M.; Giaccia, A. J. & Stork, P. J. (1999). Mitogen-activated protein kinase phosphatase-1 (MKP-1) expression is induced by low oxygen conditions found in solid tumor microenvironments. A candidate MKP for the inactivation of hypoxia-inducible stress-activated protein kinase/c-Jun N-terminal protein kinase activity. *Journal of Biological Chemistry,* Vol.274, No. 18, (Apr 30 1999), pp. 12890-12897, ISSN 0021-9258

Lakka, A.; Mylonis, I.; Bonanou, S.; Simos, G. & Tsakalof, A. (2011). Isolation of hypoxia-inducible factor 1 (HIF-1) inhibitors from frankincense using a molecularly imprinted polymer. *Investigational New Drugs*, Vol.29, No. 5, (Oct 2011), pp. 1081-1089, ISSN 1573-0646

Lancaster, D. E.; McDonough, M. A. & Schofield, C. J. (2004a). Factor inhibiting hypoxia-inducible factor (FIH) and other asparaginyl hydroxylases. *Biochemical Society Transactions*, Vol.32, No. Pt 6, (Dec 2004a), pp. 943-945, ISSN 0300-5127

Lancaster, D. E.; McNeill, L. A.; McDonough, M. A.; Aplin, R. T.; Hewitson, K. S.; Pugh, C. W.; Ratcliffe, P. J. & Schofield, C. J. (2004b). Disruption of dimerization and substrate phosphorylation inhibit factor inhibiting hypoxia-inducible factor (FIH) activity. *Biochemical Journal*, Vol.383, No. Pt. 3, (Nov 1 2004b), pp. 429-437, ISSN 1470-8728

Lee, E.; Yim, S.; Lee, S. K. & Park, H. (2002). Two transactivation domains of hypoxia-inducible factor-1alpha regulated by the MEK-1/p42/p44 MAPK pathway. *Molecules and Cells*, Vol.14, No. 1, (Aug 31 2002), pp. 9-15, ISSN 1016-8478

Lee, H. C.; Tian, B.; Sedivy, J. M.; Wands, J. R. & Kim, M. (2006). Loss of Raf kinase inhibitor protein promotes cell proliferation and migration of human hepatoma cells. *Gastroenterology*, Vol.131, No. 4, (Oct 2006), pp. 1208-1217, ISSN 0016-5085

Li, F.; Sonveaux, P.; Rabbani, Z. N.; Liu, S.; Yan, B.; Huang, Q.; Vujaskovic, Z.; Dewhirst, M. W. & Li, C. Y. (2007). Regulation of HIF-1alpha stability through S-nitrosylation. *Molecular Cell*, Vol.26, No. 1, (Apr 13 2007), pp. 63-74, ISSN 1097-2765

Lin, S. C.; Chien, C. W.; Lee, J. C.; Yeh, Y. C.; Hsu, K. F.; Lai, Y. Y. & Tsai, S. J. (2011). Suppression of dual-specificity phosphatase-2 by hypoxia increases chemoresistance and malignancy in human cancer cells. *Journal of Clinical Investigation*, Vol.121, No. 5, (May 2 2011), pp. 1905-1916, ISSN 1558-8238

Liu, C.; Shi, Y.; Du, Y.; Ning, X.; Liu, N.; Huang, D.; Liang, J.; Xue, Y. & Fan, D. (2005). Dual-specificity phosphatase DUSP1 protects overactivation of hypoxia-inducible factor 1 through inactivating ERK MAPK. *Experimental Cell Research*, Vol.309, No. 2, (Oct 1 2005), pp. 410-418, ISSN 0014-4827

Liu, F.; Wang, P.; Jiang, X.; Tan, G.; Qiao, H.; Jiang, H.; Krissansen, G. W. & Sun, X. (2008). Antisense hypoxia-inducible factor 1alpha gene therapy enhances the therapeutic efficacy of doxorubicin to combat hepatocellular carcinoma. *Cancer Science*, Vol.99, No. 10, (Oct 2008), pp. 2055-2061, ISSN 1349-7006

Liu, L.; Cao, Y.; Chen, C.; Zhang, X.; McNabola, A.; Wilkie, D.; Wilhelm, S.; Lynch, M. & Carter, C. (2006). Sorafenib blocks the RAF/MEK/ERK pathway, inhibits tumor angiogenesis, and induces tumor cell apoptosis in hepatocellular carcinoma model PLC/PRF/5. *Cancer Research*, Vol.66, No. 24, (Dec 15 2006), pp. 11851-11858, ISSN 0008-5472

Liu, Q.; Liu, L.; Zhao, Y.; Zhang, J.; Wang, D.; Chen, J.; He, Y.; Wu, J.; Zhang, Z. & Liu, Z. (2011). Hypoxia induces genomic DNA demethylation through the activation of HIF-1alpha and transcriptional upregulation of MAT2A in hepatoma cells. *Molecular Cancer Therapeutics*, Vol.10, No. 6, (Jun 2011), pp. 1113-1123, ISSN 1538-8514

Liu, Y. V.; Baek, J. H.; Zhang, H.; Diez, R.; Cole, R. N. & Semenza, G. L. (2007). RACK1 competes with HSP90 for binding to HIF-1alpha and is required for O(2)-independent and HSP90 inhibitor-induced degradation of HIF-1alpha. *Molecular Cell*, Vol.25, No. 2, (Jan 26 2007), pp. 207-217, ISSN 1097-2765

Llovet, J. M. & Bruix, J. (2003). Systematic review of randomized trials for unresectable hepatocellular carcinoma: Chemoembolization improves survival. *Hepatology,* Vol.37, No. 2, (Feb 2003), pp. 429-442, ISSN 0270-9139

Llovet, J. M.; Ricci, S.; Mazzaferro, V.; Hilgard, P.; Gane, E.; Blanc, J. F.; de Oliveira, A. C.; Santoro, A.; Raoul, J. L.; Forner, A.; Schwartz, M.; Porta, C.; Zeuzem, S.; Bolondi, L.; Greten, T. F.; Galle, P. R.; Seitz, J. F.; Borbath, I.; Haussinger, D.; Giannaris, T.; Shan, M.; Moscovici, M.; Voliotis, D. & Bruix, J. (2008). Sorafenib in advanced hepatocellular carcinoma. *New England Journal of Medicine,* Vol.359, No. 4, (Jul 24 2008), pp. 378-390, ISSN 1533-4406

Luo, J. C. & Shibuya, M. (2001). A variant of nuclear localization signal of bipartite-type is required for the nuclear translocation of hypoxia inducible factors (1alpha, 2alpha and 3alpha). *Oncogene,* Vol.20, No. 12, (Mar 22 2001), pp. 1435-1444, ISSN 0950-9232

Lyberopoulou, A.; Venieris, E.; Mylonis, I.; Chachami, G.; Pappas, I.; Simos, G.; Bonanou, S. & Georgatsou, E. (2007). MgcRacGAP interacts with HIF-1alpha and regulates its transcriptional activity. *Cellular Physiology and Biochemistry,* Vol.20, No. 6, 2007), pp. 995-1006, ISSN 1015-8987

Manach, C.; Williamson, G.; Morand, C.; Scalbert, A. & Remesy, C. (2005). Bioavailability and bioefficacy of polyphenols in humans. I. Review of 97 bioavailability studies. *American Journal of Clinical Nutrition,* Vol.81, No. 1 Suppl, (Jan 2005), pp. 230S-242S, ISSN 0002-9165

Min, L.; He, B. & Hui, L. (2010). Mitogen-activated protein kinases in hepatocellular carcinoma development. *Seminars in Cancer Biology,* Vol.21, No. 1, (Feb 2010), pp. 10-20, ISSN 1096-3650

Minet, E.; Arnould, T.; Michel, G.; Roland, I.; Mottet, D.; Raes, M.; Remacle, J. & Michiels, C. (2000). ERK activation upon hypoxia: involvement in HIF-1 activation. *FEBS Letters,* Vol.468, No. 1, (Feb 18 2000), pp. 53-58, ISSN 0014-5793

Mitsuhashi, N.; Shimizu, H.; Ohtsuka, M.; Wakabayashi, Y.; Ito, H.; Kimura, F.; Yoshidome, H.; Kato, A.; Nukui, Y. & Miyazaki, M. (2003). Angiopoietins and Tie-2 expression in angiogenesis and proliferation of human hepatocellular carcinoma. *Hepatology,* Vol.37, No. 5, (May 2003), pp. 1105-1113, ISSN 0270-9139

Mottet, D.; Michel, G.; Renard, P.; Ninane, N.; Raes, M. & Michiels, C. (2002). ERK and calcium in activation of HIF-1. *Annals of the New York Academy of Science,* Vol.973, No., (Nov 2002), pp. 448-453, ISSN 0077-8923

Mylonis, I.; Chachami, G.; Samiotaki, M.; Panayotou, G.; Paraskeva, E.; Kalousi, A.; Georgatsou, E.; Bonanou, S. & Simos, G. (2006). Identification of MAPK phosphorylation sites and their role in the localization and activity of hypoxia-inducible factor-1alpha. *Journal of Biological Chemistry,* Vol.281, No. 44, (Nov 3 2006), pp. 33095-33106, ISSN 0021-9258

Mylonis, I.; Chachami, G.; Paraskeva, E. & Simos, G. (2008). Atypical CRM1-dependent nuclear export signal mediates regulation of hypoxia-inducible factor-1alpha by MAPK. *Journal of Biological Chemistry,* Vol.283, No. 41, (Oct 10 2008), pp. 27620-27627, ISSN 0021-9258

Mylonis, I.; Lakka, A.; Tsakalof, A. & Simos, G. (2010). The dietary flavonoid kaempferol effectively inhibits HIF-1 activity and hepatoma cancer cell viability under hypoxic conditions. *Biochemical and Biophysical Research Communications,* Vol.398, No. 1, (Jul 16 2010), pp. 74-78, ISSN 1090-2104

Nakamura, K.; Zen, Y.; Sato, Y.; Kozaka, K.; Matsui, O.; Harada, K. & Nakanuma, Y. (2007). Vascular endothelial growth factor, its receptor Flk-1, and hypoxia inducible factor-1alpha are involved in malignant transformation in dysplastic nodules of the liver. *Human Pathology,* Vol.38, No. 10, (Oct 2007), pp. 1532-1546, ISSN 0046-8177

Nilsson, M. B.; Zage, P. E.; Zeng, L.; Xu, L.; Cascone, T.; Wu, H. K.; Saigal, B.; Zweidler-McKay, P. A. & Heymach, J. V. (2010). Multiple receptor tyrosine kinases regulate HIF-1alpha and HIF-2alpha in normoxia and hypoxia in neuroblastoma: implications for antiangiogenic mechanisms of multikinase inhibitors. *Oncogene,* Vol.29, No. 20, (May 20 2010), pp. 2938-2949, ISSN 1476-5594

Niu, G.; Briggs, J.; Deng, J.; Ma, Y.; Lee, H.; Kortylewski, M.; Kujawski, M.; Kay, H.; Cress, W. D.; Jove, R. & Yu, H. (2008). Signal transducer and activator of transcription 3 is required for hypoxia-inducible factor-1alpha RNA expression in both tumor cells and tumor-associated myeloid cells. *Molecular Cancer Research,* Vol.6, No. 7, (Jul 2008), pp. 1099-1105, ISSN 1541-7786

Papadakis, A. I.; Paraskeva, E.; Peidis, P.; Muaddi, H.; Li, S.; Raptis, L.; Pantopoulos, K.; Simos, G. & Koromilas, A. E. (2010). eIF2{alpha} Kinase PKR modulates the hypoxic response by Stat3-dependent transcriptional suppression of HIF-1{alpha}. *Cancer Research,* Vol.70, No. 20, (Oct 15 2010), pp. 7820-7829, ISSN 1538-7445

Patsenker, E.; Popov, Y.; Stickel, F.; Schneider, V.; Ledermann, M.; Sagesser, H.; Niedobitek, G.; Goodman, S. L. & Schuppan, D. (2009). Pharmacological inhibition of integrin alphavbeta3 aggravates experimental liver fibrosis and suppresses hepatic angiogenesis. *Hepatology,* Vol.50, No. 5, (Nov 2009), pp. 1501-1511, ISSN 1527-3350

Pearson, G.; Robinson, F.; Beers Gibson, T.; Xu, B. E.; Karandikar, M.; Berman, K. & Cobb, M. H. (2001). Mitogen-activated protein (MAP) kinase pathways: regulation and physiological functions. *Endocrine Reviews,* Vol.22, No. 2, (Apr 2001), pp. 153-183, ISSN 0163-769X

Poon, E.; Harris, A. L. & Ashcroft, M. (2009). Targeting the hypoxia-inducible factor (HIF) pathway in cancer. *Expert Reviews in Molecular Medicine,* Vol.11, No., 2009), pp. e26, ISSN 1462-3994

Poon, R. T.; Ho, J. W.; Tong, C. S.; Lau, C.; Ng, I. O. & Fan, S. T. (2004). Prognostic significance of serum vascular endothelial growth factor and endostatin in patients with hepatocellular carcinoma. *British Journal of Surgery,* Vol.91, No. 10, (Oct 2004), pp. 1354-1360, ISSN 0007-1323

Poon, R. T.; Lau, C.; Pang, R.; Ng, K. K.; Yuen, J. & Fan, S. T. (2007). High serum vascular endothelial growth factor levels predict poor prognosis after radiofrequency ablation of hepatocellular carcinoma: importance of tumor biomarker in ablative therapies. *Annals of Surgical Oncology,* Vol.14, No. 6, (Jun 2007), pp. 1835-1845, ISSN 1068-9265

Rapisarda, A.; Uranchimeg, B.; Sordet, O.; Pommier, Y.; Shoemaker, R. H. & Melillo, G. (2004). Topoisomerase I-mediated inhibition of hypoxia-inducible factor 1: mechanism and therapeutic implications. *Cancer Research,* Vol.64, No. 4, (Feb 15 2004), pp. 1475-1482, ISSN 0008-5472

Richard, D. E.; Berra, E.; Gothie, E.; Roux, D. & Pouyssegur, J. (1999). p42/p44 mitogen-activated protein kinases phosphorylate hypoxia-inducible factor 1alpha (HIF-1alpha) and enhance the transcriptional activity of HIF-1. *Journal of Biological Chemistry,* Vol.274, No. 46, (Nov 12 1999), pp. 32631-32637, ISSN 0021-9258

Rius, J.; Guma, M.; Schachtrup, C.; Akassoglou, K.; Zinkernagel, A. S.; Nizet, V.; Johnson, R. S.; Haddad, G. G. & Karin, M. (2008). NF-kappaB links innate immunity to the hypoxic response through transcriptional regulation of HIF-1alpha. *Nature,* Vol.453, No. 7196, (Jun 5 2008), pp. 807-811, ISSN 1476-4687

Rosmorduc, O. & Housset, C. (2010). Hypoxia: a link between fibrogenesis, angiogenesis, and carcinogenesis in liver disease. *Seminars in Liver Disease,* Vol.30, No. 3, (Aug 2010), pp. 258-270, ISSN 1098-8971

Salceda, S.; Beck, I.; Srinivas, V. & Caro, J. (1997). Complex role of protein phosphorylation in gene activation by hypoxia. *Kidney International,* Vol.51, No. 2, (Feb 1997), pp. 556-559, ISSN 0085-2538

Sang, N.; Stiehl, D. P.; Bohensky, J.; Leshchinsky, I.; Srinivas, V. & Caro, J. (2003). MAPK signaling up-regulates the activity of hypoxia-inducible factors by its effects on p300. *Journal of Biological Chemistry,* Vol.278, No. 16, (Apr 18 2003), pp. 14013-14019, ISSN 0021-9258

Schofield, C. J. & Ratcliffe, P. J. (2005). Signalling hypoxia by HIF hydroxylases. *Biochemical and Biophysical Research Communications,* Vol.338, No. 1, (Dec 9 2005), pp. 617-626, ISSN 1471-0072

Semenza, G. L. (2001). HIF-1, O(2), and the 3 PHDs: how animal cells signal hypoxia to the nucleus. *Cell,* Vol.107, No. 1, (Oct 5 2001), pp. 1-3, ISSN 0092-8674

Semenza, G. L. (2003). Targeting HIF-1 for cancer therapy. *Nature Reviews Cancer,* Vol.3, No. 10, (Oct 2003), pp. 721-732, ISSN 1474-175x

Semenza, G. L. (2010). Defining the role of hypoxia-inducible factor 1 in cancer biology and therapeutics. *Oncogene,* Vol.29, No. 5, (Feb 4 2010), pp. 625-634, ISSN 1476-5594

Seta, K. A.; Kim, R.; Kim, H. W.; Millhorn, D. E. & Beitner-Johnson, D. (2001). Hypoxia-induced regulation of MAPK phosphatase-1 as identified by subtractive suppression hybridization and cDNA microarray analysis. *Journal of Biological Chemistry,* Vol.276, No. 48, (Nov 30 2001), pp. 44405-44412, ISSN 0021-9258

Tanaka, H.; Yamamoto, M.; Hashimoto, N.; Miyakoshi, M.; Tamakawa, S.; Yoshie, M.; Tokusashi, Y.; Yokoyama, K.; Yaginuma, Y. & Ogawa, K. (2006). Hypoxia-independent overexpression of hypoxia-inducible factor 1alpha as an early change in mouse hepatocarcinogenesis. *Cancer Research,* Vol.66, No. 23, (Dec 1 2006), pp. 11263-11270, ISSN 0008-5472

Triantafyllou, A.; Mylonis, I.; Simos, G.; Bonanou, S. & Tsakalof, A. (2008). Flavonoids induce HIF-1alpha but impair its nuclear accumulation and activity. *Free Radical Biology and Medicine,* Vol.44, No. 4, (Feb 15 2008), pp. 657-670, ISSN 0891-5849

Villanueva, A.; Hoshida, Y.; Toffanin, S.; Lachenmayer, A.; Alsinet, C.; Savic, R.; Cornella, H. & Llovet, J. M. (2010). New strategies in hepatocellular carcinoma: genomic prognostic markers. *Clinical Cancer Research,* Vol.16, No. 19, (Oct 1 2010), pp. 4688-4694, ISSN 1078-0432

von Marschall, Z.; Cramer, T.; Hocker, M.; Finkenzeller, G.; Wiedenmann, B. & Rosewicz, S. (2001). Dual mechanism of vascular endothelial growth factor upregulation by hypoxia in human hepatocellular carcinoma. *Gut,* Vol.48, No. 1, (Jan 2001), pp. 87-96, ISSN 0017-5749

Wei, W. & Yu, X. D. (2007). Hypoxia-inducible factors: crosstalk between their protein stability and protein degradation. *Cancer Letters,* Vol.257, No. 2, (Nov 18 2007), pp. 145-156, ISSN 0304-3835

Wiesener, M. S.; Jurgensen, J. S.; Rosenberger, C.; Scholze, C. K.; Horstrup, J. H.; Warnecke, C.; Mandriota, S.; Bechmann, I.; Frei, U. A.; Pugh, C. W.; Ratcliffe, P. J.; Bachmann, S.; Maxwell, P. H. & Eckardt, K. U. (2003). Widespread hypoxia-inducible expression of HIF-2alpha in distinct cell populations of different organs. *Faseb Journal,* Vol.17, No. 2, (Feb 2003), pp. 271-273, ISSN 1530-6860

Wilhelm, S. M.; Carter, C.; Tang, L.; Wilkie, D.; McNabola, A.; Rong, H.; Chen, C.; Zhang, X.; Vincent, P.; McHugh, M.; Cao, Y.; Shujath, J.; Gawlak, S.; Eveleigh, D.; Rowley, B.; Liu, L.; Adnane, L.; Lynch, M.; Auclair, D.; Taylor, I.; Gedrich, R.; Voznesensky, A.; Riedl, B.; Post, L. E.; Bollag, G. & Trail, P. A. (2004). BAY 43-9006 exhibits broad spectrum oral antitumor activity and targets the RAF/MEK/ERK pathway and receptor tyrosine kinases involved in tumor progression and angiogenesis. *Cancer Research,* Vol.64, No. 19, (Oct 1 2004), pp. 7099-7109, ISSN 0008-5472

Wilson, W. R. & Hay, M. P. (2011). Targeting hypoxia in cancer therapy. *Nature Reviews Cancer,* Vol.11, No. 6, (Jun 2011), pp. 393-410, ISSN 1474-1768

Xiang, Z. L.; Zeng, Z. C.; Fan, J.; Tang, Z. Y.; He, J.; Zeng, H. Y. & Chang, J. Y. (2011). The expression of HIF-1alpha in primary hepatocellular carcinoma and its correlation with radiotherapy response and clinical outcome. *Molecular Biology Reports,* doi: 10.1007/s11033-011-0949-1 (Jun 7 2011), ISSN 1573-4978

Xu, D.; Yao, Y.; Lu, L.; Costa, M. & Dai, W. (2010). Plk3 functions as an essential component of the hypoxia regulatory pathway by direct phosphorylation of HIF-1alpha. *Journal of Biological Chemistry,* Vol.285, No. 50, (Dec 10 2010), pp. 38944-38950, ISSN 1083-351X

Zender, L.; Villanueva, A.; Tovar, V.; Sia, D.; Chiang, D. Y. & Llovet, J. M. (2010). Cancer gene discovery in hepatocellular carcinoma. *Journal of Hepatology,* Vol.52, No. 6, (Jun 2010), pp. 921-929, ISSN 0168-8278

Zhao, L. J.; Wang, L.; Ren, H.; Cao, J.; Li, L.; Ke, J. S. & Qi, Z. T. (2005). Hepatitis C virus E2 protein promotes human hepatoma cell proliferation through the MAPK/ERK signaling pathway via cellular receptors. *Experimental Cell Research,* Vol.305, No. 1, (Apr 15 2005), pp. 23-32, ISSN 0014-4827

13

# Gap Junction Intercellular Communication and Connexin Expression Profile in Normal Liver Cells and Hepatocarcinoma

Glaucia M. Machado-Santelli[1] and Marisa Ionta[2]
[1]*Department of Cell and Developmental Biology, Institute of Biomedical Sciences, University of Sao Paulo, Sao Paulo*
[2]*Institute of Biomedical Sciences, Federal University of Alfenas, Minas Gerais*
*Brazil*

## 1. Introduction

Gap junction intercellular communication (GJIC) is considered to play a relevant role in homeostasis of multicellular organisms by regulating processes such as cell proliferation and cell differentiation. Specialized membrane structures mediate cell-to-cell communication, the gap junctional channels, which allow the transfer of molecules less than 1000Daltons (Da) between adjacent cells such as ions, aminoacids, nucleotides, metabolites and second messengers. Gap junctional channels consist of the two juxtaposed hemichannels called connexons, each of them constituted of six proteic subunits composed of connexin (Cx). These proteins are codified by multigene family with at least 21 members and their expression is tissue specific. The different isoforms are named according to their molecular mass (kilo Dalton) and they share a similar structure of four membrane-spanning domains, two extracellular loops, one cytoplasmic loop, one cytosolic N-terminal tail and C-terminal region. The transmembrane domains and the extracellular loops are highly conserved among the family members. N-terminus is also conserved, while the cytoplasmic loop and C-terminus show great variation in terms of sequence and length. Furthermore cytoplasmic tail and loop are susceptible to various post-translational modifications (including phosphorylation), which are important to modulate functional activity of connexin (Figure 1).

The liver represents an interesting system to study gap junction intercellular communication (GJIC) and through the years, a wealth of knowledge is available about functional GJIC and connexin expression profile in different physiological conditions which include cell proliferation, cell differentiation and cell death and disruption of GJIC has been associated with hepatocarcinogenesis process.

## 2. Gap junction channels biogenesis and degradation mechanisms

The synthesis, assembly and turnover of GJ channels follow the general secretory roles for membrane proteins. Connexins are synthesized by membrane-bound ribosomes and they are cotranslationally integrated into the endoplasmic reticulum membrane. The oligomerization of connexins into connexon (hemichannel) occurs in a progressive fashion starting in the endoplasmic reticulum and ending in the trans-Golgi network, however the exact localization of oligomerization depends on the connexin type. It is thought that both Cx26 and Cx32 oligomerize in the endoplasmic reticulum, whereas Cx43 oligomerizes in the *trans*-Golgi network (Musil and Goodenough, 1993; Martin et al., 2001).

Connexons are then delivery to the cell surface via vesicles transported through microtubules, which fuse to plasma membrane. Upon arrival at the cell membrane, connexons can either reside in nonjunctional regions or docking with an opposing connexon to form fully functional channels.

Connexons can be **homomeric** (formed by a single type of connexin) or **heteromeric** (formed by more than one type of connexin). Functional channels are **homotypic** when formed by identical connexons (homomeric or heteromeric) or **heterotypic**, formed by the interaction between different connexons (Figure 1).

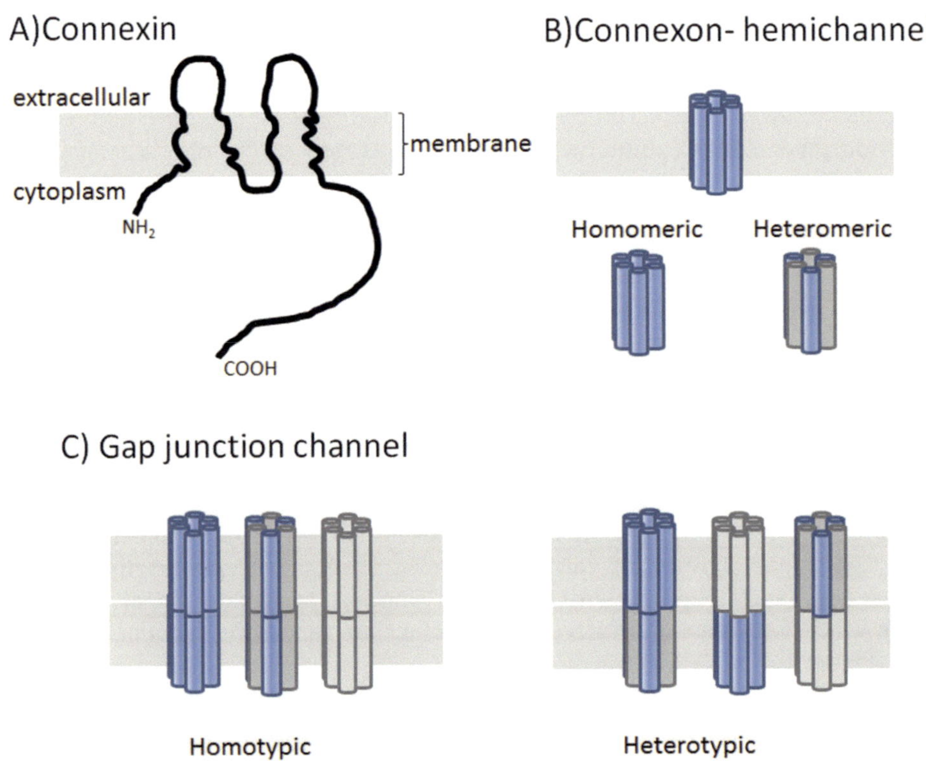


Fig. 1. A) The connexin structure consists of four membrane-spanning domains, two extracellular and one intra-cellular loops, one N-terminal tail and one C-terminal tail; B) Six connexins ( represented by cylinder) organize the connexon which can be homomeric (with a single connexin isoform) or heteromeric ( formed by more than one type of connexin); C)Two connexons dock together to form a gap junctional channel that can be homotypic if they are identical or heterotypic, if they are different.

The ability to form homotypic and heterotypic channels with homomeric and heteromeric connexons adds even greater versatility to the functional modulation of GJ channels. In liver, connexin 26 is able to form heteromeric connexon with Cx32 but did not form heteromeric connexon with connexin 43 once the isoforms need to be compatible. It is important to notice that homomeric channels formed by Cx32 or Cx26 present differences in permeability when compared to heteromeric channels formed by just Cxs 26 or Cx32 (reviewed by Mese et al., 2007).

Docking of connexons implies their insertion into gap junction plaques which comprise punctuated regions at membrane juxtaposed area (Figure 2). The formation of functional

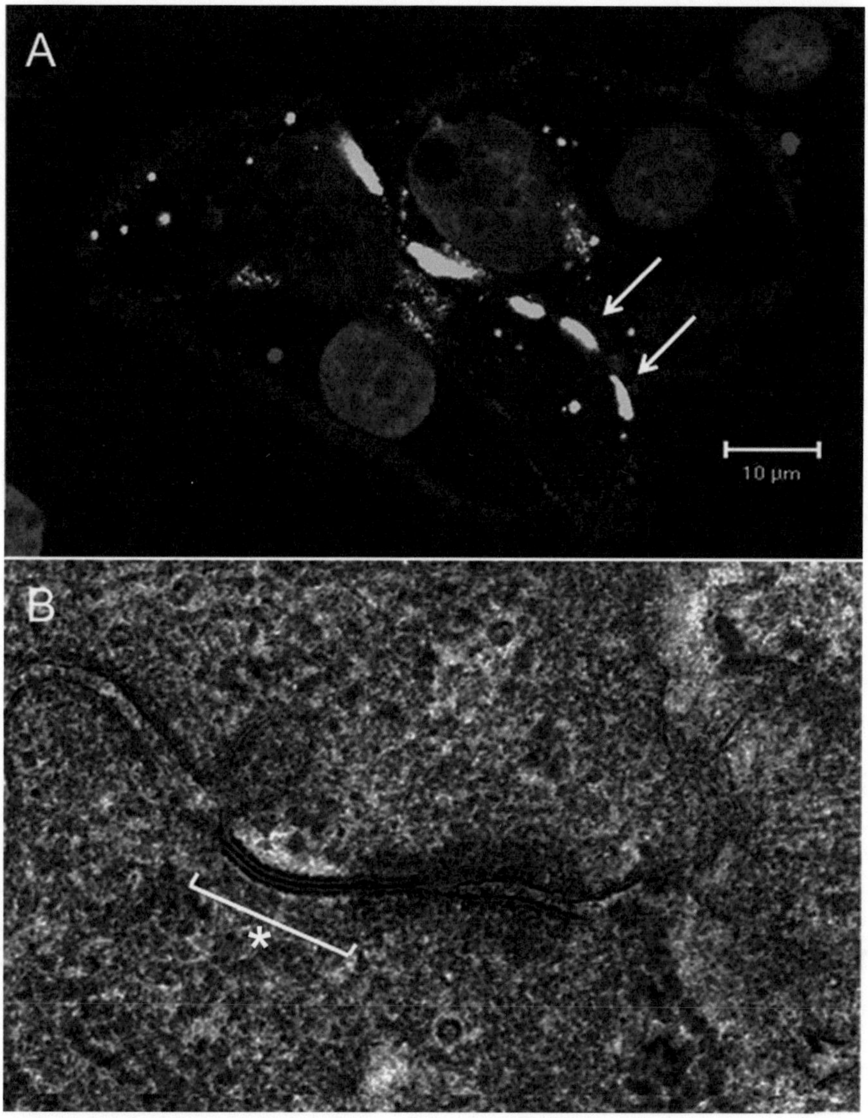


Fig. 2. Gap junctional channels clustered in plaques: A) laser scanning confocal microscopy image of Cx43/GFP-transfected HTC cells showing gap junctional plaques (arrows); B) transmission electron microphotography of gap junctional plaque (asterisk) (courtesy of Prof. Dr.Victor Arana-Chavez, FOUSP).

gap junction requires the appropriate cell-to-cell adhesion. There is evidence that interaction of Cx43 with the tight junction protein (ZO1) may play a role in regulating the size of the gap junction plaque (Hunter et al., 2003).

In general, the turnover rate of connexin is very fast in relation to other plasma membrane proteins. According to studies performed *in vivo* and *in vitro,* the half-lives of Cx26 and Cx32 are respectively 2 and 3 hours (Traub et al., 1983; 1987). The removal of gap junction from the plasma membrane occurs by endocytosis. During this process, both membranes of the gap junction are internalized into one of the adjacent cells and thereby form a double-membrane vacuole called annular gap junction. These structures are further degraded by both lysosomes and proteasomes. The preferential degradation pathway is associated to both cell and connexin type ( Laird et al., 2005; 2006). The degradation of Cx32 in the liver occurs mainly via the lysosomal pathway (Rahman et al., 1993). Furthermore the phosphorylation status of connexin is important to regulate its internalization and degradation. *In vitro* studies have been done to understand the mechanism involved in Cx43 internalization and degradation. They showed that the internalization and degradation of Cx43 gap junction is closely related to its hyperphosphorylation (via Mek/Erk pathway) and ubiquitination (Leithe and Rivedal, 2004).

## 3. Gap junctions and connexin expression in normal liver

The liver is composed of several cell types and consequently it expresses different connexin isoforms. Biliary cells, endothelial cells and oval cells (hepatic stem cells) express mainly Cx43. Hepatocytes express both Cx26 and/or Cx32 depending on the spatial localization in the hepatic lobule. For example, Cx32 is uniformly distributed throughout the liver and therefore it is expressed by hepatocytes in hepatic acinus, while Cx26 is preferentially expressed by hepatocytes localized in the periportal spaces. Thus, most non-parenchymal cells express Cx43 while hepatocytes express Cx26 or Cx32. Considering that hepatic cells establish cell-to-cell communication by channels consisted of different connexins it is not surprising that they present different permeability (permselectivity). It was demonstrated that Cx32 gap junctions had a 10-fold higher relative permeability to adenosine compared with Cx43 channels. By contrast, the phosphorylation status of the adenosine shifted its preferential selectivity from Cx32 channels towards those formed by Cx43. The Cx43 intercellular channels were eight times more permeable to AMP and ADP than Cx32 channels, and the permeability of ATP through Cx43 was more than 300-fold better than that through Cx32 channels. Thus biophysical properties of gap junctional channel depend on the type and phosphorylation status of the connexin that form the channel.

In normal conditions, adult liver display very low proliferative activity. However after injuries or partial hepatectomy, the remaining intact cells start to proliferate. During this proliferation stage, it was observed decreasing of Cx26 and Cx32 expression in hepatocytes. Similar situation was observed when hepatocytes from primary culture were stimulated by mitogen (Kojima et al., 1997). It is important to remember that during liver regeneration process there is not only cell proliferation of hepatocytes but also cell differentiation of oval cells into hepatocytes. Oval cells naturally express Cx43, however along the differentiation program this cell type switch the connexin isoform preferentially express from Cx43 to Cx32 and/or Cx26 (Zhang et al., 1994). Hepatocytes cultured *in vitro* commonly increase Cx43 expression with the concomitant decrease of Cx32 expression (Figure 3). Thus, the immortalized cell lines derived from liver express Cx43 instead of Cx32. Furthermore, hepatocarcinogenesis process leads the hepatocytes to express again Cx43, event that contributes to lose of the differentiated phenotype.

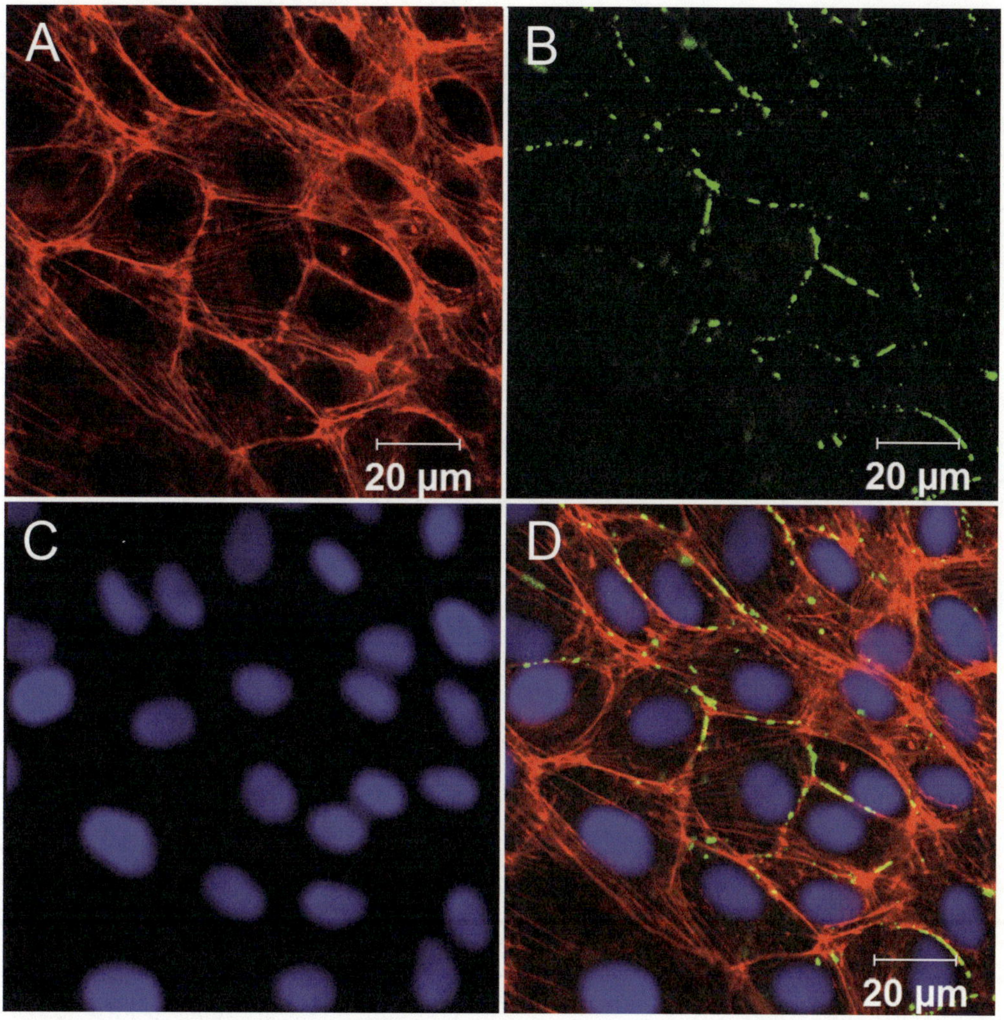


Fig. 3. Laser scanning confocal microscope images of BRL3A (Normal liver cells) submitted to immunofluorescence reaction with anti-connexin43 antibody: A) TRITC-phalloidin stained microfilaments; B) Cx43 is presented in the cytoplasm and gap junctions (green); C) nuclei in blue and D) merged channels .

Although the relationship between GJIC and cell proliferation is well established, its involvement in liver cell apoptosis is not fully understood. It was demonstrated that GJIC is induced in the early phases of apoptosis in serum-deprived rat WB-F344 liver epithelial cells parallel to the increased expression and phosphorylation of Cx43.

## 4. Modulation of connexin expression, subcellular localization and functional gap junction in HCC cells

Hepatocytes growing *in vitro* change their morphological features losing the liver-cell-specific functions. As early mentioned, the reversion of differentiated phenotype in hepatocytes growing *in vitro* is accompanied by changes in the expression profile of connexin. Under these new physiological conditions, the cells express mainly Cx43, the major isoform expressed by oval cells, instead of Cx32 or Cx26, isoforms typically expressed by hepatocytes.

Similar event occurs during malignant transformation and hepatocarcinoma cells rarely present mutation in connexin genes. Thus changes in connexin expression profile during hepatocarcinogenesis can be related to epigenetic events. For example, it was demonstrated that the reduction of Cx26 expression in hepatocarcinoma was consequence of its promoter hypermethylation. Furthermore, other events have been related to down regulation of Cx32 expression such as inappropriate phosphorylation pattern and aberrant subcellular localization in HCC cells.

Connexin phosphorylation status is very important and essential to regulate several events including intracellular trafficking, connexon assembly and disassembly, insertion in the plasma membrane, degradation and gating of gap junctional channels (Laird et al., 2005). The majority of connexins are phosphoproteins excepting the Cx26 and concerning phosphorylation process, the Cx43 has been widely studied since this molecule has different phosphorylation sites (21 serine and 2 tyrosine residues that are target of different kinase proteins) (Solan and Lamp, 2005). A number of phosphorylated Cx43 variants have been described with different patterns of electrophoretic mobility in sodium dodecyl sulfate-polyacrylamide gel. At least three forms have been described (P0, non-phosphorylated form; P1 phosphorylated form; and P2 hyper-phosphorylated form).

By comparing two rat derived cell lines, one derived from normal liver (BRL3A) and other from hepatocarcinoma (HTC), we could establish association of different phenotype with the phosphorylation pattern of Cx43. Normal liver cells grow in monolayer present contact inhibition and good cell communication capacity via gap junction channels formed by Cx43 (Figure 4 ). Meanwhile, hepatocarcinoma cell line represents a liver tumor cell line poorly differentiated that grows overlapping, and does not present functional GJIC despite expressing Cx43 (Figure 5). This difference in cell communication capacity is assumed to be due to phosphorylation status of Cx43 and its consequent intracellular localization. The major Cx43 form found in normal cells was the non-phosphorylated (P0) that was correctly inserted in plasma membrane and formed functional GJ. Meanwhile, in hepatocarcinoma cells it was observed predominantly the phosphorylated form of Cx43 (P1) which was concentrated in cytoplasm, unable to form functional gap junction in plasma membrane. These results point out to the importance of phosphorylation status of Cx43 to define its membrane insertion (Ionta et al, 2009).

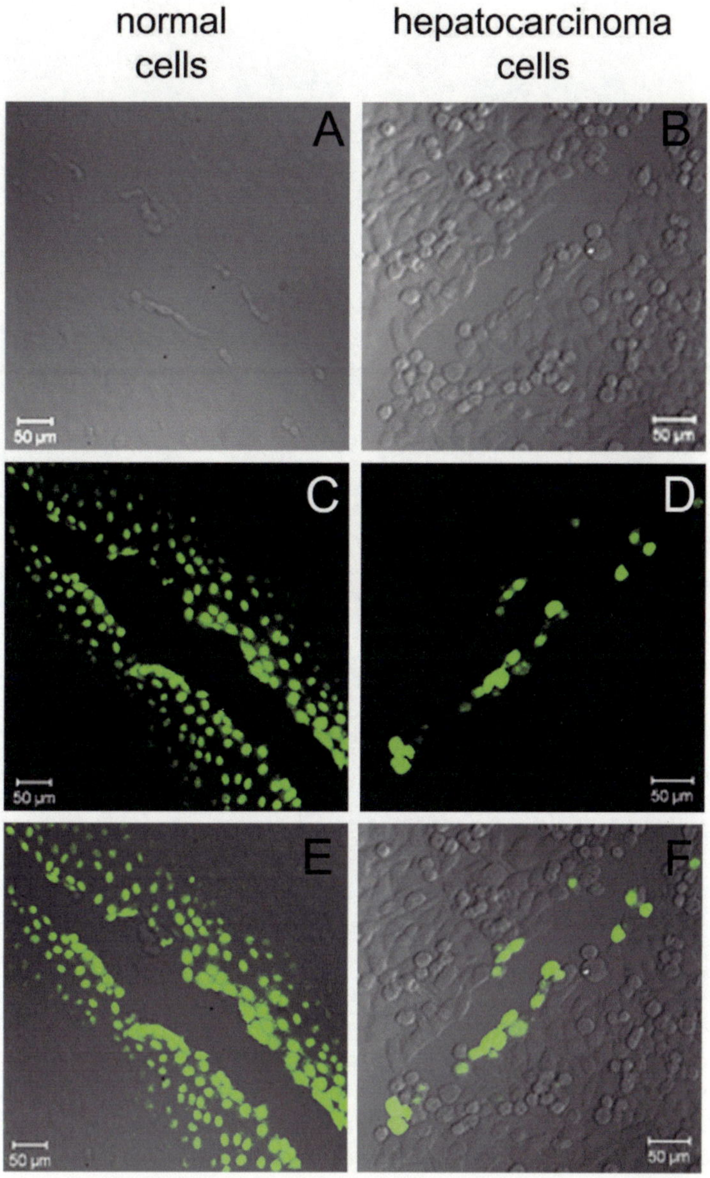


Fig. 4. Scrape loading/dye transfer* assay performed in BRL3A (A, C and E) and HTC cells and HTC cells (B, D and F).Differential interference contrast microscopy images in A and B, fluorescent images in C and D, and merge in E and F. BRL3A presented good communication capacity because it possible to observe at least 5 rows of fluorescent cells from scrape. HTC cells was deficient in GJIC, the fluorescent cells were visualized only in areas near to scrape.

*Scrape loading and dye transfer (SL/DT) is a functional assay widely used to evaluate the level of the intercellular communication and it is based in the introduction of the non-permeable fluorescent dye (Lucifer Yellow, MW= 457,2) into cells of monolayer culture through a transient cut in the cell membrane. Lucifer Yellow does not diffuse through intact membrane but it is transferred into adjacent cells via GJ in competent cells. The transference is monitored with fluorescence microscopy.

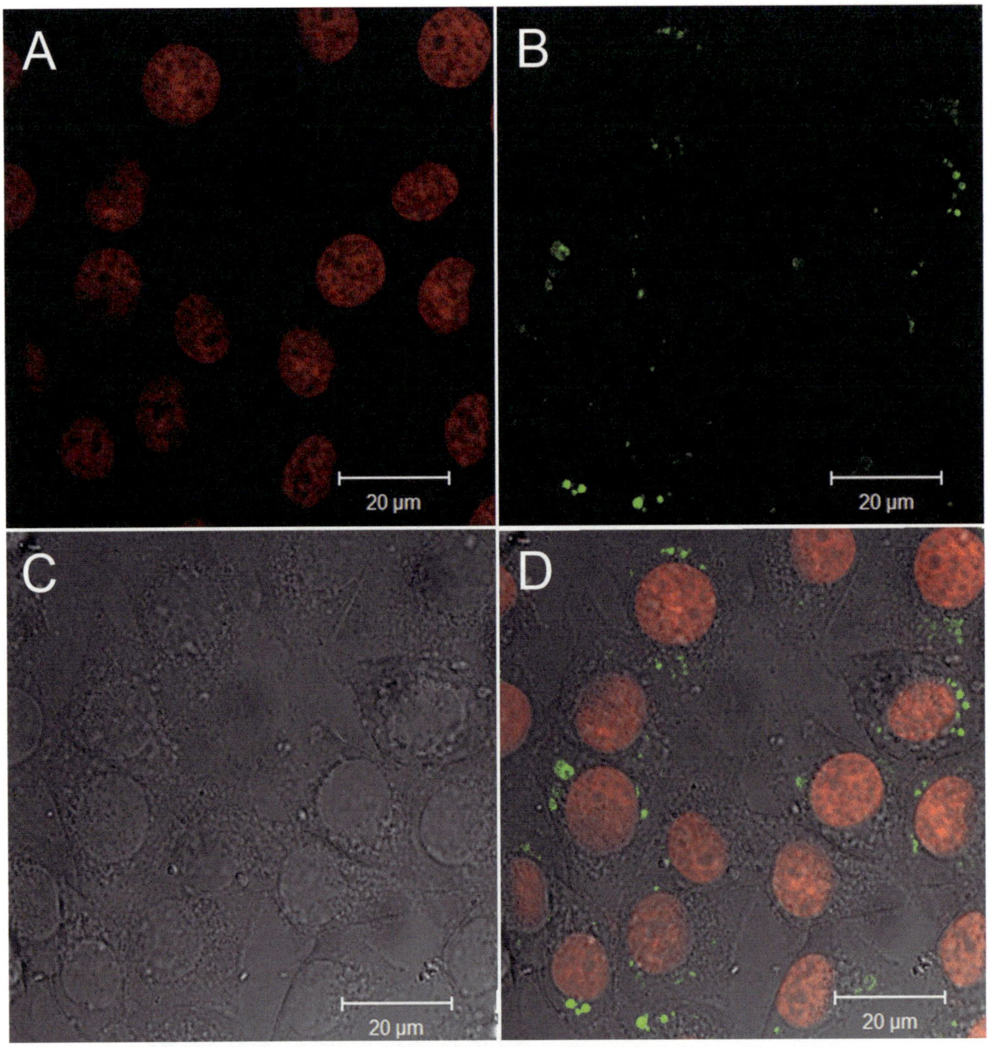


Fig. 5. Laser scanning confocal microscope images of HTC cells submitted to immunofluorescence reaction with anti-connexin43 antibody: A) Nuclei stained with propidium iodide (red); B) Cx43 is presented in the cytoplasm (green); C) differential interference contrast microscopy and D) merged channels.

## 5. Non-channel functions of connexin and tumor suppressor genes

The deficiency or absence of functional GJIC observed in most of solid tumors led Loewenstein (1979) to propose that the GJ would have a role in controlling cell proliferation. At first this function was associated with the functionality of the channels. There was then an effort to identify if GJIC deficiency was related to a specific stage of chemical carcinogenesis.

The assay performed in well established models permitted to demonstrate the tumor promoter's ability in inhibiting the GJIC. Changes in connexin isoform expressed were shown in models of chemical carcinogenesis with compounds that induce liver tumors, such as pesticides and phenobarbital. In some cases it was observed the induction of Cx43 expression, connexin isoform usually not expressed by hepatocytes. The molecular mechanism of this process is not well understood, but alterations in the expression and function of connexin are now consistently associated with the hyperproliferative response. In the earlier 1990s, connexin genes have been proposed as tumor suppressor. This idea was reinforced by experimental data that related functional GJ restoration with exogenous Cx expression. *In vivo* studies clearly showed the relevance of Cx32 in maintenance of hepatic tissue normality and in the prevention of hepatocarcinogenesis (Temme et al., 1997).

Although it is not established if there is specific connexin isoforms acting as tumor suppressor in each histological type of cancer, there are some data linking Cx43 and CX32 to liver cancer. Eghbali et al (1991) transfected Cx32 in Sk-Hep1 cells and did not observe growth inhibition *in vitro*, although they detected lower tumorigenic capacity of these cells when they were injected in animals, compared with non-transfected. Sk-Hep1cell line was established from ascitic fluid of a patient with liver hepatocellular carcinoma but it is, in fact, of endothelial origin according morphological, biochemical and immunological markers. Overexpression of Cx32 reverted to normal the transformed phenotype of a rat liver cell line deficient in GJIC derived from a GJIC-competent parental cell line (WB-344).

We studied the effect of exogenous Cx43 expression in rat hepatocarcinoma cell line (HTC) and observed that transfected cells (HTC-Cx43) presented lower proliferation rate than non-transfect cells. The Cx43 was observed forming clusters at plasma membrane in transfected cells in opposition to non-transfected cells that presented Cx43 mainly localized in cytoplasm. Exogenous Cx43 expression induced morphological changes which were compatible with differentiated phenotype. Despite of Cx43 expressed by HTC-Cx43 cells do reach plasma membrane and form cluster there was not GJIC restoration. Therefore, the exogenous Cx43 expression induced a GJ-independent down-regulation in cell proliferation of HTC cell line. We attributed this effect to changes in phosphorylation pattern of Cx43 which was essential to its delivery to plasma membrane. Cx43 expression profile of HTC-Cx43 cells exhibited P1 band intensity similar to HTC cells, P0 and P2 more intense than HTC cells. All together, the data indicate that the exogenous Cx43 was critical for decreasing growth rate in rat hepatocellular carcinoma cells and contributed to reversion of the transformed phenotype. These events were independent of the functional GJIC restoration (Ionta et al, 2009).

Connexin are able to interact direct or indirectly with several molecules related to the regulation of cell proliferation and cellular compounds such as cytoskeleton elements. These interactions were demonstrated by immunofluorescence or co-precipitation studies, approaches that do not distinguish if the interaction is direct or indirect. In fact, the action of connexin as single proteins would affect the production or activity of cell growth regulators, including p27Kip1, cyclin A, cyclin D1, cyclin D2, cdk5, cdk6, ERK1/2, signal transducer and activator of transcription protein 3, Src, human EGF receptor 2, FGF1 and FGF receptor 3 (review in Vinken et al , 2011). Cx43 seems to have a role in cellular migration by interacting with actin through the zonula occludens. On the contrary of connexin overexpression experiments, these data were observed in an RNA interference knockdown screen. Interactions between Cx43 and ZO-1 or ZO-2, both zonula occludens proteins, were demonstrated in several studies. They bind to the same region of Cx43 in a cell cycle dynamic process, so Cx43-ZO-1 interaction occurs mainly in G0 and while Cx43-ZO-2 in G0 and S phases.

A different kind of interaction with actin seems to occur in HTC-Cx43/GFP cells treated with geodiamolides, natural peptides from marine sponge usually involved with microfilament disruption. We observed that low geodiamolides concentration for short time (2 or 4 hours) treatment did not alter the organization of actin filaments but induces larger GJ plaques (Rangel et al., 2010). The effect could be related to the stabilization of GJ plaques due to both (i) improvement in the connexon exportation or (ii) inhibition of the degradation pathway. To uncouple events leading to GJ assembly from those related to GJ removal, HTC-CX43/GFP cells were treated with geodiamolides in combination or not with fungal antibiotic BrefeldinA, a drug that disrupts the Golgi and protein trafficking to plasma membrane. BrefeldinA drastically reduced the GJ plaques formation, and the same response was obtained when the cells were treated with BrefeldinA and geodiamolides simultaneously. These data indicate that the peptide affects mainly the delivery pathway of Cx43 protein, suggesting that geodiamolide increases the length of GJ plaques mainly because it improves the delivery pathway of Cx43 protein.

## 6. Acknowledgments

Supported by CNPq, Brazil.

## 7. Conclusion

Disruption of GJIC is closed associated to hepatocarcinogenesis process despite of hepatocarcinoma cells rarely present mutation in connexin genes. Epigenetic events can be involved with to lose functional GJ. Change in connexin expression profile (from Cx32 to Cx43) is frequently observed in liver tumor cells. Abnormal localization of connexin (cytoplasmatic instead plasma membrane) also is characteristic de tumor cells. Thus, many studies were employed in the past to verify if connexin could be target of therapeutic approaches. The studies about connexin biosynthesis, traffic, docking at plasma membrane and degradation were very important to understand as functional channels are formed as well as the possible protein partners related with delivery and removal of connexin at plasma membrane. The phosphorylation status of connexin is very critical in relation this issue, likewise the participation of many proteins (signaling pathways, cytoskeleton and cell-to-cell adhesion). The attention for connexins was reinforced when it was observed that functional GJIC was restored in tumor cells by forced expression of connexin. Fortunately along of time a lot of information were collected and today we know that connexins exert tumor suppressor activity on hepatocarcinoma cells dependent and independent-functional GJIC. So, in the future it is possible that connexin will be used as therapeutic target for hepatocarcinoma.

## 8. References

Eghbali B, Kessler JA, Reid LM, Roy C, Spray DC.Involvement of gap junctions in tumorigenesis: transfection of tumor cells with connexin 32 cDNA retards growth in vivo.Proc Natl Acad Sci USA 1;88(23):10701-5, 1991.

Hunter, A.W., J. Jourdan, R.G. Gourdie, Fusion of GFP to the carboxyl terminus of connexin43 increases gap junction size in HeLa cells, Cell Adhes Commun 10, 211 - 214, 2003.

Ionta, M, Ferreira RA, Pfister SC, Machado-Santelli. Exogenous Cx43 expression decrease cell proliferation rate in rat hepatocarcinoma cells independently of functional gap junction. Cancer cell Int, Aug;13;9:22, 2009.

Kojima T, Mochizuki C, Mitaka T, Mochizuki Y. Effects of melatonin on proliferation, oxidative stress and Cx32 gap junction protein expression in primary cultures of adult rat hepatocytes. Cell Struct Funct.22(3):347-56, 1997.

Laird DW. Connexin phosphorylation as a regulatory event linked to gap junction internalization and degradation. Biochim Biophys Acta, 1711:172-182, 2005.

Laird DW. Life cycle of connexins in health and disease. Biochem J 394:527–43, 2006.

Leithe E, Rivedal E.. Epidermal growth factor regulates ubiquitination, internalization and proteasome-dependent degradation of connexin43. J Cell Sci. 117(Pt 7):1211-20, 2004.

Loewestein WR. Junctional intercellular communication and the control of growth. Bioch Biophys Acta. 560:1-65, 1979.

Martin PE, Blundell G, Ahmad S, Errington RJ, Evans WH. Multiple pathways in the trafficking and assembly of connexin 26, 32 and 43 into gap junction intercellular communication channels. J Cell Sci 114: 3845-3855, 2001.

Meşe G, Richard G, White TW.Gap junctions: basic structure and function. J Invest Dermatol. 127(11):2516-24, 2007.

Musil LS, Goodenough DA. Multisubunit assembly of an integral plasma membrane channel protein, gap junction connexin43, occurs after exit from the ER. Cell 74:1065–77, 1993.

Rahman S, Carlile G, Evans WH. Assembly of hepatic gap junctions. Topography and distribution of connexin 32 in intracellular and plasma membranes determined using sequence-specific antibodies. J Biol Chem 268:1260-1265, 1993.

Rangel M, Ionta M, Pfister SC, Sant'Anna Ferreira RA and Machado-Santelli GM. Marine sponge depsipeptide increases gap junction length in HTC cells transfected with Cx43-GFP . Cell Biol Intern Rep, e0003, 2010.

Solan JL, Lampe PD.Connexin phosphorylation as a regulatory event linked to gap junction channel assembly. Biochim Biophys Acta, 10;1711(2):154-63, 2005.

Temme A, Buchmann A, Gabriel HD, Nelles E, Schwarz M, Willecke K . High incidence of spontaneous and chemically induced liver tumors in mice deficient for connexin32.Curr Biol.7(9):713-6, 1997.

Traub O, Druge PM, Willecke K. Degradation and resynthesis of gap junction protein in plasma membranes of regenerating liver after partial hepatectomy or cholestasis. Proc Natl Acad Sci U S A 80:755-759, 1983.

Traub O, Look J, Paul D, Willecke K. Cyclic adenosine monophosphate stimulates biosynthesis and phosphorylation of the 26 kDa gap junction protein in cultured mouse hepatocytes. Eur J Cell Biol43:48-54, 1987.

Vinken M, Decrock E, Leybaert L, Bultynck G, Himpens B, Vanhaecke T, Rogiers V. Non-channel functions of connexins in cell growth and cell death. Biochim Biophys Acta. 2011 (on line).

Zhang M, Thorgeirsson SS. Modulation of Connexins during Differentiation of Oval Cell into Hepatocytes. Exp Cell Res 213:37-42, 1994.

# 14

# Mechanisms of HBx Mediated Liver Cancer: Multiple Pathways and Opportunities

Mark A. Feitelson et al.*
*Department of Biology, Temple University, Philadelphia, PA USA*

## 1. Introduction

Chronic hepatitis B virus (HBV) infection is associated with a high risk for the development of chronic liver diseases (CLDs) which include hepatitis, cirrhosis and hepatocellular carcinoma (HCC). HCC is among the top five most prevalent tumor types worldwide, has few effective treatment options, and is highly lethal. The pathogenesis of CLD and HCC is immune mediated, and the virus has developed a number of defense mechanisms that essentially prevent infected cells from being effectively eliminated by the immune system. This, in part, involves the sustained, high level expression of the virus encoded protein, hepatitis B x antigen (HBx). Recent work has shown that HBx blocks pathways of innate immunity (Kumar et al., 2011; Wei et al., 2010), thereby blunting the development of adaptive immunity that is central to virus elimination. In addition, HBx inhibits immune mediated apoptosis by multiple pathways, including those mediated by Fas and tumor necrosis factor alpha (TNFα). In this context, HBx has been shown to up-regulate TNFα expression (Lara-Pezzi et al., 1998), which is thought to kill uninfected hepatocytes more readily than infected cells, thereby promoting expansion of the virus within the liver, since virus infected hepatocytes would preferentially regenerate following a bout of chronic hepatitis. HBx also switches the growth signals mediated by elevated transforming growth factor beta 1 (TGFβ1) from that of negative growth regulation to that of positive growth regulation. TGFβ1 is a transcriptional target of HBx (Yoo et al., 1996), suggesting that HBx expression in the liver promotes fibrogenesis and the development of cirrhosis. Within the infected hepatocyte, HBx blocks the action of tumor suppressors, such as p53 and Rb (Feitelson et al., 2008), and up-regulates the expression of selected host genes that strongly promote hepatocarcinogenesis even in the absence of HBx (see below). Recent work has also

---

* Alla Arzumanyan[1], Tiffany Friedman[1], N. Lale Tufan[2], Zhaorui Lian[1], Marcia M. Clayton[1], Joyce Kang[3], Helena M. G. P. V. Reis[4], Jingbo Pan[5], Jie Liu[6], Patrick Arbuthnot[7] and Michael Kew[7]
[1]*Department of Biology, Temple University, Philadelphia, PA, USA*
[2]*Department of Medical Biology, Pamukkale University School of Medicine, Kinikli Denizli, Turkey*
[3]*Division of Medical Microbiology, Guiyang Medical College, Guizhou Province, People's Republic of China*
[4]*MIT Portugal Program, Av. Antonio Jose de Almeida, Lisboa, Portugal*
[5]*Department of Pathology, Anatomy and Cell Biology, Thomas Jefferson University, Philadelphia, PA, USA*
[6]*Department of Digestive Diseases of Huashan Hospital, Fudan University, Shanghai, P. R. China*
[7]*Molecular Hepatology Research Unit, Department of Medicine, University of the Witwatersrand, Johannesburg, South Africa*

shown that HBx promotes phenotypic changes in hepatocytes characteristic of epithelial-to-mesenchymal transition (EMT). One of the molecular hallmarks of EMT, down-regulated expression of the cell adhesion molecule, E-cadherin, is blocked by sustained HBx expression via several mechanisms (Feitelson et al., 2009). HBx also overrides immune mediated apoptotic signals by constitutively activating key signaling pathways, such as nuclear factor kappa B (NF-κB), which is known to be hepatoprotective (Beg et al., 1995, 1996), and phosphatidylinositol 3-kinase (PI3K)/Akt, which is known to promote growth in many tumor types (Chung et al., 2004). The finding that HBx stabilizes β-catenin by a variety of mechanisms, and up-regulates ErbB2 (Liu et al., 2009), further underscores the importance of these actions in maintaining hepatocellular growth and survival required for virus propagation during the many years and decades that span chronic infection. Unfortunately, these same pathways are also those that contribute centrally to the development of HCC. This body of work provides many opportunities for the development of diagnostic markers that form a fingerprint of those chronically infected patients who are most likely to go on and develop HCC. These markers will serve as therapeutic targets for the repositioning of known drugs for this new indication, and/or the discovery of new drugs that will target rate limiting pathways during multi-step carcinogenesis. In doing so, this work proposes that the chemoprevention of cancer, instead of the treatment of tumor bearing patients, is worth pursuing, and could likely reduce or eliminate the morbidity and mortality associated with chronic HBV infection long before tumors appear. This represents an important challenge, since the knowledge gained will identify cause and effect relationships important for the identification of definitive biomarkers and pharmacological targets that participate decisively in tumorigenesis.

## 2. Relationship between HBx expression and the pathogenesis of CLD and (HCC): A model

HBx is one of four genes expressed by HBV during infection, and is known to have gene regulatory functions. Truncated envelope polypeptides that appear during chronic infection may also regulate gene expression and contribute to the pathogenesis of CLD and liver cancer (Chen et al., 2006; Lauer et al., 1992), but their contributions are less well characterized. HBx has been defined as a *trans*-activating protein that promotes virus gene expression and replication during infection (Belloni et al., 2009; Spandau & Lee, 1988; Tsuge et al., 2010). Experimental infection of newborn woodchucks with the related woodchuck hepatitis virus (WHV) results in the development of carriers in nearly 100% of cases, and most of these go on to develop severe chronic hepatitis and HCC (Tennant & Gerin, 2001). However, infection of neonatal woodchucks with an X protein negative clone of WHV failed to establish the chronic carrier state (Chen et al., 1993; Zoulim et al., 1994). This suggests that X protein promotes viremia. The impact of X protein on virus gene expression and replication is also supported by considerable *in vitro* data (Benhenda et al., 2009; Keasler et al., 2009; Tsuge et al., 2010). During the course of CLD, bouts of hepatitis are associated with hepatocellular destruction and regeneration. Among infected cells, the X open reading frame (ORF), which is at the end of the virus genome, becomes repeatedly integrated into host DNA at the replication forks that exist in host DNA during regeneration. This suggests that the intracellular levels of HBx increase with the severity and progression of CLD, and there is now considerable experimental evidence to support this hypothesis (Feitelson et al., 1993a; Jin et al, 2001; Wang et al., 1991a, 1991b). In fact, the highest levels of HBx expression have been observed in cirrhotic nodules (Wang et al., 1991a, 1991b). As indicated above, HBx *trans*-activates HBV enhancers and promoters, thereby promoting long term virus replication. However, it is proposed that when the levels of intracellular HBx increase with time among patients with CLD, it *trans*-regulates the expression of many cellular genes as well (Balsano et al., 1994; Twu & Schloemer, 1987) by a variety of mechanisms. It is postulated that these changes in cellular gene expression help to make cells more permissive to continued virus replication, but also protect the cells from immune responses aimed at removal of infected hepatocytes. This is accomplished by triggering EMT (Du et al., 2010; Yang et al., 2009), by promoting up-regulated expression of selected oncogene associated pathways, and by turning off tumor suppressor, senescence and apoptotic pathways (Kew, 2011; Oishi et al., 2007; Park et al., 2011; Xu et al., 2010) that are often activated by immune responses against virus infected cells. The fact that HBx promotes cell cycle progression and cell growth (Feitelson et al., 2005), means that when this happens in normal hepatocytes, negative growth regulatory (senescence and tumor suppressor) pathways are triggered to reestablish homeostasis. The latter may underlie the putative "proapoptotic" properties of HBx observed in cell lines and *in vivo*, even though there is a considerable literature showing that HBx is also "anti-apoptotic" (Assrir et al., 2010). In this model, it is proposed that apoptosis is a cellular response to inappropriate growth stimulatory signals in the liver mediated by HBx during chronic infection and not due to an inherent property of HBx. Although there is considerable literature suggesting that HBx inhibits several DNA repair systems (e.g., Cheng et al., 2010; Martin-Lluesma et al., 2008; Mathonnet et al., 2004; Qadri et al, 2011), which would promote the development of mutations in the liver prior to the appearance of tumors, it appears that a major contribution of HBx to the pathogenesis of CLD is epigenetic. This is because many natural effectors of HBx correlate with HBx expression in chronically infected human livers and because mutations are not widespread in preneoplastic hepatocytes (Feitelson et al., 2002). The finding that HBx and its natural effectors (target genes) correlate in nontumor liver, but are mostly absent from adjacent tumor tissues, suggests that HBx and its target genes drive pathogenesis prior to the appearance of tumor, but are no longer rate limiting once tumors appear. In the latter case, it is proposed that epigenetic mechanisms mediated by HBx are replaced by genetic mechanisms that are independent of HBx. If so, then HBx may play a predominant role in the pathogenesis of CLD, but a more modest role in tumor progression.

## 3. Natural targets of HBx

Early work characterized HBx as a *trans*-regulatory protein that was initially shown to up-regulate the expression of almost every target gene that was evaluated using mostly reporter gene assays in transient transfected cell lines (Rossner, 1992). It seemed that in order to better understand what HBx was doing *in vivo*, the natural effectors and targets of HBx in the infected liver had to be identified and characterized. HBx targets that were up- or down-regulated were identified by microarray analysis, miRNA arrays, chromatin immunoprecipitation, and by other techniques (e.g., Hu et al., 2006; Sung et al., 2009; Wu et al., 2001, 2002). Some of the targets include telomerase (Liu et al, 2010), the ras pathway signaling molecule, RASSF1A (Yang, et al, 2010), the metastasis associated protein, MTA (Bui-Nguyen et al, 2010), β-catenin (Lian et al., 2006; Pan et al., 2007), E-cadherin (Liu et al., 2006), c-myc (Wu et al., 2001), and DNA methyltransferase 1 (Zheng et al., 2009). HBx is a protein binding protein that also regulates gene expression by activating a number of signal transduction pathways in the cytoplasm (e.g., NF-κB, PI3K/Akt, JAK/STAT, PKC, AP-1, ras, src, Wnt and others) (Feitelson & Duan, 1997; Henkler & Koshy, 1996; Kew, 2011). Constitutive activation of these signaling pathways has been identified with up-regulated expression of specific target genes. For example, HBx mediated activation of the mitogen-activated protein kinase (MAPK) pathway has been shown to up-regulate the expression of hypoxia-inducible factor-1 alpha (HIF-1α) (Yoo et al., 2003), which promotes the survival of hepatocytes in cirrhotic nodules, where a hypoxic environment is known to exist during CLD. Further, HBx mediated constitutive activation of Wnt signaling is associated with up-regulated expression of c-myc and cyclin-D1, both of which promote hepatocellular growth. In the nucleus, HBx interacts with the basal transcription machinery (Haviv, et al., 1995, 1996), binds to the transcriptional scaffolds CBP/p300 (Cougot et al., 2007) and mSin3a (Arzumanyan et al., 2011), and alters the extent of DNA methylation and histone acetylation (Zheng et al., 2009). Further, there is increasing evidence that HBx alters the expression of host gene expression by up- or down-regulating selected miRNAs (Kong et al., 2011; Wu, et al., 2011). In many cases, the natural targets of these epigenetic changes have not been identified. The importance of doing so will provide both prognostic markers and therapeutic targets relevant to the pathogenesis of CLD and HCC, thus providing opportunities for earlier intervention.

### 3.1 HBx and fibrogenesis

#### 3.1.1 Transforming growth factor beta 1 (TGFβ1)

The close association between intrahepatic expression of HBx and the severity of CLD suggests that HBx may take a part in driving pathogenesis. TGFβ1 is an important mediator of fibrosis and apoptosis in carriers with CLD (Castilla et al., 1991; Liu et al., 1999), as indicated by the direct correlation between serum TGFβ1 levels, elevated aminotransferases, and fibrosis scored in liver biopsy specimens (Flisiak et al., 2004). HBx has been shown to transcriptionally up-regulate the expression of TGFβ1 both in cell cultures and in HBx transgenic mice (Martin-Vilchez et al., 2008; Norton et al., 2004; Yoo et al., 1996). In liver tissue with HBx protein expression, phospho-Smad2 was detectable, suggesting a functional link between viral protein expression and TGF-β1 signaling. Phospho-Smad2 staining correlated significantly with fibrotic stage in patients with HBV infection and steatosis/steatohepatitis (Weng et al., 2009). HBx mediated up-regulation of TGFβ1 was further potentiated by suppressed expression of the natural inhibitor of TGFβ1, alpha-2-macroglobulin (α2M, Figure 1) (Pan et al., 2004). HBx may suppress α2M gene expression by either activation of NF-κB, which then blocks the activation of the α2M gene by STAT3, and/or by the HBx activation of PI3K, which then blocks α2M expression. Independent work showed that HBx also shifted TGFβ1 signaling from tumor suppression to tumor promotion in the livers of patients with chronic hepatitis B, and that this involved differential phosphorylation of smad3 *in vivo* (Murata et al., 2009). HBx was also shown to enhance TGFβ signaling by stabilizing a protein complex consisting of smad4 and components of the basic transcriptional machinery (Lee et al., 2001). The fact that HBx stimulates multiple signal transduction pathways (e.g., NF-κB, PI3K, MAPK, Wnt, ras, src, etc), combined with altered smad signaling, also appear to override the homeostatic and growth inhibitory properties of TGFβ1. This results in the development of a strong profibrogenic environment in the liver (Akhurst, 2002) which may underlie the close relationship between HBx, inflammation, and fibrogenesis seen in earlier studies (Wang et al., 1991a, 1991b). In this context, hepatic inflammation, fibrosis and cell death were demonstrated in TGFβ1 transgenic mice (Sanderson et al., 1995), underscoring the contribution of elevated TGFβ1 expression to CLD. Interestingly, HBx also blocks TGFβ1 mediated growth inhibition and apoptosis, in part, through the up-regulation of PI3K (Shih et al., 2000), suggesting that HBx may confer resistance to TGFβ1 mediated growth inhibition, while uninfected cells remain sensitive, thereby favoring survival of virus infected hepatocytes. These observations are consistent with the strong correlation between HBx staining and the progression of CLD among HBV infected carriers (Jin et al, 2001; Wang et al., 1991a, 1991b).

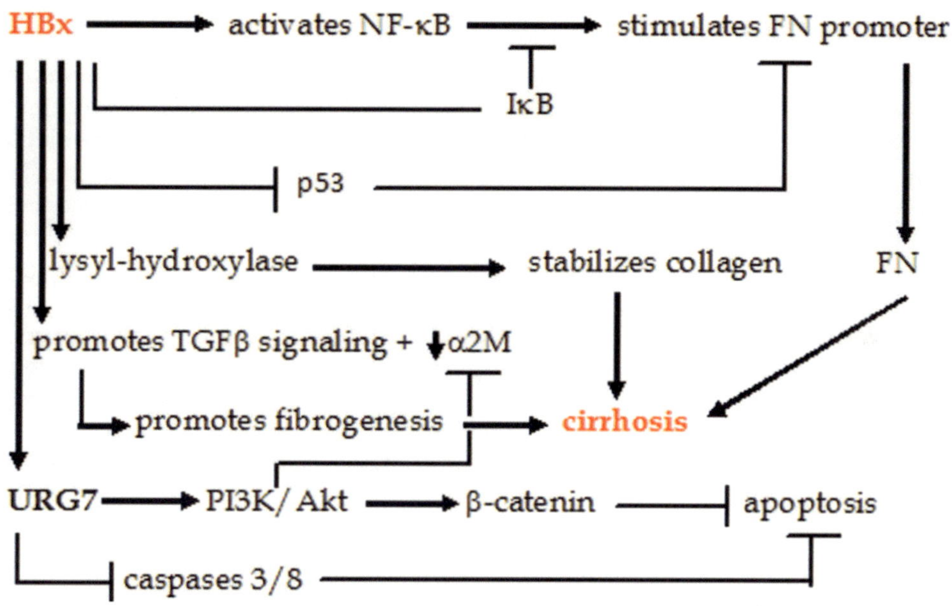


Fig. 1. Proposed model of how HBx may contribute to the development of cirrhosis. See the text for details.

### 3.1.2 Fibronectin (FN)

This close relationship is exemplified by the observations that HBx activation of NF-κB resulted in the stimulation of the fibronectin (FN) promoter (Figure 1), and that liver tissue samples from chronically infected patients showed a strong correlation between HBx and FN mRNA in hepatocytes from fibrotic and cirrhotic livers (Norton et al., 2004). In this context, the fact that HBx binds to and inactivates the tumor suppressor protein, p53, both *in vitro* and *in vivo* (Feitelson et al., 1993b; Ueda et al., 1995), and that p53 normally suppresses the FN promoter, suggest that inactivation of p53 also results in increased FN production. Interestingly, up-regulation of FN in HBx expressing cells also showed a modest (50%) decrease in adherence to FN (Lara-Pezzi et al., 2001a, 2001b) and depressed expression of the FN receptor, α5β1 integrin. There was also an observed decrease in the levels of collagen/laminin receptor α1 subunit in HBx positive compared to negative cells

(Lara-Pezzi et al., 2001a), suggesting that HBx promotes the detachment of infected cells from the extracellular matrix (ECM). This detachment was associated with increased cell migration, indicating that changes in the ECM-cell relationship probably also contributed to alterations in tissue morphology that accompany the development of cirrhosis. Since activated ras and src signaling depress $\alpha5\beta1$ expression (Varner et al., 1995), that HBx stimulates ras and src signaling (Klein & Schneider, 1997), and that HBx disrupts adherens junctions in a src dependent manner (Lara-Pezzi et al., 2001b), it is likely that the activation of these signaling pathways by HBx contribute importantly to decreased integrin expression, decreased cell adhesion, and an increased propensity for cell migration and loss of tissue morphology in the infected liver, and to metastasis in already established tumors.

### 3.1.3 Lysyl hydroxylase (LH3)

As indicated above, the accumulation and remodeling of ECM is central to the development of fibrosis and cirrhosis. In this context, the finding that HBx up-regulates the expression of the enzyme, lysyl hydroxylase 3 (LH3) in liver cells, and that LH3 co-stains with HBx in livers of HBV infected patients (unpublished observations), suggests another mechanism whereby an HBx target gene may contribute to fibrosis (Figure 1). LH3 mediates the chemical cross-linking of several collagen and collagen-like molecules (Myullyla et al., 2007). This may promote stabilization of the ECM during chronic infection. Given that LH3 knockout mice with disrupted formation of basement membranes during embryogenesis resulted in embryonic lethality (Myullyla et al., 2007), the over-expression of LH3 during chronic HBV infection may promote the development and persistence of basement membranes that are characteristic of fibrosis. This would sever the intimate relationship between hepatocytes and the bloodstream observed in normal livers. Although LH3 is associated with the endoplasmic reticulum, it has also been found in the extracellular space and in serum (Salo et al., 2006), implying that LH3 serum levels may be elevated in the blood prior to the development of HCC.

### 3.1.4 Does HBx activate stellate cells?

It is also possible that HBx expression promotes stellate cell activation. Although there is little evidence that HBV infects stellate cells, when HBx was transfected into a human stellate cell line, it promoted proliferation and up-regulated expression of fibrosis related molecules (Guo et al., 2009). Independent work showed that HBx expressing hepatocytes induced paracrine activation of human and rat hepatic stellate cells. When these cells were exposed to conditioned medium from HBx-expressing hepatocytes, they showed increased expression of collagen I, connective tissue growth factor, alpha smooth muscle actin, matrix metalloproteinase-2, and TGF$\beta$, together with an enhanced proliferation rate (Martin-Vilchez et al., 2008). More recently, hedgehog signaling and ligand production have been demonstrated to be activated in clinical samples from HBV (and hepatitis C virus) infected patients These ligands promoted the *in vitro* expansion of liver myofibroblasts, activated endothelial cells, and progenitors expressing markers of tumor stem/initiating cells (Pereira et al., 2010). Independent data has shown that hedgehog signaling is profibrogenic, in that it promotes activation and EMT in quiescent hepatic stellate cells (Choi et al., 2009), and in the context of cholestatic liver injury (Omenetti et al., 2011). Given that hedgehog signaling is also known to promote tissue remodeling in the liver (Omenetti & Diehl, 2008), it is possible that this may contribute to the progression and formation of cirrhotic nodules in the liver of chronically infected patients. Preliminary data also suggests that HBx activates hedgehog signaling in liver cancer cells (Kim et al., 2011), although the role of this activation in hepatocarcinogenesis remains to be studied. Further, it is not clear whether the up-regulation of hedgehog ligands is activated by HBx, and whether this in some way contributes to fibrogenesis.

### 3.2 HBx up-regulated genes in chronically infected liver

#### 3.2.1 Up-regulated gene, clone 7 (URG7)

Subtractive hybridization of mRNAs from HBx positive compared to negative human hepatoblastoma (HepG2) cells yielded a set of differentially expressed mRNAs that revealed additional mechanisms whereby HBx contributes to the pathogenesis of HCC. Several unique mRNAs were identified by subtractive hybridization, and among them were a number of previously uncharacterized transcripts. One of them, URG7, encoded a 99 amino acid polypeptide with no distinguishing functional motifs (Lian et al., 2001), was found to down-regulate the expression of the TGFβ1 inhibitor, α2M (Figure 1), suggesting that it contributes to the development and progression of fibrosis. It appears to do so by activation of PI3K, by stabilization of β-catenin, and by blocking the activities of caspase 8 and 3 (Pan et al., 2007) (Figures 1 and 2). Among its many activities, HBx also activates PI3K (Lee et al., 2001), stabilizes β-catenin (Lian et al., 2006), and blocks caspase 3 (Gottlob et al., 1998), suggesting that these functions may be carried out by URG7. Further data showed that both HBx and URG7 activated fragments of the β-catenin promoter, and also promoted expression of β-catenin target genes. These include c-myc (Terradillos et al., 1997), multi-drug resistance gene 1 (MDR1) (Doong et al., 1998) and cyclin D1 (Park et al., 2006). While the activation of β-catenin target genes by URG7 suggests that the latter promotes tumor formation, URG7 did not promote growth of HepG2 cells in soft agar, nor did it accelerate the outgrowth of HepG2 based tumors in SCID mice (Lian et al., 2001). Its role in blocking apoptosis, however, is shared with that of β-catenin (Chen et al., 2001). Importantly, one of the major characteristics of tumor cells is resistance to immune mediated apoptosis. The finding that URG7 is over-expressed in infected liver, but not in HCC cells from clinical specimens, suggests that resistance to apoptosis precedes the development of tumor, and that it probably protects HBV infected cells from immune damage and elimination. On the molecular level, caspase 8, which is just up-stream of caspase 3, transmits death signals from Fas (T cell) and from TNFα signaling (Figure 2). In this context, it had previously been shown that HBx blocks Fas mediated killing in primary human hepatocytes (Diao et al., 2001), which may actually be mediated by URG7. Further, the finding that HBx activates NF-κB (Su & Schneider, 1996), that activated NF-κB protects hepatocytes from cell death (Beg et al., 1995, 1996), and that NF-κB transcriptionally activates URG7 (Pan et al., 2001), suggest a pathway that promotes persistence of the carrier state (and sustained HBV replication) even in the presence of recurring immune responses spanning many years. The findings of elevated TNFα production in human hepatocytes infected with HBV, and that HBx targets this up-regulation (Lara-Pezzi et al, 1998), not only suggests that TNFα is a target for HBx, but is also consistent with the strong correlation between HBx expression and inflammatory liver disease (Jin et al., 2001; Wang et al., 1991a, 1991b).

Additionally, the observation that HBx activates the expression of Fas ligand in HCC cell lines (Shin et al., 1999), may provide a way for virus infected cells to escape direct T cell killing by inducing apoptosis in such T cells. This would not only promote chronicity, but in tumor cells, an escape from immune elimination.

### 3.2.2 Up-regulated gene 11 (URG11) and hepatocarcinogenesis

Another transcript identified by subtractive hybridization in HBx positive compared to negative HepG2 cells encoded a novel protein provisionally designated as URG11 (Lian et al., 2003). The protein product was about 70kDa (673 amino acids) in size and contained five von Willebrand factor type-C repeats and one C-type lectin domain. Functional characterization showed that over-expression of URG11 significantly stimulated cell growth in culture, anchorage-independent growth in soft agar, accelerated tumor formation, and yielded larger tumors in SCID mice injected subcutaneously with HepG2 cells. Further work showed that HBx *trans*-activated URG11, and that URG11 *trans*-activated the β-catenin promoter. URG11 specific siRNA inhibited the growth of HBx expressing liver cells in serum free medium. The latter was associated with depressed levels of β-catenin. As

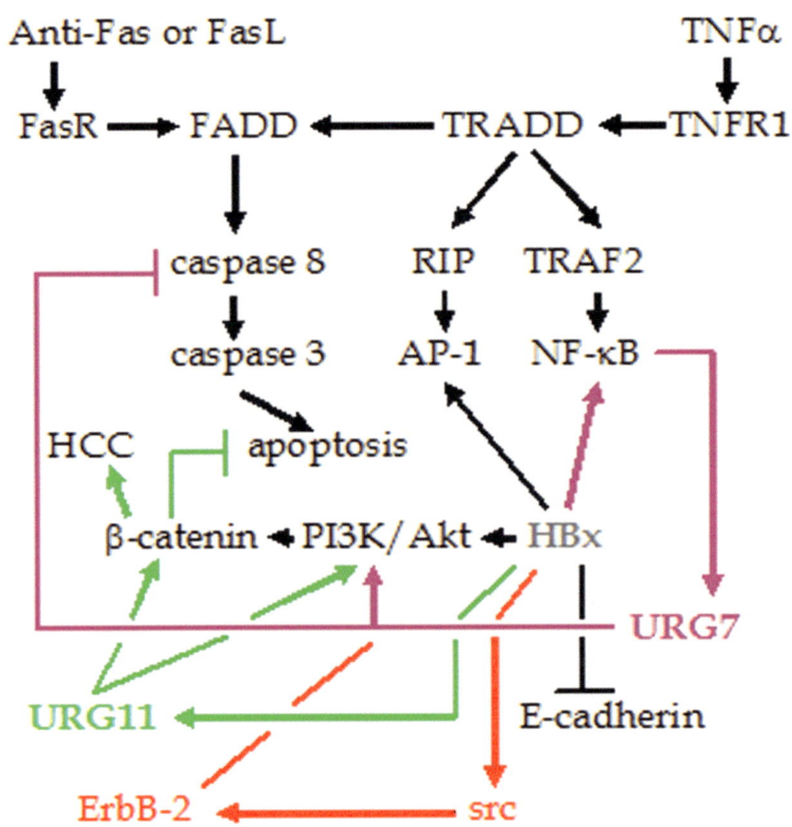


Fig. 2. Model showing selected steps of how HBx inhibits apoptosis and promotes tumorigenesis. HBx alters pathways involving URG7 (in purple), URG11 (in green), and ErbB-2 (in red). See the text for additional details.

with URG7, there was extensive co-staining between HBx and URG11 in chronically infected liver (Lian et al., 2006) but not in tumor. This suggests that URG11 promotes hepatocellular growth prior to the appearance of HCC. The ability of URG11 specific siRNA to block the growth of liver tumor cells both *in vitro* and *in vivo*, not only underscores the importance of elevated URG11 to cell growth, but also suggests that it may be a novel target for the development of specific therapeutics against HCC (Fan et al., 2011). Independent work has recently shown that URG11 was induced under hypoxic conditions in human kidney tubule cells (Du et al., 2010). The latter was associated with increased levels of HIF-1α, which is also known to be a target of HBx (Holotnakova et al., 2010). Importantly, HIF-1α is known to *trans*-activate VEGF *in vivo* (Yoo et al., 2003), suggesting that neovascularization may occur in cirrhotic nodules prior to the appearance of HCC. If this occurs during the pathogenesis of chronic hepatitis B, it would most likely be observed in cirrhotic nodules, since this represents a hypoxic environment characterized by high levels of HBx expression (Wang et al., 1991a, 1991b). Interestingly, elevated expression of URG11 in kidney tubule cells was also associated with suppression of E-cadherin, and up-regulation of the mesenchymal markers vimentin and alpha-SMA, suggesting that URG11 is associated with EMT. In chronic HBV infection, the development of cirrhosis is accompanied by considerable alterations in the tissue architecture within the liver, implying that URG11 may also play a significant role in tissue remodeling during the pathogenesis of chronic infection.

### 3.2.3 Elevated vascular endothelial growth factor receptor 3 (VEGFR-3)

Vascular endothelial growth factor receptor 3 (VEGFR-3), which is associated with angiogenesis, is a receptor tyrosine kinase that is expressed in lymphatic endothelial cells (Iljin et al., 2001). Binding of VEGFR-3 to the ligands VEGF-C or VEGF-D stimulate lymphangiogenesis (Alitalo & Carmeliet, 2002), while in carcinogenesis, the production of VEGFs by tumors promote metastases and result in decreased survival (Su et al., 2006). Elevated VEGF has been found in patients with HCC (Dahr et al., 2002, Poon et al., 2003). VEGFR-3 is also expressed in tumor cells from several tumor types (Bando et al., 2004, Su et al., 2006), including HCC (Dahr et al., 2002), implying the existence of an autocrine/paracrine loop that promotes tumor development independent of lymphangiogenesis (Su et al., 2006). In HCC, elevated VEGFR-3 is associated with portal vein invasion of tumors, increased hepatic tumor recurrence, and shorter survival (Dhar et al., 2002), suggesting that VEGFR-3 is important in the pathogenesis of HCC. In this context, differential display of HBx positive compared to negative cells showed that HBx up-regulated the expression of an mRNA which encoded a splice variant of VEGFR-3 (Lian et al., 1997). This was verified at the mRNA and protein levels in HBx positive compared to negative HepG2 cells. In infected liver, expression of VEGFR-3 was prominent in nodules of HCC and correlated with HBx expression. VEGFR-3 stimulated cell cycle in culture, anchorage independent growth in soft agar, and accelerated tumor formation and larger tumor size in SCID mice injected with HepG2 cells over-expressing VEGFR-3. Further work showed that over-expression of VEGFR-3 in the absence of HBx resulted in activation of PI3K/Akt, which then activated β-catenin gene expression (Figure 2), and with inactivation of the tumor suppressor, PTEN. Interestingly, HBx also mediates these changes, suggesting that they may be actually carried out by up-regulation of VEGFR-3. These findings also suggest that in addition to lymphangiogenesis, VEGFR-3 may promote tumorigenesis in HBx associated HCC.

### 3.2.4 Elevation of β-catenin and suppression of E-cadherin

Constitutive activation of β-catenin is characteristic of many tumor types (Fukuchi et al., 1998; Morin et al., 1997). This results in constitutive Wnt signaling, where β-catenin translocates to the nucleus and stimulates the expression of genes that promote tumorigenesis (Clevers & van de Wetering, 1997; Peifer & Polakis, 2000; Terradillos et al., 1997). Importantly, β-catenin mutations are found in small HCCs and in preneoplastic liver (Calvisi et al., 2001; Terris et al., 1999,), suggesting they occur early in tumor development. The finding of frequent β-catenin mutations in a subset of human HCC (de La Costa et al., 1998, Miyoshi et al., 1998), especially in HBV-negative tumors (Hsu et al., 2000), implies that the majority of β-catenin activation must occur by mechanisms other than mutation. In the chronically infected liver, HBx has been shown to be associated with the constitutive activation of wild type β-catenin. The finding that the activation of wild type β-catenin was associated with URG11 (Lian et al., 2006) and URG7 (Pan et al., 2007), underscores the importance of this activation in hepatocarcinogenesis. Moreover, β-catenin appears to be stabilized by a number of mechanisms, including *trans*-activation of the β-catenin promoter (Lian et al., 2006; Pan et al., 2007), inhibition of proteasomal degradation (Cui et al., 2006; Zhang et al., 2000), and suppression of E-cadherin expression (Arzumanyan et al., 2011; Lee et al., 2005; Liu et al., 2006) (Figure 2). The latter is of particular importance because suppression of the cell adhesion protein, E-cadherin, is a hallmark of EMT, which is important to the pathogenesis of CLD and HCC. The importance of suppressed E-cadherin expression is further underscored by the findings that this occurs by DNA methylation of the E-cadherin promoter (Lee et al., 2005; Liu et al., 2006), by the inhibition miR-373 expression by HBx, and by HBx mediated stimulation of histone deacetylase (HDAC) at the E-cadherin promoter (Arzumanyan et al., 2011). Independent of the mechanism involved, suppression of E-cadherin has important ramifications upon β-catenin. Normally, β-catenin participates in cell adhesion by serving as a link between E-cadherin and the cytoskeleton. When E-cadherin expression is suppressed, β-catenin is released from this role and translocates to the nucleus where it activates genes that promote cell growth. Thus, in the presence of HBx, there is an inverse correlation with E-cadherin expression, and a direct correlation with the accumulation of cytoplasmic and nuclear β-catenin at the expense of membranous β-catenin, both in cultured cells and in clinical specimens (Arzumanyan et al., 2011; Lian et al., 2006; Liu et al., 2006). This suggests a tight coupling between EMT and the promotion of hepatocellular growth prior to the development of HCC (Du et al., 2010).

### 3.2.5 Elevated expression of ErbB-2

Another natural effector of HBx is ErbB-2 (Liu et al., 2009). ErbB-2 (HER2 or neu) is a member of the epidermal growth factor receptor tyrosine kinases that is involved in the transmission of differentiation and proliferation signals (Olayioye et al., 2000, Yarden & Sliwkowski, 2001). High levels of ErbB-2 have been shown in various types of cancers (Sauter et al., 1993; Slamon et al., 1987; Tanner et al., 1996), and in some tumors, over-expression is associated with poor prognosis. In breast cancer, up-regulated ErbB-2 appears to be an early event, since it appears in tumor and nontumor tissue (Menard et al., 2002). In HCC, elevated ErbB-2 has been reported in hyperplastic nodules (Niu & Wang, 2005) and in 30-40% of HCCs (Chen et al., 2002; Neo et al., 2004). However, ErbB-2 was not found in HCC tissues from other studies (Alitalo & Carmeliet, 2002; Hsu et al., 2002; Vlasoff et al., 2002). The finding that HBx up-regulates and stabilizes β-catenin (Lian et al., 2006), which in some tumors is activated by elevated levels of ErbB-2, suggested that constitutive expression of β-catenin may be associated with elevated ErbB2. Accordingly, when HBx positive and negative cells were subjected to proteomics analysis, ErbB-2 was up-regulated in HBx expressing but not control cells. ErbB-2 was also strongly up-regulated in HBV infected liver, where it correlated with HBx expression, and weakly in some HCC nodules (Liu et al., 2009). Among tumor bearing patients, strong ErbB-2 staining in the liver was associated with dysplasia, and a shorter survival after tumor diagnosis. This implies that elevated ErbB-2 is an early marker of HCC. Treatment of HBx expressing cells with ErbB-2 specific siRNA not only reduced ErbB2 expression, but also reduced the expression of β-catenin, suggesting that ErbB-2 contributed to the stabilization of β-catenin. ErbB-2 specific siRNA also partially blocked the ability of HBx to promote DNA synthesis and growth of cells *in vitro* (Liu et al., 2009). These results suggested that ErbB-2/β-catenin up-regulation contributed to HBx mediated hepatocellular growth. The additional finding that HBx stimulates expression of the epidermal growth factor receptor (EGFR or ErbB1) (Menzo et al.,1993), and that EGFR signaling stabilizes β-catenin (Takahashi et al., 1997), suggested that EGF signaling may be strongly activated in patients at high risk for HCC or with already established tumors. This suggests that elevated ErbB-2 may be rate limiting in tumor formation, and if so, may be a therapeutic target (Altimari et al., 2003). Further, the accumulation of wild type β-catenin in the presence of elevated ErbB-2 correlated with the activation of PI3K/Akt signaling, which is known to be activated by HBx and ErbB-2 (Lian et al., 2006; Shih et al., 2000; Yarden & Sliwkowski, 2001) (Figure 2). PI3K/Akt activity may also be stimulated by src, the latter of which is activated by HBx, early in tumor development (Lara-Pezzi et al., 2001b; Shih et al., 2003). Further, the peptidyl prolyl isomerase, Pin1, is up-regulated in HCC, and is known to stabilize both HBx (Pang et al., 2007) and ErbB-2 (Lam et al., 2008), suggesting a variety of possible mechanisms underlying the close HBx/ErbB-2 relationship.

### 3.2.6 Other natural target genes of HBx

In addition to transcriptional regulation of gene expression, HBx up-regulates expression of the ribosomal protein, S15a (Lian et al., 2004) and down-regulates expression of the translation initiation factor, Sui1 (Lian et al., 1999). S15a is a highly conserved protein (Chan et al., 1994; Reed, 1980; Schaap et al., 1995) that promotes mRNA/ribosome interactions early in translation (Lavoie et al., 1994). S15a also stimulates growth in yeast (Pringle et al., 1981; Reed, 1980,), in plants (Bonhan-Smith & Moloney, 1994; Bonham-Smith et al., 1992) and in human lung carcinoma cells (Akiyama et al., 2000). The observation that S15a stimulates hepatocellular growth and survival *in vitro*, and tumor formation *in vivo*, suggests that it also plays a role in hepatocarcinogeneis, and that HBx contributes to transformation, in part, at the level of protein translation by up-regulated expression of S15a (Lian et al., 2004). As stated above,, HBx was also shown to depress the expression of the translation initiation factor, sui1. Sui1, whose function is to work with eIF-2 to enable the initiator tRNA$^{MET}$ to establish ribosomal recognition of an AUG codon (Yoon and Donahue, 1992), suggests that the expression of hu-sui1 contributes to the regulation of protein translation. *In vivo* work showed that sui1 was expressed in nontumor liver but not in tumor cells from patients with HCC. Sui1 inhibited cell growth in culture, in soft agar, and partially inhibited tumor formation in nude mice, suggesting that suppression of sui1 may result in the abrogation of negative growth regulation that contributes to the development of HCC (Lian et al., 1999). Given that S15a and sui1 are both involved in regulating translation, it is likely that HBx also contributes to HCC by altering gene expression at multiple steps within translation, although the mRNAs that are differentially translated remain to be identified.

HBx also stimulates the expression of the novel protein, URG4 (Tufan et al., 2002). URG4, encodes a protein of about 104 kDa that was strongly expressed in HBV- infected liver and in HCC cells, where it co-stained with HBx, and was weakly expressed in uninfected liver, suggesting URG4 was an effector of HBx *in vivo*. Over-expression of URG4 without HBx in human hepatoblastoma cells promoted hepatocellular growth and survival in tissue culture and in soft agar, and accelerated tumor development in nude mice (Tufan et al., 2002). URG4 over-expression was associated with elevated cyclin D1 expression, and treatment of such cells with URG4 specific siRNA reduced both cyclin D1 expression and inhibited cell cycle progression (Tufan et al., 2010). These observations suggest that URG4 may be an oncogene that contributes to HBV associated HCC. Independent work showed that over-expression of URG4 in osteosarcoma tissues directly correlated with tumor recurrence and metastasis, as well as with the proliferative activity of osteosarcoma cells. Patients with high expression of URG4 had shorter survival time, suggesting that URG4 might be rate limiting in carcinogenesis and a valuable prognostic marker in osteosarcoma patients (Huang et al., 2009). Thus, URG4 may contribute to carcinogenesis outside of the liver.

HBx also appears to up-regulate the expression of insulin - like growth factor 2 (IGF-2) and the IGF-1 receptor in HCC (Kim et al., 1996; Su et al., 1994). The finding that insulin-like growth factor-2 expression, which is normally observed only in fetal liver (Soares et al., 1985), is elevated in HCCs (D'Arville et al., 1991, Cariani et al., 1991), and in premalignant proliferative nodules in the liver (Cariani et al., 1988; D'Arville et al., 1991), suggest that its reactivation may be an early step in the development of this tumor type. The elevation of IGF-2 expression in HCCs from HBV infected but not uninfected patients, combined with the finding of a strong correlation between IGF-2 and HBx in the liver by immunohistochemical staining (Su et al., 1994), suggest that IGF-2 may be a natural target of HBx during chronic infection. In human hepatoma cell lines, IGF-2 was expressed strongly in growing cells, but was undetectable in confluent cultures (Su et al., 1994), suggesting that it was associated with cell proliferation. At the molecular level, the tumor suppressor, PTEN normally suppresses IGF-2 expression (Kang-Park et al., 2003), but in the presence of HBx, PTEN expression is blocked, resulting in activation of IGF-2 (Chung et al., 2003). Normally, PTEN is up-regulated by another tumor suppressor, p53, but since HBx binds to and inactivates p53 (Feitelson et al., 1993b; Wang et al., 1994), PTEN expression also drops (Chung et al., 2003). In addition, HBx activation of Sp1 via protein kinase C (PKC) and p44/p42MAPK signaling pathways are also operative in promoting IGF-2 gene expression (Kang-Park et al., 2001). These multiple pathways underscore the importance of IGF-2 up-regulation in hepatocarcinogenesis. Finally, the finding that HBx stimulates the expression of the IGF-1 receptor in human HCC cell lines (Kim et al., 1996), which binds both IGF-1 and IGF-2, suggests that HBx may set up an autocrine loop that enhances cell growth. Thus, the up-regulated expression of IGF-2, which appears to be a target of HBx *in vivo*, may promote hepatocarcinogenesis.

The finding that HBx interacts with and inhibits the function of the proteasome (Huang et al., 1996) suggests another mechanism whereby HBx could alter gene expression at a post-translational level. This inhibition appears to be important in supporting HBx *trans*-activation activity (Hu et al., 1999). Given that HBx *trans*-activates virus gene expression and replication, when mutants of the X protein that bound to and inhibit the proteasome were introduced into WHV, and the resulting virus used for experimental infection, no or transient viremia was observed. In contrast to wild type WHV, which resulted in a high carrier rate among experimentally infected woodchucks, none of the animals infected with the X mutant developed the carrier state (Zhang et al., 2001). Further work *in vitro* showed that in the presence of proteasome inhibitors, replication of the wild-type virus was not affected, while the replication of the X-negative HBV or WHV was enhanced and restored to the wild-type levels. Similar results were obtained in mouse models replicating wild type and X mutant HBV (Zhang et al., 2010). Thus, HBx appears to affect hepadnavirus replication through a proteasome-dependent pathway (Zhang et al., 2004). Moreover, in the livers of transgenic mice where the levels of HBx expression increased with age, there was a parallel age related decreases in the peptidase activities of the proteasome in the liver (Hu et al., 2006). Microarray analysis showed that many of the genes affected involved transcription and cell growth. For example, insulin-like growth factor-binding protein 1 was down-regulated in the HBx mouse liver (Hu et al., 2006), while *in vitro*, HBx stabilized c-myc (Kalra & Kumar, 2006) and the protooncoprotein, pituitary tumor-transforming gene 1 (PTTG1) (Molina-Jimenez et al., 2010), by blocking ubiquitination and proteasomal degradation. HBx also differentially regulated the level of β-catenin through two ubiquitin-dependent proteasome pathways depending upon the status of p53 (Jung et al., 2007). Given that HBx expression is dominant in liver compared to HCC tissue (Wang et al., 1991a, 1991b), it was not surprising to find an elevated proteasomal activity in HCC compared to surrounding nontumor liver, both in HBx transgenic mice that developed tumors, and in clinical samples from patients with HCC (Cui et al., 2006). These observations suggest that changes in proteasome function accompany the pathogenesis of CLD and HCC, and that these changes appear to be related to the levels of HBx .

## 4. Conclusions

Tumorigenesis is a multi-step process, and as outlined above, HBx impacts upon this process by targeting selected pathways and genes in natural infection. For most of the target genes presented here, up-regulated or down-regulated expression was established by comparison of gene expression profiles in HBx positive compared to negative cells, suggesting that they were due to the properties of HBx. Clinical validation was carried out on liver and tumor tissues obtained from HBV infected patients. For up-regulated genes, there was strong co-staining between HBx and the putative target, while for down-regulated genes, there was an inverse relationship by immunohistochemistry, and in many cases, northern blotting or RT/PCR analyses as well. Moreover, many of the natural targets of HBx discussed herein were characterized to gain at least a preliminary outline as to their contribution to the pathogenesis of HCC. The overall results show that HBx contributes to multiple steps in hepatocarcinogenesis, and that the pleiotrophic nature of HBx, known for many years, is now being better understood by the functions of the proteins encoded by these target genes. These data provide crucial information as to the steps in the pathogenesis of HCC that are likely to be rate limiting, which is very important for the application of therapeutic approaches to known targets and for the development of therapeutics to novel targets. The hope embodied in these studies is that they will lead to the development of diagnostic/prognostic biomarkers and/or therapies that will specifically target gene products whose functions appear to be rate limiting in tumorigenesis. The fact that most of the up-regulated genes are over-expressed in liver, and much less often in tumor, means that specific therapies could be devised to ultimately reduce the risk for development of HCC, and if this is achieved, this would open up the probability that chemoprevention could become a realistic approach to treating patients at high risk for the appearance of cancer. This approach will not only be useful, for approaching cancer prevention in the liver, but if one or more of the URGs described above are also elevated in precancerous lesions from other tissue types, the approach would become more widespread in preventing the development of other tumors. In doing so, this has the possibility of establishing a different paradigm for therapeutic approaches against cancer.

## 5. Acknowledgements

This work was supported by grants CA111427, CA104025, and AI076535 awarded to Dr. Mark Feitelson

## 6. References

Akhurst, R.J. (2002). TGF-beta antagonists: why suppress a tumor suppressor?. *J Clin Invest* 109:1533-1536.

Akiyama, N., Matsuo, Y., Sai, H., Noda, M. & Kizaka-Kondoh S. (2000). Identification of a series of transforming growth factor beta-responsive genes by retrovirus-mediated gene trap screening. *Mol Cell Biol* 9:3266-3273.

Alitalo, K. & Carmeliet. P. (2002). Molecular mechanisms of lymphangiogenesis in health and disease. *Cancer Cell* 1:219-227.

Altimari, A., Fiorentino, M., Gabusi, E., Gruppioni, E., Corti, B., D'Errico, A. & Grigioni, W.F. (2003). Investigation of ErbB1 and ErbB2 expression for therapeutic targeting in primary liver tumours. *Dig Liver Dis* 25:332-338.

Arzumanyan, A., Friedman, T., Kotei, E., Ng, I.O.L., Lian, Z. & Feitelson, M.A. (2011). Epigenetic repression of E-cadherin expression by hepatitis B x antigen (HBx) in liver cancer. *Oncogene* in press.

Assrir, N., Soussan, P., Kremsdorf, D. & Rossignol, J.M. Role of the hepatitis B virus proteins in pro- and anti-apoptotic processes. *Frontiers in Bioscience* 15:12-24, 2010.

Balsano, C., Billet, O., Bennoun, M., Cavard, C., Zider, A., Grimber, G., Natoli, G., Briand, P. & Levrero, M. (1994). Hepatitis B virus X gene product acts as a transactivator in vivo. *J Hepatol* 21:103-109.

Bando, H., Brokelmann, M., Toi, M., Alitalo, K., Sleeman, J.P., Sipos, B, Gröne, H.J. & Weich, H.A. (2004). Immunodetection and quantification of vascular endothelial growth factor receptor-3 in human malignant tumor tissues. *Int J Cancer* 11:184-191.

Beg, A. & Baltimore, D. (1996). An essential role for NF-κB in preventing TNF-α-induced cell death. *Science* 274:782-784.

Beg, A., Sha, W., Bronson, R., Ghosh, S. & Baltimore, D. (1995). Embryonic lethality and liver regeneration in mice lacking the RelA component of NF-κB. *Nature* 376:167-170.

Belloni, L., Pollicino, T., De Nicola, F., Guerrieri F., Raffa, G., Fanciulli, M., Raimondo, G. & Levrero M. (2009). Nuclear HBx binds the HBV minichromosome and modifies the epigenetic regulation of cccDNA function. *Proc Natl Acad Sci USA* 106:19975-199799.

Benhenda, S., Cougot, D., Buendia, M.A. & Neuveut, C. (2009). Hepatitis B virus X protein molecular functions and its role in virus life cycle and pathogenesis. *Adv Cancer Res* 103:75-109.

Bonham-Smith, P.C. & Moloney, M.M. (1994). Nucleotide and protein sequences of a cytoplasmic ribosomal protein S15a gene from Arabidopsis thaliana. *Plant Physiol* 106:401-402.

Bonham-Smith, P.C., Oancia, T.L. & Moloney, M.M. (1992). Cytoplasmic ribosomal protein S15a from Brassica napus: molecular cloning and developmental expression in mitotically active tissues. *Plant Mol Biol* 18:909-919.

Bui-Nguyen, T.M., Pakala, S.B., Sirigiri, R.D., Xia, W., Hung, M.C., Sarin, S.K., Kumar, V., Slagle, B.L. & Kumar, R. (2010). NF-kappaB signaling mediates the induction of MTA1 by hepatitis B virus transactivator protein HBx. *Oncogene* 29:1179-1189.

Calvisi, D.F., Factor, V.M., Loi, R. & Thorgeirson, S.S. (2001). Activation of β-catenin during hepatocarcinogenesis in transgenic mouse models: Relationship to phenotype and tumor grade. *Cancer Res* 61:2085-2091.

Cariani, E., Lasserre, C., Kemeny, F., Franco, D. & Brechot, C. (1991). Expression of insulin-like growth factor II, α-fetoprotein and HBV transcripts in human primary liver cancer. *Hepatology* 13:644-649.

Cariani, E., Lasserre, C., Seurin, D., Hamelin, B., Kemeny, F., Franco, D., Czech, M.P., Ullrich, A. & Brechot, C. (1988). Differential expression of insulin-like growth factor II mRNA in human primary liver cancers, benign liver tumors, and liver cirrhosis. *Cancer Res* 48:6844-6849.

Castilla, A., Prieto, J. & Fausto, N. Transforming growth factors beta 1 and alpha in chronic liver disease. (1991). Effects of interferon alpha therapy. *N Engl J Med* 324:933-940.

Chan, Y.L., Olvera, J., Paz, V. & Wool, I.G. (1994). The primary structure of rat ribosomal protein S15a. *Biochem Biophys Res Commun* 200:1498-1504.

Chen, B.F., Liu, C.J., Jow, G.M., Chen, P.J., Kao, J.H. & Chen, D.S. (2006). High prevalence and mapping of pre-S deletion in hepatitis B virus carriers with progressive liver diseases. *Gastroenterology* 130:1153-1168.

Chen, H.S., Kaneko, S., Girones, R., Anderson, R.W., Hornbuckle, W.E., Tennant, B.C., Cote, P.J., Gerin, J.L., Purcell, R.H. & Miller, R.H. (1993). The woodchuck hepatitis virus X gene is important for establishment of virus infection in woodchucks. *J Virol* 67:1218-1226.

Chen, S., Guttridge, D.C., You, Z.. Zhang, Z.. Fribley, A.. Mayo, MW., Kitajewski, J. & Wang, C.Y. (2001). Wnt-1 signaling inhibits apoptosis by activating beta-catenin/T cell factor-mediated transcription. *J Cell Biol* 152:87-96.

Chen, X., Cheung, S.T., So, S., Fan, S.T., Barry, C., Higgins, J., Lai, K.M., Ji, J., Dudoit, S., Ng, I.O., van de Rijn, M., Botstein, D., et al. (2002). Gene expression patterns in human liver cancers. *Mol Biol Cell* 13:1929-1939.

Cheng, B., Zheng, Y., Guo, X., Wang, Y. & Liu, C. (2010). Hepatitis B viral X protein alters the biological features and expressions of DNA repair enzymes in LO2 cells. *Liver Intl* 30:319-326.

Choi, S.S., Omenetti, A,. Witek, R.P., Moylan, C.A., Syn, W.K., Jung, Y,. Yang, L., Sudan, D.L., Sicklick, J.K., Michelotti, G.A., Rojkind, M. & Diehl, A.M. (2009). Hedgehog pathway activation and epithelial-to-mesenchymal transitions during myofibroblastic transformation of rat hepatic cells in culture and cirrhosis. *Am J Physiol - GI & Liver Physiol* 297:G1093-G1106.

Chung, T.W., Lee, Y.C. & Kim, C.H. (2004). Hepatitis B viral HBx induces matrix metalloproteinase-9 gene expression through activation of ERK and PI-3K/AKT pathways: involvement of invasive potential. *FASEB J* 18:1123-1125.

Chung, T.W., Lee, Y.C., Ko, J.H. & Kim, C.H. (2003). Hepatitis B virus X protein modulates the expression of PTEN by inhibiting the function of p53, a transcriptional activator in liver cells. *Cancer Res* 63:3453-3458.

Clevers, H. & van de Wetering, M. (1997). TCF/LEF factor earn their wings. *Trends Genet* 13:485-489.

Cougot, D., Wu, Y., Cairo, S., Caramel, J., Renard, C.A., Lévy, L., Buendia, M.A. & Neuveut, C. (2007). The hepatitis B virus X protein functionally interacts with CREB-binding protein/p300 in the regulation of CREB-mediated transcription. *J Biol Chem* 282:4277-4287.

Cui, F., Wang, Y., Wang, J., Wei, K., Hu, J., Liu, F., Wang, H., Zhao, X., Zhang, X. & Yang, X. (2006). The up-regulation of proteasome subunits and lysosomal proteases in hepatocellular carcinomas of the HBx gene knockin transgenic mice. *Proteomics* 6:498-504, 2006.

D'Arville, C.N., Nouri-Aria, K.T., Johnson, P. & Williams, R. (1991). Regulation of insulin-like growth factor II gene expression by hepatitis B virus in hepatocellular carcinoma. *Hepatology* 13:310-315.

de La Coste, A., Romannolo, B., Billuart, P., Renard, C.A., Buendia, M.A., Soubrane, O., Fabre, M., Chelly, J., Beldjord, C., Kahn, A. & Perret, C. (1998). Somatic mutations of the beta-catenin gene are frequent in mouse and human hepatocellular carcinoma. *Proc Natl Acad Sci USA* 95:8847-8851.

Dhar, D.K., Naora, H., Yamanoi, A., Ono, T., Kohno, H., Otani, H. & Nagasue, N. (2002). Requisite role of VEGF receptors in angiogenesis of hepatocellular carcinoma: a comparison with angiopoietin/Tie pathway. *Anticancer Res* 22:379-386.

Diao, J., Khine, A.A., Sarangi, F., Hsu, E., Iorio, C., Tibbles, L.A., Woodgett, J.R., Penninger, J. & Richardson, C.D. (2001). X protein of hepatitis B virus inhibits Fas-mediated apoptosis and is associated with up-regulation of the SAPK/JNK pathway. *J Biol Chem* 276:8328-8340.

Doong, D.L., Lin M.H., Tsai, M.M., Li T.R., Chuang, S.E. & Cheng, A.L. (1998). Transactivation of the human MDR1 gene by hepatitis B X gene product. *J Hepatol* 29:872-878.

Du, R., Huang, C., Bi, Q., Zhai, Y., Xia, L., Liu, J., Sun, S. & Fan, D. (2010). URG11 mediates hypoxia-induced epithelial-to-mesenchymal transition by modulation of E-cadherin and beta-catenin. *Biochem Biophys Res Commun* 391:135-141.

Fan, R., Li, X., Du, W., Zou, X., Du, R., Zhao, L., Luo, G., Mo, P., Xia, L., Pan, Y., Shi, Y., Lian, Z., Feitelson, M.A., Nie, Y., Liu, J. & Fan D. (2011). Adenoviral-mediated RNA interference targeting URG11 inhibits growth of human hepatocellular carcinoma. *Intl J Cancer* 128:2980-2993.

Feitelson, M.A. & Duan, L.X. (1997). Hepatitis B virus X antigen in the pathogenesis of chronic infections and the development of hepatocellular carcinoma. *Am J Pathol* 150:1141-1157.

Feitelson, M.A., Lega, L., Duan, L.X., & Clayton, M. (1993a). Characteristics of woodchuck hepatitis X antigen in the livers and sera from chronically infected animals. *J Hepatol* 17(Suppl. 3):S24-S34.

Feitelson, M.A., Reis, H., Liu, J., Lian, Z. & Pan, J. (2005). Hepatitis B virus X antigen (HBxAg) and cell cycle control in chronic infection and hepatocarcinogenesis. In: *Frontiers in Bioscience. Viral Infection and Cell Cycle Control*, Zhao R., ed., Frontiers in Bioscience, Albertson, N.Y., USA, pp. 1558-1572.

Feitelson, M.A., Reis, H., Tufan, L.S., Liu, J., Zhu, M., Pan, J. & Lian, Z. (2008). Hepatitis B x antigen interference with tumor suppressor pathways in hepatocarcinognesis. In: *The Pleiotropic Functions of the Viral protein HBx in HBV Infection and the Development of Liver Cancer*, Kobarg, J., ed., Research Signpost, Kerala, India, pp. 1-18.

Feitelson MA, Reis HMGPV, Tufan NL, Sun B, Pan J, Lian Z. (2009). Putative roles of hepatitis B x antigen in the pathogenesis of chronic liver disease. *Cancer Letters* 286:69–79.

Feitelson, M.A., Sun, B., Tufan, N L., Liu, J., Pan, J. & Lian, Z. (2002). Genetic mechanisms of hepatocarcinogenesis. *Oncogene* 21:2593-2604.

Feitelson, M.A., Zhu, M., Duan, L.X. & London, W.T. (1993b). Hepatitis B X antigen and p53 are associated *in vitro* and in liver tissues from patients with primary hepatocellular carcinoma. *Oncogene* 8:1109-1117.

Flisiak, R., Al-Kadasi, H., Jaroszewicz, J., Prokopowicz, D. & Flisiak, I. (2004). Effect of lamivudine treatment on plasma levels of transforming growth factor beta1, tissue inhibitor of metalloproteinases-1 and metalloproteinase-1 in patients with chronic hepatitis B. *World J. Gastroenterol* 10:2661-2665.

Fukuchi, T., Sakamoto, M., Tsuda, H., Maruyama, K., Nozawa, S. & Hirohashi, S. (1998). β-Catenin mutation in carcinoma of the uterine endometrium. *Cancer Res* 58:3526-3528.

Gottlob, K., Fulco, M., Levrero, M. & Graessmann, A. (1998). The hepatitis B virus HBx protein inhibits caspase 3 activity. *J Biol Chem* 273:33347-33353.

Guo, G.H., Tan, D.M., Zhu, P.A. & Liu, F. (2009). Hepatitis B virus X protein promotes proliferation and upregulates TGF-beta1 and CTGF in human hepatic stellate cell line, LX-2. *Hepatobil Panc Dis Intl* 8:59-64.

Haviv, I., Vaizel, D. & Shaul, Y. (1995). The X protein of hepatitis B virus coactivates potent activation domains. *Mol Cell Biol* 15:1079-1085.

Haviv, I., Vaizel, D. & Shaul, Y. (1996). pX, the HBV-encoded coactivator, interacts with components of the transcription machinery and stimulates transcription in a TAF-independent manner. *EMBO J* 15:3413-3420.

Henkler, F. & Koshy, R. (1996). Hepatitis B virus transcriptional activators: mechanisms and possible role in oncogenesis. *J Viral Hepat* 3:109-121.

Holotnakova, T.,Tylkova, L., Takacova, M., Kopacek, J., Petrik, J., Pastorekova, S. & Pastorek, J. (2010). Role of the HBx oncoprotein in carbonic anhydrase 9 induction. *J Med Virol* 82:32-40.

Hsu, C., Huang, C.L., Hsu, H.C., Lee, P.H., Wang, S.J. & Cheng, A.L. (2002). HER-2/neu overexpression is rare in hepatocellular carcinoma and not predictive of anti-HER-2/neu regulation of cell growth and chemosensitivity. *Cancer* 94:415-420.

Hsu, H.C., Jeng, Y.M., Mao, T.L., Chu, J.S., Lai, P.L. & Peng, S.Y. (2000). β-Catenin mutations as associated with a subset of low stage hepatocellular carcinoma negative for hepatitis B virus with favorable prognosis. *Am J Pathol* 157:763-770.

Hu, Z., Zhang, Z., Doo, E., Coux, O., Goldberg, A.L. & Liang, T.J. (1999). Hepatitis B virus X protein is both a substrate and a potential inhibitor of the proteasome complex. *J Virol* 73:7231-7240.

Hu, Z., Zhang, Z., Kim, J.W., Huang, Y. & Liang, T.J. (2006). Altered proteolysis and global gene expression in hepatitis B virus X transgenic mouse liver. *J Virol* 80:1405-1413.

Huang, J., Kwong, J., Sun, E.C. & Liang, T.J. (1996). Proteasome complex as a potential cellular target of hepatitis B virus X protein. J Virol 70:5582-5591.

Huang, J., Zhu, B., Lu, L., Lian, Z., Wang, Y., Yang, X., Tufan, N.L.S., Liu, J. & Luo, Z. (2009). The expression of novel gene URG4 in osteosarcoma: Correlation with patients' prognosis. *Pathology* 41:149-154.

Iljin, K., Karkkainen, M.J., Lawrence, E.C., Kimak, M.A., Uutela, M., Taipale, J., Pajusola, K., Alhonen, L., Halmekyto, M., Finegold, D.N., Ferrell, R.E. & Alitalo, K. (2001). VEGFR3 gene structure, regulatory region, and sequence polymorphisms. *FASEB J* 15:1028-1036.

Jin, Y.M., Yun, C., Park, C., Wang, H.J., & Cho, H. (2001). Expression of hepatitis B virus X protein is closely correlated with the high periportal inflammatory activity of liver diseases. *J Viral Hepat* 8:322-330.

Jung, J.K., Kwun, H.J., Lee, J.O., Arora, P. & Jang, K.L. (2007). Hepatitis B virus X protein differentially affects the ubiquitin-mediated proteasomal degradation of beta-catenin depending on the status of cellular p53. *J Gen Virol* 88:2144-2154.

Kalra, N. & Kumar, V. (2006). The X protein of hepatitis B virus binds to the F box protein Skp2 and inhibits the ubiquitination and proteasomal degradation of c-Myc. FEBS Lett 580:431-436.

Kang-Park, S., Lee, J.H., Shin, J.H. & Lee, Y.I. (2001). Activation of the IGF-II gene by HBV-X protein requires PKC and p44/p42 map kinase signalings. *Biochem Biophys Res Commun* 283:303-307.

Kang-Park, S., Lee, Y.I. & Lee, Y.I. (2003). PTEN modulates insulin-like growth factor II (IGF-II)-mediated signaling; the protein phosphatase activity of PTEN downregulates IGF-II expression in hepatoma cells. *FEBS Lett* 545:203-208.

Keasler, V.V., Hodgson, A.J., Madden, C.R. & Slagle, B.L. (2009). Hepatitis B virus HBx protein localized to the nucleus restores HBx-deficient virus replication in HepG2 cells and in vivo in hydrodynamically-injected mice. *Virology* 390:122-129.

Kew, M.C. (2011). Hepatitis B virus x protein in the pathogenesis of hepatitis B virus-induced hepatocellular carcinoma. *J Gastroenterol Hepatol* 26(Suppl 1):144-152.

Kim, H.Y., Cho, H.K., Hong, S.P. & Cheong, J. (2011). Hepatitis B virus X protein stimulates the Hedgehog-Gli activation through protein stabilization and nuclear localization of Gli1 in liver cancer cells. *Cancer Lett* 309:176-184.

Kim, S.O,, Park, J.G. & Lee, Y.I. (1996). Increased expression of the insulin - like growth factor I (IGF - I) receptor gene in hepatocellular carcinoma cell lines: implications of IGF - I receptor gene activation by hepatitis B virus X gene product. *Cancer Res* 56:3831 – 3836.

Klein, N.P. & Schneider, R.J. (1997). Activation of src family kinases by hepatitis B virus HBx protein and coupled signaling to ras. *Mol Cell Biol* 17:6427-6436.

Kong, G., Zhang, J., Zhang, S., Shan, C., Ye, L. & Zhang, X. (2011). Up-regulated microRNA-29a by hepatitis B virus X protein enhances hepatoma cell migration by targeting PTEN in cell culture model. *PLoS One* 6:e19518

Kumar, M., Jung, S.Y., Hodgson, A.J., Madden, C.R., Qin, J. & Slagle, B.L. (2011). Hepatitis B virus regulatory HBx protein binds to adaptor protein IPS-1 and inhibits the activation of beta interferon. *J Virol* 85:987-995.

Lam, P.B., Burga, L.N., Wu, B.P., Hofstatter, E.W., Lu, K.P. & Wulf, G.M. (2008). Prolyl isomerase Pin1 is highly expressed in Her2-positive breast cancer and regulates erbB2 protein stability. *Mol Cancer* 7:91-102.

Lara-Pezzi, E., Majano, P.L., Gómez-Gonzalo, M., García-Monzón, C., Moreno-Otero, R., Levrero, M. & López-Cabrera, M. (1998). The hepatitis B virus X protein up-regulates tumor necrosis factor alpha gene expression in hepatocytes. *Hepatology* 8:1013-1021.

Lara-Pezzi, E., Majano, P.L., Yanez-Mo, M., Gomez-Gonzalo, M., Carretero, M., Moreno-Otero, R., et al, (2001a). Effect of the hepatitis B virus HBx protein on integrin-mediated adhesion to and migration on extracellular matrix. *J Hepatol* 34:409-415.

Lara-Pezzi, E., Roche, S., Andrisani, O.M., Sanchez-Madrid, F. & Lopez-Cabrera, M. (2001b). The hepatitis B virus protein induces adherens junction disruption in a src-dependent manner. *Oncogene* 20:3323-3331.

Lauer, U., Weissm L., Hofschneiderm P.H. & Kekule, A.S. (1992). The hepatitis B virus pre-S/S(t) transactivator is generated by 3' truncations within a defined region of the S gene. *J Virol* 66:5284-5289.

Lavoie, C., Tam, R., Clark, M., Lee, H., Sonenberg, N. & Lasko, P. (1994). Suppression of a temperature-sensitive cdc33 mutation of yeast by a multicopy plasmid expressing a Drosophila ribosomal protein. *J Biol Chem* 269:14625-14630.

Lee, D.K., Park, S.H., Yi, Y., Choi, S.G., Lee, C., Parks, W.T., Cho H.S., de Caestecker, M.P., Shaul, Y., Roberts, A.B. & Kim, S.J. (2001). The hepatitis B virus encoded oncoprotein pX amplifies TGF-β family signaling through direct interaction with Smad4: potential mechanism of hepatitis B virus-induced liver fibrosis. *Genes Dev* 15:455-466.

Lee, J.O., Kwun, H.J., Jung, J.K., Choi, K.H., Min, D.S. & Jang, K.L. (2005). Hepatitis B virus X protein represses E-cadherin expression via activation of DNA methyltransferase 1. *Oncogene* 24:6617-6625.

Lee, Y.I., Kang-Park, S., Do, S.I. & Lee, Y.I. (2001). The hepatitis B virus-X protein activates a phosphatidylinositol 3-kinase-dependent survival signaling cascade. *J Biol Chem* 276:16969-16977.

Lian, Z., Liu, J., Li, L., Li, X., Arbuthnot, P., Kew, M. & Feitelson, M.A. (2004). Human S15a is an effector which is up-regulated by HBV X protein. *Mol Carcinogen* 40:34-46.

Lian, Z., Liu, J., Li, L., Li, X., Clayton, M., Wu, M. C., Wang, H. Y., Arbuthnot, P., Kew, M. & Feitelson, M.A. (2006). Enhanced cell survival of Hep3B cells by the hepatitis B x antigen effector, URG11, is associated with up-regulation of β-catenin. *Hepatology* 43:415-424.

Lian Z. Liu J. Li, L. Li, X. Tufan, N.L., Clayton, M., Wu, M.C., Wang, H.Y., Arbuthnot, P.. Kew, M. & Feitelson, M.A. (2003). Up-regulated expression of a unique gene by hepatitis B x antigen promotes hepatocellular growth and tumorigenesis. *Neoplasia* 5:229-244.

Lian, Z., Liu, J., Pan, J., Tufan, N.L.S., Zhu, M., Arbuthnot, P., Kew, M., Clayton, M.M. & Feitelson M.A. (2001). A cellular gene up-regulated by hepatitis B virus encoded X antigen promotes hepatocellular growth and survival. *Hepatology* 34:146-157.

Lian, Z., Pan, J., Liu, J., Zhu, M., Arbuthnot, P., Kew, M.C. & Feitelson, M.A. (1999). The translation initiation factor, SUI1, may be a target of hepatitis B x antigen in hepatocarcinogenesis. *Oncogene* 18:1677-1687.

Liu, F., Li, B. & Nan, Y. (1999). The effect of serum TGFβ1 of patients with chronic hepatitis B in liver fibrosis. *Chin J Hepatol* 7:196-198.

Liu, J., Ahiekpor, A., Li, L., Li, X., Arbuthnot, P., Kew, M. & Feitelson, M.A. (2009). Increased expression of c-*erb*B-2 in liver is associated with HBxAg expression and shorter survival in patients with hepatocellular carcinoma. *Intl J Cancer* 125:1894-1901.

Liu, J., Lian, Z., Han, S., Waye, M.M.Y., Wang, H., Wu, M.C., Wu, K., Ding, J., Arbuthnot, P., Kew, M., Fan, D. & Feitelson, M.A. (2006). Down-regulation of E-cadherin by hepatitis B virus x antigen in hepatocellular carcinoma. *Oncogene* 25:1008-1017.

Liu, H., Shi, W., Luan, F., Xu, S., Yang, F., Sun, W., Liu, J. & Ma, C. (2010). Hepatitis B virus X protein up-regulates transcriptional activation of human telomerase reverse transcriptase. *Virus Genes* 40:174-182.

Martin-Lluesma, S., Schaeffer, C., Robert, E.I., van Breugel, P.C., Leupin, O., Hantz, O. & Strubin, M. (2008). Hepatitis B virus X protein affects S phase progression leading to chromosome segregation defects by binding to damaged DNA binding protein 1. *Hepatology* 48:1467-1476.

Martin-Vilchez, S., Sanz-Cameno, P., Rodriguez-Munoz, Y., Majano, P.L., Molina-Jimenez, F., Lopez-Cabrera, M., Moreno-Otero, R. & Lara-Pezzi, E. (2008). The hepatitis B virus X protein induces paracrine activation of human hepatic stellate cells. *Hepatology* 47:1872-1883.

Mathonnet, G., Lachance, S.. Alaoui-Jamali, M. & Drobetsky, E.A. (2004). Expression of hepatitis B virus X oncoprotein inhibits transcription-coupled nucleotide excision repair in human cells. *Mutat Res* 554:305-318.

Menard, S., Casalini, P., Campiglio, M., Pupa, S.M. & Tagliabue, E. (2002). Role of HER2/neu in tumor progression and therapy. *Cell Mol Life Sci* 61:2965-2978.

Menzo, S., Clementi, M., Alfani, E., Bagnarelli, P., Iacovacci, S., Manzin, A., Dandri, M., Natoli, G., Levrero, M. & Carloni, G. (1993). *Trans*-activation of epidermal growth factor receptor gene by the hepatitis B virus X-gene product. *Virology* 196:878-882.

Miyoshi, Y., Iwao, K., Nagasawa, Y., Aihara, T., Sasaki, Y., Imaoka, S., Murata, M., Shimano, T. & Nakamura, Y. (1998). Activation of the beta-catenin gene in primary hepatocellular carcinoma by somatic alterations involving exon 3. *Cancer Res* 58:2524-2527.

Molina-Jimenez, F., Benedicto, I., Murata, M., Martin-Vilchez, S., Seki T., Antonio Pintor-Toro, J., Tortolero, M., Moreno-Otero, R., Okazaki, K., Koike, K., Barbero, J.L., Matsuzaki, K., Majano, P.L. & Lopez-Cabrera, M. (2010). Expression of pituitary tumor-transforming gene 1 (PTTG1)/securin in hepatitis B virus (HBV)-associated liver diseases: evidence for an HBV X protein-mediated inhibition of PTTG1 ubiquitination and degradation. *Hepatology* 51:777-787.

Morin, P.J., Sparks, A.B., Korinek, V., Barker, N., Clevers, H., Vogelstein, B. & Kinzler, K.W. (1997). Activation of β-catenin-Tcf signaling in colon cancer by mutations in β-catenin or APC. *Science* 275:1787-1790.

Murata, M., Matsuzaki, K., Yoshida, K., Sekimoto, G., Tahashi, Y., Mori, S., Uemura, Y., Sakaida, N., Fujisawa, J., Seki, T., Kobayashi, K., Yokote, K., Koike, K. & Okazaki, K. (2009). Hepatitis B virus X protein shifts human hepatic transforming growth factor (TGF)-β signaling from tumor suppression to oncogenesis in early chronic hepatitis B. *Hepatology* 49:1203-1217.

Myullyla, R., Wang, C., Keikkinen, J., Juffer, A., Lampela, O. Risteli, M., Ruotsalainen, H., Salo, A. & Sipilä, L. (2007). Expanding the lysyl hydroxylase toolbox: New insights into the localization and activities of lysyl hydroxylase 3 (LH3). *J Cell Physiol* 212:323-329.

Neo, S.Y., Leow, C.K., Vega, V.B., Long, P.M., Islam, A.F.M., Lai, P.B.S., Liu, E.T. & Ren, E.C. (2004). Identification of discriminators of hepatoma by gene expression profiling using a minimal dataset approach. *Hepatology* 39:944-953.

Niu, Z.S. & Wang, M. (2005). Expression of c-erbB-2 and glutathione S-transferase-pi in hepatocellular carcinoma and its adjacent tissue. *World J Gastroenterol* 11:4404-4408.

Norton, P.A., Reis, M., Prince, S., Larkin, J., Pan, J., Liu, J., Gong, Q., Zhu, M. & Feitelson, M.A. (2004). Activation of fibronection gene expression by hepatitis B virus X antigen. *J Viral Hepat* 11:332-341.

Oishi, N., Shilagardi, K., Nakamoto, Y., Honda, M., Kaneko, S. & Murakami, S. (2007). Hepatitis B virus X protein overcomes oncogenic RAS-induced senescence in human immortalized cells. *Cancer Sci.* 98:1540-1548.

Olayioye, M.A., Neve, R.M., Lane, H.A. & Hynes, N.E. (2000). The ErbB signaling network: receptor heterodimerization in development and cancer. *EMBO J* 19:3159-3167.

Omenetti, A., Bass, L.M., Anders, R.A., Clemente, M.G., Francis, H.. Guy, C.D., McCall, S., Choi, S.S., Alpini, G.. Schwarz, K.B., Diehl, A.M. & Whitington, P.F. (2011). Hedgehog activity, epithelial-mesenchymal transitions, and biliary dysmorphogenesis in biliary atresia. *Hepatology* 53:1246-1258.

Omenetti, A. & Diehl, A.M. (2008). The adventures of sonic hedgehog in development and repair. II. Sonic hedgehog and liver development, inflammation, and cancer. *Am J Physiol - GI & Liver Physiol* 294:G595-G598.

Pan, J., Clayton, M.M. & Feitelson, M.A. (2004). Hepatitis B x antigen promotes transforming growth factor β1 (TGFβ1) activity by up-regulation of TGFβ1 and down-regulation of alpha 2- macroglobulin. *J Gen Virol* 85:275-282.

Pan, J., Duan, L.X., Sun, B.S. & Feitelson, M.A. (2001). Hepatitis B virus X protein decreases the anti-Fas induced apoptosis in human liver cells by inducing NF-κB. *J Gen Virol* 82(Part 1):171-182.

Pan, J., Lian, Z., Wallett, S. & Feitelson, M.A. (2007). The hepatitis B x antigen effector, URG7, blocks tumour necrosis factor alpha-mediated apoptosis by activation of phosphoinositol 3-kinase and beta-catenin. *J Gen Virol* 8:3275-3285.

Pang, R., Lee, T.K., Poon, R.T., Fan, S.T., Wong, K.B., Kwong, Y.L. & Tse, E. (2007). Pin1 interacts with a specific serine-proline motif of hepatitis B virus X-protein to enhance hepatocarcinogenesis. *Gastroenterology* 132:1088-1103.

Park, S.G., Chung, C., Kang, H., Kim, J.Y. & Jung, G. (2006). Up-regulation of cyclin D1 by HBx is mediated by NF-kappaB2/BCL3 complex through kappaB site of cyclin D1 promoter. J Biol Chem 281:31770-31777.

Park, S.H., Jung, J.K., Lim, J.S., Tiwari, I. & Jang, K.L. (2011). Hepatitis B virus X protein overcomes all-*trans*-retinoic acid-induced cellular senescence by down-regulating levels of p16 and p21 via DNA methylation. *J Gen Virol* 92:1309-1317.

Peifer, M. & Polakis, P. (2000). Wnt signaling in oncogenesis and embryogenesis—a look outside the nucleus. *Science* 287:1606-1609.

Pereira, T.A., Witek, R.P., Syn, W.K., Choi, S.S., Bradrick, S.. Karaca, G.F., Agboola, K.M., Jung, Y., Omenetti, A.. Moylan, C.A., Yang, L., Fernandez-Zapico, M.E., Jhaveri, R.. Shah, V.H., Pereira, F.E. & Diehl, A.M. (2010). Viral factors induce Hedgehog pathway activation in humans with viral hepatitis, cirrhosis, and hepatocellular carcinoma. *Lab Invest* 90:1690-1703.

Poon, R.T.P., Lau, C.P.K., Cheung, S.T., Yu, W.C. & Fan, S.T. (2003). Quantitative correlation of serum levels and tumor expression of vascular endothelial growth factor in patients with hepatocellular carcinoma. *Cancer Res* 63:3121-3126.

Pringle, J.R. & Hartwell, L.H. (1981). The Saccharomyces cerevisiae cell cycle. In: *The Molecular Biology of the Yeast Saccharomyces cerevisiae: Life Cycle and Inheritance.* Strathern, J.N., Jones, E.W. & Broach, J.R., eds. Cold Spring Harbor Laboratory Press, Cold Spring Harbor, N.Y., USA, p. 97-142.

Qadri, I., Fatima, K. & AbdeL-Hafiz, H. (2011). Hepatitis B virus X protein impedes the DNA repair via its association with transcription factor, TFIIH. *BMC Microbiol* 11:48.

Reed, S.I. (1980). The selection of S. cerevisiae mutants defective in the start event of cell division. *Genetics* 95, 561-577.

Rossner, M.T. (1992). Hepatitis B virus X-gene product: a promiscuous transcriptional activator. *J Med Virol* 36:101-117.

Salo, A.M., Wang, C., Sipila, L., Sormunen, R., Vapola, M., Kervinen, P., Ruotsalainen, H., Heikkinen, J. & Myllylä, R. (2006). Lysyl hydroxylase 3 (LH3) modifies proteins in the extracellular space, a novel mechanism for matrix remodeling. *J Cell Physiol* 207:644-653.

Sanderson, N., Factor, VB., Nagy, P., Kopp, J., Kondaiah, P., Wakefield, L., Roberts, A.B., Sporn, M.B. & Thorgeirsson, S.N. (1995). Hepatic expression of mature transforming growth factor β1 in transgenic mice results in multiple tissue lesions. *Proc Natl Acad Sci USA* 92:2572-2576.

Sauter, G., Moch, H., Moore, D., Carroll, P., Kerschmann, R. & Chew, K. (1993). Heterogeneity of erbB-2 gene amplification in bladder cancer. *Cancer Res* 53:2199-2203.

Schaap, P.J., de Groot, P.W., Muller, Y., van Griensven, L.J. & Visser, J. (1995). Molecular cloning and sequence of the cytoplasmic ribosomal protein S15a gene from Agaricus bisporus. *Exp Mycol* 19:160-162.

Shih, W.L., Kuo, M.L., Chuang, S.E., Cheng, A.L. & Doong, S.L. (2000). Hepatitis B virus X protein inhibits transforming growth factor-beta -induced apoptosis through the activation of phosphatidylinositol 3-kinase pathway. *J Biol Chem* 275:25858-25864.

Shih, W.L., Kuo, M.L., Chuang, S.E., Cheng, A.L. & Doong, S.L. (2003). Hepatitis B virus X protein activates a survival signaling by linking SRC to phosphatidylinositol 3-kinase. *J Biol Chem* 278:31807-31813.

Shin, E.C., Shin, J.S., Park, J.H., Kim, H. & Kim, S.J. (1999). Expression of Fas ligand in human hepatoma cell lines: role of hepatitis B virus X (HBx) in induction of Fas ligand. *Int J Cancer* 82:587-591.

Slamon, D.J., Clark, G.M., Wong, S.G., Levin, W.J., Ullrich, A. & McGuire, W.L. (1987). Human breast cancer: correlation of relapse and survival with amplification of the HER-2/neu oncogene. *Science* 235:177-182.

Soares, M.B., Ishii, D.N. & Efstratiadis, A. (1985). Developmental and tissue-specific expression of a family of transcripts related to rat insulin-like growth factor II mRNA. *Nucleic Acids Res* 14:1119-1134.

Spandau, D.F. & Lee, C.H. (1988). *Trans*-activation of viral enhancers by the hepatitis B virus X protein. *J Virol* 62:427-434.

Su, F. & Schneider, R.J. (1996). Hepatitis B virus HBx protein activates transcription factor NF-kappaB by acting on multiple cytoplasmic inhibitors of rel-related proteins. *J Virol* 70:4558-4566.

Su, J.L., Yang, P.C., Shih, J.Y., Yang, C.Y., Wei, L.H., Hsieh, C.Y., Chou, C.H., Jeng, Y.M., Wang, M.Y., Chang, K.J., Hung, M.C. & Kuo, M.L. (2006). The VEGF-C/Flt-4 axis promotes invasion and metastasis of cancer cells. *Cancer Cell* 9:209-223.

Su, Q., Liu, J.F., Zhang, S.X., Li, D.F. & Yang, J.J. (1994). Expression of insulin-like growth factor II in hepatitis B, cirrhosis and hepatocellular carcinoma: Its relationship with hepatitis B virus antigen expression. *Hepatology* 19:788-799.

Sung, W.K., Lu, Y., Lee, C.W., Zhang, D., Ronaghi, M &, Lee, C.G. (2009). Deregulated direct targets of the hepatitis B virus (HBV) protein, HBx, identified through chromatin immunoprecipitation and expression microarray profiling. *J Biol Chem* 284:21941-21954.

Takahashi, K., Suzuki, K. & Tsukatani, Y. (1997). Induction of tyrosine phosphorylation and association of β-catenin with EGF receptor upon tryptic digestion of quiescent cells at confluence. *Oncogene* 15:71-78.

Tanner, B., Kreutz, E., Weikel, W., Meinert, R., Oesch, F., Knapstein, P.G. & Becker, R. (1996). Prognostic significance of c-erbB-2 mRNA in ovarian cancinoma. *Gynecol Oncol* 62:268-77.

Tennant, B.C. & Gerin, J.L. (2001). The woodchuck model of hepatitis B virus infection. *Ilar J* 42:89-102.

Terradillos, O., Billet, O., Renard, C.A., Levy, R., Molina, T., Briand, P. & Buendia, M.A. (1997). The hepatitis B virus X gene potentiates c-myc-induced liver oncogenesis in transgenic mice. *Oncogene* 14:395-404.

Terris, B., Pineau, P., Bregeaud, L., Valla, D., Belghiti, J., Tiollais, P., Degott, C. & Dejean A. (1999). Close correlation between beta-catenin gene alterations and nuclear accumulation of the protein in human hepatocellular carcinoma. *Oncogene* 18:6583-6588.

Tsuge, M., Hiragam, N., Akiyamam, R., Tanakam, S., Matsushitam, M., Mitsuim, F., Abem, H., Kitamura, S., Hatakeyama, T., Kimura, T., Miki, D., Mori, N., Imamura, M., Takahashi, S., Hayes, C.N. & Chayama K. (2010). HBx protein is indispensable for development of viraemia in human hepatocyte chimeric mice. *J Gen Virol* 91:1854-1864.

Tufan, N.L.S, Dodurga, Y., Gok, D., Cetinkaya, A. & Feitelson, M.A. (2010). RNA interference-mediated URG4 gene silencing diminishes cyclin D1 mRNA expression in HepG2 cells. *Genet Mol Res* 9:1557-1567.

Tufan, N.L.S., Lian, Z., Liu, J., Pan, J., Arbuthnot, P., Kew, M., Clayton, M.M. & Feitelson, M.A. (2002). Hepatitis B x antigen stimulates expression of a novel cellular gene, URG4, that promotes hepatocellular growth and survival. *Neoplasia* 4:355-368.

Twu, J.S. & Schloemer, R.H. (1987). Transcriptional *trans*-activating function of hepatitis B virus. *J Virol* 61:3448-3453.

Ueda, H., Ullrich, S.J., Ngo, L., Gangemi, D., Kappel, C.A., Feitelson, M.A. & Jay, G. (1995). Functional inactivation but not structural mutation of p53 causes liver cancer. *Nat Genet* 9: 41-47.

Varner, J.A., Emerson, D.A. & Juliano, R.L. (1995). Integrin alpha 5 beta 1 expression negatively regulates cell growth: reversal by attachment to fibronectin. *Mol Biol Cell* 6:725-740.

Vlasoff, D.M., Baschinsky, D.D.Y., De Young, B.R., Morrison, C.D., Nuovo, G.J. & Frankel, W.L. (2002). C-erb B2 (HER2/neu) is neither over-expressed nor amplified in hepatic neoplasms. *Applied Immunohistochem Mol Morphol* 10:237-241.

Wang, W., London, W.T., Lega, L. & Feitelson, M.A. (1991a). Hepatitis B x antigen in liver from carrier patients with chronic hepatitis and cirrhosis. *Hepatology* 14:29-37.

Wang, W., London, W.T., & Feitelson, M.A. (1991b). Hepatitis B x antigen in hepatitis B virus carrier patients with liver cancer. *Cancer Res* 51:4971-4977.

Wang, X.W., Forrester, K., Yeh, H., Feitelson, M.A., Gu, J.-r. & Harris, C.C. (1994). Hepatitis B virus X protein inhibits p53 sequence-specific DNA binding, transcriptional activity and association with ERCC3. *Proc Natl Acad Sci (USA) 91:2230-2234.*

Wei, C., Ni, C., Song, T., Liu, Y., Yang, X., Zheng, Z., Jia, Y., Yuan, Y., Guan, K., Xu, Y., Cheng, X., Zhang, Y., Yang, X., Wang, Y., Wen, C., Wu, Q., Shi, W. & Zhong, H. (2010). The hepatitis B virus X protein disrupts innate immunity by down-regulating mitochondrial antiviral signaling protein. *J Immunol* 185:1158-1168.

Weng, H.L., Liu, Y., Chen, J.L., Huang, T., Xu, L.J., Godoy, P.. Hu, J.H., Zhou, C., Stickel, F., Marx, A., Bohle, R.M., Zimmer, V., Lammert, F., Mueller, S., Gigou, M., Samuel, D., Mertens, P.R., Singer, M.V., Seitz, H.K. & Dooley, S. (2009). The etiology of liver damage imparts cytokines transforming growth factor beta1 or interleukin-13 as driving forces in fibrogenesis. *Hepatology* 50:230-243.

Wu, G.C., Forgues, M., Siddique, S., Farnsworth, J., Valerie, K. & Wang, X.W. (2002). SAGE transcript profiles of normal primary human hepatocytes expressing oncogenic hepatitis B virus X protein. *FASEB J* 16:1665-1667.

Wu, G.C., Salvay, D.M., Forgues, M., Valerie, K., Farnsworth, J., Markin, R.S. & Wang, X.W. (2001). Distinctive gene expression profiles associated with hepatitis B x protein. *Oncogene* 20:3674-3682.

Wu, G., Yu, F., Xiao, Z., Xu, K., Xu, J., Tang, W., Wang, J. & Song, E. (2011). Hepatitis B virus X protein down-regulates expression of the miR-16 family in malignant hepatocytes *in vitro*. *Br J Cancer* 105:146-153.

Xu, J., Yun, X., Jiang, J., Wei, Y., Wu, Y., Zhang, W., Liu, Y., Wang, W., Wen,Y. & Gu, J. (2010). Hepatitis B virus X protein blunts senescence-like growth arrest of human hepatocellular carcinoma by reducing Notch1 cleavage. *Hepatology* 52:142-154.

Yang, L., Ma, Z., Wang, D., Zhao, W., Chen, L., Wang, G. (2010). MicroRNA-602 regulating tumor suppressive gene RASSF1A is overexpressed in hepatitis B virus-infected liver and hepatocellular carcinoma. *Cancer Biol Ther* 9:803-808.

Yang, S.Z., Zhang, L.D., Zhang, Y.. Xiong, Y.. Zhang, Y.J., Li, H.L., Li, X.W. & Dong, J.H. (2009). HBx protein induces EMT through c-Src activation in SMMC-7721 hepatoma cell line. *Biochem Biophys Res Commun* 382:555-560.

Yarden, Y. & Sliwkowski, M.X. (2001). Untangling the ErbB signaling network. *Nat Rev Mol Cell Biol* 2:127-137.

Yoo, Y.D., Ueda, H., Park, K., Flanders, K.C., Lee, Y.I., Jay, G. & Kim, S.J. (1996). Regulation of transforming growth factor-beta 1 expression by the hepatitis B virus (HBV) X transactivator. Role in HBV pathogenesis. *J Clin Invest* 97:388-395.

Yoo, Y.G., Oh, S.H., Park, E.S., Cho, H., Lee, N., Park, H., Kim, D.K., Yu, D.Y,, Seong, J.K. & Lee, M.O. (2003). Hepatitis B virus X protein enhances transcriptional activity of hypoxia-inducible factor-1alpha through activation of mitogen-activated protein kinase pathway. *J Biol Chem* 278:39076-39084.

Yoon, H. & Donahue, T.F. (1992). The suil suppressor locus in Saccharomyces cerevisiae encodes a translation factor that functions during tRNA(iMet) recognition of the start codon. *Mol Cell Biol* 12:248-260.

Zhang, Z., Sun, E., Ou, J.H. & Liang, T.J. (2010). Inhibition of cellular proteasome activities mediates HBX-independent hepatitis B virus replication in vivo. *J Virol* 84:9326-9331.

Zhang, Z., Torii, N., Furusaka, A., Malayaman, N., Hu, Z. & Liang, T.J. (2000). Structural and functional characterization of interaction between hepatitis B virus X protein and the proteasome complex. *J Biol Chem* 275:15157-15165.

Zhang Z. Torii N. Hu Z. Jacob J. Liang TJ. (2001). X-deficient woodchuck hepatitis virus mutants behave like attenuated viruses and induce protective immunity *in vivo*. *J Clin Invest* 108:1523-1531.

Zhang Z. Protzer U. Hu Z. Jacob J. Liang TJ. (2004). Inhibition of cellular proteasome activities enhances hepadnavirus replication in an HBX-dependent manner. *J Virol* 78:4566-4572.

Zheng, D.L., Zhang, L., Cheng, N., Xu, X., Deng, Q., Teng, X.M., Wang, K.S., Zhang, X., Huang, J. & Han, Z.G. (2009). Epigenetic modification induced by hepatitis B virus X protein via interaction with de novo DNA methyltransferase DNMT3A. *J Hepatol* 50:377-387.

Zoulim, F., Saputelli, J. & Seeger, C. (1994). Woodchuck hepatitis virus X protein is required for viral infection in vivo. *J Virol* 68:2026-2030.

# 15

# Molecular Mechanism of DNA Damage Response Pathway During Hepatic Carcinogenesis

Yasunobu Matsuda[1] and Toshifumi Wakai[2]
[1]*Department of Medical Technology, Niigata University Graduate School of Health Sciences*
[2]*Division of Digestive and General Surgery, Niigata University Graduate School of Medical and Dental Sciences*
*Japan*

## 1. Introduction

Hepatocellular carcinoma (HCC) is one of the most common cancers worldwide. The prevalence of HCC is still increasing in Asia and Africa, and represents a leading cause of death among patients with chronic liver diseases in industrial countries including Europe and North America (Llovet et al., 2003). The prognosis of HCC is considerably poor for following reasons: (1) aggressive treatment for HCC is not usually possible because most of the patients have impaired liver function, (2) hepatoma cells are refractory to standard chemotherapy drugs and radiation, and (3) HCC frequently recurs even after curative resection (Poon et al., 2009). Moreover, owing to the lack of reliable clinical HCC markers, fewer than 20% of patients are diagnosed at a stage where curative treatment can be performed (Llovet et al., 2003).

HCC is unique among the various types of malignancies, in that it frequently arises in individuals with hepatitis B virus (HBV)- and C virus (HCV)-related liver cirrhosis. Although the precise mechanism of the relationship between the hepatitis viruses and hepatocarcinogenesis is unknown, recent studies have suggested that an aberrant response against DNA damage might be involved in HBV- and HCV-induced carcinogenesis, as observed in many types of cancer cells. Therefore, for future development of treatments against HCC, understanding the functional role of the DNA damage response (DDR) in HCC-prone individuals would be of value.

## 2. Impact of oxidative DNA damage during hepatocarcinogenesis

Many previous studies have indicated a close relationship between metal overload and oxidative DNA damage (Imlay et al., 1988). For example, when DNA is exposed to hydrogen peroxide with iron, the Fenton reaction, in which hydrogen peroxide ($H_2O_2$) is catalysed to hydroxyl radicals (OH•) by iron (II) (Lloyd et al., 1998), causes the production of carcinogenic malondialdehyde, 4-hydroxynonenal (4-HNE) and other exocyclic DNA adducts including 8-hydroxy-2'-deoxyguanosine (8-OHdG) (Jomova et al., 2011). Among these products, 8-OHdG is considered to be an oxidative DNA marker produced by reactive oxygen species (ROS), because the numbers of 8-OHdG-positive hepatocytes are significantly increased with progression of the severity of chronic hepatitis activity (Kitada et al., 2001; Ichiba et al., 2003) with iron content (Tanaka et al., 2008). Kato et al. (2001) investigated whether therapeutic iron reduction by phlebotomy with a low-iron diet could decrease the risk of HCC development in patients with chronic HCV. They found that patients treated with phlebotomy for 6 years showed significantly decreased levels of 8-OHdG in the liver, with improved severity of chronic hepatitis. Interestingly, all the patients who received phlebotomy did not develop HCC, suggesting a strong correlation between oxidative DNA damage and hepatocarcinogenesis. Subsequent studies reported that the level of hepatic 8-OHdG can be a predictive factor for the risk of recurrence in HCC patients after surgery (Matsumoto et al., 2003; Tanaka et al., 2008) and for individuals with naive chronic HCV infection (Chuma et al., 2008).

Intracellular ROS not only induce DNA damage but also regulate various types of intracellular signaling. In hepatoma cells, ROS potentiate cell growth by activating the signaling pathways of the stress kinases Akt, extracellular signal-regulated kinase (ERK) and Jun N-terminal kinase (JNK) (Liu et al., 2002). On the other hand, ROS accelerate tumor invasiveness in many types of cancers. In the case of hepatoma cells, Lim et al. (2008) reported tight correlations among ROS induction, E-cadherin downregulation, Snail upregulation and E-cadherin promoter methylation (Lim et al., 2008). Since E-cadherin is a master regulator of the epithelial-to-mesenchymal transition in HCC cells, it is plausible that tumor invasiveness is significantly accelerated by ROS. Importantly, recent studies have revealed that hepatitis viruses might have the property of producing ROS, supporting the idea that oxidative DNA damage might be directly induced in viral hepatitis.

### 2.1 Causative risk for HCC and ROS

#### 2.1.1 HBV and ROS

Chronic HBV infection is still prevalent in Asia and Africa, and is one of the most important risk factors for HCC. HBV encodes HBV X (HBx), surface (HBs), core (HBc) and pol genes, and among these, HBx is widely considered to be a potent inducer of HCC. Many studies have reported that HBx transactivates the host genome (Twu et al., 1989; Feitelson et al., 1999), leading to deregulation of the cell cycle checkpoints. Intriguingly, a crucial role of HBx in oxidative DNA damage has recently been reported. Lee et al. (2004) reported that HBx downregulates the mitochondrial enzymes involved in electron transport in oxidative phosphorylation. They found that HBx increases the levels of mitochondrial ROS and lipid peroxide production, suggesting that HBx-induced mitochondrial dysfunction might be one of the main reasons for HCC development. A close relationship between iron metabolism and the ROS level in HBX-expressing cells was reported by Gu et al. (2008), who showed that HBx decreases transferrin receptor 1 expression through downregulation of iron regulatory protein 1 and upregulation of ferritin heavy chain expression with ROS production. Intriguingly, HBx-mediated ROS induction also causes DNA hypermethylation. HBx of genotype D HBV causes hypermethylation of the gene promoter of glutathione S-transferase GSTP1, which is a candidate enzyme for protecting cells against ROS with related toxic products (Niu et al., 2009). In turn, ROS stimulate HBx expression (Ha et al., 2010), suggesting that ROS may be an autocrine transducer of HBx-mediated carcinogenesis. Very recently, HBX was shown to activate the transcriptional activity of Forkhead box class O 4 (Foxo4) via JNK, leading to enhancement of the resistance to oxidative stress-induced cell death (Srisuttee et al., 2011).

### 2.1.2 HCV and ROS

HCV infection is a leading cause of HCC development throughout the world. Several lines of evidence have suggested that HCV plays a critical role in the state of oxidative stress in the liver. HCV is constructed of core, E1, E2 and nonstructural (NS2, NS3, NS4A, NS4B, NS5, NS5A, NS5B) proteins, and each of these encoded proteins has been shown to be essential for the pathogenesis of HCV. HCV core protein plays a role in cell proliferation, while NS5A interacts with the double-stranded RNA-dependent PKR to promote viral replication. Many studies have revealed that chronic HCV infection leads to double-stranded DNA breaks and enhances the mutation frequency of whole cellular genes (Machida et al., 2004). Okuda et al. (2002) reported that HCV core protein localizes to mitochondria, leading to redistribution of cytochrome c from the mitochondria to the cytoplasm. Their data clearly indicate that HCV can be a direct source of ROS production. Moreover, HCV core protein has been shown to be strongly associated with the outer membrane of mitochondria to increase $Ca^{2+}$ uptake, leading to oxidation of the glutathione pool and a decrease in the NADPH content in vivo (Korenaga et al., 2005). Recently, the mechanism by which hepatic iron overload develops in patients with HCV-associated chronic liver disease has been elucidated. Miura et al. (2008) reported that hepcidin, which plays a pivotal role as a negative regulator of iron absorption, was significantly decreased in HCV replicon cells and HCV core-expressing cells. Their findings should be important, because the decreased level of hepcidin may lead to increased duodenal iron transport as well as macrophage iron release, thereby causing hepatic iron accumulation. Since increased activity of histone deacetylase (HDAC) was found to be the main reason for the decreased levels of hepcidin (Miura et al., 2008), HDAC may play a critical role in HCV-related hepatocarcinogenesis.

### 2.1.3 Alcohol consumption and ROS

It is widely known that ethanol is a strong inducer of DNA damage. The ethanol derivative acetaldehyde causes DNA damage by directly binding to DNA and inhibiting DNA repair systems (Seitz et al., 2006). Furthermore, ethanol treatment increases the production of intracellular ROS and lowers the levels of antioxidants, leading to enhancement of oxidative stress (Wu et al., 2009). Ethanol-induced oxidative stress plays a critical role in the pathogenesis of DNA damage as well as liver injury, and mitochondrial dysfunction is also induced by oxidation of various mitochondrial proteins (Suh et al., 2004). One of the most well-known mediators of alcohol-induced ROS is cytochrome P450 2E1 (CYP2E1) (Lu et al., 2008; Wu et al., 2009; Beier et al., 2010). CYP2E1 is an important enzyme for the conversion of ethanol to acetaldehyde and acetate, and is involved in the metabolism of xenobiotics. Ethanol intoxication increases CYP2E1 not only in the endoplasmic reticulum but also in mitochondria, leading to oxidative stress in these compartments (Robin et al., 2005). Intriguingly, Wang et al. (2009) reported that both protein-bound 4-HNE and etheno-DNA adducts were strongly correlated with cytochrome P450 2E1 (CYP2E1) expression in patients with alcoholic liver diseases. More importantly, Tsutsumi et al. (2003) reported the mechanism of the synergic enhancement of ROS production by HCV infection and alcohol consumption. They reported that HCV core protein cooperates with ethanol for activation of ERK and p38 mitogen-activated protein kinase (MAPK) pathways, leading to a decreased level of glutathione S-transferase (GST). Since GST plays a key role in protecting cells against oxidative stress, it is plausible that ethanol consumption would worsen the pathogenesis of the liver disease in HCV-infected patients. Thus, there is no doubt that alcohol consumption enhances DNA damage and is a strong promoter of hepatocarcinogenesis in individuals with chronic viral hepatitis.

### 2.1.4 Nonalcoholic steatohepatitis and ROS

To date, the prevalence of nonalcoholic fatty liver disease (NAFLD), including its aggressive type nonalcoholic steatohepatitis (NASH), has been increasing in developed countries. NASH may account for a large proportion of idiopathic or cryptogenic cirrhosis, as well as HCC in individuals with non-B non-C hepatitis (Mori et al., 2004; Starley et al., 2010). It has been suggested that ROS induced by mitochondrial dysfunction may play a key role in the mechanism of NAFLD (Pérez-Carreras et al., 2003), and growing evidence suggests that the ethanol-inducible cytochrome CYP2E1 is involved in the pathological conditions of NASH (Lieber, 2004). CYP2E1 expression and activities are frequently increased in the livers of NASH patients (Weltman et al., 1998; Chalasani et al., 2003), indicating that CYP2E1 may promote cellular injury (Robertson et al., 2001). However, since CYP2E1 is an ethanol-inducible enzyme, the reason why this enzyme is induced in NAFLD patients remains unknown. In this regard, Baker et al. (2010) reported that the genes for alcohol dehydrogenase, catalase and aldehyde dehydrogenase were elevated in the liver of NASH patients. They suggested that these genes may be partly induced by certain intestinal bacteria, especially in obese individuals. Further studies are awaited for more understanding of the mechanism of the cancer development in NASH patients.

## 3. DDR machinery

As mentioned above, intracellular ROS are potent inducers of oxidative DNA damage. ROS are produced by a variety of types of environmental stimuli, including ultraviolet light, ionizing radiation and chemical agents (Bertram et al., 2008). When organisms are exposed to such stimuli during cell division, genomic instability and DNA replication errors are easily caused, which may be the first step for cancer development or premature aging. To prevent such errors of DNA replication, a strict DDR system is highly conserved among mammals and induces cell cycle arrest or apoptosis. The DDR is mainly regulated by two phosphatidylinositol-3-related kinases, ataxia telangiectasia mutated (ATM) and ATM-Rad3-related (ATR), and the cell cycle checkpoint kinases Chk1 and Chk2 (Poehlmann et al., 2010). ATM is exclusively activated by DNA double-strand breaks induced by ionizing irradiation, whereas ATR is mainly stimulated by disrupted DNA replication forks caused by stimuli such as ultraviolet light and hydroxyurea (Abraham, 2001). During the process of DDR or stalled DNA replication, the ATM and ATR-mediated pathways interact with each other to phosphorylate histone H2AX, and MDC1, 53BP1, BRCA1 and MRE11 are recruited for phosphorylation. The Chk1 and Chk2 kinases are activated to regulate

Cdc25, Weel and p53, and finally cyclin-dependent kinases (Cdks) are inactivated to induce cell cycle arrest (Kawabe, 2004; Iliakis et al., 2008). To date, there have been many studies showing that these DDR-associated proteins are functionally deregulated in cancer cells. Of note, recent studies revealed that hepatitis viruses are considerably involved in the regulation of the DDR machinery.

### 3.1 HBV and the DDR

It is well known that HBX has the capacity to transform cells both in vitro and in vivo (Shirakata et al., 1989; Kim et al., 1991). Although the precise mechanism of HBx-mediated carcinogenesis is unclear, recent studies have suggested that HBV directly interferes with the DDR (Groisman et al., 1999; Matsuda et al., 2009). Zhao et al. (2008) reported that HBV infection stimulates the steady state of ATR with downstream targets including Chk1, p53 and gamma-H2AX, while the activity of ATM-Chk2 signaling is unchanged. Along with the ATR-mediated response to the replication stress, HBV-infected cells may acquire survival potential toward DNA damage. Wang et al. (2008) reported that HBX activates p38 MAPK and its Cdk4 and Cdk2, leading to phosphorylation of Rb and transcription of ARF. Accordingly, HBx-mediated p38 MAPK signaling sensitizes the cells to p53-mediated apoptosis by activating ATR, which leads to phosphorylation of p53. Wu et al. (2008) reported that HBx-transformed cells show defective S-phase arrest and consequent G2/M arrest after DNA damage induced by mitomycin C. Importantly, they also found that HBx impairs the ATR-dependent phosphorylation of Chk1 and monoubiquitination of FANCD2, suggesting that the defect in the intra-S-phase checkpoint may be the reason for genomic instability. Studach et al. (2009) reported that HBx-induced polyploid cells showed continued DNA damage after long repopulation, which was associated with loss of p53 function. They suggested that polo-like kinase 1 (Plk1), which is frequently overexpressed in human HCC, might play an important role in the acquisition of HBx-induced DNA damage. Interestingly, HBX-mediated Plk1 activation reduces claspin, an adaptor of ATR-mediated Chk1 phosphorylation, leading to inactivation of Chk1 and finally allowing the propagation of DNA damage (Studach et al., 2010). These lines of evidence may explain why Chk1 is inactivated in the presence of ATR activation in HBV-infected cells. Interestingly, Zheng et al. (2011) reported that HBV exploits the activated DDR, and that ATR and ATM kinase inhibitors, such as theophylline, significantly reduce the yield of HBV DNA. Collectively, HBx and DDR are closely linked in a tight loop, not only from the viewpoint of hepatocarcinogenesis but also from the viral life cycle.

When normal cells are exposed to stimuli that cause DNA damage, the well-known tumor suppressor p53 is transcriptionally activated to stimulate DNA damage repair proteins or induce apoptosis. Prost et al. (1998) suggested that HBx might inhibit the p53-dependent DNA repair system, since the efficiency of DNA repair is decreased in HBx-expressing p53-wild-type cells to the level of p53-null hepatocytes. Jia et al. (1999) reported that HBx functionally binds to p53 as well as p53-associated DNA repair factors, leading to impaired p53-downstream signaling. They also found that HBx not only binds to p53 but also to p53 partners, and TFIIH transcription-nucleotide excision repair factors such as the DNA helicases XPB and XPD. Since HBx strongly induces DNA damage via multiple pathways (Fig. 1), it is plausible that other DNA-damaging agents could significantly promote the tumorigenesis in individuals with chronic HBV infection (Lee et al., 2005).

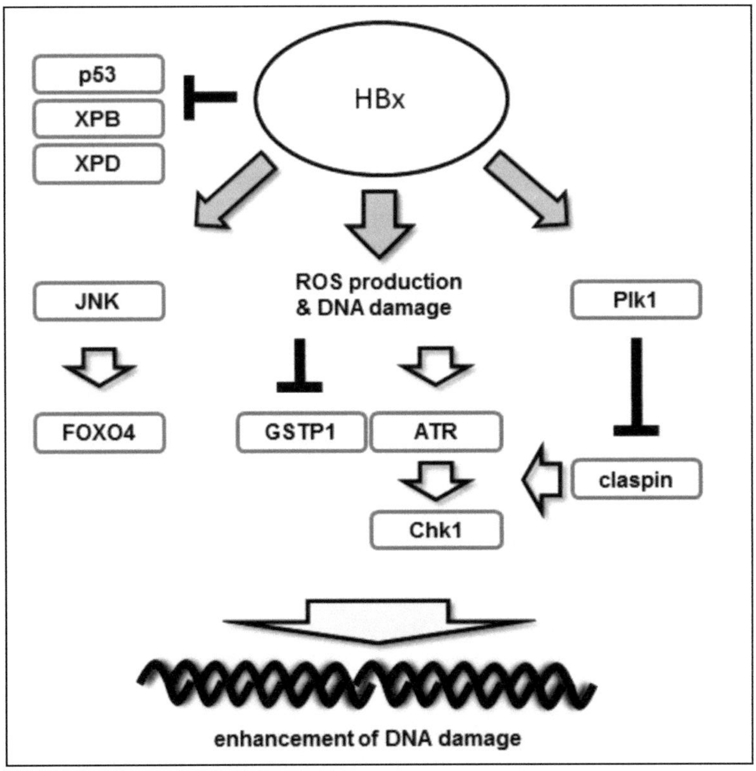


Fig. 1. Functional role of HBx in the DNA repair machinery.

HBx induces mitochondrial ROS production, followed by oxidative DNA damage. HBx inactivates claspin via Plk, modulates the GSTP1 gene promoter and activates FOXO4, thereby weakening the DNA damage repair response. Moreover, HBx binds to p53, leading to inhibition of p53-mediated antitumor activity.

### 3.2 HCV and the DDR

Recently, the functional role of HCV in DNA repair processes has been clarified, and its mechanism appears to be more complex than that of HBV. Lai et al. (2008) reported that HCV nonstructural proteins NS3 and NS4A translocate ATM into the cytoplasm. In the presence of DNA damage, NS3A and NS4A were shown to delay the dephosphorylation of activated ATM and gamma-H2AX. As a result, ATM-mediated DNA repair might be impaired in HCV-infected cells, leading to an increase in double-stranded DNA breaks. Similarly, Machida et al. (2010) reported that peripheral blood mononuclear cells from HCV-infected patients show frequent chromosomal aberrations with impaired nonhomologous end-joining repair, suggesting that HCV NS3 might be partly responsible for the inhibition of DNA repair. Taken together, HCV may directly inhibit the DNA repair processes not only in hepatocytes but also in monocytes, where HCV-associated lymphoma could develop. On the other hand, HCV core protein was shown to bind to the DNA repair protein NBS1 to inhibit the formation of the Mre11/NBS1/Rad50 complex, a keystone complex connecting the ATM-mediated DNA repair machinery (Machida et al., 2010). Intriguingly, Ariumi et al. (2008) reported that replication of HCV RNA was suppressed in ATM- or Chk2-knockdown cells, suggesting that the ATM signaling pathway is critical for HCV RNA replication. These lines of evidence strongly indicate that a tight relationship between HCV and the ATM-mediated DDR machinery may exist.

Although the mechanism of HCV-DNA damage is unclear, some studies have suggested that this might be partly caused by aberrant function of p53. Nishimura et al. (2009) reported that HCV induces overexpression of 3beta-hydroxysterol Delta24-reductase (DHCR24), which causes accumulation of the MDM2-p53 complex in the cytoplasm and inhibits the acetylation and activation of p53 in the nucleus. Their findings may explain how HCV-infected cells acquire resistance to oxidative stress-induced apoptosis. Recently, HCV-encoding proteins were shown to independently interact with p53. One of the most potent candidates for p53 inactivation is HCV NS5A. NS5A physiologically associates with p53, leading to localization of the p53-NS5A complex in the perinuclear membrane. In this setting, the NS5A-p53 complex inhibits p53-mediated transcriptional activation from a synthetic promoter containing multiple p53-binding sites, leading to transcriptional repression of the p21/waf1 gene (Majumder et al., 2001). Moreover, NS5A forms a heteromeric complex with TATA box binding protein (TBP) and p53. The binding of NS5A to p53 and TBP may abrogate their interaction with the DNA consensus, and the formation of p53-TBP and p53-excision repair cross complementing factor 3 (ERCC3) protein-protein complex would be impaired (Qadri et al., 2002; Gong et al., 2004). Similar to NS5A, the HCV core was also shown to colocalize with p53 in subnuclear granular structures and in the perinuclear area, and to repress the activity of p53 (Smirnova et al., 2006). It has been suggested that the HCV core can interfere with p53-mediated signaling in several ways, such as physical interactions, modulation of p53 gene regulatory activity and post-translational modification (Kao et al., 2004). Collectively, HCV should be regarded as a direct inhibitor of DNA repair by inducing intracellular ROS, abrogating the ATM-mediated DDR and inhibiting p53 activity (Fig. 2).

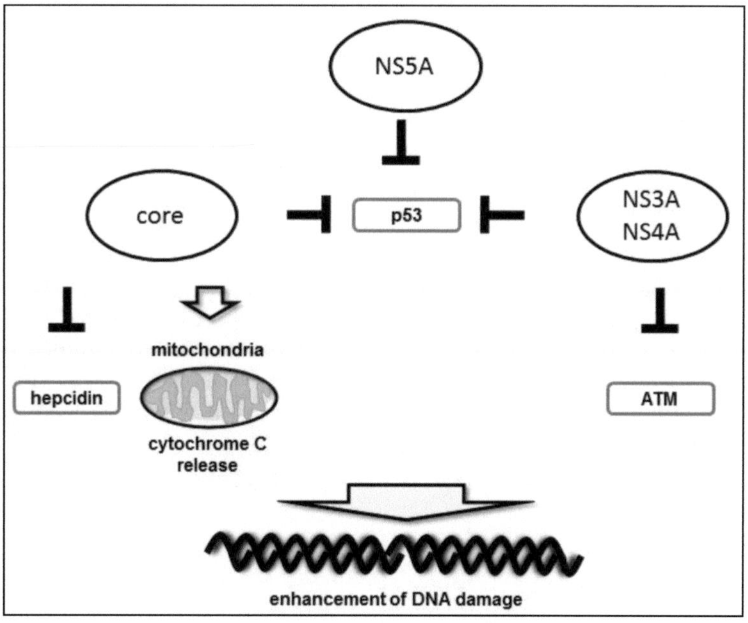


Fig. 2. Functional role of HCV in the DNA repair machinery.

HCV-encoded proteins independently interfere with the DNA damage repair machinery. The NS3A and NS4A proteins inhibit ATM signaling through cytoplasmic sequestration, while the NS5A protein binds and inhibits p53. The core protein induces mitochondrial ROS, while inhibiting hepcidin, leading to an increased iron load. **ATM**, ataxia telangiectasia mutated.

## 4. Conclusions

To date, newly developed antiviral drugs, such as nucleotide analogs and interferon, have been introduced in the management of individuals with chronic HBV or HCV infection. Unfortunately, the clinical evidence suggests that their therapeutic efficacy is still less than satisfactory. Many patients have to discontinue the antiviral therapy owing to side effects or lower efficacy of the treatment, implying that they face the risk of cancer development. Even when not infected with hepatitis viruses, some obese individuals have a high risk of HCC development induced by NASH. Since there are no useful curative treatments for HCC, the need to prevent the early step of hepatocarcinogenesis is inevitable. Many studies have shown that the DNA damage repair system might be considerably involved in HCC development, irrespective of the different etiologies. Novel treatments for preventing DNA damage and/or potentiating the cellular capacity of DNA damage repair are under investigation and the results are awaited.

## 5. References

Abraham, RT. (2001). Cell cycle checkpoint signaling through the ATM and ATR kinases. *Genes Dev*, Vol.15, No.17, pp. 2177–2196

Ariumi, Y., Kuroki, M., Dansako, H., Abe, K., Ikeda, M., Wakita, T. & Kato, N. (2008). The DNA damage sensors ataxia-telangiectasia mutated kinase and checkpoint kinase 2 are required for hepatitis C virus RNA replication. *J Virol*, Vol.82, No.19, 9639-9646

Baker, SS., Baker, RD., Liu, W., Nowak, NJ. & Zhu, L. (2010). Role of alcohol metabolism in non-alcoholic steatohepatitis. *PLoS One*, Vol.5, No.3, pp. e9570

Beier, JI. & McClain, CJ. (2010). Mechanisms and cell signaling in alcoholic liver disease. *Biol Chem*, Vol.391, No.11, pp. 1249-1264

Bertram, C.& Hass, R. (2008). Cellular responses to reactive oxygen species-induced DNA damage and aging. *Biol Chem*, Vol.389, No.3, pp. 211-220

Chalasani, N., Gorski, JC., Asghar, MS., Asghar, A., Foresman, B., Hall, SD. & Crabb, DW. (2003). Hepatic cytochrome P450 2E1 activity in nondiabetic patients with nonalcoholic steatohepatitis. *Hepatology*, Vol.37, No.3, pp. 544-550

Chuma, M., Hige, S., Nakanishi, M., Ogawa, K., Natsuizaka, M., Yamamoto, Y. & Asaka, M. (2008). 8-Hydroxy-2'-deoxy-guanosine is a risk factor for development of hepatocellular carcinoma in patients with chronic hepatitis C virus infection. *J Gastroenterol Hepatol*, Vol.23, No.9, pp. 1431-1436

Feitelson, MA. (1999). Hepatitis B virus in hepatocarcinogenesis. *J Cell Physiol*, Vol.181, No.2, pp. 188–202

Gong, GZ., Jiang, YF., He, Y., Lai, LY., Zhu, YH. & Su, XS. (2004). HCV NS5A abrogates p53 protein function by interfering with p53-DNA binding. *World J Gastroenterol*, Vol.10, No.15, pp. 2223-2227

Groisman, IJ., Koshy, R., Henkler, F., Groopman, JD. & Alaoui-Jamali, MA. (1999). Downregulation of DNA excision repair by the hepatitis B virus-x protein occurs in p53-proficient and p53-deficient cells. *Carcinogenesis*, Vol.20, No.3, pp. 479-483

Gu, JM., Lim, SO., Oh, SJ., Yoon, SM., Seong, JK. & Jung, G. (2008). HBx modulates iron regulatory protein 1-mediated iron metabolism via reactive oxygen species. *Virus Res*, Vol.133, No.2, pp. 167-177

Ha, HL. & Yu, DY. (2010). HBx-induced reactive oxygen species activates hepatocellular carcinogenesis via dysregulation of PTEN/Akt pathway. *World J Gastroenterol*, Vol.16, No.39, pp. 4932-4937

Ichiba, M., Maeta, Y., Mukoyama, T., Saeki, T., Yasui, S., Kanbe, T., Okano, J., Tanabe, Y., Hirooka, Y., Yamada, S., Kurimasa, A., Murawaki, Y. & Shiota G. (2003). Expression of 8-hydroxy-2'-deoxyguanosine in chronic liver disease and hepatocellular carcinoma. *Liver Int*, Vol.23, No.5, pp. 338-345

Iliakis, G., Wu, W. & Wang, M. (2008). DNA double strand break repair inhibition as a cause of heat radiosensitization: re-evaluation considering backup pathways of NHEJ. *Int J Hyperthermia*, Vol.24, No.1, pp. 17-29

Imlay, JA. & Linn, S. (1988). DNA damage and oxygen radical toxicity. *Science*, Vol.240, No.4857, pp. 1302-1309"

Jia, L., Wang, XW. & Harris, CC. (1999). Hepatitis B virus X protein inhibits nucleotide excision repair. *Int J Cancer*, Vol.80, No.6, pp. 875-879

Jomova, K. & Valko, M. (2011). Advances in metal-induced oxidative stress and human disease. *Toxicology*, Vol.283, No.2-3, pp. 65-87

Kao, CF., Chen, SY., Chen, JY. & Wu Lee, YH. (2004). Modulation of p53 transcription regulatory activity and post-translational modification by hepatitis C virus core protein. *Oncogene*, Vol.23, No.14, pp. 2472-2483

Kato, J., Kobune, M., Nakamura, T., Kuroiwa, G., Takada, K., Takimoto, R., Sato, Y., Fujikawa, K., Takahashi, M., Takayama, T., Ikeda, T. & Niitsu, Y. (2001). Normalization of elevated hepatic 8-hydroxy-2'-deoxyguanosine levels in chronic hepatitis C patients by phlebotomy and low iron diet. *Cancer Res*, Vol.61, No.24, pp. 8697-8702

Kawabe, T. (2004). G2 checkpoint abrogators as anticancer drugs. *Mol Cancer Ther*, Vol.3, No.4, pp. 513-519

Kim, CM., Koike, K., Saito, I., Miyamura, T. & Jay, G. (1991). HBX gene of hepatitis B virus induces liver cancer in transgenic mice. *Nature*, Vol.351, No.6324, pp. 317–320

Kitada, T., Seki, S., Iwai, S., Yamada, T., Sakaguchi, H. & Wakasa, K. (2001). In situ detection of oxidative DNA damage, 8-hydroxydeoxyguanosine, in chronic human liver disease. *J Hepatol*,Vol.35, No.5, pp. 613-618

Korenaga, M., Wang, T., Li, Y., Showalter, LA., Chan, T., Sun, J. & Weinman, SA. (2005). Hepatitis C virus core protein inhibits mitochondrial electron transport and increases reactive oxygen species (ROS) production. *J Biol Chem*, Vol.280, No.45, pp. 37481-37488

Lai, CK., Jeng, KS., Machida, K., Cheng, YS. & Lai, MM. (2008). Hepatitis C virus NS3/4A protein interacts with ATM, impairs DNA repair and enhances sensitivity to ionizing radiation. *Virology*, Vol.370, No.2, pp. 295-309

Lee, AT., Ren, J., Wong, ET., Ban, KH., Lee, LA. & Lee, CG. (2005). The hepatitis B virus X protein sensitizes HepG2 cells to UV light-induced DNA damage. *J Biol Chem*, Vol.280, No.39, pp. 33525-33535

Lee, YI., Hwang, JM., Im, JH., Lee, YI., Kim, NS., Kim, DG., Yu, DY., Moon, HB. & Park, SK. (2004). Human hepatitis B virus-X protein alters mitochondrial function and physiology in human liver cells. *J Biol Chem*, Vol.279, No.15, pp. 15460-15471

Lieber, CS. (2004). CYP2E1: from ASH to NASH. Hepatol Res, Vol.28, No.1, pp. 1-11

Lim, SO., Gu, JM., Kim, MS., Kim, HS., Park, YN., Park, CK., Cho, JW., Park, YM. & Jung, G. (2008). Epigenetic changes induced by reactive oxygen species in hepatocellular carcinoma: methylation of the E-cadherin promoter. *Gastroenterology*, Vol.135, No.6, pp. 2128-2140

Liu, SL., Lin, X., Shi, DY., Cheng, J., Wu, CQ. & Zhang, YD. (2002). Reactive oxygen species stimulated human hepatoma cell proliferation via cross-talk between PI3-K/PKB and JNK signaling pathways. *Arch Biochem Biophys*, Vol.406, No.2, pp. 173-182

Llovet, JM., Burroughs, A. & Bruix J. (2003). Hepatocellular carcinoma. *Lancet*, Vol.362, No.9399, pp. 1907-1917

Lloyd, DR., Carmichael, PL. & Phillips, DH. (1998). Comparison of the formation of 8-hydroxy-2'-deoxyguanosine and single- and double-strand breaks in DNA mediated by fenton reactions. *Chem Res Toxicol*, Vol.11, No.5, pp. 420-427

Lu, Y. & Cederbaum, AI. (2008). CYP2E1 and oxidative liver injury by alcohol. *Free Radic Biol Med*, Vol.44, No.5, pp. 723-738

Machida, K., Cheng, KT., Sung, VM., Shimodaira, S., Lindsay, KL., Levine, AM., Lai, MY. & Lai, MM. (2004). Hepatitis C virus induces a mutator phenotype: enhanced mutations of immunoglobulin and protooncogenes. *Proc Natl Acad Sci USA*, Vol.101, No.12, pp. 4262-4267

Machida, K., McNamara, G., Cheng, KT., Huang, J., Wang, CH., Comai, L., Ou, JH. & Lai, MM. (2010). Hepatitis C virus inhibits DNA damage repair through reactive oxygen and nitrogen species and by interfering with the ATM-NBS1/Mre11/Rad50 DNA repair pathway in monocytes and hepatocytes. *J Immunol*, Vol.185, No.11, pp. 6985-6998

Majumder, M., Ghosh, AK., Steele, R., Ray, R., Ray, RB. (2001). Hepatitis C virus NS5A physically associates with p53 and regulates p21/waf1 gene expression in a p53-dependent manner. *J Virol*, Vol.75, No.3, pp. 1401-1407

Matsuda, Y. & Ichida, T. (2009). Impact of hepatitis B virus X protein on the DNA damage response during hepatocarcinogenesis. *Med Mol Morphol*,Vol.42, No.3, pp. 138-142

Matsumoto, K., Satoh, Y., Sugo, H., Takamori, S., Kojima, K., Fukasawa, M., Beppu, T. & Futagawa, S. (2003). Immunohistochemical study of the relationship between 8-hydroxy-2'-deoxyguanosine levels in noncancerous region and postoperative recurrence of hepatocellular carcinoma in remnant liver. *Hepatol Res*, Vol.25, No.4, pp. 435-441

Miura, K., Taura, K., Kodama, Y., Schnabl, B. & Brenner, DA. (2008). Hepatitis C virus-induced oxidative stress suppresses hepcidin expression through increased histone deacetylase activity. *Hepatology*, Vol.48, No.5, pp. 1420-1429

Mori, S., Yamasaki, T., Sakaida, I., Takami, T., Sakaguchi, E., Kimura, T., Kurokawa, F., Maeyama, S. & Okita, K. (2004). Hepatocellular carcinoma with nonalcoholic steatohepatitis. *J Gastroenterol*, Vol.39, No.4, pp. 391-396

Nishimura, T., Kohara, M., Izumi, K., Kasama, Y., Hirata, Y., Huang, Y., Shuda, M., Mukaidani, C., Takano, T., Tokunaga, Y., Nuriya, H., Satoh, M., Saito, M., Kai, C. & Tsukiyama-Kohara, K. (2009). Hepatitis C virus impairs p53 via persistent overexpression of 3beta-hydroxysterol Delta24-reductase. *J Biol Chem*, Vol.284, No.52, pp. 36442-36452

Niu, D., Zhang, J., Ren, Y., Feng, H. & Chen, WN. (2009). HBx genotype D represses GSTP1 expression and increases the oxidative level and apoptosis in HepG2 cells. *Mol Oncol*, Vol.3, No.1, pp. 67-76

Okuda, M., Li, K., Beard, MR., Showalter, LA., Scholle, F., Lemon, SM. & Weinman, SA. (2002). Mitochondrial injury, oxidative stress, and antioxidant gene expression are induced by hepatitis C virus core protein. *Gastroenterology*, Vol.122, No.2, pp. 366-375

Pérez-Carreras, M., Del Hoyo, P., Martín, MA., Rubio, JC., Martín, A., Castellano, G., Colina, F., Arenas, J. & Solis-Herruzo, JA. (2003). Defective hepatic mitochondrial respiratory chain in patients with nonalcoholic steatohepatitis. *Hepatology*, Vol.38, No.4, pp. 999-1007

Poehlmann, A. & Roessner, A. (2010). Importance of DNA damage checkpoints in the pathogenesis of human cancers. *Pathol Res Pract*, Vol.206, No.9, pp. 591-601

Poon, D., Anderson, BO., Chen, LT., Tanaka, K., Lau, WY., Van Cutsem, E., Singh, H., Chow, WC., Ooi, LL., Chow, P., Khin, MW. & Koo, WH (2009). Asian Oncology Summit. Management of hepatocellular carcinoma in Asia: consensus statement from the Asian Oncology Summit 2009. *Lancet Oncol*, Vol.10, No.11, pp. 1111-1118

Prost, S., Ford, JM., Taylor, C., Doig, J. & Harrison, DJ. (1998). Hepatitis B x protein inhibits p53-dependent DNA repair in primary mouse hepatocytes. *J Biol Chem*, Vol.273, No.50, pp. 33327-33332

Qadri, I., Iwahashi, M. & Simon, F. (2002). Hepatitis C virus NS5A protein binds TBP and p53, inhibiting their DNA binding and p53 interactions with TBP and ERCC3. *Biochim Biophys Acta*, Vol.1592, No.2, pp. 193-204

Robertson, G., Leclercq, I. & Farrell, GC. (2001). Nonalcoholic steatosis and steatohepatitis. II. Cytochrome P-450 enzymes and oxidative stress. *Am J Physiol Gastrointest Liver Physiol*, Vol.281, No.5, pp. G1135-1139

Robin, MA., Sauvage, I., Grandperret, T., Descatoire, V., Pessayre, D. & Fromenty, B. (2005). Ethanol increases mitochondrial cytochrome P450 2E1 in mouse liver and rat hepatocytes. *FEBS Lett*, Vol.579, No.30, pp. 6895-6902

Seitz, HK. & Stickel, F. (2006). Risk factors and mechanisms of hepatocarcinogenesis with special emphasis on alcohol and oxidative stress. *Biol Chem*, Vol.387, No.4, pp. 349-360

Shirakata, Y., Kawada, M., Fujiki, Y., Sano, H., Oda, M., Yaginuma, K., Kobayashi, M. & Koike, K. (1989). The X gene of hepatitis B virus induced growth stimulation and tumorigenic transformation of mouse NIH3T3 cells. *Jpn J Cancer Res*, Vol.80, No.7, pp. 617–621

Smirnova, IS., Aksenov, ND., Kashuba, EV., Payakurel, P., Grabovetsky, VV., Zaberezhny, AD., Vonsky, MS., Buchinska, L., Biberfeld, P., Hinkula, J. & Isaguliants, MG. (2006). Hepatitis C virus core protein transforms murine fibroblasts by promoting genomic instability. *Cell Oncol*, Vol.28, No.4, pp. 177-190

Srisuttee, R., Koh, SS., Park, EH., Cho, IR., Min, HJ., Jhun, BH., Yu, DY., Park, S., Park, do Y., Lee, MO., Castrillon, DH., Johnston, RN. & Chung, YH. (2011). Up-regulation of

Foxo4 mediated by hepatitis B virus X protein confers resistance to oxidative stress-induced cell death. *Int J Mol Med*, Vol.28, No.2, pp. 255-260

Starley, BQ., Calcagno, CJ. & Harrison, SA. (2010). Nonalcoholic fatty liver disease and hepatocellular carcinoma: a weighty connection. *Hepatology*, Vol.51, No.5, pp. 1820-1832

Studach, L., Wang, WH., Weber, G., Tang, J., Hullinger, RL., Malbrue, R., Liu, X. & Andrisani, O. (2010). Polo-like kinase 1 activated by the hepatitis B virus X protein attenuates both the DNA damage checkpoint and DNA repair resulting in partial polyploidy. *J Biol Chem*, Vol.285, No.39, pp. 30282-30293

Studach, LL., Rakotomalala, L., Wang, WH., Hullinger, RL., Cairo, S., Buendia, MA. & Andrisani, OM. (2009). Polo-like kinase 1 inhibition suppresses hepatitis B virus X protein-induced transformation in an in vitro model of liver cancer progression. *Hepatology*, Vol.50, No.2, pp. 414-423

Suh, SK., Hood, BL., Kim, BJ., Conrads, TP., Veenstra, TD. & Song, BJ. (2004). Identification of oxidized mitochondrial proteins in alcohol-exposed human hepatoma cells and mouse liver. *Proteomics*, Vol.4, No.11, pp. 3401-3412

Tanaka, H., Fujita, N., Sugimoto, R., Urawa, N., Horiike, S., Kobayashi, Y., Iwasa, M., Ma, N., Kawanishi, S., Watanabe, S., Kaito, M. & Takei, Y. (2008). Hepatic oxidative DNA damage is associated with increased risk for hepatocellular carcinoma in chronic hepatitis C. *Br J Cancer*, Vol.98, No.3, pp. 580-586

Tsutsumi, T., Suzukim T., Moriyam K., Shintanim Y., Fujiem H., Miyoshim H., Matsuuram Y., Koikem K., & Miyamura, T. (2003). Hepatitis C virus core protein activates ERK and p38 MAPK in cooperation with ethanol in transgenic mice. Hepatology, Vol.38, No.4, pp. 820-828

Twu, JS. & Robinson, WS. (1989). Hepatitis B virus X gene can trans-activate heterologous viral sequences. *Proc Natl Acad Sci USA*, Vol.86, No.6, pp.2046–2050

Wang, WH., Hullinger, RL. & Andrisani, OM. (2008). Hepatitis B virus X protein via the p38MAPK pathway induces E2F1 release and ATR kinase activation mediating p53 apoptosis. *J Biol Chem*, Vol.283, No.37, pp. 25455-25467

Wang, Y., Millonig, G., Nair, J., Patsenker, E., Stickel, F., Mueller, S., Bartsch, H. & Seitz, HK. (2009). Ethanol-induced cytochrome P4502E1 causes carcinogenic etheno-DNA lesions in alcoholic liver disease. *Hepatology*, Vol.50, No.2, pp. 453-461

Weltman, MD., Farrell, GC., Hall, P., Ingelman-Sundberg, M. & Liddle, C. (1998). Hepatic cytochrome P450 2E1 is increased in patients with nonalcoholic steatohepatitis. *Hepatology*, Vol.27, No.1, 128-133

Wu, D. & Cederbaum, AI. (2009). Oxidative stress and alcoholic liver disease. *Semin Liver Dis*, Vol.29, No.2, pp. 141-154

Wu, XY., Qian, JJ., Lin, Y. & Zheng, MH. (2008). Hepatitis B virus X protein disrupts DNA interstrand crosslinking agent mitomycin C induced ATR dependent intra-S-phase checkpoint. *Eur J Cancer*, Vol.44, No.11, pp. 1596-1602

Zhao, F., Hou, NB., Yang, XL., He, X., Liu, Y., Zhang, YH., Wei, CW., Song, T., Li, L., Ma, QJ. & Zhong, H. (2008). Ataxia telangiectasia-mutated-Rad3-related DNA damage checkpoint signaling pathway triggered by hepatitis B virus infection. *World J Gastroenterol*, Vol.14, No.40, pp. 6163-6170

Zheng, Z., Li, J., Sun, J., Song, T., Wei, C., Zhang, Y., Rao, G., Chen, G., Li, D., Yang, G., Han, B., Wei, S., Cao, C. & Zhong, H. (2011). Inhibition of HBV replication by theophylline. *Antiviral Res*, Vol.89, No.2, pp. 149-155

# Part 3

## Detection / Prevention / Prevalence

# 16

# Hepatocellular Carcinoma: Methods of Circulating Tumor Cells (CTC) Measurements

Natalia Olaya[1] and Franck Chiappini[2]
[1]*Laboratorio clínico, de patología y banco de sangre/ Fundación Valle del Lili Cali*
[2]*Beth Israel Deaconess Medical Center, Center of Life Science, Division of Endocrinology, Diabetes and Metabolism, Boston,*
[1]*Colombia*
[2]*USA*

## 1. Introduction

Hepatocellular carcinoma (HCC) is responsible for significant morbidity and mortality in cirrhosis and also accounts for between 85% and 90% of primary liver cancer (Caldwell & Park 2009; Hussain & El-Serag 2009; Tandon & Garcia-Tsao 2009). Most of HCC in the world occur in the setting of cirrhosis and over half-million of people develop liver cancer every year and an almost equal number die of it (Caldwell & Park 2009; Hussain & El-Serag 2009). Liver cancer prognosis is determined by factors related to the tumor (etiologies) and factors related to the cirrhosis i.e. parameters of liver dysfunction (CLIP 1998; Llovet et al., 1999; Okuda et al., 1985; Tandon & Garcia-Tsao 2009). During the last 30 years the HCC-incidence rate increased dramatically, despite the development of the HBV-vaccine and the program for newborn vaccination against HBV, developed in European and Asian countries (El-Serag et al., 2003; Hussain & El-Serag 2009).

Since 1997, and after implementing a program for vaccination of newborns against HBV, Chinese and Japanese populations began to show a decrease in HCC incidence, especially among males (Plymoth et al., 2009; Yu S. Z. 1995). In the other hand, HCV-infection is rising around the world (Davila et al., 2004; Kong S. Y. et al., 2009; Min et al., 2009; Yoon et al., 2009; Yu M. L. & Chuang 2009) counter balancing the benefit effects of HBV-vaccination. This increase in incidence rate is observed through the world and it does not belong to a specific region. For example, the USA and Europe have the same positive incidence slope (Davila et al., 2004; Donato et al., 2006; El-Serag 2002; El-Serag 2004; El-Serag et al., 2003; Hassan et al., 2002; Hussain & El-Serag 2009; Scatton et al., 2009; Wu et al., 2000). The etiologies of HCC remain the same; the most important causes are the HBV and HCV infections, heavy alcohol consumption, aflatoxin B1, age and gender (males are more susceptible than females), race (Asian and African over 20 years old) , tobacco consumption and obesity associated with non-alcoholic fatty liver disease and the increase of the Diabetes II mellitus that rise the risk factor between 2 and 3, genetic hemochromatosis, primary biliary cirrhosis, alpha1-antitrypsin deficiency and autoimmune hepatitis (Banks et al., 2006; Borgen et al., 1998; Bostick et al., 1998; Caldwell & Park 2009; CLIP 1998; Collier & Sherman

1998; Davila et al., 2004; Donato et al., 2006; El-Serag 2002; El-Serag 2004; El-Serag et al., 2003; Hassan et al., 2002; Hussain & El-Serag 2009; Idilman et al., 1998; Ishikawa et al., 1998; Jung et al., 1998; Llovet et al., 1999; Luzzi et al., 1998; Mendizabal & Reddy 2009; Mocellin & Hoon & et al., 2006; Mocellin & Keilholz & et al., 2006; Naume 1998; Naume et al., 1998; Okuda et al., 1985; Racila et al., 1998; Schutte et al., 2009; Wu et al., 2000; Yao D. F. et al., 2007; Yu M. C. et al., 2000; Yu S. Z. 1995).

Usually, HCC develops during a long process of inflammation and fibrosis, eventually leading to cirrhosis. (Britto et al., 2000; Hussain & El-Serag 2009; Idilman et al., 1998; McMahon 2009). The majority of liver masses are detected incidentally in asymptomatic patients. These lesions are identified using imaging tools such as ultrasonography (US), computed tomography (CT), and magnetic resonance imaging (MRI). A diagnostic approach to HCC has been developed based on the literature and expert consensus, and incorporates serology, cytohistology and radiology/imaging characteristics. (Assy et al., 2009; Bruix & Sherman 2005; Bruix et al., 2001; Byrnes et al., 2007; Durand et al., 2001; Gomaa et al., 2009; Hussain & El-Serag 2009; Mendizabal & Reddy 2009).

HCC is one of the most aggressive cancers. Patients who show progress over the terminal stage have a 1-year survival of less than 10%. In the other hand, patients presenting as early-stage HCC with preserved liver function, a solitary HCC or up to three nodules, each less than 3cm have 5-years survival figures up to 75%. The choice of the therapy and the prognosis are dictated by the severity of the liver function, portal hypertension and medical co-morbidities. National and internationals consensus were established to choose the best treatment adapted for each case and obtain the best prognostic. Milan, Barcelona Clinic Liver Cancer, Cancer of the Liver Italian Program, and San Francisco criteria had determined the prognosis of patients based on the number and size of nodules, the metastasis and the state of liver function leading to the best choice for the patient (Banks et al., 2006; Borgen et al., 1998; Bostick et al., 1998; Caldwell & Park 2009; CLIP 1998; Collier & Sherman 1998; Davila et al., 2004; Donato et al., 2006; El-Serag 2002; El-Serag 2004; El-Serag et al., 2003; Freeman R. B. et al., 2006; Hassan et al., 2002; Idilman et al., 1998; Ishikawa et al., 1998; Jung et al., 1998; Llovet et al., 1999; Luzzi et al., 1998; Naume 1998; Naume et al., 1998; Racila et al., 1998; Sanchez Antolin et al., 2009; Yao D. F. et al., 2007).

Based on these data, the physician can choose resection, orthotopic liver transplantation (OLT), percutaneous ethanol injection or radiofrequency ablation, chemoembolisation, systemic chemotherapy and symptomatic therapy. The first 3 treatments are potentially curative, the second following treatments are palliative and the last one usually is applied at the terminal stage of the disease (Mendizabal & Reddy 2009). At the time the HCC will be treated an important question that the physician has to face is the risk of recurrence and metastasis. To answer this question the best approach would be able to detect the circulating tumor cells in the bloodstream.

## 2. Definition of CTC and HCC

In the field of biology of tumors, some expressions have been coined for the different types of circulating cellular elements. The term *circulating tumor cells* (CTC) defines specifically the tumor cells detected in blood or lymphatic vessels. Circulating cells in the bloodstream or in the lymphatic system are considered to be tumoral microemboli (CTM) and represent a collective migration. The terms disseminated tumor cells (DTC) and isolated tumor cell (ITC) can be also found in the literature, but are usually used to define the cells that can be detected in both the organs and the bloodstream. The word micrometastasis is usually used to indicate tumor cells found in distant organs. (Luzzi et al., 1998; Schuler & Dolken 2006; Zieglschmid et al., 2005). The presence of circulating tumor cells reflects the aggressiveness nature of a solid tumor. Many attempts have been made to develop assays that reliably detect and enumerate these cells. The clinical results obtained with such assays suggest that in some tumor types, CTC detection and identification can be used to estimate prognosis and may serve as an early marker to assess anti-tumor activity of treatment. In addition, CTC can be used to predict progression-free survival and overall survival. CTC are an interesting source of biological information in order to understand dissemination, drug resistance and treatment-induced cell death. (Alix-Panabieres et al., 2008; Braun et al., 2005; Curry et al., 2004; Mocellin & Hoon & et al., 2006; Mocellin & Keilholz & et al., 2006; Muller et al., 2005; Nakagawa et al., 2007; Pantel et al., 2008; Pantel & Woelfle 2005; Paterlini-Brechot & Benali 2007; Riethdorf et al., 2008; Sleijfer et al., 2007; Strijbos et al., 2008; Willipinski-Stapelfeldt et al., 2005).

In general, intra- or extrahepatic metastases appear at a late tumor stage or after treatment suggesting that earlier during the development of the HCC, the tumor spread circulating of liver-derived cells or circulating tumoral cells also named in literature "micrometastasis". In HCC animal models showed that 10 to 10 000 CTC are capable to initiate new metastasis (Groom et al., 1999; Hermanek et al., 1999; Liotta et al., 1974; Luzzi et al., 1998). Even after curative resection, the tumor recurrence rate remains high. Although CTC detection has been applied and well documented in different types of cancer, especially breast cancer, CTC detection is not routinely performed in HCC follow-up and remains in the experimental field. However, CTC detection might bring new interesting information of metastatic process, might be used as diagnostic tool of early recurrence and may allow a better patient selection for liver transplantation. Mechanisms of tumor recurrence are still poorly understood. Several arguments point out that HCC tumor cells can infiltrate the blood system as shown by the presence of alpha-fetoprotein mRNA (Aselmann et al., 2001; Kamiyama et al., 1996; Kienle et al., 2000; Komeda et al., 1995; Lemoine et al., 1997; Matsumura 2001; Matsumura et al., 2001; Matsumura et al., 1995; Matsumura et al., 1994; Matsumura et al., 1999; Morimoto et al., 2005). CTC seem to be correlated with poor survival in many types of tumors (Aselmann et al., 2001; Kamiyama et al., 1996; Komeda et al., 1995; Lemoine et al., 1997; Matsumura et al., 1994; Morimoto et al., 2005).

However, HCC circulating cells are still difficult to detect, and their presence and amount are poorly correlated with either long-term survival or recurrence in the setting of HCC. Given the lack of specific biological markers, few studies focused on CTC detection. The challenge of CTC detection is related to the requirement of both high sensitivity and specificity. A wrong labeling of "non-tumor cells" (epithelial non tumor cells or normal hepatocytes, for instance) as "tumor cells' could generate poor clinical interest.

Methods of CTC detection have to be highly sensitive and specific. The first technical challenge in this field consists of finding exceptional cells. Just a few CTC are mixed with the approximately 10 million leukocytes and 5 billion erythrocytes in 1 ml of blood. To be useful, the method used to identify circulating tumor cells must also detect all tumor cells and discriminate them from non-tumor cells. (Alix-Panabieres et al., 2008; Becker et al., 2005; Braun et al., 2005; Curry et al., 2004; Mocellin & Hoon & et al., 2006; Nakagawa et al., 2007; Paterlini-Brechot & Benali 2007; Ross et al., 1993; Schuler & Dolken 2006; Smerage & Hayes 2006). Before considering the technical problems, it is important to have circulating hepatoma-specific biomarkers to be able to detect the CTC and further to be useful to early diagnosis, monitoring metastasis or post treatment recurrences of HCC.

Currently, CTC detection is mainly based on alpha-fetoprotein (AFP) messenger RNA (mRNA) assessment or quantification, and in few reported cases using cytomorphometric technology, especially the ISET devise. A high sensibility could be obtained using flow cytometry assays but high blood volumes (200 ml) and long analysis time (40 h for one sample) are required. Consequently, its use has been discouraged as a routine technique (Mejean et al., 2000).

## 3. HCC markers and their application for CTC

The hepatocellular carcinomas can synthesize various tumor-related proteins, polypeptides and isoenzymes more or less specific of the hepatoma tissues. It is important to detect CTC in the bloodstream or lymphatic system to have tumor specific markers of HCC. Finding one of these circulating proteins does not mean that there circulating tumor cells.

### 3.1 Secreted proteins

#### 3.1.1 Relevance of cytokines in HCC circulating tumor cells

Hepatocellular carcinoma tumor has shown to secret a lot of cytokines related to the development of the tumor, like vascular endothelial growth factor (VEGF), transforming growth factor-beta 1 (TGF-β1), Interleukin 8 (IL-8) or tumor-specific growth factor (TSGF). These serum markers are useful to follow-up the development and the prognosis of the HCC but useless to follow-up circulating tumor cells in blood (Zhou et al., 2006).

#### 3.1.2 The case of the serum AFP

The serum α-fetoprotein (AFP) levels show high levels in newborns and then declines progressively below 10 ng/ml in 300 days of life. An increase of serum AFP levels can be observed during pregnancy, and in patients with mucovicidosis, acute hepatitis (30%-50%), chronic hepatitis (15%-50%), cirrhosis (11%-47%) and other cancers (gastrointestinal, pancreatic, biliary, non-seminomatous germ-cell testicular, and germ cell ovarian). Serum level AFP sensitivity is between 39% to 64% with approximately 60% for a cutoff of 20 ng/mL, and decrease to 22% if higher cutoff of 200 ng/mL is used (Bruix et al., 2001; Collier & Sherman 1998; Fujiyama et al., 2002; Okuda 1986; Saffroy et al., 2007; Trevisani et al., 2001). AFP specificity is around 76%-91% with a low predictive value between 9%-32% (Bruix et al., 2001; Collier & Sherman 1998; Okuda 1986; Saffroy et al., 2007).

In addition, the serum AFP level is correlated with the tumor size. 80% of small HCCs (<2cm) do not express AFP. In the other hand, AFP level can be elevated in patients with chronic liver disease with high degree of hepatocytes regeneration such as HCV-infection that show a high level of AFP in absence of malignancy (Toyoda et al., 2004; Vejchapipat et al., 2004). For these reasons, some additional serological markers used in combination with AFP seem to improve the performance of this biomarker, especially in terms of sensitivity.

Studies were done by using one or two more markers like des-γ carboxyprothrombin (DCP) also called prothrombin induced by vitamin K absence II (PIVKAII) and glycosylated AFP-L3 (*Lens culinaris* Agglutinin-Reactive AFP) fraction serum levels to diagnose earlier HCC and increasing the sensitivity especially when HCC is associate with cirrhosis, HCV or HBV infection (Dohmen et al., 2003; Fujiyama et al., 2002; Gonzalez & Keeffe 2011; Lok et al., 2009; Min et al., 2009; Saffroy et al., 2007; Suehiro et al., 1994). But there is no study that correlates their serum levels and the circulating tumor cell during the HCC development.

### 3.2 The mRNA markers

In the next sections, we focus on and describe the most specific markers of messenger RNA used to detect CTC in hepatocellular carcinoma.

#### 3.2.1 Relevance of α-fetoprotein (AFP) messenger RNA (mRNA)

Initially, the albumin gene has been proposed as a biological marker to track CTC during HCC development but has been rapidly abandoned since many groups have reported illegitimate transcription of albumin gene in peripheral-blood leukocytes. The relevance of AFP mRNA as a marker of circulating tumor cells is better but is also controversial because these cells have not been further characterized and it has been shown that they may correspond to normal circulating hepatocytes (Lemoine et al., 1997; Louha et al., 1999; Minata et al., 2001). Furthermore, these tumor cells have mostly been sought and detected shortly after liver resection (Kienle et al., 2000; Lemoine et al., 1997; Louha et al., 1999; Matsumura et al., 1994; Minata et al., 2001). This finding suggests that CTC could spread following liver mobilization or manipulation. Although the mechanisms leading to intra and extrahepatic recurrences are still unknown, some observations suggest that bone marrow (BM) could also be a specific reservoir of CTC. Indeed, several reports have suggested that tumor cells are of BM origin (Agarwal et al., 2004; Houghton et al., 2004; Sell 2002). Hepatic tumor stem cells may take advantage of the potential for stem cell support of the BM microenvironment. The amplification of AFP mRNA by means of reverse transcription (RT) and a nested polymerase chain reaction (PCR) is the highly sensitive method for the detection of residual HCC cells in peripheral blood. The qualitative (positive versus negative) detection of HCC circulating tumor cells in blood samples from individual patients is of limited value in predicting the risk of disease progression. Because the level of AFP mRNA is increased in HCC tissue compared with in normal hepatocytes, the quantification of AFP transcripts seems to be a more reliable indicator of disease progression. A more highly sensitive assay based on TaqMan® technology to quantify AFP mRNA in "real time" should be preferred (Cheung et al., 2006; Gross-Goupil et al., 2003; Lu Y. et al., 2007; Matsumura 2001). Even using this methodology, reported results are not homogeneous and contradictory (Bruix et al., 2001). The main studies which have evaluated AFP mRNA are summarized in Table 1. The false-positive results can be obtained using AFP mRNA.

| Author | PCR | Sensitivity | Cases | Samples | Positivity | Predictability of recurrence |
|---|---|---|---|---|---|---|
| (Kamiyama et al., 1996) | qRT-PCR | 1 CHC/ $10^7$ | 37<br>136 | Blood<br>BM | 18%<br>28% | No<br>Yes |
| (Morimoto et al., 2005) | qRT-PCR | 1 CHC/$10^6$ | 38<br>25 | Blood<br>BM | 10 %<br>48% | Yes<br>No |
| (Kienle et al., 2000) | nRT-PCR | 5 cells/ 1mL | 24 | Blood<br>BM | 29%<br>43% | Suspect |
| (Aselmann et al., 2001) | Competitive RT | 10 cells/ 9 mL | 22<br>11 | Blood<br>BM | 26%<br>45% | NA |
| (Sutcliffe et al., 2005) | RT-PCR | NA | 18 | BM | 93% | No |
| (Matsumura et al., 1995; Matsumura et al., 1994) | nRT-PCR | | 33 | Blood | 52% | Extrahepatic metastases |
| (Komeda et al., 1995) | nRT-PCR | 15 cells/mL | 64 | Blood | 36% | Extrahepatic metastases |
| (Lemoine et al., 1997) | nRT-PCR | 1CHC/$10^5$ mono | 20 | Blood | 25% | No |
| (Miyazono et al., 2001) | nRT-PCR | $10^{-6}$µg/µLof RNA | 33 | Blood | 54% | Yes |
| (Ijichi et al., 2002) | nRT-PCR | 1CHC/$10^5$ mono | 87 | Blood | 36% | Yes |
| (Witzigmann et al., 2002) | nRT-PCR | 1 CHC/$10^7$ mono | 85 | Blood | 26-45% | No |
| (Gross-Goupil et al., 2003) | RT-PCR | 1 CHC/$10^6$ | 52 | Blood | 25% | No |

Table 1. Evaluation of serum alpha-fetoprotein as a marker of circulation tumor cell in different hepatocellular carcinoma studies. nRT-PCR, nested RT-PCR; qRT-PCR, quantitative RT-PCR.

### 3.2.2 Transforming growth factor beta-1 (TGF-β1) mRNA

The levels of circulating TGF-β1 and TGF-β1 mRNA were significantly higher in the HCC patients than any other group of patients. The sensitivity and specificity of circulating TGF-β1 level (>1.2 μg/L) were 90% and 94% for HCC diagnosis, but no significant correlation was found between TGF-β1 expression an AFP levels or tumor size. The combined detection of TGF-β1 and serum AFP could raise the detection rate of HCC up to 97%. Both of circulating TGF-β1 and TGF-β1 mRNA could be used as sensitive biomarkers for diagnosis and prognosis of HBV-induced HCC (Dong et al., 2008; Wang Y. L. et al., 2007). Unfortunately, TGF-β1 mRNA was poor studied and further investigations have to be done to use circulating TGF-β1 mRNA as a marker of circulating tumor cells in HCC.

### 3.2.3 Insulin-like growth factor (IGF)-II mRNA

Studies using amplified fragments of IGF-II mRNA by RT-PCR showed that the lowest sensitivity with 2 ng/L of total RNA. Dong et al., showed that the positive frequencies of IGF-II mRNA were 100% in HCC, around 50% in paracancerous and 0% in noncancerous tissues respectively. But, the positive frequency of circulating IGF-II mRNA was 34% in HCC, and no amplification was found in other liver diseases, extrahepatic tumors, and normal control, meaning that IGF-II is specific of the HCC but nor really sensitive. Associated to other circulating markers IGF-II can be helpful to detect CTC. The circulating IGF-II mRNA was correlated with the stage of HCC (incidence=100%) with extrahepatic metastasis, and 35% with AFP-negative. No difference was found between tumor size and circulating IGF-II mRNA (Dong et al., 2005; Wang Y. L. et al., 2007) but these results are controversial (Qian et al., 2010).

### 3.2.4 Alpha-albumin (ALF) mRNA

For more than a decade, we know that mRNAs of hepatocytes-specific albumin genes are detected in peripheral blood by RT-PCR. It was shown that there is evidence that detection of albumin mRNA associated with the detection of AFP mRNA is strongly associated with the presence of metastases (Hillaire et al., 1994; Kar & Carr 1995; Komeda et al., 1995; Matsumura et al., 1995). Wong et al., showed that circulating hepatocellular carcinoma cells can be detected and be semi-quantified by albumin RT-PCR (Wong et al., 1997). On the other hand, Wu et al., showed that, the down regulation of alpha-albumin (ALF) specifically in HCC circulating cells can be used has a specific marker to discriminate the normal hepatocellular circulating cells that express abundantly ALF. RT-PCR ALF in association with RT-PCR AFP have been proposed to distinguish normal or malignant hepatocytes in peripheral blood, but the interpretation of the results is still debated (Resto et al., 2000).

### 3.2.5 Prostate-specific antigen (PSA) and mRNA PSA

The Prostate-Specific Antigen (PSA) had shown to be well-established reliability marker and remained a valid prostate marker in patients with acute hepatitis and HCC (Malavaud et al., 1999). But these results are controversial, PSA and mRNA PSA seem to don't be specific to the tissue and frequently detected in peripheral blood cells from healthy patients (Ishikawa et al., 1998). In addition, like the cytokines, serum PSA cannot be used as hepatocellular carcinoma marker for circulating tumor cells.

### 3.2.6 Heat shock protein (HSP)

Heat shock proteins (HSP) are stimulated under perturbation or stressors by the tissue. HSP are ubiquitous molecules and can be also expressed during carcinogenesis. Different HSP have been related to the development of the hepatocellular carcinoma like gp96 or GRP94, HSP70 and HSP27, but none of them were used as a specific marker of circulating tumor cell (Wang Y. L. et al., 2007).

### 3.2.7 Human telomerase reverse transcriptase mRNA or hTERT mRNA

Human telomerase is a ribonucleic protein composed by the association of three structures: human telomerase RNA component (hTERC); human telomerase-associated protein 1 (hTEP1); and human telomerase reverse transcriptase (hTERT). hTERT is the catalytic unit of the complex. Also, telomerase is expressed in embryonic cells, in most human cancer cells or immortal cell lines, but not in normal somatic cell lines or tissues. For these reasons, hTERT was investigated as a marker of diagnosis and prognosis of HCC, but the results are controversial and appear that false-positive results can be observed because of lymphocytes, precancerous liver parenchymal cells and micrometastasis maybe responsible (for review (Grizzi et al., 2007; Wang Y. L. et al., 2007; Zhou et al., 2006)). Recently, Kong et al., investigated hTERT in peripheral blood in HCC from 343 Korean patients. There is no association between hTERT expression and clinical features and nor relationship between AFP and hTERT mRNA. Their conclusion is that AFP and hTERT mRNA expression in peripheral blood is useless as HCC prognostic markers (Kong S. Y. et al., 2009).

### 3.2.8 Cancer-testis antigens (CTA)

Cancer-testis antigens (CTA) represent a category of tumor-associated antigens normally expressed in male germ cells but not in adult somatic tissues (Scanlan et al., 2002). CTA are heterogeneous group of antigens. Actually, more than 44 distinct CT "gene" or "antigen" families have been reported in literature. Certain CT gene families contain multiple members, as well as splice variants and today more than 89 distinct transcripts are known to be encoded by CT genes (Scanlan et al., 2002). A number of CT antigens have been found expressed with high percentage and specificity in HCC. The expression of the CT antigens mRNA was investigated by Wu et al., in the HCC and corresponding peripheral blood of 37 patients with HCC, 15 samples of cirrhotic tissues and 15 normal tissues with the same method. Two CT antigens SSX-2 and SSX-5 showed in this study high specific and high frequent expression only in HCC tissues. In corresponding peripheral blood of HCC tissues, the positive expressions rate of these two CT antigens mRNA was not very high (Benoy et al., 2006). The same group of researchers used another two CT antigens SSX-1 and NY-ESO1 in the same group of patients and with the same methods (RT-PCR) with the corresponding peripheral blood. They showed that SSX-1 can be potential used in peripheral blood, with short term recurrence rat at 46% (6/13) in patients whose peripheral blood expressed SSX-1 mRNA, while the recurrence rate in patients with negative SSX-1 mRNA was 28.6% (4/14) (Bergamaschi et al., 2008). In another study, Peng et al., showed that specific expression of CT antigens was observed in AFP-negative HCC, suggesting the application of their mRNA as tumor markers to detect circulating HCC cells (Peng J. R. et al., 2005). Yang et al., showed that FATE/BJ-HCC-2 (another CTA) mRNA expression was detected in the peripheral blood mononuclear cells (PBMCs) of 46.67% patients, whose HCC tissue samples were cut off and positive for FATE/BJ-HCC-2 mRNA, which implicated tumor cell dissemination in blood circulation and related to the metastasis of HCC. These studies suggest that CT antigens expressions can be used in peripheral blood to detect HCC circulating cells, but also can be associated to the research of AFP mRNA to increases the specificity and the frequency of the method. This group of markers seems promising and further studies have to be done first to determine the panel of CT antigens to be used as markers of HCC circulating cells.

### 3.3 New approaches

To attempt the lack of CTC markers, new techniques and technologies are used such as microarray/mRNA large analyses, proteomic and "secretome" analyses and finally microRNA testing.

#### 3.3.1 Microarray/mRNA large analyses

DNA chips were used to measure and find new markers to diagnose HCC, but also to use these as CTC markers. The studies showed the expression of mRNAs for members of the glypican and syndecan families of heparin sulfate proteoglycans such as GPC3 can be a good CTC marker that can be used in human or in mouse models (Suzuki et al., 2010; Yao M. et al., 2011). Another interesting marker was discovered called Snail. Snail mRNA was study in blood of patients with HCC and metastasis (Min et al., 2009). But further investigation has to be done to figure out the specificity and the sensitivity of those markers.

#### 3.3.2 Proteomic and secretome analyzes

In the process to find new markers for CTC, a number of teams started to work with proteomic analysis such as quadrupol IT-TOF, SELDI- TOF MALDI-TOF/TOF mass spectrometry. Their objective is tracking earlier the development and the progression of the HCC. Few markers or group of markers were identified by these methods such as the usual markers AFP, AFP-L3, TGF-β1, and PIVKA-II but also vitronectin, alpha-1-fucosidase (AFU) and DCP, Golgi protein-73 (GP73), hepatocyte growth factor (HGF), and nervous growth factor (NGF) (Dai et al., 2009; Donati et al., 2010; Liu X. & Wan & et al., 2011; Paradis et al., 2005; Peng X. Q. et al., 2009; Poon et al., 2003; Zinkin et al., 2008).

Interestingly, the proteomic analyses were able to detect new markers in the serum secreted (which is called "secretome") by the carcinoma cells (Makridakis & Vlahou 2010; Malaguarnera et al., 2010; Niu et al., 2010). Over 90 proteins in some studies compiled with high powerful biocomputational analysis where identified and used to diagnose HCC early (Dai et al., 2009; Paradis et al., 2005; Poon et al., 2003; Zinkin et al., 2008). Unfortunately these studies did not analyze the real usefulness of these markers to identify CTC in the patients with HCC.

A sub-group of HCC was identified by these techniques expressing stem cell markers (CD133, CD90, CD44, EpCAM, CD13 or neural cell adhesion molecule; NCAM) defining what is called now liver cancer stem cell but unfortunately these markers were not studied in the area of circulating tumor cells (Chiba et al., 2009; Huang & Geng 2010; Liu L. L. & Fu & et al., 2011). They are very promising markers. Another group of markers very promising to detect CTC belongs to the chemokine receptors such as CXCR4, CX3CR1 and CCR6 express during HCC progression (Huang & Geng 2010; Li et al., 2010), but none of them were tested during a clinical trial.

### 3.3.3 MicroRNA markers: A new hope

Around 28 years ago, microRNA (miRNA) was discovered and showed the regulation of genes (Lee et al., 1993; Reinhart et al., 2000) such as oncogenes or tumor suppressor genes at the level of the mRNA. More than 35 studies focused on the identification of miRNA or a group of miRNAs to be used as marker of early diagnosis or metastasis. miR-122/-122a, miR-221/222, miR-145, miR-146a, miR-26 (NFκB pathway), miR-199a-3p (mTOR pathway) and miR-26 (MYC pathway) were strongly linked to the development and metastasis of the HCC. Also a group of miRNAs were used to identify and classify HCC (Hoshida et al., 2010; Ji & Wang 2009; Kerr et al., 2011; Kojima et al., 2011; Kong G. et al., 2011; Sato et al., 2011), but non of them were used as a CTC marker and tested during a clinical trial.

### 3.4 Conclusion

In Conclusion, we can observe that not too many specific HCC markers are available and useful for the detection of the CTC. This is certainly due to the heterogeneity of the hepatocellular carcinoma. The most important marker used in clinical routine is the detection of serum AFP mRNA expression (Table 1). But this marker is not expressed in all HCC and by consequence in all CTC leading false negative results. Some propose to combine the research of more than one marker to increase the specificity and the sensitivity of CTC detection method. One of promising marker is Cancer-Testis Antigens but more studies need to be done to select one or more CTA combined (or not) with the detection of the AFP mRNA expression. As we notice previously, CTC are very rare in peripheral blood. We saw also that real-time polymerase chain reaction is a method that in addition to be specific by the nature of the primers used, it can amplify the signal by increasing the number of copies of mRNA originally presents in the sample. But before using RT-PCR, it's necessary to concentrate the number of CTC from the peripheral blood in a smaller volume. The next chapter will describe these methods.

## 4. Enrichment of the sample

CTC are usually detected in the peripheral circulation, but we can find CTC in other body fluids like the cerebrospinal fluids or the urines. The limitations to discover the CTC in these fluids are the same than in the blood circulation. However, it is possible to extract a relatively big amount of blood without harming the patient and much easier.

We will focus on the methods of CTC detection in the blood. As we describe above, CTC in the peripheral circulation occur at an estimated number of one CTC per $10^{5-7}$ peripheral blood mononuclear cell or PBMC. Because of the scarcity of the target cells, it is necessary to concentrate the sample. Since enrichment will inevitably be accompanied by some loss of CTC, irrespective of the method, some essays are performed directly in whole blood (Lu Y. et al., 2007).

Two different groups of techniques can be used to enrich samples, the non-specific and the specific enrichment techniques. The non-specific enrichment techniques use physico-chemical CTC properties (size, density, etc). The specific enrichment technique use markers expressed by the CTC. The advantages of the non-specific and specific enrichment techniques are summarized in the Table 2 and described in the following paragraphs.

| Methods of Enrichment | Advantages | Disadvantages | References |
|---|---|---|---|
| | | **Non-Specific** | |
| **Density** (OncoQuick®, Ficoll, UNI-Set®) | 1. Isolation of whole and living CTC,<br>2. Can use another method of enrichment more specific (immunomagnetic beads),<br>3. Cytopathology, Cytological staining, ICH, FISH...etc can be performed,<br>4. RNA, DNA extractions followed by RT-PCR or PCR respectively can be done. | 1. Non-specific,<br>2. Rare CTC can be lost in the plasma fraction or trapped among erythrocyte and neutrophils,<br>3. Low and variable sensitivity,<br>4. Depends of the type of CTC, temperature, centrifuge,<br>5. Expensive. | (Balic et al., 2005; Becker et al., 2005; Mankin et al., 2002; Paterlini-Brechot & Benali 2007) |
| **Size** (MEMS, ISET) | 1. Easy<br>2. Precise counting of the cells per ml of blood, independently of the volume of the blood treated,<br>3. Allows Cytopathology, Cytological staining, ICH, FISH...etc,<br>4. Allows Microdissection followed by<br>5. RNA, DNA extraction follow by RT-PCR or PCR respectively<br>6. Avoids multiple steps,<br>7. Increases sensitivity (1 single CTC can be detect from 1ml of blood). | 1. Non-specific,<br>2. CTC can go through the filter,<br>3. Cells can be damaged,<br>4. Expensive, but less than the immunomagnetic beads. | (Li et al., 2010; Mejean et al., 2000; Paterlini-Brechot & Benali 2007; Pinzani et al., 2006; Vona et al., 2004) |
| **Cytospin** | 1. Easy,<br>2. Allows Cytopathology, Cytological staining, ICH, FISH...etc,<br>3. Allows Microdissection follow by<br>4. RNA, DNA extraction follow by RT-PCR or PCR respectively. | 1. Increase the mortality of the CTC. | (Becker et al., 2005; Farina et al., 2004; Kallergi et al., 2008; Kollermann et al., 1999; Saraiva-Romanholo et al., 2003) |
| **Lysis Buffer** (Qiagen) | 1. Easy,<br>2. The cells harvested by this method can be re-enriched or analysed by the methods already described,<br>3. Low cost. | 1. Increase the mortality of the CTC,<br>2. Low sensitivity. | (Aryal et al., 2004; Khan et al., 2000; Wharton et al., 1999) |

| Specific | | | |
|---|---|---|---|
| **ImmunoMagnetic Beads** (MACS system, CellSearch) | 1. Specific<br>2. Morphological analysis of CTC, Cytopathology, Cytological staining, ICH, FISH...etc,<br>3. Multiple labelling of antigens on CTC,<br>4. Direct quantification of CTC. | 1. Subjective analyses for CTC identification,<br>2. Time-consuming screening of tumor cells,<br>3. Need specific marker(s) and antibody available,<br>4. Expensive. | (Alix-Panabieres et al., 2005; Alix-Panabieres et al., 2008; Alix-Panabieres et al., 2007; Czerkinsky et al., 1983) |
| **EPISPOT** | 1. High sensitivity,<br>2. Detection of viable CTC,<br>3. Detection of secreted proteins. | 1. Protein must be actively secreted, shed, or released,<br>2. No identification and isolation of secreting cell possible. | (Alix-Panabieres et al., 2005; Alix-Panabieres et al., 2008; Alix-Panabieres et al., 2007; Czerkinsky et al., 1983) |
| **FACS** | 1. High sensitivity,<br>2. Technique for counting, examining, and sorting microscopic particles (CTC) suspended,<br>3. Simultaneous multiparametric analyses of the physical and/or chemical characteristics. | 1. Need the apparatus,<br>2. High cost. | (Lobodasch et al., 2007; Mankin et al., 2002; Pachmann et al., 2005) |
| **FAST** | 1. High sensitivity,<br>2. Can detect rare events. | 1. Fluorescent dye-conjugated antibodies,<br>2. Specificity depend of the antibodies,<br>3.Very expensive. | (Curry et al., 2004; Hsieh et al., 2006; Lu Y. et al., 2007; Pinzani et al., 2006) |
| **CTC-Chip** | 1. High sensitivity,<br>2. Detection of viable CTC. | 1. Detect only cytokeratin+-CTC,<br>2. Need to control precisely laminar flow conditions,<br>3. Expensive. | (Alix-Panabieres et al., 2008; Nagrath et al., 2007) |

Table 2. Summary of advantages and disadvantages of the methods of CTC enrichment. CTC, circulating tumor cell; CTC-Chip, circulating tumor cell chip; EPIPSPOT, epithelial immunospot; FACS, Fluorescence-activated cell sorting = flow cytometric; FAST, fiber-optic array scanning technology; ICH, immunocytochemistry; ISET, isolation by size of epithelial tumor cells; MACS, magnetic cell sorting; MEMS, micro-electro-mechanical system.

### 4.1 The non-specific enrichment techniques

#### 4.1.1 Density gradient(s) centrifugation

The tumor cells, epithelial cells, platelets and low density leukocytes from leukocytes and erythrocytes can be separated by the propriety of their particular density (Table 2). Briefly, each cell type has their own density and the assumption of the methods is to put the cells in a buffer with a specific kind of density that usually corresponds to the density of the cells (CTC) that we want to isolate. Density gradient centrifugation is the preferred method to purify cells, subcellular organelles and macromolecules. Density gradients can be generated by placing layer after layer of gradient media such as sucrose in a tube with the heaviest layer at the bottom and the lightest at the top in either a discontinuous or continuous mode. The cell fraction to be separated is placed on top of the layer and centrifuged. Density gradient separation can be classified into two categories: 1). Rate-zonal (size) separation. 2). Isopycnic (density) separation.

Rate-zonal separation takes advantage of particle size and mass instead of particle density for sedimentation. The examples of common applications include separation of cells, cellular organelles such as endosomes or separation of proteins, such as antibodies (Rickwood D; Grahm J. M. 2001).

Criteria for successful rate-zonal centrifugation are:

- Density of the sample solution must be less than that of the lowest density portion of the gradient.
- Density of the sample particle (CTC) must be greater than that of the highest density portion of the gradient.
- The pathlength of the gradient must be sufficient for the separation to occur. However, if too long runs are performed, particles may all pellet at the bottom of the tube.

In isopycnic separation, a particle of a particular density will sink during centrifugation until a position is reached where the density of the surrounding solution is exactly the same as the density of the particle. Once this quasi-equilibrium is reached, the length of centrifugation does not have any influence on the migration of the particle. A common example for this method is separation of nucleic acids in a CsCl gradient. A variety of gradient media can be used for isopycnic separations (Rickwood D; Grahm J. M. 2001).

Criteria for successful isopycnic separation:

- Density of the sample particle must fall within the limits of the gradient densities.
- Any gradient length is acceptable.
- The run time must be sufficient for the particles to band at their isopycnic point. Excessive run times have no adverse effect (Ford 1991; Graham 1997; Rickwood David. 1992; Rickwood David, Ford T., Steensgaard Jens. 1994; Rickwood D; Grahm J. M. 2001).

In the context of the CTC enrichment by centrifugation the isopycnic separation is the method usually used. The cells that have a density higher than the density of the buffer will stay in the bottom of the tube. If the density of the cells is lower than the buffer, they will remain on the top of the liquid, forming a ring. On the contrary, if the density of the cells is the same than the buffer, the cells will form a ring in the middle of the tube. A well known example of the method is the commercial buffer FICOLL™ tube (Amersham

Biosciences AB) or Lymphoprep® (Nicomed) to separate the red blood cells from the other cells including CTC (Table 2).

OncoQuick® (Greiner) method uses a specific buffer able to isolate the CTC (Balic et al., 2005; Mankin et al., 2002; Paterlini-Brechot & Benali 2007). These methods are usually fast but expensive and found in a context of clinical laboratory used in routine diagnosis (Table 2). Alternative and cheaper methods can be used by preparing in the laboratory the gradient/density buffers. The same tube can contain one, two or three gradient buffers to increase the specificity of the separation between the different cells present in the blood (Gertler et al., 2003; Paterlini-Brechot & Benali 2007; Racila et al., 1998; Zach & Lutz 2006).

#### 4.1.2 Lysis buffers

The content of different cells has different osmotic pressures. It is possible to expose the samples to buffer(s) that can be hypo-or hyper osmotic to any cell different to the target cells. After the lysis step the mix is centrifuged and the pellets will contain the CTC. Some companies provide a kit with lysis buffers ready to use. After lysis, the next step is the extraction of DNA or RNA (e.g. Red Lysis Buffer from Qiagen or Panomics) or the extracted cells can be purified by immunomagnetic beads enrichment (Aryal et al., 2004; Khan et al., 2000; Wharton et al., 1999). However, lysis buffer can induce the death of a lot of cells including the CTC and it is not appropriate if the sample contains few CTC leading to false negative results.

#### 4.1.3 Cytocentrifugation (cytospin)

The cytocentrifugation was designed for hypocellular fluids; it spins at lower speeds and has more gradual acceleration and deceleration than normal centrifuges. Some are able to deposit cells directly onto a slide for examination. Cytocentrifugation could be used in research purposes and is also widely used in the routine surgical pathology practice. This method is fast and affordable (Becker et al., 2005; Kallergi et al., 2008; Kollermann et al., 1999; Molnar et al., 2001).

Methods to identify CTC can after be used (see below). As it occurs with magnetic beads, cytospin increases mortality of the target cells (Table 2). Because enrichment by cytocentrifugation is a critical step, addition of 10 % buffered formaldehyde solution added to the blood sample can preserve morphology of the cells and will certainly preserve nucleic acids integrity (Farina et al., 2004), but the disadvantage of this method is that formaldehyde kills the cells (Table 2). Liquid based cytology (LBC) using a filtration process and computer assisted thin layer deposition of cells has been developed as a replacement for cytocentrifugation and/or smearing, owing to its improved cell recovery capabilities and better cell preservation. In most published series, LBC allows a good interobserver reproducibility. In the urine, processing by the Cytyc ThinprepH 2000 system (Cytyc Corp, Boxborough, Massachusetts, USA) is a method that combines centrifugation and filter transfer methods. The vial containing CTC is placed into a processor (the machine which prepares the smears) together with a glass slide and filter mechanism. The processor immerses the filter assembly into the vial and spins it at a high speed to ensure an even mix of the cells and to break up large cell groups. The fixative is then sucked through a filter membrane which traps the cells but allows fluid through. When an adequate number of cells have been deposited on the filter, the processor detects a drop in the suction pressure and stops drawing fluid through the filter. It then applies the filter to a specially prepared glass slide and transfers the cells across. The slide is deposited into a vial of fixative (paraffin 10%) from which it is subsequently taken out and stained. It results in increased cellularity and a pronounced reduction of debris, red blood cells (RBC), and crystals (Papillo & Lapen 1994; Piaton et al., 2004; Wright & Halford 2001).

There are several advantages to this system. One is that it produces a thin layer of cells which is easier to evaluate than a thick smear. The morphology of the cells is also better. In addition, the entire cell sample is captured in the fixative vial which leads to a more representative smear being prepared. One of the most important advantages of this test is that the material that is left over after a smear has been prepared can be used for adjunctive testing. A further advantage is that the smears may be initially subjected to image analysis. Computer software "reads" the smears and registers the co-ordinates of the fields with what it regards as the most abnormal cells. On review the system directs the cytotechnologists to these fields where they are evaluated. This can cut down on technologists' screening time (Table 2).

There are also some disadvantages, which include increased manpower needed to prepare the smears, and the dependence of smear preparation on the instrument. This technique cannot be used directly from blood samples. The red blood cells need to be eliminated by FICOLL® method for example and after the sample can be processed by this technique (Table 2). This method is usually used for urine or ascites samples. However, optimization of cell capture and fixation can be achieved by methods other than Cytyc Thinprep LBC, particularly while using meticulous modern cytocentrifugation methods in the study of hypocellular fluids like in urine for the bladder cancer (Piaton et al., 2004; Wright & Halford 2001). In their study, Piaton et al., conclude that Cytyc Thinprep LBC and modern cytocentrifugation techniques are appropriate methods for cytology based molecular studies. From an economical point of view (standard cytocentrifugation are around $ 538 compared to Cytyc ThinprepH $ 1,278 ), and taking into account the value of a meticulous technique, cytocentrifugation with disposable sample chambers remains the quality standard for current treatment of urinary samples for example (Piaton et al., 2004).

#### 4.1.4 Filters

A non-specific method of enrichment using filters can captured the cells with a certain size. The cells captured on the filter can after be transferred and analyzed on a slide. In this case the samples can come from blood or body fluids (urines, cerebrospinal fluid or ascites). We will describe two kinds of methods using this technology and usually used to isolate CTC (Table 2): the Isolation by Size of Epithelial Tumor Cells (ISET) method and the Micro-Electro-Mechanical System (MEMS).

**The Isolation by Size of Epithelial Tumor Cells** (ISET) method (Metagenex, Paris, France, www.metagenex.fr) separates cells by size with a filter. Cells larger than 10 μm, including tumor cells from carcinomas, are enriched from leukocytes (erythrocytes are lysed, see above) on a filter. Enriched cells are stained on the filter and CTC are precisely counted after cytopathological evaluation. The cells on the filter can be also studied by immunolabelling,

FISH, TUNEL and molecular analysis. Molecular analysis can be performed specifically to CTC after laser microdissection. The filter can be also mounted between slide and coverslip for routine microscope observation and storage. Although promising, this method is expensive, time consuming and the filters are not easily available (Mejean et al., 2000; Paterlini-Brechot & Benali 2007; Pinzani et al., 2006). Cells should be better characterized using morphological methods that allow both detection and characterization. A second potential main advantage is that CTC could be compared to the primary tumor in order to better understand the mechanism of metastatic process. However, this approach has been rarely performed and neither firm recommendation nor conclusion could be drawn. This method has a high sensibility since one tumoral cell could be detect in 1 ml of blood. The technique also avoids damaging the tumor cell which can be diagnosed using a simple pathologist analysis. However, the pathologist should get used to this technique to avoid a misinterpretation with others types of cells. The use of ISET technology to detect and characterize CTC in HCC has been reported in one study. Vona et al., (Vona et al., 2004) reported that microemboli and isolated CTC could be detected in HCC patient. Presence of CTC was associated with a shorter survival. This work also showed the feasibility of molecular studies of individual circulating cells. Indeed, β-Catenin mutations were searched in samples of 60 single microdissected CTC. β-Catenin mutations were found in only 3 CTC that highlighted the weak impact of these mutations in the initial step of tumor cell invasion. Further studies are needed.

**The Micro-Electro-Mechanical System (MEMS)**-based is a parylene membrane microfilter device for single stage capture and electrolysis of circulating tumor cells in human blood, and the potential of this device to allow genomic analysis. After the CTC are captured in the filter, electrical lysis of cells on membrane filter is applied and the DNA as well as RNA can be extracted and analyzed by PCR or RT-PCR respectively. CTC enrichment is performed by either gradient centrifugation of CTC based on their buoyant density or magnetic separation of epithelial CTC, both of which are laborious procedures with variable efficiency, and CTC identification is typically done by trained pathologists through visual observation of stained cytokeratin-positive epithelial CTC. These processes may take hours, if not days. The Micro-Electro-Mechanical System (MEMS)-based makes the process simpler, faster and better to separate CTC (~90% recovery) from blood cells. Since enrichment will inevitably be accompanied by loss of CTC, irrespective of the exact method, some essays are performed directly in whole blood (Lu Y. et al., 2007). But the disadvantages of this technique are that morphology of the cells is lost, besides markers also and the capacity to count exactly the number of CTC (Table 2).

### 4.2 The specific enrichment techniques

The specific enrichment techniques can use specifically protein tumoral markers expressed by the CTC. These methods use antibodies against the protein tumoral markers coupled to steel beads, by applying a magnetic field the cells expressing the marker can be captured. Several immune-magnetic methods (MACS system, Deanabeads® Invitrogen, macro-iron beads, ferrofluid(colloidal iron)-based systems) to enrich the sample have been used successfully (Sergeant et al., 2008). We will describe the methods and their advantages and their disadvantages. Another approach to enrich the sample is to use the properties of CTC to grow-up in a specific culture cell medium. A method (EPISPOT) that combines the capacity of CTC to secret specific markers and grow-up in specific cell medium was developed (see Table 2).

### 4.2.1 Magnetic separation

To use immune-magnetic detection system the first step is to deplete the whole blood of the red cells (by lysis buffers or density gradient) to obtain the PBMC. After, the magnetic particles coated and surrounded by a specific antibody are added to the PBMC supposing containing the CTC. Labeled cells are then collected by applying a magnetic force while non labeled cells are containing in the supernatant and are discerned. This use of magnetic beads to catch specifically CTC is called "positive selection" (Alix-Panabieres et al., 2008; Paterlini-Brechot & Benali 2007; Sleijfer et al., 2007).

Since a large number of leukocytes (potential source of false negative CTC) still remain trapped with the cells, some methods include a "negative selection" of leukocytes (with anti-CD 45 beads for example) followed with a "positive selection" with antibodies specific to epithelial cells (EpCAM, CK) (Allard et al., 2004; Paterlini-Brechot & Benali 2007; Smirnov et al., 2005). The problem of this procedure is that gets ride the majority of leukocytes but still hold in non-malignant epithelial cells and loses tumor cells which do not express epithelial antigens and/or are lysed during the first step (Paterlini-Brechot & Benali 2007; Zigeuner et al., 2003).

The methods using antibodies like immune-magnetic methods (MACS system, Deanabeads® Invitrogen, macro-iron beads, ferrofluid(colloidal iron)-based systems) to enrich the sample will induce false-positive extraction (Sergeant et al., 2008). For example, antibodies against cytokeratin (CK) or other epithelial-specific antigens have been reported to bind both specifically and non-specifically to macrophages, plasma cells and nucleated hematopoietic cells precursors. The non-specific binding of the antibodies involves Fc receptor-bearing leukocytes and monocytes or illegitimate expression of epithelial antigens in normal hematopoietic cells. Some of these positive cells are morphologically difficult to distinguish from CTC. Variable numbers of epithelial cells have been found in peripheral blood of subject without malignancy in some physio-pathological conditions like benign epithelial proliferative diseases, inflammation, surgeries and tissue trauma (Allard et al., 2004; Becker et al., 2005; Goeminne et al., 2000; Naume et al., 2004; Naume & Espevik 1991; Paterlini-Brechot & Benali 2007). Moreover, epithelial CTC may lose epithelial markers during dissemination through the process called epithelial-to-mesenchymal transition (EMT). Since the epithelial markers that get lost during EMT may include markers used for CTC measurement, underestimation of the actual CTC number may occur, inducing de facto false negative results (Christiansen & Rajasekaran 2006; Paterlini-Brechot & Benali 2007; Sleijfer et al., 2007; Wang J. Y. et al., 2006; Willipinski-Stapelfeldt et al., 2005). In the case that the method induce false positive, the problem can be diminished avoided using a second marker or a full panel of markers and techniques (see below) to characterize the CTC, like RT-PCR, immunocytochemistry or immunefluorescence, morphology by optical microscopy (Paterlini-Brechot & Benali 2007; Schuler & Dolken 2006; Sleijfer et al., 2007). In another hand, in the case of the false negative results the doubt persist, and only strict follow-up of the patient by repeating the detection of the CTC can potentially eliminate this doubt. No available antibodies are 100% tumor or tissue-specific (El-Serag 2004; Goeminne et al., 2000;

Paterlini-Brechot & Benali 2007). To isolate CTC a method using a ligand biotinylated was used. Biotinylated asialofetuin, a ligand of asialoglycoprotein receptor, was experimented and followed by magnetic separation or density gradient (Ficoll-Paque PLUS; GE Healthcare). The cells were identified by microscopy, FISH, immunofluorescence staining, flux cytometry and RT-PCR. This technique shows 81% specificity and 20 cells/5ml for the sensitivity (Xu et al., 2011). This promising approach has to be confirmed in a larger cohort of patients and still depend on the receptors expressed at the surface of the CTC.

#### 4.2.2 Culture of CTC

After isolation of the CTC by the different methods described above, to increase the number of CTC, the primary tumor cells can be cultured in the specific culture medium (Allard et al., 2004). The optimal conditions of culture growth and specially the culture medium leading the growth of the CTC, but not the other epithelial or non epithelial cells, have to be determined through an experiment. Some companies propose commercial kits. For example, The Cancer Cell Isolation Kit® from Panomics includes lysis buffer to increase the number of CTC. One of the main problems is that cultured cells can lose their original markers and derive. Mimicry of tumoral microenvironment *in vitro* is particularly difficult because for most tumors it is largely unknown. Another problem is that the samples containing the CTC are usually contaminated by stromal cells like fibroblasts, which create competition in the Petri dish. After few days, only the fibroblasts are present in the flask.

#### 4.2.3 Epithelial immunoSPOT (EPISPOT)

A technique that allows the detection of only viable cells after a $CD45^+$ cell depletion was introduced for CTC analysis from bone marrow aspirates and blood samples (Alix-Panabieres et al., 2008; Alix-Panabieres et al., 2007; Braun et al., 2005). This technique was designated EPISPOT (epithelial ImmunoSPOT). It is a protein-secreting profiling based on the secretion or active release of specific marker proteins using an adaptation of the enzyme-linked immunospot technology. As immunospots are the protein fingerprint left only by the viable releasing epithelial cells, a cell culture is needed to accumulate a sufficient amount of the released marker proteins (Table 2). The dying cells do not secrete adequate amounts of protein and are not detected (Alix-Panabieres et al., 2005; Alix-Panabieres et al., 2008; Alix-Panabieres et al., 2007; Czerkinsky et al., 1983). This assay can also provide important information on the profile of secreted proteins potentially relevant for metastasis formation. However, this technique has still to be validated in large-scale clinical studies on cancer patients (Alix-Panabieres et al., 2008; Alix-Panabieres et al., 2007). After the enrichment and isolation of the CTC, the next step is to identify, characterize and finally enumerate them. The CTC can be identified by indirect or direct methods. But these important steps need tumor markers specific to the CTC seeked.

## 5. Experimental models

### 5.1 HCC mouse models

Over decades, different HCC mouse models have been developed.

Chemically induced HCC-models are diverse and not always reproducible. The chemicals usually used are diethylnitrosamine (DEN), peroxisome proliferators, aflatoxine, carbon tetrachloride ($CCl_4$), choline deficient diet or thiacetamide (Heindryckx et al., 2009; Weylandt et al., 2011). Transgenic mouse models were also developed, for example mice that contained HBV or HCV viruses or expressed specifically oncogenes (c-myc, c-myc + E2F1) or growth factors (TGF-α, TGF-α + c-myc, EGF, FGF19, GMNT, PDGF, α1-antitrypsin) (Heindryckx et al., 2009). Circulating tumor cells were not looked for in any of these animal models. One reason is the huge differences between models and the presence of specific markers for each situation.

In order to solve these problems, researchers developed ectopic implantation that is fast and easy to perform. However, there is still many differences between the cell lines, no direct interaction with the liver tissues and difficulty to export to humans (Heindryckx et al., 2009).

### 5.2 Orthotopic implantation

Orthotopic implantation is a more suitable model because the cells are directly implanted in the liver tissue. Nevertheless, the procedure is challenging. There are big differences between cell lines and the choice of the markers is still limited (Heindryckx et al., 2009). Mechanisms leading to tumoral cells spreading are ill known. Currently, there are few models of orthotopic implantation of human tumoral cells (Scatton et al., 2008; Scatton et al., 2006). An experimental model of human orthotopic HCC transplantation in NOD/SCID (non-obese diabetic/several compromise immuno-deficient) mice allows to generate and to modulate CTC (Scatton et al., 2008; Scatton et al., 2006). In this mouse model, tumoral spreading is an early event during tumoral development and the number of CTC is directly correlated to the tumor size.

When injected under the liver capsule, a primary tumor develops and continuously yields circulating tumor cells. In addition, the CTC could be modulated after tumor removal. Liver tumor removal led to a very low level of tumoral cells in blood 30 days later. After complete tumor removal, the number of CTC significantly decreases but still remains detectable even at a low level. The FACS was used to detect CTC (detection of human HLA marker in mouse bloodstream). The reality of CTC was then demonstrated. An important finding is that the bone marrow could be early and permanently colonized by CTC (Scatton et al., 2006).

### 5.3 Small imaging animal models

With the recent development of the small imaging apparatus (example: IVIS Lumina II XR Imaging System, positron emission tomography) to study development and the progression of diseases in the live animals like rheumatism, a new area to study CTC in live animals is open. This technique was applied to study the CTC in ectopic or orthotopic HCC cell lines implantation. As we discuss above, the lack of specific HCC markers makes CTC studies very challenging. The idea is to bind luminescence tag (luciferase, yellow fluorescence or red fluorescence proteins) in the hepatoma cell lines injected in the liver that be detected by bioluminescence machine. For example, thymidine kinase-luciferase was placing under the transcriptional control of endogenous AFP promoter to develop a transgenic mouse model that injected with DEN will develop HCC (Lu X. et al., 2011). The development of the HCC was followed in the live animal by bioluminescence and PET analyses. The inconvenient of this method is that the HCC model has to express AFP. To avoid this problem hepatoma cell lines where engineered with luciferease (HCC-LM3) (Ma et al., 2011) or red luminescence protein (Xiao et al., 2011). This approach to study CTC in the context of HCC is very promising, but the major problem is the sensitivity of the bioluminescence machine. This approach has not yet studied in the context of CTC in the blood or in organs other than liver.

## 6. Conclusion

There are two major problems to detect circulating hepatocarcinoma cells in the human blood. The first problem is the low number of specific markers known. The second problem is that few cells are present in the bloodstream. To overcome these problems, few years ago new approaches have been developed such as the techniques to study membrane proteins by mass spectrometry and the development of fluorescent hepatoma cells.

Nowadays, these procedures are not suitable in clinical practice. However, it is undeniable that early detection of tumors and metastasis is urgently needed in medicine and these new exciting techniques and findings are changing our point of view of carcinogenesis very fast. In the future, CTC detection will certainly be an important diagnostic tool in cancer patients, providing a new and accurate assessment of lesion staging.

## 7. Acknowledgment

We are grateful to Pr. Olivier Scatton for useful criticisms and discussion.

## 8. References

Agarwal, S. K., Lee Burns, A., et al. (2004). Molecular pathology of the MEN1 gene. *Ann N Y Acad Sci*, Vol. 1014, No. pp. 189-198

Alix-Panabieres, C., Brouillet, J. P., et al. (2005). Characterization and enumeration of cells secreting tumor markers in the peripheral blood of breast cancer patients. *J Immunol Methods*, Vol. 299, No. 1-2, pp. 177-188

Alix-Panabieres, C., Riethdorf, S. & Pantel, K. (2008). Circulating tumor cells and bone marrow micrometastasis. *Clin Cancer Res*, Vol. 14, No. 16, pp. 5013-5021

Alix-Panabieres, C., Vendrell, J. P., et al. (2007). Detection and characterization of putative metastatic precursor cells in cancer patients. *Clin Chem*, Vol. 53, No. 3, pp. 537-539

Allard, W. J., Matera, J., et al. (2004). Tumor cells circulate in the peripheral blood of all major carcinomas but not in healthy subjects or patients with nonmalignant diseases. *Clin Cancer Res*, Vol. 10, No. 20, pp. 6897-6904

Aryal, K. R., Lengyel, A. J., et al. (2004). Nipple core biopsy for the deformed or scaling nipple. *Breast*, Vol. 13, No. 4, pp. 350-352

Aselmann, H., Wolfes, H., et al. (2001). Quantification of alpha 1-fetoprotein mRNA in peripheral blood and bone marrow: a tool for perioperative evaluation of patients with hepatocellular carcinoma. *Langenbecks Arch Surg*, Vol. 386, No. 2, pp. 118-123

Assy, N., Nasser, G., et al. (2009). Characteristics of common solid liver lesions and recommendations for diagnostic workup. *World J Gastroenterol*, Vol. 15, No. 26, pp. 3217-3227

Balic, M., Dandachi, N., et al. (2005). Comparison of two methods for enumerating circulating tumor cells in carcinoma patients. *Cytometry B Clin Cytom*, Vol. 68, No. 1, pp. 25-30

Banks, E., Reeves, G., et al. (2006). Hormone replacement therapy and false positive recall in the Million Women Study: patterns of use, hormonal constituents and consistency of effect. *Breast Cancer Res*, Vol. 8, No. 1, pp. R8

Becker, S., Becker-Pergola, G., et al. (2005). Image analysis systems for the detection of disseminated breast cancer cells on bone-marrow cytospins. *J Clin Lab Anal*, Vol. 19, No. 3, pp. 115-119

Benoy, I. H., Elst, H., et al. (2006). Real-time RT-PCR detection of disseminated tumor cells in bone marrow has superior prognostic significance in comparison with circulating tumor cells in patients with breast cancer. *Br J Cancer*, Vol. 94, No. 5, pp. 672-680

Bergamaschi, A., Tagliabue, E., et al. (2008). Extracellular matrix signature identifies breast cancer subgroups with different clinical outcome. *J Pathol*, Vol. 214, No. 3, pp. 357-367

Borgen, E., Beiske, K., et al. (1998). Immunocytochemical detection of isolated epithelial cells in bone marrow: non-specific staining and contribution by plasma cells directly reactive to alkaline phosphatase. *J Pathol*, Vol. 185, No. 4, pp. 427-434

Bostick, P. J., Chatterjee, S., et al. (1998). Limitations of specific reverse-transcriptase polymerase chain reaction markers in the detection of metastases in the lymph nodes and blood of breast cancer patients. *J Clin Oncol*, Vol. 16, No. 8, pp. 2632-2640

Braun, S., Vogl, F. D., et al. (2005). A pooled analysis of bone marrow micrometastasis in breast cancer. *N Engl J Med*, Vol. 353, No. 8, pp. 793-802

Britto, M. R., Thomas, L. A., et al. (2000). Hepatocellular carcinoma arising in non-cirrhotic liver in genetic haemochromatosis. *Scand J Gastroenterol*, Vol. 35, No. 8, pp. 889-893

Bruix, J. & Sherman, M. (2005). Management of hepatocellular carcinoma. *Hepatology*, Vol. 42, No. 5, pp. 1208-1236

Bruix, J., Sherman, M., et al. (2001). Clinical management of hepatocellular carcinoma. Conclusions of the Barcelona-2000 EASL conference. European Association for the Study of the Liver. *J Hepatol*, Vol. 35, No. 3, pp. 421-430

Byrnes, V., Shi, H., et al. (2007). The clinical outcome of small (<20 mm) arterially enhancing nodules on MRI in the cirrhotic liver. *Am J Gastroenterol*, Vol. 102, No. 8, pp. 1654-1659

Caldwell, S. & Park, S. H. (2009). The epidemiology of hepatocellular cancer: from the perspectives of public health problem to tumor biology. *J Gastroenterol*, Vol. 44 Suppl 19, No. pp. 96-101

Cheung, S. T., Liu, C. L., et al. (2006). Preoperative plasma transcript AA454543 level is an independent prognostic factor for hepatocellular carcinoma after partial hepatectomy. *Neoplasia*, Vol. 8, No. 9, pp. 696-701

Chiba, T., Kamiya, A., Yokosuka, O. & Iwama, A. (2009). Cancer stem cells in hepatocellular carcinoma: Recent progress and perspective. *Cancer Lett*, Vol. 286, No. 2, pp. 145-153

Christiansen, J. J. & Rajasekaran, A. K. (2006). Reassessing epithelial to mesenchymal transition as a prerequisite for carcinoma invasion and metastasis. *Cancer Res*, Vol. 66, No. 17, pp. 8319-8326

CLIP. (1998). A new prognostic system for hepatocellular carcinoma: a retrospective study of 435 patients: the Cancer of the Liver Italian Program (CLIP) investigators. *Hepatology*, Vol. 28, No. 3, pp. 751-755

Collier, J. & Sherman, M. (1998). Screening for hepatocellular carcinoma. *Hepatology*, Vol. 27, No. 1, pp. 273-278

Curry, D. N., Krivacic, R. T., et al. (2004). High-speed detection of occult tumor cells in peripheral blood. *Conf Proc IEEE Eng Med Biol Soc*, Vol. 2, No. pp. 1267-1270

Czerkinsky, C. C., Nilsson, L. A., et al. (1983). A solid-phase enzyme-linked immunospot (ELISPOT) assay for enumeration of specific antibody-secreting cells. *J Immunol Methods*, Vol. 65, No. 1-2, pp. 109-121

Dai, Z., Zhou, J., et al. (2009). Lectin-based glycoproteomics to explore and analyze hepatocellular carcinoma-related glycoprotein markers. *Electrophoresis*, Vol. 30, No. 17, pp. 2957-2966

Davila, J. A., Morgan, R. O., et al. (2004). Hepatitis C infection and the increasing incidence of hepatocellular carcinoma: a population-based study. *Gastroenterology*, Vol. 127, No. 5, pp. 1372-1380

Dohmen, K., Shigematsu, H., Irie, K. & Ishibashi, H. (2003). Clinical characteristics among patients with hepatocellular carcinoma according to the serum levels of alpha-fetoprotein and des-y-carboxy prothrombin. *Hepatogastroenterology*, Vol. 50, No. 54, pp. 2072-2078

Donati, M., Brancato, G. & Donati, A. (2010). Clinical biomarkers in hepatocellular carcinoma (HCC). *Front Biosci (Schol Ed)*, Vol. 2, No. pp. 571-577

Donato, F., Gelatti, U., Limina, R. M. & Fattovich, G. (2006). Southern Europe as an example of interaction between various environmental factors: a systematic review of the epidemiologic evidence. *Oncogene*, Vol. 25, No. 27, pp. 3756-3770

Dong, Z. Z., Yao, D. F., et al. (2005). Expression and alteration of insulin-like growth factor II-messenger RNA in hepatoma tissues and peripheral blood of patients with hepatocellular carcinoma. *World J Gastroenterol*, Vol. 11, No. 30, pp. 4655-4660

Dong, Z. Z., Yao, D. F., et al. (2008). Clinical impact of plasma TGF-beta1 and circulating TGF-beta1 mRNA in diagnosis of hepatocellular carcinoma. *Hepatobiliary Pancreat Dis Int*, Vol. 7, No. 3, pp. 288-295

Durand, F., Regimbeau, J. M., et al. (2001). Assessment of the benefits and risks of percutaneous biopsy before surgical resection of hepatocellular carcinoma. *J Hepatol*, Vol. 35, No. 2, pp. 254-258

El-Serag, H. B. (2002). Hepatocellular carcinoma: an epidemiologic view. *J Clin Gastroenterol*, Vol. 35, No. 5 Suppl 2, pp. S72-78

El-Serag, H. B. (2004). Hepatocellular carcinoma: recent trends in the United States. *Gastroenterology*, Vol. 127, No. 5 Suppl 1, pp. S27-34

El-Serag, H. B., Davila, J. A., Petersen, N. J. & McGlynn, K. A. (2003). The continuing increase in the incidence of hepatocellular carcinoma in the United States: an update. *Ann Intern Med*, Vol. 139, No. 10, pp. 817-823

Farina, A., Sekizawa, A., et al. (2004). Total cell-free DNA (beta-globin gene) distribution in maternal plasma at the second trimester: a new prospective for preeclampsia screening. *Prenat Diagn*, Vol. 24, No. 9, pp. 722-726

Ford, T. C., Graham, J.M. (1991). *An Introduction to Centrifugation*, BIOS Scientific Publishers, Ltd., 1 872748 40 6

Freeman, R. B., Jr. (2006). Transplantation for hepatocellular carcinoma: The Milan criteria and beyond. *Liver Transpl*, Vol. 12, No. 11 Suppl 2, pp. S8-13

Freeman, R. B., Mithoefer, A., et al. (2006). Optimizing staging for hepatocellular carcinoma before liver transplantation: A retrospective analysis of the UNOS/OPTN database. *Liver Transpl*, Vol. 12, No. 10, pp. 1504-1511

Fujiyama, S., Tanaka, M., et al. (2002). Tumor markers in early diagnosis, follow-up and management of patients with hepatocellular carcinoma. *Oncology*, Vol. 62 Suppl 1, No. pp. 57-63

Gertler, R., Rosenberg, R., et al. (2003). Detection of circulating tumor cells in blood using an optimized density gradient centrifugation. *Recent Results Cancer Res*, Vol. 162, No. pp. 149-155

Goeminne, J. C., Guillaume, T. & Symann, M. (2000). Pitfalls in the detection of disseminated non-hematological tumor cells. *Ann Oncol*, Vol. 11, No. 7, pp. 785-792

Gomaa, A. I., Khan, S. A., et al. (2009). Diagnosis of hepatocellular carcinoma. *World J Gastroenterol*, Vol. 15, No. 11, pp. 1301-1314

Gonzalez, S. A. & Keeffe, E. B. (2011). Diagnosis of hepatocellular carcinoma: role of tumor markers and liver biopsy. *Clin Liver Dis*, Vol. 15, No. 2, pp. 297-306

Graham, J. M. R., D. (1997). *Subcellular Fractionation: A Practical Approach*, Oxford Univ Press, 0199634947

Grizzi, F., Franceschini, B., et al. (2007). Usefulness of cancer-testis antigens as biomarkers for the diagnosis and treatment of hepatocellular carcinoma. *J Transl Med*, Vol. 5, No. pp. 3

Groom, A. C., MacDonald, I. C., et al. (1999). Tumor metastasis to the liver, and the roles of proteinases and adhesion molecules: new concepts from in vivo videomicroscopy. *Can J Gastroenterol*, Vol. 13, No. 9, pp. 733-743

Gross-Goupil, M., Saffroy, R., et al. (2003). Real-time quantification of AFP mRNA to assess hematogenous dissemination after transarterial chemoembolization of hepatocellular carcinoma. *Ann Surg*, Vol. 238, No. 2, pp. 241-248

Hassan, M. M., Frome, A., Patt, Y. Z. & El-Serag, H. B. (2002). Rising prevalence of hepatitis C virus infection among patients recently diagnosed with hepatocellular carcinoma in the United States. *J Clin Gastroenterol*, Vol. 35, No. 3, pp. 266-269

Heindryckx, F., Colle, I. & Van Vlierberghe, H. (2009). Experimental mouse models for hepatocellular carcinoma research. *Int J Exp Pathol*, Vol. 90, No. 4, pp. 367-386

Hermanek, P., Hutter, R. V., Sobin, L. H. & Wittekind, C. (1999). International Union Against Cancer. Classification of isolated tumor cells and micrometastasis. *Cancer*, Vol. 86, No. 12, pp. 2668-2673

Hillaire, S., Barbu, V., et al. (1994). Albumin messenger RNA as a marker of circulating hepatocytes in hepatocellular carcinoma. *Gastroenterology*, Vol. 106, No. 1, pp. 239-242

Hoshida, Y., Toffanin, S., et al. (2010). Molecular classification and novel targets in hepatocellular carcinoma: recent advancements. *Semin Liver Dis*, Vol. 30, No. 1, pp. 35-51

Houghton, J., Stoicov, C., et al. (2004). Gastric cancer originating from bone marrow-derived cells. *Science*, Vol. 306, No. 5701, pp. 1568-1571

Hsieh, H. B., Marrinucci, D., et al. (2006). High speed detection of circulating tumor cells. *Biosens Bioelectron*, Vol. 21, No. 10, pp. 1893-1899

Huang, F. & Geng, X. P. (2010). Chemokines and hepatocellular carcinoma. *World J Gastroenterol*, Vol. 16, No. 15, pp. 1832-1836

Hussain, K. & El-Serag, H. B. (2009). Epidemiology, screening, diagnosis and treatment of hepatocellular carcinoma. *Minerva Gastroenterol Dietol*, Vol. 55, No. 2, pp. 123-138

Idilman, R., De Maria, N., Colantoni, A. & Van Thiel, D. H. (1998). Pathogenesis of hepatitis B and C-induced hepatocellular carcinoma. *J Viral Hepat*, Vol. 5, No. 5, pp. 285-299

Ijichi, M., Takayama, T., et al. (2002). alpha-Fetoprotein mRNA in the circulation as a predictor of postsurgical recurrence of hepatocellular carcinoma: a prospective study. *Hepatology*, Vol. 35, No. 4, pp. 853-860

Ishikawa, T., Kashiwagi, H., et al. (1998). Expression of alpha-fetoprotein and prostate-specific antigen genes in several tissues and detection of mRNAs in normal circulating blood by reverse transcriptase-polymerase chain reaction. *Jpn J Clin Oncol*, Vol. 28, No. 12, pp. 723-728

Ji, J. & Wang, X. W. (2009). New kids on the block: diagnostic and prognostic microRNAs in hepatocellular carcinoma. *Cancer Biol Ther*, Vol. 8, No. 18, pp. 1686-1693

Jung, R., Kruger, W., et al. (1998). Specificity of reverse transcriptase polymerase chain reaction assays designed for the detection of circulating cancer cells is influenced by cytokines in vivo and in vitro. *Br J Cancer*, Vol. 78, No. 9, pp. 1194-1198

Kallergi, G., Agelaki, S., et al. (2008). Phosphorylated EGFR and PI3K/Akt signaling kinases are expressed in circulating tumor cells of breast cancer patients. *Breast Cancer Res*, Vol. 10, No. 5, pp. R80

Kamiyama, T., Miyakawa, H., et al. (1996). Ischemic hepatitis in cirrhosis. clinical features and prognostic implications. *J Clin Gastroenterol*, Vol. 22, No. 2, pp. 126-130

Kar, S. & Carr, B. I. (1995). Detection of liver cells in peripheral blood of patients with advanced-stage hepatocellular carcinoma. *Hepatology*, Vol. 21, No. 2, pp. 403-407

Kerr, T. A., Korenblat, K. M. & Davidson, N. O. (2011). MicroRNAs and liver disease. *Transl Res*, Vol. 157, No. 4, pp. 241-252

Khan, Z. A., Jonas, S. K., et al. (2000). P53 mutations in primary and metastatic tumors and circulating tumor cells from colorectal carcinoma patients. *Clin Cancer Res*, Vol. 6, No. 9, pp. 3499-3504

Kienle, P., Weitz, J., et al. (2000). Detection of isolated disseminated tumor cells in bone marrow and blood samples of patients with hepatocellular carcinoma. *Arch Surg*, Vol. 135, No. 2, pp. 213-218

Kojima, K., Takata, A., et al. (2011). MicroRNA122 is a key regulator of alpha-fetoprotein expression and influences the aggressiveness of hepatocellular carcinoma. *Nat Commun*, Vol. 2, No. pp. 338

Kollermann, J., Heseding, B., et al. (1999). Comparative immunocytochemical assessment of isolated carcinoma cells in lymph nodes and bone marrow of patients with clinically localized prostate cancer. *Int J Cancer*, Vol. 84, No. 2, pp. 145-149

Komeda, T., Fukuda, Y., et al. (1995). Sensitive detection of circulating hepatocellular carcinoma cells in peripheral venous blood. *Cancer*, Vol. 75, No. 9, pp. 2214-2219

Kong, G., Zhang, J., et al. (2011). Upregulated MicroRNA-29a by Hepatitis B Virus X Protein Enhances Hepatoma Cell Migration by Targeting PTEN in Cell Culture Model. *PLoS One*, Vol. 6, No. 5, pp. e19518

Kong, S. Y., Park, J. W., et al. (2009). Alpha-fetoprotein and human telomerase reverse transcriptase mRNA levels in peripheral blood of patients with hepatocellular carcinoma. *J Cancer Res Clin Oncol*, Vol. 135, No. 8, pp. 1091-1098

Lee, R. C., Feinbaum, R. L. & Ambros, V. (1993). The C. elegans heterochronic gene lin-4 encodes small RNAs with antisense complementarity to lin-14. *Cell*, Vol. 75, No. 5, pp. 843-854

Lemoine, A., Le Bricon, T., et al. (1997). Prospective evaluation of circulating hepatocytes by alpha-fetoprotein mRNA in humans during liver surgery. *Ann Surg*, Vol. 226, No. 1, pp. 43-50

Li, N., Guo, W., et al. (2010). Expression of the chemokine receptor CXCR4 in human hepatocellular carcinoma and its role in portal vein tumor thrombus. *J Exp Clin Cancer Res*, Vol. 29, No. pp. 156

Liotta, L. A., Kleinerman, J. & Saidel, G. M. (1974). Quantitative relationships of intravascular tumor cells, tumor vessels, and pulmonary metastases following tumor implantation. *Cancer Res*, Vol. 34, No. 5, pp. 997-1004

Liu, L. L., Fu, D., Ma, Y. & Shen, X. (2011). The Power and the Promise of Liver Cancer Stem Cell Markers. *Stem Cells Dev*, Vol. No. pp.

Liu, X., Wan, X., et al. (2011). Golgi protein 73(GP73), a useful serum marker in liver diseases. *Clin Chem Lab Med*, Vol. No. pp.

Llovet, J. M., Bru, C. & Bruix, J. (1999). Prognosis of hepatocellular carcinoma: the BCLC staging classification. *Semin Liver Dis*, Vol. 19, No. 3, pp. 329-338

Lobodasch, K., Frohlich, F., et al. (2007). Quantification of circulating tumor cells for the monitoring of adjuvant therapy in breast cancer: an increase in cell number at completion of therapy is a predictor of early relapse. *Breast*, Vol. 16, No. 2, pp. 211-218

Lok, A. S., Sterling, R. K., et al. (2009). Des-gamma-Carboxy Prothrombin and alpha-Fetoprotein as Biomarkers for the Early Detection of Hepatocellular Carcinoma. *Gastroenterology*, Vol. No. pp.

Louha, M., Nicolet, J., et al. (1999). Liver resection and needle liver biopsy cause hematogenous dissemination of liver cells. *Hepatology*, Vol. 29, No. 3, pp. 879-882

Lu, X., Guo, H., et al. (2011). Alpha-fetoprotein-thymidine kinase-luciferase knockin mice: A novel model for dual modality longitudinal imaging of tumorigenesis in liver. *J Hepatol*, Vol. 55, No. 1, pp. 96-102

Lu, Y., Wu, L. Q., et al. (2007). Expression of SSX-1 and NY-ESO-1 mRNA in tumor tissues and its corresponding peripheral blood expression in patients with hepatocellular carcinoma. *Chin Med J (Engl)*, Vol. 120, No. 12, pp. 1042-1046

Luzzi, K. J., MacDonald, I. C., et al. (1998). Multistep nature of metastatic inefficiency: dormancy of solitary cells after successful extravasation and limited survival of early micrometastases. *Am J Pathol*, Vol. 153, No. 3, pp. 865-873

Ma, X., Liu, Z., et al. (2011). Dual-modality monitoring of tumor response to cyclophosphamide therapy in mice with bioluminescence imaging and small-animal positron emission tomography. *Mol Imaging*, Vol. 10, No. 4, pp. 278-283

Makridakis, M. & Vlahou, A. (2010). Secretome proteomics for discovery of cancer biomarkers. *J Proteomics*, Vol. 73, No. 12, pp. 2291-2305

Malaguarnera, G., Giordano, M., et al. (2010). Serum markers of hepatocellular carcinoma. *Dig Dis Sci*, Vol. 55, No. 10, pp. 2744-2755

Malavaud, B., Miedouge, M., et al. (1999). Prostate-specific antigen in acute hepatitis and hepatocellular carcinoma. *Prostate*, Vol. 41, No. 4, pp. 258-262

Mankin, H. J., Fondren, G., et al. (2002). The use of flow cytometry in assessing malignancy in bone and soft tissue tumors. *Clin Orthop Relat Res*, Vol. No. 397, pp. 95-105

Matsumura, M. (2001). [AFP mRNA in the circulation]. *Nippon Rinsho*, Vol. 59 Suppl 6, No. pp. 377-382

Matsumura, M., Ijichi, M., et al. (2001). Simple quantitative assay of alpha-fetoprotein mRNA in liver tissue using the real-time detection polymerase chain reaction assay - its application for clinical use. *Hepatol Res*, Vol. 20, No. 1, pp. 84-96

Matsumura, M., Niwa, Y., et al. (1995). Sensitive assay for detection of hepatocellular carcinoma associated gene transcription (alpha-fetoprotein mRNA) in blood. *Biochem Biophys Res Commun*, Vol. 207, No. 2, pp. 813-818

Matsumura, M., Niwa, Y., et al. (1994). Detection of alpha-fetoprotein mRNA, an indicator of hematogenous spreading hepatocellular carcinoma, in the circulation: a possible predictor of metastatic hepatocellular carcinoma. *Hepatology*, Vol. 20, No. 6, pp. 1418-1425

Matsumura, M., Shiratori, Y., et al. (1999). Presence of alpha-fetoprotein mRNA in blood correlates with outcome in patients with hepatocellular carcinoma. *J Hepatol*, Vol. 31, No. 2, pp. 332-339

McGlynn, K. A., Tsao, L., et al. (2001). International trends and patterns of primary liver cancer. *Int J Cancer*, Vol. 94, No. 2, pp. 290-296

McMahon, B. J. (2009). The natural history of chronic hepatitis B virus infection. *Hepatology*, Vol. 49, No. 5 Suppl, pp. S45-55

Mejean, A., Vona, G., et al. (2000). Detection of circulating prostate derived cells in patients with prostate adenocarcinoma is an independent risk factor for tumor recurrence. *J Urol*, Vol. 163, No. 6, pp. 2022-2029

Mendizabal, M. & Reddy, K. R. (2009). Current management of hepatocellular carcinoma. *Med Clin North Am*, Vol. 93, No. 4, pp. 885-900, viii

Min, A. L., Choi, J. Y., et al. (2009). High expression of Snail mRNA in blood from hepatocellular carcinoma patients with extra-hepatic metastasis. *Clin Exp Metastasis*, Vol. 26, No. 7, pp. 759-767

Minata, M., Nishida, N., et al. (2001). Postoperative detection of alpha-fetoprotein mRNA in blood as a predictor for metastatic recurrence of hepatocellular carcinoma. *J Gastroenterol Hepatol*, Vol. 16, No. 4, pp. 445-451

Miyazono, F., Natsugoe, S., et al. (2001). Surgical maneuvers enhance molecular detection of circulating tumor cells during gastric cancer surgery. *Ann Surg*, Vol. 233, No. 2, pp. 189-194

Mocellin, S., Hoon, D., et al. (2006). The prognostic value of circulating tumor cells in patients with melanoma: a systematic review and meta-analysis. *Clin Cancer Res*, Vol. 12, No. 15, pp. 4605-4613

Mocellin, S., Keilholz, U., Rossi, C. R. & Nitti, D. (2006). Circulating tumor cells: the 'leukemic phase' of solid cancers. *Trends Mol Med*, Vol. 12, No. 3, pp. 130-139

Molnar, B., Ladanyi, A., et al. (2001). Circulating tumor cell clusters in the peripheral blood of colorectal cancer patients. *Clin Cancer Res*, Vol. 7, No. 12, pp. 4080-4085

Morimoto, O., Nagano, H., et al. (2005). Association between recurrence of hepatocellular carcinoma and alpha-fetoprotein messenger RNA levels in peripheral blood. *Surg Today*, Vol. 35, No. 12, pp. 1033-1041

Muller, V., Stahmann, N., et al. (2005). Circulating tumor cells in breast cancer: correlation to bone marrow micrometastases, heterogeneous response to systemic therapy and low proliferative activity. *Clin Cancer Res*, Vol. 11, No. 10, pp. 3678-3685

Nagrath, S., Sequist, L. V., et al. (2007). Isolation of rare circulating tumor cells in cancer patients by microchip technology. *Nature*, Vol. 450, No. 7173, pp. 1235-1239

Nakagawa, T., Martinez, S. R., et al. (2007). Detection of circulating tumor cells in early-stage breast cancer metastasis to axillary lymph nodes. *Clin Cancer Res*, Vol. 13, No. 14, pp. 4105-4110

Naume, B. (1998). [New methods for early detection of breast cancer metastasis]. *Tidsskr Nor Laegeforen*, Vol. 118, No. 3, pp. 354

Naume, B., Borgen, E., et al. (1998). Increased sensitivity for detection of micrometastases in bone-marrow/peripheral-blood stem-cell products from breast-cancer patients by negative immunomagnetic separation. *Int J Cancer*, Vol. 78, No. 5, pp. 556-560

Naume, B., Borgen, E., et al. (2004). Detection of isolated tumor cells in peripheral blood and in BM: evaluation of a new enrichment method. *Cytotherapy*, Vol. 6, No. 3, pp. 244-252

Naume, B. & Espevik, T. (1991). Effects of IL-7 and IL-2 on highly enriched CD56+ natural killer cells. A comparative study. *J Immunol*, Vol. 147, No. 7, pp. 2208-2214

Niu, D., Feng, H. & Chen, W. N. (2010). Proteomic analysis of HBV-associated HCC: insights on mechanisms of disease onset and biomarker discovery. *J Proteomics*, Vol. 73, No. 7, pp. 1283-1290

Okuda, K. (1986). Early recognition of hepatocellular carcinoma. *Hepatology*, Vol. 6, No. 4, pp. 729-738

Okuda, K., Ohtsuki, T., et al. (1985). Natural history of hepatocellular carcinoma and prognosis in relation to treatment. Study of 850 patients. *Cancer*, Vol. 56, No. 4, pp. 918-928

Pachmann, K., Clement, J. H., et al. (2005). Standardized quantification of circulating peripheral tumor cells from lung and breast cancer. *Clin Chem Lab Med*, Vol. 43, No. 6, pp. 617-627

Pantel, K., Brakenhoff, R. H. & Brandt, B. (2008). Detection, clinical relevance and specific biological properties of disseminating tumor cells. *Nat Rev Cancer*, Vol. 8, No. 5, pp. 329-340

Pantel, K. & Woelfle, U. (2005). Detection and molecular characterisation of disseminated tumor cells: implications for anti-cancer therapy. *Biochim Biophys Acta*, Vol. 1756, No. 1, pp. 53-64

Papillo, J. L. & Lapen, D. (1994). Cell yield. ThinPrep vs. cytocentrifuge. *Acta Cytol*, Vol. 38, No. 1, pp. 33-36

Paradis, V., Degos, F., et al. (2005). Identification of a new marker of hepatocellular carcinoma by serum protein profiling of patients with chronic liver diseases. *Hepatology*, Vol. 41, No. 1, pp. 40-47

Paterlini-Brechot, P. & Benali, N. L. (2007). Circulating tumor cells (CTC) detection: clinical impact and future directions. *Cancer Lett*, Vol. 253, No. 2, pp. 180-204

Peng, J. R., Chen, H. S., et al. (2005). Expression of cancer/testis (CT) antigens in Chinese hepatocellular carcinoma and its correlation with clinical parameters. *Cancer Lett*, Vol. 219, No. 2, pp. 223-232

Peng, X. Q., Wang, F., Geng, X. & Zhang, W. M. (2009). Current advances in tumor proteomics and candidate biomarkers for hepatic cancer. *Expert Rev Proteomics*, Vol. 6, No. 5, pp. 551-561

Piaton, E., Hutin, K., et al. (2004). Cost efficiency analysis of modern cytocentrifugation methods versus liquid based (Cytyc Thinprep) processing of urinary samples. *J Clin Pathol*, Vol. 57, No. 11, pp. 1208-1212

Pinzani, P., Salvadori, B., et al. (2006). Isolation by size of epithelial tumor cells in peripheral blood of patients with breast cancer: correlation with real-time reverse transcriptase-polymerase chain reaction results and feasibility of molecular analysis by laser microdissection. *Hum Pathol*, Vol. 37, No. 6, pp. 711-718

Plymoth, A., Viviani, S. & Hainaut, P. (2009). Control of hepatocellular carcinoma through hepatitis B vaccination in areas of high endemicity: perspectives for global liver cancer prevention. *Cancer Lett*, Vol. 286, No. 1, pp. 15-21

Poon, T. C., Yip, T. T., et al. (2003). Comprehensive proteomic profiling identifies serum proteomic signatures for detection of hepatocellular carcinoma and its subtypes. *Clin Chem*, Vol. 49, No. 5, pp. 752-760

Qian, J., Yao, D., et al. (2010). Characteristics of hepatic igf-ii expression and monitored levels of circulating igf-ii mRNA in metastasis of hepatocellular carcinoma. *Am J Clin Pathol*, Vol. 134, No. 5, pp. 799-806

Racila, E., Euhus, D., et al. (1998). Detection and characterization of carcinoma cells in the blood. *Proc Natl Acad Sci U S A*, Vol. 95, No. 8, pp. 4589-4594

Reinhart, B. J., Slack, F. J., et al. (2000). The 21-nucleotide let-7 RNA regulates developmental timing in Caenorhabditis elegans. *Nature*, Vol. 403, No. 6772, pp. 901-906

Resto, V. A., Caballero, O. L., et al. (2000). A putative oncogenic role for MPP11 in head and neck squamous cell cancer. *Cancer Res*, Vol. 60, No. 19, pp. 5529-5535

Rickwood, D. (1992). *Centrifugation : A Practical Approach.*, 090414755X,

Rickwood, D., Ford T., Steensgaard Jens. (1994). *Centrifugation: Essential Data.*, John Wiley & Son Ltd., 0471942715,

Rickwood, D. G. J. M. (2001). *Biological Centrifugation*, Springer Verlag, 0387915761,

Riethdorf, S., Wikman, H. & Pantel, K. (2008). Review: Biological relevance of disseminated tumor cells in cancer patients. *Int J Cancer*, Vol. 123, No. 9, pp. 1991-2006

Ross, A. A., Cooper, B. W., et al. (1993). Detection and viability of tumor cells in peripheral blood stem cell collections from breast cancer patients using immunocytochemical and clonogenic assay techniques. *Blood*, Vol. 82, No. 9, pp. 2605-2610

Saffroy, R., Pham, P., et al. (2007). New perspectives and strategy research biomarkers for hepatocellular carcinoma. *Clin Chem Lab Med*, Vol. 45, No. 9, pp. 1169-1179

Sanchez Antolin, G., Garcia Pajares, F., et al. (2009). Milan criteria versus San Francisco criteria in hepatocellular carcinoma: our center's experience. *Transplant Proc*, Vol. 41, No. 3, pp. 1012-1013

Saraiva-Romanholo, B. M., Barnabe, V., et al. (2003). Comparison of three methods for differential cell count in induced sputum. *Chest*, Vol. 124, No. 3, pp. 1060-1066

Sato, F., Hatano, E., et al. (2011). MicroRNA profile predicts recurrence after resection in patients with hepatocellular carcinoma within the Milan Criteria. *PLoS One*, Vol. 6, No. 1, pp. e16435

Scanlan, M. J., Gure, A. O., et al. (2002). Cancer/testis antigens: an expanding family of targets for cancer immunotherapy. *Immunol Rev*, Vol. 188, No. pp. 22-32

Scatton, O., Chiappini, F., et al. (2008). Generation and modulation of hepatocellular carcinoma circulating cells: a new experimental model. *J Surg Res*, Vol. 150, No. 2, pp. 183-189

Scatton, O., Chiappini, F., et al. (2006). Fate and characterization of circulating tumor cells in a NOD/SCID mouse model of human hepatocellular carcinoma. *Oncogene*, Vol. 25, No. 29, pp. 4067-4075

Scatton, O., Liddo, G. & Belghiti, J. (2009). Liver transplantation for hepatocellular carcinoma: current topics in France. *J Hepatobiliary Pancreat Surg*, Vol. No. pp.

Schuler, F. & Dolken, G. (2006). Detection and monitoring of minimal residual disease by quantitative real-time PCR. *Clin Chim Acta*, Vol. 363, No. 1-2, pp. 147-156

Schutte, K., Bornschein, J. & Malfertheiner, P. (2009). Hepatocellular carcinoma--epidemiological trends and risk factors. *Dig Dis*, Vol. 27, No. 2, pp. 80-92

Sell, S. (2002). Cellular origin of hepatocellular carcinomas. *Semin Cell Dev Biol*, Vol. 13, No. 6, pp. 419-424

Sergeant, G., Penninckx, F. & Topal, B. (2008). Quantitative RT-PCR detection of colorectal tumor cells in peripheral blood--a systematic review. *J Surg Res*, Vol. 150, No. 1, pp. 144-152

Sleijfer, S., Gratama, J. W., et al. (2007). Circulating tumor cell detection on its way to routine diagnostic implementation? *Eur J Cancer*, Vol. 43, No. 18, pp. 2645-2650

Smerage, J. B. & Hayes, D. F. (2006). The measurement and therapeutic implications of circulating tumor cells in breast cancer. *Br J Cancer*, Vol. 94, No. 1, pp. 8-12

Smirnov, D. A., Zweitzig, D. R., et al. (2005). Global gene expression profiling of circulating tumor cells. *Cancer Res*, Vol. 65, No. 12, pp. 4993-4997

Strijbos, M. H., Gratama, J. W., et al. (2008). Circulating endothelial cells in oncology: pitfalls and promises. *Br J Cancer*, Vol. 98, No. 11, pp. 1731-1735

Suehiro, T., Sugimachi, K., et al. (1994). Protein induced by vitamin K absence or antagonist II as a prognostic marker in hepatocellular carcinoma. Comparison with alpha-fetoprotein. *Cancer*, Vol. 73, No. 10, pp. 2464-2471

Sutcliffe, R., Maguire, D., et al. (2005). Detection and clinical significance of bone marrow micrometastases in patients undergoing liver transplantation for hepatocellular carcinoma. *Transplantation*, Vol. 80, No. 1, pp. 88-94

Suzuki, M., Sugimoto, K., et al. (2010). Up-regulation of glypican-3 in human hepatocellular carcinoma. *Anticancer Res*, Vol. 30, No. 12, pp. 5055-5061

Tandon, P. & Garcia-Tsao, G. (2009). Prognostic indicators in hepatocellular carcinoma: a systematic review of 72 studies. *Liver Int*, Vol. 29, No. 4, pp. 502-510

Toyoda, H., Kumada, T., et al. (2004). Changes in the characteristics and survival rate of hepatocellular carcinoma from 1976 to 2000: analysis of 1365 patients in a single institution in Japan. *Cancer*, Vol. 100, No. 11, pp. 2415-2421

Trevisani, F., D'Intino, P. E., et al. (2001). Serum alpha-fetoprotein for diagnosis of hepatocellular carcinoma in patients with chronic liver disease: influence of HBsAg and anti-HCV status. *J Hepatol*, Vol. 34, No. 4, pp. 570-575

Vejchapipat, P., Tangkijvanich, P., et al. (2004). Association between serum hepatocyte growth factor and survival in untreated hepatocellular carcinoma. *J Gastroenterol*, Vol. 39, No. 12, pp. 1182-1188

Vona, G., Estepa, L., et al. (2004). Impact of cytomorphological detection of circulating tumor cells in patients with liver cancer. *Hepatology*, Vol. 39, No. 3, pp. 792-797

Wang, J. Y., Wu, C. H., et al. (2006). Molecular detection of circulating tumor cells in the peripheral blood of patients with colorectal cancer using RT-PCR: significance of the prediction of postoperative metastasis. *World J Surg*, Vol. 30, No. 6, pp. 1007-1013

Wang, Y. L., Li, G., et al. (2007). Analysis of alpha-fetoprotein mRNA level on the tumor cell hematogenous spread of patients with hepatocellular carcinoma undergoing orthotopic liver transplantation. *Transplant Proc*, Vol. 39, No. 1, pp. 166-168

Weylandt, K. H., Krause, L. F., et al. (2011). Suppressed liver tumorigenesis in fat-1 mice with elevated omega-3 fatty acids is associated with increased omega-3 derived lipid mediators and reduced TNF-{alpha}. *Carcinogenesis*, Vol. 32, No. 6, pp. 897-903

Wharton, R. Q., Jonas, S. K., et al. (1999). Increased detection of circulating tumor cells in the blood of colorectal carcinoma patients using two reverse transcription-PCR assays and multiple blood samples. *Clin Cancer Res*, Vol. 5, No. 12, pp. 4158-4163

Willipinski-Stapelfeldt, B., Riethdorf, S., et al. (2005). Changes in cytoskeletal protein composition indicative of an epithelial-mesenchymal transition in human

micrometastatic and primary breast carcinoma cells. *Clin Cancer Res*, Vol. 11, No. 22, pp. 8006-8014
Witzigmann, H., Geissler, F., et al. (2002). Prospective evaluation of circulating hepatocytes by alpha-fetoprotein messenger RNA in patients with hepatocellular carcinoma. *Surgery*, Vol. 131, No. 1, pp. 34-43
Wong, I. H., Leung, T., et al. (1997). Semiquantification of circulating hepatocellular carcinoma cells by reverse transcriptase polymerase chain reaction. *Br J Cancer*, Vol. 76, No. 5, pp. 628-633
Wright, R. G. & Halford, J. A. (2001). Evaluation of thin-layer methods in urine cytology. *Cytopathology*, Vol. 12, No. 5, pp. 306-313
Wu, G. X., Lin, Y. M., et al. (2000). Significant down-regulation of alpha-albumin in human hepatoma and its implication. *Cancer Lett*, Vol. 160, No. 2, pp. 229-236
Xiao, C. L., Tao, Z. H., et al. (2011). Isomalto oligosaccharide sulfate inhibits tumor growth and metastasis of hepatocellular carcinoma in nude mice. *BMC Cancer*, Vol. 11, No. pp. 150
Xu, W., Cao, L., et al. (2011). Isolation of circulating tumor cells in patients with hepatocellular carcinoma using a novel cell separation strategy. *Clin Cancer Res*, Vol. 17, No. 11, pp. 3783-3793
Yao, D. F., Dong, Z. Z. & Yao, M. (2007). Specific molecular markers in hepatocellular carcinoma. *Hepatobiliary Pancreat Dis Int*, Vol. 6, No. 3, pp. 241-247
Yao, M., Yao, D. F., et al. (2011). Oncofetal antigen glypican-3 as a promising early diagnostic marker for hepatocellular carcinoma. *Hepatobiliary Pancreat Dis Int*, Vol. 10, No. 3, pp. 289-294
Yoon, Y. J., Han, K. H. & Kim do, Y. (2009). Role of serum prothrombin induced by vitamin K absence or antagonist-II in the early detection of hepatocellular carcinoma in patients with chronic hepatitis B virus infection. *Scand J Gastroenterol*, Vol. 44, No. 7, pp. 861-866
Yu, M. C., Yuan, J. M., Govindarajan, S. & Ross, R. K. (2000). Epidemiology of hepatocellular carcinoma. *Can J Gastroenterol*, Vol. 14, No. 8, pp. 703-709
Yu, M. L. & Chuang, W. L. (2009). Treatment of chronic hepatitis C in Asia: when East meets West. *J Gastroenterol Hepatol*, Vol. 24, No. 3, pp. 336-345
Yu, S. Z. (1995). Primary prevention of hepatocellular carcinoma. *J Gastroenterol Hepatol*, Vol. 10, No. 6, pp. 674-682
Zach, O. & Lutz, D. (2006). Tumor cell detection in peripheral blood and bone marrow. *Curr Opin Oncol*, Vol. 18, No. 1, pp. 48-56
Zhou, L., Liu, J. & Luo, F. (2006). Serum tumor markers for detection of hepatocellular carcinoma. *World J Gastroenterol*, Vol. 12, No. 8, pp. 1175-1181
Zieglschmid, V., Hollmann, C. & Bocher, O. (2005). Detection of disseminated tumor cells in peripheral blood. *Crit Rev Clin Lab Sci*, Vol. 42, No. 2, pp. 155-196
Zigeuner, R. E., Riesenberg, R., et al. (2003). Isolation of circulating cancer cells from whole blood by immunomagnetic cell enrichment and unenriched immunocytochemistry in vitro. *J Urol*, Vol. 169, No. 2, pp. 701-705
Zinkin, N. T., Grall, F., et al. (2008). Serum proteomics and biomarkers in hepatocellular carcinoma and chronic liver disease. *Clin Cancer Res*, Vol. 14, No. 2, pp. 470-477

# 17

# Use of a Human–Derived Liver Cell Line for the Detection of Protective Effect of Dietary Antioxidants Against Food Mutagens

Paloma Morales* and A.I. Haza
*Departamento de Nutrición, Bromatología y Tecnología de los Alimentos, Facultad de Veterinaria, Universidad Complutense de Madrid, Madrid Spain*

## 1. Introduction

Hepatocellular carcinoma is the most frequent form of primary liver cancer, it is one of the most common life threatening solid tumors with global annual diagnosis exceeding one million new cases and remains the third leading cause of cancer death (Ahmedin et al., 2007). Human diet often contains compounds that cause DNA damage. Common dietary mutagens would include N-nitroso compounds (Tricker & Preussmann, 1991), fungal toxins (Gelderblom et al., 2001), or cooked meat carcinogens (Layton et al., 1995). High nitrate levels in processed foods may be a risk factor, possibly through their ability to form N-nitroso compounds in vivo (Ferguson et al., 2004). N-nitroso compounds are known hepatocarcinogenic agents and have been implicated in the etiology of several human cancers Bansal et al., 2005). N-Nitrosamines are mutagenic and carcinogenic compounds widely present in the human diet and have been detected at ppb levels in a wide variety of matrices such as bacon, ham, frankfurters, sausages, cheese, beer, rubber, ground water, smoked tobacco and cosmetics (Filho et al., 2003). N-nitrosopiperidine (NPIP) is a potent extrahepatic carcinogen inducing tumours mainly in the esophagus and the nasal cavity (Gray et al., 1991). N-nitrosodibutylamine (NDBA) produces tumours in the esophagus and urinary bladder in rat, although the liver is its major target tissue for carcinogenesis (Williams et al., 1993). N-nitrosopyrrolidine (NPYR) induce mainly liver tumors in rats (Gray et al., 1991) and is a weak pulmonary carcinogen in mice (Wong et al., 2003) and N-nitrosodimethylamine (NDMA) is the most commonly encountered volatile N-nitrosamine in food samples and is a potent liver, lung and kidney carcinogen (Preussmann & Stewart, 1984).

Heterocyclic amines (HCAs) and polycyclic aromatic hydrocarbons (PAHs) are formed during the high-temperature cooking of meat and fish. To date, more than 20 different heterocyclic amines (HCAs) have been identified in cooked foods and they can be classified into two main groups called carbolines and aminoimidazoazaarenes (AIAs) (Toribio et al., 2007). AIAs are formed at the normal cooking temperatures of 100–225°C while heating

* Corresponding Author

foodstuffs in the presence of creatinine, amino-acids and sugars, involving Maillard reaction (Ristic et al., 2004). Among those, 2-amino-3,8-dimethylimidazo[4,5-f]quinoxaline (8-MeIQx), 2-amino- 3,4,8-trimethylimidazo[4,5-f]-quinoxaline (4,8-diMeIQx) and 2-amino-1-methyl-6-phenyl-imidazo[4,5-b]pyridine (PhIP) are the most abundant (Skog et al., 1998). Benzo(a)pyrene (BaP), an important PAH, is a potent systemic and local carcinogen known to induce skin, lung, and stomach tumours in animal models (Ueng et al., 2001). NPIP, NDBA, NPYR and HCAs were categorized as Group 2B: possible causative agents in human cancer, while NDMA and B(a)P as Group 2A: probable causative agents in human cancer (IARC, 1993).

N-nitrosamines, HCAs and B(a)P are DNA reactive chemicals that require metabolic activation, usually by various cytochrome P450 (CYP) enzymes for interaction with DNA (Ingelman-Sundberg, 2002). It has been suggested that DNA damage and free radical damage are in part involved in the carcinogenic action induced by N-nitrosamines (Bartsch et al., 1989). Strand breaks or alkali labile sites, including abasic sites, may be results of the action of reactive oxygen species that arise during the metabolism of food mutagens in the cell. In a previous work we showed that N-nitrosamines (Arranz et al., 2007; García et al., 2008a,b), benzo(a)pyrene (Delgado et al., 2009) and heterocyclic amines (Haza et al., 2011) were able to generate DNA strand breaks and oxidized bases. The increasing appreciation of the importance of food mutagens as potential human carcinogens stimulated intense research on protective dietary factors in chemical carcinogenesis.

Current evidence strongly supports a contribution of polyphenols to the prevention of various diseases associated with oxidative stress, such as cancer and cardiovascular, neurodegenerative and age-related diseases (Kanazawa et al., 2006). Phenolics have been reported to have a capacity to scavenge free radicals (Havsteen, 2002). Gallic acid (3,4,5-trihydroxybenzoicacid, GA) is a polyhydroxyphenolic compound, which can be found in various natural products, like gallnuts, tea leaves, bark, green tea, apple-peels, grapes, strawberries, pineapples, bananas, lemons, and in red and white wine (Madlener, et al., (2007). GA is a strong antioxidant that possesses antimutagenic and anticarcinogenic activities (Inoue, et al., 1994; Stich, et al., 1982) and exerts antiproliferative effects on cancer cells by generating hydrogen peroxide (Lapidot, et al., 2002). It inhibits melanogenesis which may be related to GA's antioxidant activity in scavenging reactive oxygen species (Seo et al., 2003).

Piceatannol (3-hydroxyresveratrol or astringinine, PCA) is a phenolic compound that occurs naturally in grapes and red wine (McDonald et al., 1998). The total amount of PCA in red-grape wine has been reported to be up to 15 mg/l (Cantos et al., 2003), however the biotransformation of the abundant red wine component, resveratrol (*trans*-3,5,4-trihydroxystilbene), contributes to increase PCA concentrations at tissue level (Piver et al., 2004). Both substances are synthesized in plants in response to fungal or other environmental stress, classifying them as phytoalexins. Piceatannol has been identified as the active ingredient of *Melaleucaleucadendron* (white tea tree), *Cassia garretiana* (Asian legume) and *Rheum undulatum* (Korean rhubarb), which are used in traditional herbal medicine (Tsuruga, et al., 1991; Matsuda, et al., 2000) and as the antileukemic compound in the seeds of *Euphorbia lagascae*, which is used in folk medicine to treat cancer, tumors and warts (Ferrigni et al., 1984). Teguo et al. 2001 also detected piceatannol in cell suspension cultures of *Vitis vinifera* (wine grapes).

Several studies established the single cell gel electrophoresis (SCGE) or Comet assay as a suitable method for assessing the ability of phytochemicals to protect cells against genotoxic effect of several xenobiotics (Collins, 2005). In this study, the Comet assay was modified to permit the detection of oxidized bases by including a step in which DNA is digested with formamidopyrimidine-DNA glycosylase (Fpg) or endonuclease III (Endo III) to uncover oxidized purines and pyrimidines, respectively (Figure 1).

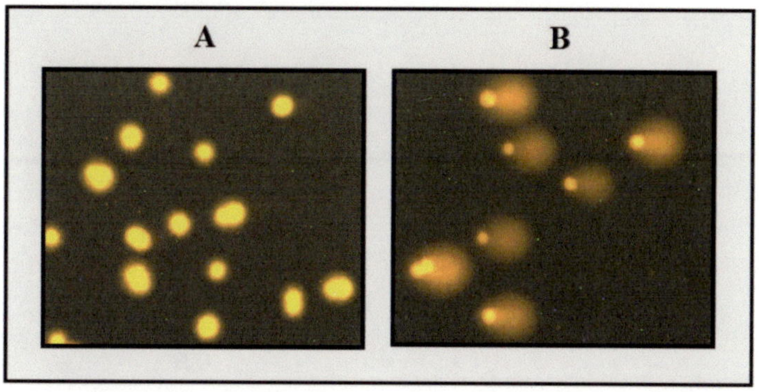


Fig. 1. HepG2 cells untreated (A) and treated (B) with N-nitrosopyrrolidine (NPYR) and incubated with Fpg enzyme, visualized under fluorescence microscopy and using comet assay.

As part of our program to evaluate the protective effects of dietary polyphenols with different chemical structure (previously we have evaluated, flavonols and flavanols) we sought to determine whether galic acid (as representative of phenolic acids) or piceatannol (stilbenes) could protect human hepatoma cells (HepG2) from oxidative DNA damage induced by food mutagens.

## 2. Material and methods

### 2.1 Chemicals

Galic acid (GA), piceatannol (PCA) and food mutagens used in this study are shown in Figures 2 and 3. N-nitrosodimethylamine (NDMA), N-nitrosodibutylamine (NDBA), N-nitrosopyrrolidine (NPYR), N-nitrosopiperidine (NPIP), benzo(a)pyrene (BaP), dimethyl sulfoxide (DMSO) and low melting point agarose (LMP) were purchased from Sigma-Aldrich (St. Louis, MO). 2-amino-3,8-dimethylimidazo[4,5-f]quinoxaline (8-MeIQx), 2-amino-3,4,8-trimethyl-3H-imidazo[4,5-f]quinoxaline (4,8-diMeIQx) and 2-amino-1-methyl-6-phenyl- imidazo[4,5-b]pyridine (PhIP), were purchased from Toronto Research Chemicals Inc. (North York, On. Canada). Formamidopyrimidine-DNA glycosylase (Fpg) and endonuclease III (Endo III) were obtained from Trevigen Inc. (Gaithersburg, MD). All other chemicals and solvents were of the highest grade commercially available. Food carcinogens and polyphenols were dissolved in sterile DMSO. The stock solutions were stored deep frozen (-80°C).

### 2.2 HepG2 cells

Human hepatocellular carcinoma (HepG2) cells were purchased from Biology Investigation Center Collection (BIC, Madrid, Spain). Only cells of passage 10-17 were used in the experiments. The cells were cultured as monolayer in Dulbecco's Modified Eagle Medium supplemented with 10% v/v heat inactivated foetal calf serum, 50 U/ml penicillin and 50 μg/ml streptomycin and 1% v/v L-glutamine. Culture medium and supplements required for the growth of the cells were purchased from Gibco Laboratories (Life Technologies, Inc., Gaithersburg, MD 20884-9980). Cell cultures were incubated at 37°C and 100% humidity in a 5% $CO_2$ atmosphere.

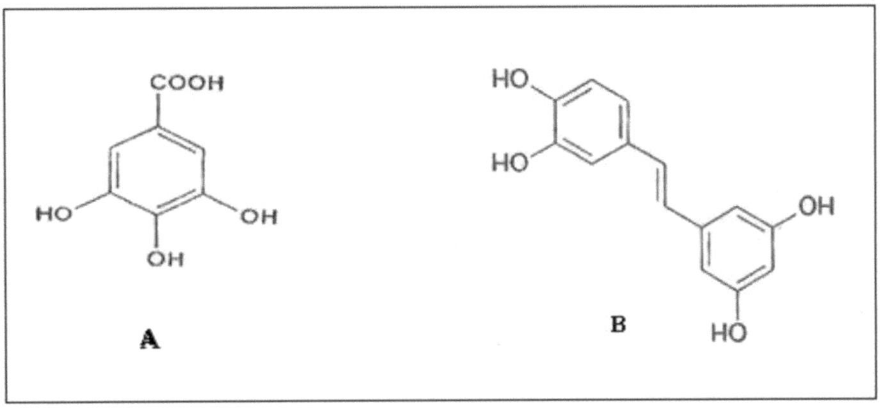


Fig. 2. Chemical structures of gallic acid (A) and piceatannol (B).

### 2.3 Analysis of DNA damage (strand breaks and oxidized purines/pyrimidines) induced by galic acid or piceatannol in the Alkaline Comet assay

Cell viability was routinely determined by the MTT (3-(4,5-dimethylthiazol-2-yl)-2,5-diphenyltetrazolium bromide) assay in order to select non-toxic concentrations of galic acid and piceatannol. The SCGE assay was carried out according to the protocol of Olive et al. (1992) with minor modifications.

Briefly, HepG2 cells were plated on to multiwell systems at a density of $1.5x10^5$ cells/ml culture medium. 24 hr after seeding, cells were exposed to galic acid (0.1-5 μM), or piceatannol (0.1-5 μM) or solvent, for another 24 h at 37 °C and 5% $CO_2$. The solvent concentration in the incubation medium never exceeds 0.1%. After treatments, 10μl of a suspension of $1x10^5$ cells were mixed with 70μl of LMP agarose type VII (0.75% concentration in PBS), distributed on slides that had been pre-coated with LMP agarose type VII (0.30% concentration in PBS), and left to set on an ice tray. Three slides were prepared for each concentration of the compound tested, one slide for control and the other slides to be treated with Fpg or Endo III. After solidification, the cells were lysed in darkness for 1 hour in a high salt alkaline buffer (2.5M NaCl, 0.1M EDTA, 0.01M Tris, 1% Triton X-100, pH 10). The slides were then equilibrated 3x5 minutes in enzyme buffer (0.04M HEPES, 0.1M of Fpg or Endo III at 1μg/ml in enzyme buffer for 30 min at 37°C in a humid dark chamber. Control slides were incubated with 30μl of enzyme buffer only. Following enzyme treatment, the slides were placed in electrophoresis buffer (0.3M NaOH, 1mM EDTA, pH 13, cooled in a refrigerator) in darkness for 40 min. Electrophoresis was performed in a cold-storage room, in darkness, in a Bio-Rad subcell GT unit containing the same buffer, for 30 min at 25V. After electrophoresis, the slides were neutralized using 0.4M Tris pH 7.5 and KCl, 0.5mM EDTA, 0.2 mg/ml BSA, pH 8). After this time, slides were incubated with 30μl fixed in methanol. Subsequently, the DNA was stained with ethidium bromide (10 μg/ml) in Tris acetate EDTA (TAE 1X) during 5 minutes and examined in a fluorescence microscope (OLYMPUS BH-2) connected to a computerized image analysis system (Comet Score 5.5). Olive tail moment (OTM) as defined by Olive et al. (1992) was determined and expressed as arbitrary units (AU). OTM= I x L, where I is the fractional amount of DNA in the comet tail (%DNA in the tail) and L is the distance from the centre of the comet head to the centre of tail distribution.

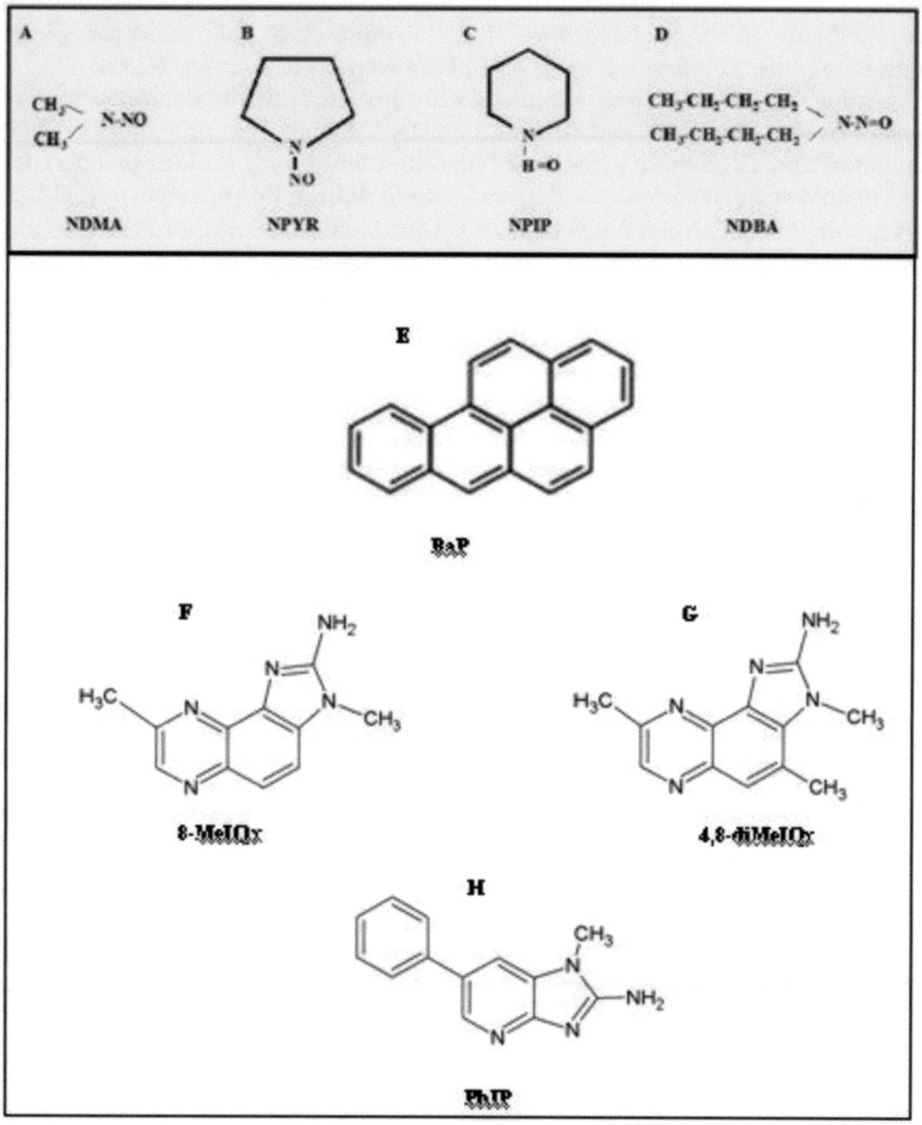


Fig. 3. Chemical structures of food mutagens used in this study: (A) N-nitrosodimethylamine (NDMA),(B) N-nitrosopyrrolidine (NPYR), (C) N-nitrosopiperidine (NPIP), (D) N-nitrosodibuthylamine (NDBA), (E) benzo(a)pyrene (BaP), (F) 2-amino-3,8-dimethylimidazo[4,5-f]quinoxaline (8-MeIQx), (G) 2-amino-3,4,8-trimethyl-3H-imidazo[4,5-f]quinoxaline (4,8-diMeIQx) and (H) 2-amino-1-methyl-6-phenylimidazo [4,5-b]pyridine (PhIP).

### 2.4 Analysis of DNA damage (strand breaks and oxidized purines/pyrimidines) induced by a simultaneous treatment of food mutagens and galic acid or piceatannol in the Alkaline Comet assay

Induction of DNA damage (strand breaks and oxidative DNA damage) by NDMA, NPYR (Arranz et al., 2007) NPIP, NDBA (García et al., 2008), B(a)P (Delgado et al., 2008), 8-MeIQx, 4,8-diMeIQx and PhIP (Haza and Morales, 2010) have been previously evaluated by our laboratory. HepG2 cells were plated on to multiwell systems at a density of $1.5x10^5$ cells/ml culture medium. 24 h after seeding, the corresponding galic acid or piceatannol concentrations were added to the wells and plates were incubated for 24hr at 37°C and 5% $CO_2$. After incubation, cells were simultaneously treated with the concentrations of food mutagens that caused a significant increased on DNA damage and previously evaluated by our laboratory. NPYR (50mM without enzymes and 5mM with EndoIII or Fpg enzymes), NDMA (135mM without enzymes and 27mM with EndoIII or Fpg enzymes), NDBA (3 mM), NPIP (44 mM), BaP (50 μM), Me IQx (500 μM), 4,8-diMeIQx (200 μM) or PhIP (300 μM), and different concentrations of galic acid (0.1-5μM) or piceatannol (0.1-5μM) for another 24 hours at 37°C and 5% $CO_2$. After the treatments, the cells were processed as described above (Figure 4.)

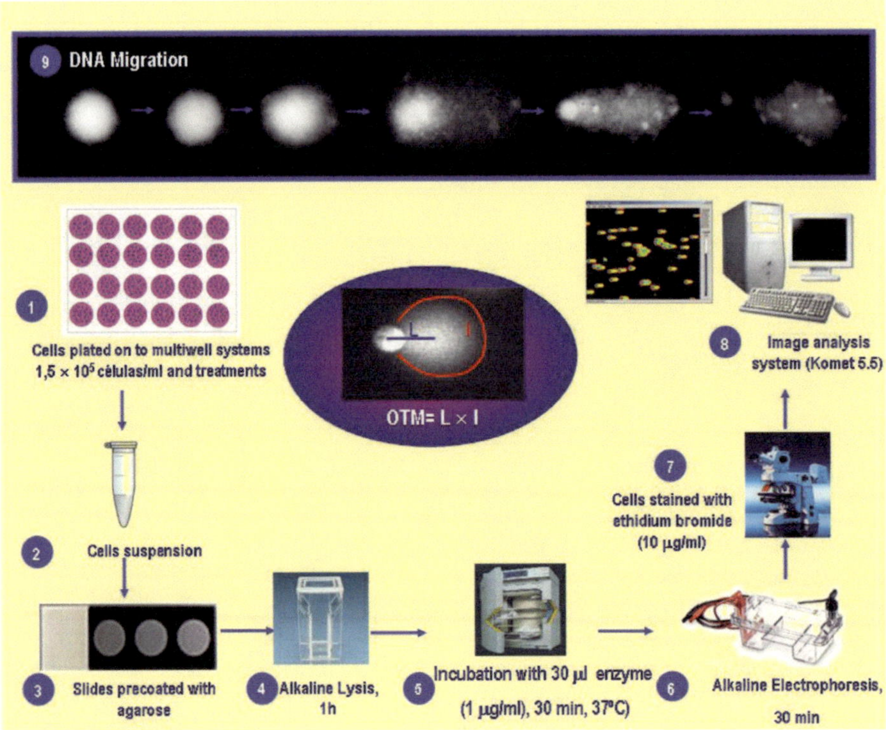


Fig. 4. Comet assay procedure.

### 2.5 Statistical analysis

Images of 50 randomly selected cells per concentration were evaluated and the test was carried out three times. The reported OTM is the mean ± standard deviation (S.D.) of three independent experiments. Thus, we compare three means of OTM from 3 different experiments. Cultures without N-nitrosamines or polyphenols were considered as negative controls. In all experiments the following negative controls have been included: cells treated with solvents and treated without enzymes, cells incubated with Endo III and cells incubated with Fpg. Induction of DNA damage by N-nitrosamines was defined as 100% of genotoxicity. The Student's t-test was used for statistical comparison between simultaneous treatments and controls, and differences were considered significant at $p \leq 0.05$.

## 3. Results

### 3.1 DNA damage (strand breaks and oxidized purines/pyrimidines) induced by galic acid or piceatannol in the Alkaline Comet assay

No cytotoxicity has been previously found at the concentrations of galic acid or piceatannol tested (data not shown). Cell viability was always above 80% of control viability. At non-cytotoxic concentrations (0.1-5μM) piceatannol and gallic acid did not induce DNA strand breaks and oxidative DNA damage (**Table 1**). For this reason this concentration range was used in subsequent studies. DNA damage was not measured at cytotoxic concentrations (> 5 μM) because under these conditions DNA damage is caused as a consequence of necrosis or apoptosis (Henderson et al., 1998).

| Compound | Concentration (μM) | DNA damage (OTM)[b] | | |
|---|---|---|---|---|
| | | DNA strand breaks | Endo III | Fpg |
| Control[a] | 0 | 1.3 ± 0.3 | 1.4 ± 0.2 | 1.9 ± 0.5 |
| **GA** | 0.1 | 1.1 ± 0.4 | 1.2 ± 0.8 | 2.1 ± 0.6 |
| | 1.0 | 1.3 ± 0.6 | 1.2 ± 0.4 | 1.8 ± 0.3 |
| | 5.0 | 1.4 ± 0.3 | 1.4 ± 0.7 | 1.6 ± 0.5 |
| **PCA** | 0.1 | 1.3 ± 0.6 | 1.2 ± 0.6 | 2.1 ± 0.7 |
| | 1.0 | 1.4 ± 0.4 | 1.3 ± 0.8 | 1.8 ± 0.8 |
| | 5.0 | 1.5 ± 0.3 | 1.5 ± 0.7 | 1.8 ± 0.7 |

[a] OTM median values in control cells without enzymes or incubated with Endo III or Fpg
[b] OTM expressed as arbitrary units. The mean DNA damage were calculated from the respective values of three independent experiments.

Table 1. Effect of different concentrations of GA and PCA on DNA strand breaks and on the formation of Endo III and Fpg sensitive sites of human hepatoma cells.

### 3.2 DNA damage induction by simultaneous treatment of food carcinogens and galic acid or piceatannol in the Alkaline Comet assay

Protection afforded by piceatannol and gallic acid towards NDBA and NPIP-induced oxidative DNA damage was shown in **Table 2**. No protective effect was shown by piceatannol and gallic acid against NDBA or NPIP-induced DNA strand breaks in HepG2 cells. Gallic acid, but not piceatannol, weakly reduced the Endo III sensitive sites induced by NDBA (28.5%, 0.1 μM). However, piceatannol reduced the NPIP-induced Endo III sensitive sites at all concentrations tested (28-36%, 0.1-5 μM) and no effect was shown by gallic acid. The maximum reduction of Fpg sensitive sites induced by NDBA was found at the highest concentration of piceatannol (5 μM, 56%). However, the maximum reduction of Fpg sensitive sites induced by NPIP was at the lowest concentration (0.1 μM, 34.2%). Gallic acid only exerted its protective effect against NPIP-induced Fpg sensitive sites (42.1-23.6%, 0.1-5 μM).

| Compound | Concentration (μM) | DNA damage (OTM)[a] | | |
|---|---|---|---|---|
| | | DNA strand breaks | Endo III | Fpg |
| **NDBA** | | 1.8±0.4 | 2.1±0.3 | 2.5±0.2 |
| GA | 0.1 | 1.5±0.6 | 1.5±0.4* (28.5) | 2.4±0.6 |
| | 1.0 | 1.5±0.4 | 1.8±0.4 | 3.0±0.3 |
| | 5.0 | 1.6±0.3 | 1.9±0.5 | 3.0±0.5 |
| PCA | 0.1 | 1.7±0.6 | 1.9±0.6 | 3.0±0.4 |
| | 1.0 | 1.6±0.5 | 1.8±0.5 | 2.0±0.3* (20.0) |
| | 5.0 | 1.8±0.3 | 1.9±0.7 | 1.1±0.5** (56.0) |
| **NPIP** | | 1.7±0.4 | 2.5±0.6 | 3.8±0.4 |
| GA | 0.1 | 1.7±0.3 | 2.3±0.5 | 2.2±0.4** (42.1) |
| | 1.0 | 1.7±0.4 | 2.3±0.3 | 2.5±0.2** (34.1) |
| | 5.0 | 1.9±0.4 | 2.3±0.5 | 2.9±0.4** (23.6) |
| PCA | 0.1 | 1.7±0.6 | 1.8±0.5** (28.0) | 2.5±0.3** (34.2) |
| | 1.0 | 1.6±0.5 | 1.8±0.5** (28.0) | 2.9±0.5** (23.6) |
| | 5.0 | 1.8±0.3 | 1.6±0.6** (36.0) | 3.0±0.6* (21.0) |

[a] OTM expressed as arbitrary units. The mean DNA damage were calculated from the respective values of three independent experiments. The values in parentheses (%) were defined as the percentage of protection of NDBA or NPIP-induced DNA damage by tested compounds. Asterisks indicate significant difference from control ** P≤0.01, * P≤0.05.

Table 2. Protective effect of GA and PCA on DNA strand breaks, the formation of Endo III and Fpg sensitive sites of human hepatoma cells induced by 3 mM of NDBA and 44 mM of NPIP.

**Table 3** shows the effect of piceatannol and gallic acid against NPYR and NDMA-induced oxidative DNA damage. Results revealed that piceatannol at the lowest concentration reduced the DNA strand breaks induced by NPYR and NDMA (0.1 μM, 32.2% and 47.6%, respectively). On the contrary, gallic acid did not shown any protective effect against NPYR or NDMA-induced DNA strand breaks. The formation of Endo III sensitive sites induced by NPYR was prevented only by piceatannol at all the concentrations (0.1-5 μM, 12.5-25%), whereas, both compounds, PCA (0.1-5 μM, 30.7-19.2%) and GA (0.1-1 μM, 23%) protected against the formation of Endo III sensitive sites induce by NDMA, respectively. On the other hand, the formation of Fpg sensitive sites induced by NPYR and NDMA were reduced by PCA and GA. At a dose of 0.1 μM, PCA exhibited the maximum reduction (38.8%) on Fpg sensitive sites induced by NPYR, whereas GA exhibited it at 5.0 μM (18.5%). PCA and GA also reduced the formation of Fpg sensitive sites induced by NDMA at concentrations of 0.1-1 μM, respectively (30.9% and 23.8-14.2%).

The effect of piceatannol and gallic acid against BaP and PhIP-induced oxidative DNA damage was shown in **Table 4**.

| Compound | Concentration (μM) | DNA damage (OTM)[a] | | |
|---|---|---|---|---|
| | | DNA strand breaks | Endo III | Fpg |
| **NDMA** | | 2.1 ±0.6 | 2.6 ±0.2 | 4.2 ±0.5 |
| GA | 0.1 | 2.5 ±0.5 | 2.0 ±0.3** (23.0) | 3.2 ±0.2** (23.8) |
| | 1.0 | 2.2 ±0.6 | 2.0 ±0.4** (23.0) | 3.6 ±0.4* (14.2) |
| | 5.0 | 2.1 ±0.3 | 2.5 ±0.5 | 4.9 ±0.7 |
| PCA | 0.1 | 1.1 ±0.6** (47.6) | 1.8 ±0.4** (30.7) | 2.9 ±0.4** (30.9) |
| | 1.0 | 2.0 ±0.4 | 2.0 ±0.4** (23.0) | 2.9 ±0.3** (30.9) |
| | 5.0 | 2.1 ±0.5 | 2.1 ±0.6** (19.2) | 4.3 ±0.6 |
| **NPYR** | | 3.1 ±0.5 | 4.0 ±0.5 | 5.4 ±0.4 |
| GA | 0.1 | 3.2 ±0.3 | 4.0 ±0.3 | 4.8 ±0.4* (11.1) |
| | 1.0 | 3.4 ±0.5 | 4.8 ±0.4 | 4.5 ±0.2** (16.6) |
| | 5.0 | 3.4 ±0.3 | 5.6 ±0.5 | 4.4 ±0.4** (18.5) |
| PCA | 0.1 | 2.1 ±0.3** (32.2) | 3.5 ±0.1** (12.5) | 3.3 ±0.3** (38.8) |
| | 1.0 | 3.3 ±0.3 | 3.2 ±0.3** (20.0) | 4.0 ±0.4** (25.9) |
| | 5.0 | 4.1 ±0.5 | 3.0 ±0.3** (25.0) | 6.1 ±0.7 |

[a] OTM expressed as arbitrary units. The mean DNA damage were calculated from the respective values of three independent experiments. The values in parentheses (%) were defined as the percentage of protection of NDMA or NPYR-induced DNA damage by tested compounds. Asterisks indicate significant difference from control ** P≤0.01, * P≤0.05.

Table 3. Protective effect of GA and PCA on DNA strand breaks, the formation of Endo III and Fpg sensitive sites of human hepatoma cells induced by NDMA (135 mM without enzymes and 27 mM with Endo III or Fpg enzymes) and NPYR (50 mM without enzymes and 5 mM with Endo III or Fpg enzymes).

Piceatannol protected against DNA strand breaks induced by BaP and PhIP at all concentrations tested (0.1-5 μM, 60.0-65.3% and 34.7-12.5%, respectively). However, gallic acid only exerted protection against BaP-induced DNA strand breaks at the highest concentrations (1-5 μM, 18.-36%). An important decrease of the formation of BaP-induced Endo III sensitive sites was also shown by piceatannol at the lowest concentration (0.1 μM, 60.5%), whereas gallic acid drastically reduced the formation of Endo III sensitive sites at all the concentrations tested (0.1-5 μM, 79.6-63.9%). On the other hand, only gallic acid showed a weakly protective effect against the PhIP-induced Fpg sensitive sites (0.1-1 μM, 17.7%).

The protective effect of gallic acid and piceatannol against MeIQx and diMeIQx-induced oxidative DNA damage was shown in **Table.5**. No effect was shown by piceatannol and gallic acid against DNA strand breaks and the formation of Endo III sensitive sites induced by MeIQx and diMeIQx. Fpg sensitive sites induced by MeIQx (41.1-31.3%) and diMeIQx (41.1-23.5%) were prevented by gallic acid at all the concentrations tested (0.1-5 μM). However, piceatannol only reduced the formation of Fpg sensitive sites at the lowest concentrations (MeIQx, 25.4% and diMeIQx, 27.4%).

| Compound | Concentration (μM) | DNA damage (OTM)ᵃ | | |
|---|---|---|---|---|
| | | DNA strand breaks | Endo III | Fpg |
| **BaP** | 50 | 15.0 ± 0.5 | 26.1 ± 0.4 | 21.2 ± 0.7 |
| GA | 0.1 | 15.2 ± 0.7 | 5.3 ± 0.3*** (79.6) | 32.1 ± 0.2 |
| | 1.0 | 12.3 ± 0.6** (18.0) | 5.2 ± 0.4*** (80.0) | 34.2 ± 0.7 |
| | 5.0 | 9.6 ± 0.6** (36.0) | 9.4 ± 0.5*** (63.9) | 34.2 ± 0.7 |
| PCA | 0.1 | 6.0 ± 0.6*** (60.0) | 10.3 ± 0.4** (60.5) | 32.3 ± 0.7 |
| | 1.0 | 6.1 ± 0.5*** (59.3) | 18.6 ± 0.4** (28.7) | 34.2 ± 0.6 |
| | 5.0 | 5.2 ± 0.5*** (65.3) | 19.1 ± 0.6** (26.8) | 39.3 ± 0.6 |
| **PhIP** | 300 | 3.2 ± 0.5 | 3.9 ± 0.7 | 4.5 ± 0.7 |
| GA | 0.1 | 3.3 ± 0.6 | 3.9 ± 0.3 | 3.7 ± 0.3* (17.7) |
| | 1.0 | 3.0 ± 0.5 | 4.3 ± 0.7 | 3.7 ± 0.4* (17.7) |
| | 5.0 | 3.0 ± 0.6 | 4.5 ± 0.7 | 4.2 ± 0.4 |
| PCA | 0.1 | 2.1 ± 0.4* (34.7) | 3.0 ± 0.2* (23.0) | 4.0 ± 0.5 |
| | 1.0 | 2.3 ± 0.3* (28.1) | 2.8 ± 0.4** (28.2) | 4.2 ± 0.5 |
| | 5.0 | 2.8 ± 0.5* (12.5) | 2.6 ± 0.4** (33,3) | 5.8 ± 0.4 |

ᵃ OTM expressed as arbitrary units. The mean DNA damage were calculated from the respective values of three independent experiments. The values in parentheses (%) were defined as the percentage of protection of BaP or PhIP-induced DNA damage by tested compounds. Asterisks indicate significant difference from control *** P ≤ 0.001, ** P≤0.01, * P≤0.05.

Table 4. Protective effect of GA and PCA on DNA strand breaks, the formation of Endo III and Fpg sensitive sites of human hepatoma cells induced by BaP and PhIP.

## 4. Discussion

The aim of the present study was to evaluate the protective effect of galic acid and piceatannol towards food mutagens-induced oxidative DNA damage (strand breaks and oxidized purines/pyrimidines) in human hepatoma cells (HepG2), using the single-cell gel electrophoresis (SCGE) assay. There is speculation that oxidative DNA damaged is involved in cancer development (Mastaloudis et al., 2004). Otherwise, metabolism of food mutagens in cells could generate reactive oxygen species that arise in DNA strand breaks or alkali labile sites, including abasic sites. Previous studies in our research group showed that NDBA, NPIP (García et al., 2008), NDMA and NPYR (Arranz et al., 2007) were able to generate oxidized bases. In addition, during the metabolic process, BaP also produces reactive oxygen species (ROS) via cytochrome P4501A1 (Burczynski and Penning 2000). In a previous investigation we also showed that HepG2 cells treated with BaP or HCAs induced Fpg and Endo III sensitive sites, indicating the presence of oxidized purines and pyrimidines, respectively (Delgado et al., 2009, Haza et al., 2010).

Polyphenols have an important activity as antioxidants and also a remarkable role on carcinogen activation in vivo and on carcinogenesis (Dolara et al., 2005; Lambert et al., 2005). However, some flavonoids such as galic acid, piceatannol, resveratrol, quercetin and myricetin showed cytotoxicity for a number of cell lines or even induced oxidative DNA strand breakage in human lymphotcytes or in HepG2 cells at concentrations higher than 100 μM (Hadi et al., 2007; Johnson and Loo, 2000). The mechanism by which these flavonoids induce DNA damage at higher concentrations might be due to the pro-oxidant properties of these compounds (Wu et al., 2004). Thus, it is important to evaluate whether the adverse effect of GA and PCA on DNA in human hepatoma cells, as shown in Table 1. Our results indicate that none of the dietary polyphenols (GA, PCA) concentrations tested (0.1-5 μM) caused DNA strand breaks, or oxidized purine or pyrimidine bases per se in HepG2 cells (Table 1), although at concentrations higher than 5 μM induced DNA strand breaks and oxidative DNA damage in HepG2 cells (data not shown). Approximately, people in the Unites States ingest each day 1g of tannic acid (TA) (Sanyal et al., 1997). As one of the food additives, TA is probably hydrolyzed in the acidic pH in the stomach, releasing the 10 potentially reactive GA residues (Brune et al., 1989). GA concentration in the stomach could achieve a maximum of 1.5mmol/L. GA from tablets and tea was rapidly absorbed, but the highest GA concentration observed in plasma was only 1.83 μmol/L and 2.09 μmol/L, respectively (Shahrzad et al., 2001). Thus, considering the uptake of hydrolysable TA, the concentrations of GA used in this study would not be absurd.

In the present study, we observed that, GA was less efficient that piceatannol to reduce DNA damage induced by food mutagens tested. The presence of three or four hydroxyl groups present in GA and PCA respectively, results in differing protective effects against food mutagens.

| Compound | Concentration (μM) | DNA damage (OTM)[a] | | |
|---|---|---|---|---|
| | | DNA strand breaks | Endo III | Fpg |
| **MeIQx** | 500 | 3.9 ± 0.6 | 5.0 ± 0.2 | 5.1 ± 0.5 |
| GA | 0.1 | 3.8 ± 0.3 | 5.0 ± 0.4 | 3.0 ± 0.2** (41.1) |
| | 1.0 | 3.8 ± 0.4 | 5.4 ± 0.4 | 3.2 ± 0.3** (37.2) |
| | 5.0 | 3.7 ± 0.4 | 6.0 ± 0.5 | 3.5 ± 0.6** (31.3) |
| PCA | 0.1 | 3.8 ± 0.4 | 5.9 ± 0.4 | 3.8 ± 0.1** (25.4) |
| | 1.0 | 4.0 ± 0.3 | 5.1 ± 0.5 | 4.2 ± 0.4** (17.6) |
| | 5.0 | 4.2 ± 0.5 | 5.0 ± 0.6 | 6.1 ± 0.6 |
| **diMeIQx** | 200 | 3.9 ± 0.2 | 4.8 ± 0.5 | 5.1 ± 0.5 |
| GA | 0.1 | 3.9 ± 0.4 | 4.6 ± 0.5 | 3.0 ± 0.3** (41.1) |
| | 1.0 | 3.8 ± 0.6 | 5.4 ± 0.6 | 3.5 ± 0.3** (31.3) |
| | 5.0 | 3.9 ± 0.5 | 6.2 ± 0.5 | 3.9 ± 0.5** (23.5) |
| PCA | 0.1 | 3.8 ± 0.4 | 5.8 ± 0.3 | 3.7 ± 0.4** (27.4) |
| | 1.0 | 4.5 ± 0.3 | 5.4 ± 0.3 | 4.8 ± 0.3 |
| | 5.0 | 5.1 ± 0.6 | 5.0 ± 0.5 | 6.3 ± 0.5 |

[a] OTM expressed as arbitrary units. The mean DNA damage were derived from three independent experiments. The values in parentheses (%) were defined as the percentage of protection of MeIQx or diMeIQx-induced DNA damage by tested compounds. Asterisks indicate significant difference from control, ** P≤0.01.

Table 5. Protective effect of GA and PCA on DNA strand breaks, the formation of Endo III and Fpg sensitive sites of human hepatoma cells induced by MeIQx and diMeIQx.

Our results revelaled that GA only prevented the DNA strand breaks induced by BaP. However, it protected cells against oxidative DNA damage-induced by food mutagens. GA removed oxidized pyrimidines induced by NDBA and BaP and oxidized purines induced by NDMA, NPYR, NPIP, MeIQx, diMeIQx and PhIP. This may be due to the antioxidant property of GA (Gali et al., 1992). Phenolic hydroxyl groups are known to be potent in scavenging free radicals and the OH group at the para position to the carboxylic group is especially effectual for the antioxidant activity (Son and Lewis, 2002). Thus the three hydroxyl groups present in GA may be responsible for its antioxidant activity. Although, Lu et al (2006) showed that the protective effect of GA derivatives seemed to depend more on their molecular polarities rather than antioxidant activities.

Our results also showed that DNA strand breaks induced by NDMA, NPYR, BaP and PhIP were reduced by PCA. In addition, PCA also removed the oxidized pyrimidines induced by NDMA, NPYR, NPIP, BaP and PhIP and the oxidized purines induced by NDMA, NPYR, NDBA, NPIP, MeIQx and diMeIQx. Supporting that, an additional hydroxyl group in the chemical structure of the PCA would significantly affect the biological activity against the mutagen. Shahidi and Wanasundara (1992) and Makena and Chung (2007) reported that the position and number of hydroxyl groups are crucial in the inhibitory effects of polyphenols. Moreover, it has been found that the biological activity of trans-Resveratrol (t-RES) and its analogues (PCA) significantly depends on the structural determinants, which are i) the number and position of hydroxyl groups(Wolter et al., 2002) ii) intramolecular hydrogen bonding (Fang et al., 2002), iii) stereoisomery and iv) double bond (Wright et al., 2001). Thus, the protective effect of GA and PCA against food mutagens may vary with the structure and dose of the individual compounds and the mutagenic compound.

Taking together our results PCA was more efficient against DNA strand breaks induced by NDMA, NPYR, BaP and PhIP that GA .GA only prevent DNA strand breaks induced by BaP. Comparing the protective effect of both compounds against BaP, PCA showed higher protective effect (60-65%) than GA (18-36%). In addition PCA was also the most active against oxidized pyrimidines induced by NDMA, NPYR, NPIP, BaP and PhIP. GA only showed reduction of the oxidized pyrimidines induced by NDMA and BaP. This reduction was higher (23%, NDMA and 80-63%, BaP) than the observed by PCA against these two compounds. On the contrary, we also showed that GA and PCA at all concentrations increased oxidized purines induced by BaP. This effect could be attributed to the excess of reactive oxygen species (ROS) produced by BaP. They might cause irreparable oxidative DNA damage (Johnson and Loo, 2000). In addition, phenolic compounds have both antioxidant and prooxidant effects depending on the experimental conditions [28]. However, GA and PCA were very efficient to remove oxidized purines induced by all the mutagens tested with the exception of NDBA (GA) and PhIP (PCA). Therefore, although there is a general structure-activity relationship (López-Lázaro, 2002) that shows that some subclasses of polyphenols can be more potent antimutagens, these structural considerations can change depending on the substitution pattern of the molecule and/or the kind of compound used to induce DNA damage.

## 5. Conclusion

Our results indicate that, PCA was more efficient that GA to reduce DNA damage induced by food mutagens tested. PCA at the concentrations tested protect human hepatoma derived cells against DNA strand breaks induced by NDMA, NPYR, BaP and PhIP, oxidized pyrimidines induced by NDMA NPYR, NPIP, BaP, PhIP and oxidized purines induced by

NDBA, NDMA, NPYR, NPIP, MeIQx and diMeIQx.. However, GA at the concentrations tested only protects human hepatoma cells against DNA strand breaks induced by BaP, oxidized pyrimidines induced by NDMA and BaP and oxidized purines induced by NDMA, NPYR, NPIP, PhIP, MeIQx and diMeIQx.

## 6. Acknowledgments

This work has been supported by Grant ALI2005-01517 from the Ministerio de Educación y Ciencia (Spain) and by Grant 910177 from the BSCH and the Universidad Complutense (UCM).

## 7. References

Ahmedin D.V.M., Rebecca, M.P.H., Murray, T., Xu, J. & Thun M.J. (2007). Cancer statistic.*CA: A Cancer Journal for Clinicians*, 57: 43-66.

Arranz, N., Haza, A.I., García, A., Rafter, J & Morales, P. (2007). "Protective Effects of Organosulfur Compounds towards N-nitrosamines-induced DNA Damage in the Single-Cell Gel Electrophoresis (SCGE/HepG2 Assay," *Food and Chemical Toxicology*, 45: 1662-1669.

Bansal, A.K., Bansal, M., Soni, G. & Bhatnagar, D. (2005). Protective role of vitamin E pre-treatment on N-nitrododiethylamine induced oxidative stress in rat liver. *Chemico Biological Interactions*, 156: 101-111.

Bartsch H, Hietanen E & Malaveille C. (1989). Carcinogenic nitrosamines: free radical aspects of their action. *Free Radical Biological and Medicine*, 7: 637–644.

Brune, M., Rossander, L. & Hallberg, L. (1989). Iron absorption and phenolic compounds: importance of different phenolic structures. *European Journal of Clinical Nutrition*, 43: 547-558.

Burczynski ME & Penning TM (2000). Genotoxic polycyclic aromatic hydrocarbon orthoquinones generated byaldo-keto reductases induce CYP1A1via nuclear translocation of the aryl 30 the formation of 8-OHdG in HepG2 cells. *Archives of. Biochemistry and. Biophysics*, 455: 197-203.

Cantos, E., Espin, J.C., Fernández, M.J., Oliva, J. & Tomás-Barberan, F.A. (2003). Postharvest UV-C-irradiated grapes as a potential source for producing stilbene-enriched red wine. *Journal of Agricultural and Food Chemistry*, 51: 1208-1214.

Collins, A.R. (2005). Assays for oxidative stress and antioxidant status: applications to research into the biological effectiveness of polyphenols. *American Journal of Clinical Nutrition*, 81: 261S-267S.

Delgado, E., Haza, A.I., Arranz, N., García, A. & P. Morales. (2008). Dietary polyphenols protect against N-nitrosamines and benzo(a)pireno-induced DNA damage (strand breaks and oxidized purines/pyrimidines) in HepG2 human hepatoma cells. *European Journal of Nutrition*, 47: 479-490.

Dolara, P., Luceri, C., Filippo, C.D., Femia, A.P., Giovannelli, L., Caderni, G., Cecchini, C., Silvi, S., Orpianesi, C. & Cresci, A. (2005). Red wine polyphenols influence carcinogenesis, intestinal microflora, oxidative damage and gene expression profiles of colonic mucosa in F344 rats. *Mutation Research/Fundamental and Molecular Mechanisms of Mutagenesis*, 591: 237-246.

Fang , J.G., Lu, M., Chen, Z.H. Zhu, H.H., Li, Y., Yang, L., Wu, L.M. & Liu, Z.L. (2002). Antioxidant effects of resveratrol and its analogues against the free-radical - induced peroxidation of linoleic acid in micelles. *Chemistry European Journal*, 8: 4191-4198.

Ferguson, L.R., Philpott, M. & Karunasinghe, N. (2004). Dietary cancer and prevention using antimutagens. *Toxicology*, 198: 147–159.

Ferrigni, N. R., McLaughlin, J. L., Powell, R. G. & Smith, C. R., Jr (1984). Use of potato disc and brine shrimp bioassays to detect activity and isolate piceatannol as the antileukemic principle from the seeds of *Euphorbia lagascae*. *Journal of Natural Products*, 47: 347-352.

Filho, P.J.S., Rios, A., Valcárcel, M. & Caramao, E.B. (2003). Development of a new method for the determination of nitrosamines by micellar electrokinetic capillary chromatography. *Water Research*, 37: 3837–3842.

Galli,, H.U., Perchellet, E.M., Klish, D.S., Hohnson, J.M.& Perchelet, J.P. (1992). Hydrolizable tannins: potent inhibitors of hydroperoxide production and tumor promotion in mouse skin treated with 12-Otetradecanoylphorbol-13-acetate in vivo. *International Journal of Cancer*, 51: 425-432.

García, A., Haza, A.I., Arranz, N., Delgado, E. Rafter, J. & Morales, P. (2008b). Organosulfur compounds alone or in combination with vitamin C protect against N-nitrosodibutylamine and N-nitrosopiperidine-induced oxidative DNA damage in HepG2 cells. *Chemico-Biological Interactions*, 173: 9-18.

García, A., Haza, A.I., Arranz, N., Rafter, J. &. Morales, P. (2008a). Protective effects of isothiocyanates alone or in combination with vitamin C towards N-nitrosodibutylamine or N-nitrosopiperidine-induced oxidative DNA damage in the single-cell gel electophoresis (SCGE)/HepG2 assay. *Journal of Applied Toxicology*, 28: 196-204.

Gelderblom, W.C., Abel, S., Smuts, C.M., Marnewick, J., Marasas, W.F., Lemmer, E.R. & Ramljak, D. (2009). Fumonisin-induced hepatocarcinogenesis: mechanisms related to cancer initiation and promotion. *Environmmental Health Perspectives*, 109: 291-300.

Gray, R., Peto, R., Branton, P.& Grasso, P. (1991). Chronic nitrosamine ingestion in 1040 rodents the effect of the choice of nitrosamine, the species studied, and the age of starting exposure. *Cancer Research*, 51, 6470–6491.

Hadi, S.M., Bhat, S.H., Azmi, A.S., Hanif, S., Shamim, U. & Ullah, M.F. (2007). Oxidative breakage of cellular DNA by plant polyphenols: A putative mechanism for anticancer properties. *Seminars in Cancer Biology*, 17: 370-376.

Havsteen, B.H. (2002). The biochemistry and medical significance of the flavonoids. *Pharmacology &. Therapeutics*, 96: 67-202.

Haza, A.I. & P. Morales. (2011). Effects of (+)catechin and (-) epicatechin on heterocyclic amines-induced oxidativeDNA damage. *Journal of Applied Toxicology*, 31(1): 53-62.

IARC. (1993). Some natural occurring substances: food items and constituents Heterocyclic Amines and Mycotoxins. In Monographs on the evaluation of carcinogenic risks to humans. International Agency for Research on Cancer 56, Lyon, 165-231.

Ingelman-Sundberg M. (2002). Polymorphism of cytochrome P450 and xenobiotic toxicity. *Toxicology*, 181-182: 447-52.

Inoue, M., Suzuki, R., Koide, T., Sakaguchi, N., Ogihara, Y. & Yabu, Y. (1994). Antioxidant gallic acid induces apoptosis in HL-60RG cells. *Biochemical and Biophysics Research Communications*, 204: 898-904.

Johnson, M, K. & Loo, G. (2000). Effects of epigallocatechin gallate and quercetin on oxidative damage to cellular DNA. *Mutation Research.*, 459: 211 - 218.

Kanazawa K, Uehara M, Yanagitani H. & Hashimoto T. (2006). Bioavailable flavonoids to suppress hydrocarbon receptor. *Cancer Research*, 60: 908–915.

Lambert, J.D., Hong, J., Yang, G., Liao, J. & Yang, C.S. (2005). Inhibition of carcinogenesis by polyphenols: Evidence from laboratory investigations. *The American Journal of Clinical Nutrition*, 81: S284-S291.

Lapidot, T., Walker, M.D. & Kanner, J. (2002). Can apple antioxidants inhibit tumor cell proliferation? Generation of $H_2O_2$ during interaction of phenolic compounds with cell culture media. *Journal of Agricultural and Food Chemistry*, 50: 3156-3160.

Layton, D.W., Bogen, K.T., Knize, M.G., Hatch, F.T., Johnson, V.M. & Felton, J.S. (1995). Cancer risk of heterocyclic amines in cooked foods: an analysis and implications for research. *Carcinogenesis*, 16(1): 39-52

López-Lázaro, M. (2002). Flavonoids as anticancer agents: Structure-activity relationship study. *Current Medicinal Chemistry -Anti-Cancer Agents* 2: 691-714.

Lu, Z., Nie, G., Belton, P.S., Tang, H. & Zhao, B. (2006). Structure activity relationship analysis of antioxidant ability and neuroprotective effect of gallic acid derivatives. Neurochemistry International, 48: 263-274.

Madlener, S., Illmer, C. & Horvath, Z. (2007). Gallic acid inhibits ribonucleotide reductase and cyclooxygenases in human HL-60 promyelocytic leukemia cells. *Cancer Letters*, 245:156-162.

Makena, P. & Chung, K. (2007). Effects of various plant polyphenols on bladder carcinogen benzidine-induced mutagenicity. *Food and Chemical Toxicology*, 45: 1899-1909.

Mastaloudis, A., Yu, T., O'Donnell, R.P., Frei, B., Dashwood, R.H. & Traber, M.G. (2004). Endurance exercise results in DNA damage as detected by the comet assay. *Free Radical Biology and Medicine*, 36: 966-975.

Matsuda, H., Kageura, T., Morikawa, T., Toguchida, I., Harima, S. & Yoshikawa, M. (2000). Effects of stilbene constituents from rhubarb on nitric oxide production in lipopolysaccharide-activated macrophages. *Bioorganic and Medicinal Chemistry Letters*, 10: 323-327.

McDonald, M.S., Hughes, M., Burns, J., lean, M.E., Matthews, D. & Crozier, A. (1998). Survey of the free and conjugated myricetin and quercetin content of red wines of different geographical origins. *Journal of Agricultural and Food Chemistry*, 46: 368-375.

Olive, P.L., Wlodek, D., Durand, R.E. & Banáth, J.P. (1992). Factors influencing DNA migration from individual cells subjected to gel electrophoresis. *Experimental Cell Research*, 198: 259-267.

Piver, B., Fer, M., Vitrac, X., Merillon, J.M., Dreano, Y., Berthou, F. & Lucas, D. (2004). Involvement of cytochrome P450 1A2 in the biotransformation of trans-resveratrol in human liver microsomes. *Biochemical Pharmacology*, 68: 773-782.

Preussmann R & Stewart BW (1984). N-Nitroso carcinogens. Chemical Carcinogens. American Chemical Society, pp 643-828.

Sanyal, R., Darroudi, F., Parzefall, W., Nagao, M. & Knasmuller, S. (1997). Inhibition of the genotoxic effects of heterocyclic amines in human derived hepatoma cells by dietary bioantimutagens. *Mutagenesis* 12, 297-303.

Seo, S.Y., Sharma, V.K.& Sharma, N.J. (2003).Mushroom tyrosinase: Recent prospects. *Journal of Agricultural and Food Chemistry*, 51: 2837-2853.

Shahidi, F., Wanasundara, P.K.(1992). Phenolic antioxidants. *Critical Reviews in Food Science and Nutrition*, 32: 67-103.

Shahrzad, S., Aoyagi, K., Winter, A., Koyama, A. & Bitsch, I. (2001). Pharmacokinetics of gallic acid and its relative bioavility from tea in healthy humans. *Journal of Nutrition*, 1207-1210.

Skog KI., Johansson MAE & Jägerstad MI. (1998). Carcinogenic Heterocyclic Amines in Model Systems and Cooked Foods: A Review on Formation, Occurrence and Intake. *Food and Chemical Toxicology*, 36: 879-896.

Son, S. & Lewis, B.A. (2002). Free radical scavenging and antioxidative activity of caffeic acid amide and ester analogues: structure activity relationship. *Journal of Agricultural and Food Chemistry*, 50: 468-472.

Stich, H.F., Rosin., M.P. & Brison, L. (1982). Inhibition of mutagenicity of a model nitrosation reaction by naturally occurring phenolics, coffee and tea. *Mutation Research*, 95: 119-128.

Teguo, P. W., Decendit, S., Krisa, S., Deffieux, G., Vercauteren, J. & and Mérillon, J. M. (2001). The accumulation of stilbene glycosides in *Vitis vinifera* cell suspension cultures. *Journal of Natural Products*, 59: 1189-1191.

Toribio F, Busquets R, Puignou L & Galceran M.T. (2007). Heterocyclic amines in griddled beef steak analysed using a single extract clean-up procedure. *Food and Chemical Toxicology*, 45: 667-675.

Tricker, A.R. & Preussmann, R. (1991). Carcinogenic N-nitrosamines in the diet: occurrence, formation, mechanisms and carcinogenic potential, *Mutation Research*, 259: 277-289.

Tsuruga, T., Chun, Y. T., Ebizuka, Y. & Sankawa, U. (1991). Biologically active constituents of *Melaleuca leucadendron*: inhibitors of induced histamine release from rat mast cells. *Chemical and Pharmaceutical Bulletin*, 39: 3276-3278.

Ueng Y., Shyu C., Liu T., Oda, Y., Liao, J & Chen, C. (2001). Protective effects of baicalein and wogonin against benzo[a]pyrene- and aflatoxin B1-induced genotoxicities. *Biochemical Pharmacology*, 62: 1653-1660.

Williams, G.M., Gebhardt, R., Sirma, H. & Stenback, F. (1993). Non-linearity of neoplastic conversion induced in rat liver by low exposures to diethylnitrosamine. *Carcinogenesis*, 14: 2149–2156.

Wolter, F., Clausnitzer, A., Akoglu, B. & Stein, J. (2002). Piceatannol, a natural analog of resveratrol, inhibits progression through the s phase of the cell cycle in colorectal cancer cell lines. *Journal of. Nutrition*, 132: 298-302.

Wong, H.L., Murphy, S.E. & Hecht, S.S. (2003). Comparative Metabolism of N-nitrosopiperidine and N-nitrosopyrrolidine by Rat Liver and Esophageal Microsomes and Cytochrome P450 2A3. *Carcinogenesis*, 24(2): 291-300.

Wright, J.S., Johnson, E.R.& DiLabio, G.A. (2001). Predicting the activity of phenolic antioxidants: theorical method, analysis of substituent effects and application to major families of antioxidants. *Journal of the American Chemical. Society*, 123: 1173-1183.

Wu, L.T., Chu, C.C., Chung, J.G., Chen, C.H., Hsu, L.S., Liu, J.K. & Chen, S.C. (2004). Effects of tannic acid and its related compounds on food mutagens or hydrogen peroxide-induced DNA strand breaks in human lymphocytes. *Mutation Research*, 556 (1-2):75-82.

# 18

# Reviews on the Epidemiology, Quality of Life, and Management of Chronic Hepatitis B (CHB)

Elegance T.P. Lam and Cindy L.K. Lam
*The University of Hong Kong*
*Hong Kong*

## 1. Introduction

Chronic hepatitis B (CHB) remains a major global health problem. About 400 million people are chronic hepatitis B carriers. CHB can affect health-related quality of life (HRQOL). Several anti-viral drugs are available for CHB patients.

## 2. Reviews on the epidemiology, Quality of Life, and management of Chronic Hepatitis B (CHB)

This chapter first reviews the epidemiology of hepatitis B virus (HBV) and recommended management for CHB to identify the health problems and service needs of these patients. The findings from studies on health-related quality of life (HRQOL) and CHB is highlighted to identify any knowledge gaps. Finally, available HRQOL measures are reviewed to determine which one is the most suitable for applications for the evaluation of Chinese CHB patients in Hong Kong.

### 2.1 Epidemiology and management for Chronic Hepatitis B (CHB)

#### 2.1.1 Epidemiology and natural history of CHB

Hepatitis B is one of the most common infectious diseases and a leading cause of death in the world (Lai, Ratziu, Yuen, & Roynard, 2003; Lavanchy, 2004, 2005; Maynard, 1990; Wright, 2006). Approximately 2 billion are infected and more than 400 million people of those are chronically infected with hepatitis B virus (HBV) (Fattovich, Bortolotti, & Donato, 2008; Lai et al., 2003). Chronically infected individuals defined as those who have diagnosed with hepatitis B surface antigen (HBsAg) for more than six months (A S Lok & McMahon, 2009; Maddrey, 2000). It was estimated that 75% of chronic hepatitis B (CHB) carriers were found in Asia and the Western Pacific regions (Gust, 1996; Maddrey, 2000; Maynard, 1990; Merican et al., 2000). HBV results in 500,000 to 1.2 million deaths per year caused by cirrhosis, liver failure or hepatocellular carcinoma (HCC) (Lavanchy, 2004, 2005). The incidence of HCC is increasing and is the fifth most common cancer worldwide killing 300,000-500,000 people per year (Lavanchy, 2004). Worldwide, approximately 30% of cirrhosis was attributable to HBV and over half (53%) of HCC was due to HBV (Perz, Armstrong, Farrington, Hutin, & Bell, 2006). HBV infection accounted for more than 50% of HCC (65%) and cirrhosis (57%) in Western Pacific regions (Perz et al., 2006).

In Hong Kong, HCC is the fourth common cancer and the third leading cause of cancer deaths (H. A. Hong Kong Cancer Registry, 2008). In 2006, there were 1745 (1462) new cases (deaths) of liver cancer registered in Hong Kong, representing 7.3% (12.1%) of all cancers in total (H. A. Hong Kong Cancer Registry, 2008). There was a male predominance with a male-to-female ratio of 3:1 (Hong Kong Cancer Registry, 2006), and the age of onset is earlier in males (Department of Health HKSAR, 1998). The age-standardized incidence (mortality) rates for males and females were 29.3 (23.3) and 8.0 (6.7) per 100,000 population, respectively (Hong Kong Cancer Registry, 2006). HBV was significantly contributed to HCC, with 80% of HCC patients found to be hepatitis B carriers (Department of Health HKSAR, 1998). Therefore, HBV infection accounts for the majority of both cirrhosis and HCC worldwide (Perz et al., 2006).

The prevalence of HBV varies notably between and within countries (Custer et al., 2004; Gust, 1996; Lavanchy, 2004, 2005; Maddrey, 2000; Maynard, 1990). It could be categorized as high, intermediate and low HBV endemicity (Custer et al., 2004; Lavanchy, 2004; Maddrey, 2000). In areas of high endemicity, ≥8% are CHB carriers and account for a total of 45% of the global population (Lavanchy, 2004). They include South East Asia, China including Hong Kong, sub-Saharan Africa and the Amazon Basin (Custer et al., 2004; Lavanchy, 2004; Maddrey, 2000). In areas of intermediate endemicity, such as eastern and southern Europe, the Middle East, Japan and part of South America, 2-7% of the population are chronic carriers (Custer et al., 2004; Lavanchy, 2004; Maddrey, 2000). The endemicity of HBV is low in most developed countries, such as North America, Northern and Western Europe and Australia, where less than 2% of the population are chronic carriers (Custer et al., 2004; Maddrey, 2000).

Hepatitis B virus (HBV) is present in the blood, saliva, semen, vaginal secretions, menstrual blood, and to a lesser degree sweat, breast milk, tears and urine of infected individuals (Lavanchy, 2004; Wright, 2006). Since HBV is resistant to breakdown outside the body, it is easily transmitted through contact with infected body fluids (Lavanchy, 2004; Wright, 2006). Three modes of HBV transmission have been categorized as: perinatal (from an infected mother to her child), horizontal transmission through mucosal contact with infected blood or bodily fluid secretions and parenteral or percutaneous transmission (such as injection drug use and needlestick injury) (C. J. Chen, Wang, & Yu, 2000; Gust, 1996; Lavanchy, 2004; Maddrey, 2000; Wright, 2006).

Routes of HBV transmission vary depending on the prevalence of HBV infection (Lavanchy, 2004; Maddrey, 2000). In areas of high endemicity, perinatal transmission is the most common route and the majority of HBV infection is acquired during the preschool years (Lavanchy, 2004; Maddrey, 2000). The lifetime risk of HBV infection is greater than 60% (Lavanchy, 2004; Maddrey, 2000). In areas of intermediate endemicity, most HBV infection occurs in infant or childhood, with lifetime risk of 20-60% (Lavanchy, 2004; Maddrey, 2000). In areas of low endemicity, HBV infection is acquired primarily by horizontal transmission (between individuals) in adolescents or early adulthood, for instance, through intravenous drug use or unprotected sexual transmission (Lavanchy, 2004; Maddrey, 2000). The lifetime risk of acquiring HBV is <20% (Lavanchy, 2004; Maddrey, 2000).

The natural history of HBV infection has three phases including immune tolerance, immune clearance and a residual phase (Lai et al., 2003; McMahon, 2008; Wright, 2006). The first phase of HBV is immune tolerance (Lai et al., 2003; McMahon, 2008; Merican et al., 2000;

Wright, 2006). During this phase, patients are hepatitis B e-antigen (HBeAg) positive and have high levels of serum HBV DNA (ranges between $10^7$-$10^{11}$ copies/mL) (Lai et al., 2003; McMahon, 2008; Merican et al., 2000; Wright, 2006). However, liver inflammatory disease is minimal or absent, with normal or minimally elevated alanine aminotransferase (ALT) level and minimal histological activity in the liver (Lai et al., 2003; McMahon, 2008; Merican et al., 2000; Wright, 2006). It usually occurs in children and young adults and may last for 10-30 years in Asian patients who acquired HBV infection during the perinatal period (Lai et al., 2003; Merican et al., 2000; Yuen, 2007). Patients in this phase are highly contagious and can transmit the disease easily (Yuen, 2007).

The second phase is immune clearance and it usually occurs when patients are aged between 15-35 years old (Lai et al., 2003; McMahon, 2008; Merican et al., 2000). It is characterized by HBeAg positive, lower level of viral replication (presented by low serum HBV DNA level), evaluated or fluctuating levels of ALT, moderate or severe liver necroinflammation and more rapid progression of fibrosis compared to the previous phase (Lai et al., 2003; McMahon, 2008; Merican et al., 2000). This phase may last for several weeks to several years (Merican et al., 2000). Liver damage has been established and the progression of the disease to a more advanced stage of illness such as cirrhosis depends on the duration of this stage (McMahon, 2008; Wright, 2006; Yuen, 2007).

In the third phase, patients undergo HBeAg seroconversion, with loss of HBeAg and appearance of an antibody to HBeAg, namely anti-HBe (European Association For the study of the liver, 2008; Keeffe et al., 2008; Lai et al., 2003; McMahon, 2008; Merican et al., 2000; Wright, 2006; Yuen, 2007). This phase is usually characterized by very low or undetectable serum HBV DNA levels (usually $10^3$-$10^5$ copies/mL), persistent normal ALT level and inactive liver histology with minimal fibrosis (European Association For the study of the liver, 2008; Keeffe et al., 2008; McMahon, 2008; Wright, 2006; Yuen, 2007).

Some patients may progress to the immune phase (phase 4), with clearance of HBsAg and appearance of an antibody to HBsAg (anti-HBs) (Merican et al., 2000). It indicates the development of full immunity to HBV (Merican et al., 2000). Serum HBV DNA tends to become undetectable and risk of re-infection or reactivation is low (Merican et al., 2000). However, this phase is rare in Asian patients, but it may occur in Caucasians at the rate of 1-2% annually which increase with time (Merican et al., 2000).

Understanding the epidemiology and natural history of CHB infection helps us to prevent HBV infection and to use anti-viral treatment more effectively. There is little benefit to treat patients in phase 1 or phase 3 (Merican et al., 2000). Based on current clinical guidelines, the goal of treatment for CHB is to reduce the risk of disease progression in phase 2, aiming to eliminate the viral replication of HBV (Merican et al., 2000).

Most patients with hepatitis B have no symptoms until they have developed cirrhosis or HCC, both of which are very debilitating conditions that can markedly decrease HRQOL. Patients in the advanced stages of illness often have fatigue, pain, poor appetite, jaundice, ascites, variceal bleeding, and impaired cognitive function(L. M. Martin, Dan, & Younossi, 2006; L. M. Martin & Younossi, 2005), all of which may affect the patient's physical functioning, work, activities of daily living, social functioning and emotions. These domains should be included in the evaluation of the HRQOL of CHB patients. Anti-viral treatments for phase 2 CHB to prevent or delay disease progression not only reduce mortality but can preserve HRQOL through the prevention of morbidity.

## 2.2 Health service needs of CHB patients and HRQOL

Chronic hepatitis B (CHB) is a chronic disease that can lead to very disabling and even lethal complications, which require different health care services at different stages of the illness.

### 2.2.1 Monitoring

Individuals who are chronically infected with HBV require lifetime monitoring of the status of infection and follow-up for the development of liver complications, for instance active chronic hepatitis, cirrhosis and HCC (Keeffe et al., 2008; Y F Liaw et al., 2008; A S Lok & McMahon, 2009). International guidelines recommend the initial evaluation of patients with CHB infection should include a thorough history, physical examination and laboratory tests to identify the current stage and the phases of HBV infection (Keeffe et al., 2008; Y F Liaw et al., 2008; A S Lok & McMahon, 2009). We also need to take into consideration family history of HBV and liver cancer, risk factors for co-infection and alcohol consumption (Keeffe et al., 2008; Y F Liaw et al., 2008; A S Lok & McMahon, 2009). Laboratory investigations should comprise HBsAg, HBeAg and anti-HBe, quantification of viral replication by levels of HBV DNA, tests for co-infection with other types of hepatitis (hepatitis C virus and hepatitis D virus), and HIV in high-risk group (Keeffe et al., 2008; Y F Liaw et al., 2008; A S Lok & McMahon, 2009). Liver biopsy should be considered in those infected individuals with elevated ALT or HBV DNA levels (Keeffe et al., 2008; Y F Liaw et al., 2008; A S Lok & McMahon, 2009). Patients should be counseled on preventive measures against transmission of HBV infection through household or sexual contacts (Keeffe et al., 2008; Y F Liaw et al., 2008). Abstinence from alcohol is highly recommended (Keeffe et al., 2008). Negative impacts on psychological, physical and social well being should be considered (Y F Liaw et al., 2008). Previous studies showed that patients with CHB had lower HRQOL scores even in the absence of cirrhosis or cancer (Y F Liaw et al., 2008; S C Ong, Mak, Aung, Li, & Lim, 2008). All infected individuals with HBV infection who are not immuned to hepatitis A should be vaccinated according to Centers for Disease Control and Prevention (CDC) recommendations (Keeffe et al., 2008; A S Lok & McMahon, 2009). After initial evaluation, the frequency and tests of monitoring depends on the stage of illness.

Patients with persistently normal ALT levels often have minimal histological changes and poor response to currently available anti-viral drugs (Y F Liaw et al., 2008). Therefore, no anti-viral drug therapy is recommended for this patient group (Y F Liaw et al., 2008). However, they should be monitored regularly and HCC surveillance may be needed. There is currently no consensus on frequency or type of test for monitoring. The updated Asia-Pacific consensus statements recommends patients with active viral replication should have HBV DNA level, ALT and HBeAg testing every 3 months for the first year and then every 3-6 months, but this is rarely feasible because of limitation in resources (Y F Liaw et al., 2008). The American Association for the Study of Liver Disease (AASLD) guidelines recommend individuals in the immune tolerant phase (stage 2) who are HBeAg-positive but with normal ALT should have ALT and AST tests every 3 months for the first year and then every 6 months (A S Lok & McMahon, 2009). Screening for HCC is particularly important for high-risk group, such as Asian men aged >40 years old or Asian women aged >50 years old, with cirrhosis and family history of severe liver disease (Keeffe et al., 2008; A S Lok & McMahon, 2009).

### 2.2.2 Anti-viral drug treatment

If patients have higher serum HBV DNA levels and increased ALT levels, drug treatment is recommended (Keeffe et al., 2008; Y F Liaw et al., 2008; A S Lok & McMahon, 2009). A liver biopsy is suggested before receiving drug therapy in order to evaluate the necroinflammatory grade and stage of fibrosis and exclude other reasons of elevated ALT levels (Y F Liaw et al., 2008). The ideal goal of CHB therapy is the complete eradication of HBV but this is still impossible. The short-term goals of CHB treatment include suppression of serum HBV DNA, normalization of ALT, HBeAg seroconversion and improvement in liver histology (European Association For the study of the liver, 2008; Keeffe et al., 2008; Y F Liaw et al., 2008; A S Lok & McMahon, 2009). The ultimate goal of long term treatment is to prevent or delay the onset of liver complications including cirrhosis and HCC, and to prolong survival (European Association For the study of the liver, 2008; Keeffe et al., 2008; Y F Liaw et al., 2008; A S Lok & McMahon, 2009). Current clinical guidelines and treatment algorithms focus on the suppression of viral replication to maintain serum HBV DNA at the lowest possible levels (European Association For the study of the liver, 2008; Keeffe et al., 2008; Y F Liaw et al., 2008; A S Lok & McMahon, 2009). This has been shown to prevent and slow the progression to cirrhosis, liver failure or HCC (European Association For the study of the liver, 2008; Keeffe et al., 2008; Y F Liaw et al., 2008; A S Lok & McMahon, 2009).

Currently, seven drugs are available for management of CHB infection including lamivudine (LVD), adefovir (ADV), entecavir (ETV), telbivudine (LdT), and tenofovir (TDF) and interferon (IFN-α), and pegylated IFN (peg-IFN) (European Association For the study of the liver, 2008; Keeffe et al., 2008; Y F Liaw et al., 2008; A S Lok & McMahon, 2009). The choice of treatment should take into account treatment efficacy, risk of developing drug resistance, long term safety profile, side effects, mode of administration and cost of drug (Fung, Lai, & Yuen, 2008).

Interferon (IFN-α) is the first drug used for the treatment of CHB (Lai & Yuen, 2008; Yuen & Lai, 2001). It has to be given by injection which limits its acceptability (Jacobson, 2006). Standard IFN-α has been used for treatment of CHB for more than two decades (Y F Liaw et al., 2008; Marcellin, Asselah, & Boyer, 2005). This treatment stimulates the immune system to eradicate HBV (Ayoub & Keeffe, 2008; Jacobson, 2006; Y F Liaw et al., 2008; A S Lok & McMahon, 2009; Marcellin et al., 2005). The efficacy of standard IFN-α has been demonstrated to be effective in suppression of HBV replication and in inducing remission of liver disease in Western populations (Fung et al., 2008; Jacobson, 2006; Y F Liaw et al., 2008; A S Lok & McMahon, 2009; A. S. Lok et al., 1992; Yuen & Lai, 2001). Peg-IFN, in a newer generation of IFN, has been shown to be superior in terms of HBeAg clearance, normalization of ALT and HBV DNA suppression (Ayoub & Keeffe, 2008; Cooksley et al., 2003; Fung et al., 2008; Keeffe et al., 2008; Y F Liaw et al., 2008; A S Lok & McMahon, 2009; Zoulim & Perrillo, 2008). The advantage of standard IFN-α or peg-IFN is a definite duration of treatment (Ayoub & Keeffe, 2008; Fung et al., 2008; Jacobson, 2006; Lai & Yuen, 2008; Y F Liaw et al., 2008). Long-term effectiveness of standard IFN has shown to be inconclusive (Fung et al., 2008; Y F Liaw et al., 2008; A S Lok & McMahon, 2009; Marcellin et al., 2005; Yuen & Lai, 2001). The efficacy of IFN is limited to CHB patients with high pretreatment ALT levels (Jacobson, 2006; A S Lok & McMahon, 2009), which is uncommon for Asian CHB patients (Fung et al., 2008). Some studies in Japanese and Chinese patients failed to demonstrate a long-term benefit of standard IFN therapy. However, a recent study of Taiwanese patients with a high ALT pretreatment level has shown a beneficial effect on reduction of liver-related complications, for instance, cirrhosis and HCC (Fung et al., 2008). The occurrence of adverse event is the main concern. Standard IFN and peg-IFN have similar side effect profiles but is less common in peg-IFN (A S Lok & McMahon, 2009). The most common side effect is influenza-like symptoms consisting of fever, chills, headache, malaise and myalgia (Jacobson, 2006; Y F Liaw et al., 2008; A S Lok & McMahon, 2009). Other side effects comprise fatigue, anorexia, weight loss and hair loss (Y F Liaw et al., 2008). Patients receiving IFN should have regular follow-up for mood deterioration (Jacobson, 2006). Recently, studies have focused on combination or sequential therapy with LVD (Y F Liaw et al., 2008). No superior effects have been found with combination therapy of IFN and lamivudine (LVD) (Jacobson, 2006; Y F Liaw et al., 2008). It reduced the risk of developing resistance.

Lamivudine (LVD) is a nucleoside analog and the first oral anti-viral drug licensed since 1998 for the treatment of CHB infection (Ayoub & Keeffe, 2008; Lai & Yuen, 2008). It has an excellent safety profile (Ayoub & Keeffe, 2008; Fung et al., 2008; Jacobson, 2006; Leung, 2008; Y F Liaw et al., 2008) and is the least expensive of all nucleoside analogs approved for the treatment of CHB (Dan, Aung, & Lim, 2008; Zoulim & Perrillo, 2008). It is effective in suppressing HBV DNA, normalizing ALT and HBeAg seroconversion (Dienstag et al., 1999; Fung et al., 2008; Lai et al., 1998; Y F Liaw et al., 2008; A S Lok & McMahon, 2009). Previous studies showed that LVD led to significant histological improvement and reduction in the progression of liver fibrosis (Ayoub & Keeffe, 2008; Dienstag et al., 1999; Lai et al., 1998; Leung, 2008). Long-term LVD therapy reduces the risk of developing cirrhosis and HCC in precirrhotic/cirrhotic and non-cirrohotic patients (Y. F. Liaw et al., 2004; Yuen et al., 2007). Duration of LVD therapy remains controversial in HBeAg negative CHB patients (A S Lok & McMahon, 2009). For patients who are HBeAg positive, LVD can be stopped 6-9 months after HBeAg seroconversion (A S Lok & McMahon, 2009). Hepatic flares, defined as increased serum ALT levels to ≥ 5 times upper normal limit, may develop on stopping LVD and result in hepatic decompensation (Fung et al., 2008; Y F Liaw et al., 2008). Earlier studies demonstrated about 50% of the patients achieved a sustained response after stopping LVD treatment (Y F Liaw et al., 2008). In one of the studies by Chan et al, 89 Chinese CHB patients with HBeAg negative received two years of LVD treatment resulted in 56% complete response (defined as normalization of ALT and HBV DNA level of $< 10^4$ copies/mL) (Y F Liaw et al., 2008). The response was sustained in 26% of patients 6 months after stopping LVD treatment (Y F Liaw et al., 2008). The main drawback of LVD is development of drug resistance (Jacobson, 2006; Y F Liaw et al., 2008; Nguyen & Keeffe, 2009; Yuen & Lai, 2001; Zoulim & Perrillo, 2008). According to a recent review, LVD drug resistance rates are approximately 50% after 3 years and 76% after 8 years (Ayoub & Keeffe, 2008; Fung et al., 2008; Leung, 2008; Nguyen & Keeffe, 2009; Yuen et al., 2007). The incidence of drug resistance increased with the duration of therapy (Ayoub & Keeffe, 2008; Fung et al., 2008; Jacobson, 2006; Leung, 2008). Benefits induced by LVD therapy are reduced once drug resistance occurs (Fung et al., 2008; Jacobson, 2006). However, even those who develop LVD-resistance, their treatment outcome is still better than untreated patients.

Adedovir (ADV) is the second oral nucleoside analog approved for CHB and has been shown to be effective, irrespective of HBeAg status or LVD-resistance (Hadziyannis et al., 2006; Hadziyannis et al., 2003; Lampertico et al., 2005; Leung, 2008; Marcellin et al., 2003). Although ADV has fairly slow action compared with other oral anti-viral treatments (in terms of HBAg seroconversion, normalization of ALT and suppression of HBV DNA), treatment with ADV up to 5 years results in significant histologic, virologic and biochemical improvement (Hadziyannis et al., 2005). Currently, ADV is primarily used in patients who have developed resistance to LVD (Fung et al., 2008; Zoulim & Perrillo, 2008). Some studies have shown the addition of ADV to LVD rather than switchover to ADV monotherapy produced a lower rate of resistance to ADV (Lampertico et al., 2007; Manolakopoulos et al., 2008; Rapti, Dimou, Mitsoula, & Hadziyannis, 2007; van der Poorten et al., 2007; Zoulim & Perrillo, 2008). Other studies have shown that ADV monotherapy in patients with LVD-resistant was as effective for HBV DNA suppression as combination therapy (Fung et al., 2007; Fung et al., 2008; Y F Liaw et al., 2008; Peters et al., 2004). Most guidelines recommended to add on ADV in LVD-resistant patients in order to minimize the development of ADV-resistance and maintain HBV DNA suppression in the long term (European Association For the study of the liver, 2008; Keeffe et al., 2008; Y F Liaw et al., 2008; A S Lok & McMahon, 2009). ADV has a higher genetic barrier than LVD resulting in lower rates of resistance (Fung et al., 2008). The cumulative incidence of ADV-resistance is 29% after 5 years of treatment in patients with HBeAg negative and about 20% in HBeAg positive patients (Hadziyannis et al., 2006; A S Lok & McMahon, 2009). According to a large trial, ADV in 10-mg doses was well tolerated and had similar safety profile as placebo (Hadziyannis et al., 2006). However, renal abnormalities were reported with 30 mg of ADV (Marcellin et al., 2003). Continued treatment of ADV up to 5 years induces a reversible increase in serum creatinine of more than 0.5 mg/dL (Hadziyannis et al., 2006). Therefore, renal function should be monitored regularly and closely (A S Lok & McMahon, 2009).

Entecavir (ETV) is the third oral nucleoside analog licensed for CHB (Lai & Yuen, 2008). It was superior to LVD and ADV in rates of histologic, biochemical and virologic responses, irrespective of HBeAg status (T. T. Chang et al., 2006; Lai et al., 2002; Lai et al., 2006; Leung, 2008). In a viral kinetic study ETV showed a more dramatic decline in HBV DNA levels than ADV (Y F Liaw et al., 2008). After 2 years of ETV treatment, no virological breakthrough from ETV resistance has been found (Fung et al., 2008; Lai & Yuen, 2008; Y F Liaw et al., 2008). The rate of resistance to ETV was very low at 1.2% in treatment-naïve patients after 5 years (Ayoub & Keeffe, 2008; European Association For the study of the liver, 2008; Lai & Yuen, 2008; Y F Liaw et al., 2008; A S Lok & McMahon, 2009; Nguyen & Keeffe, 2009). ETV has demonstrated to be effective in LVD-resistant patients, but was associated with a lower response rate and a higher resistance rate of 39.5% after 4 years (Ayoub & Keeffe, 2008; Keeffe et al., 2008; Y F Liaw et al., 2008; A S Lok & McMahon, 2009; Nguyen & Keeffe, 2009). Therefore, LVD should be discontinued when patients are switched to ETV in order to reduce the risk of ETV resistance (Fung et al., 2008; A S Lok & McMahon, 2009). ADV add-on therapy may be better than ETV switching therapy for patients with LVD-resistance (Fung et al., 2008; Keeffe et al., 2008; A S Lok & McMahon, 2009). ETV therapy is best given to treatment naïve patients (Leung, 2008).

Telbivudine (LdT) is more potent than LVD and ADV in HBV DNA suppression (H. L. Chan et al., 2007; Keeffe et al., 2008; Lai et al., 2005; A S Lok & McMahon, 2009). A phase III controlled trial showed that 60% of patients who received LdT had an undetectable HBV DNA level compared to those who received LVD (40%) after 2 years of treatment (Keeffe et al., 2008; Y. F. Liaw et al., 2009). Resistance rate increases dramatically after one year of LdT to 25.1% in HBeAg positive and 10.8% in HBeAg negative patients after 2 years of treatment (Y F Liaw et al., 2008; A S Lok & McMahon, 2009). LdT was well tolerated when used as a monotherapy and has a similar safety profile to LVD (Keeffe et al., 2008; Leung, 2008; A S Lok & McMahon,

2009). Increase in creatine kinase levels (a level of >7 times upper limit of normal (ULN)) was more commonly found in patients receiving LdT than LVD (7.5% vs. 3.1%) (Leung, 2008; Y F Liaw et al., 2008). However, it improved spontaneously with continued drug therapy. Cases of reversible myopathy and peripheral neuropathy have been reported (Leung, 2008; Y F Liaw et al., 2008; A S Lok & McMahon, 2009). Although LdT is more potent than LVD, its high resistance rate and cost limit its use as the first line treatment for CHB (Keeffe et al., 2008; Leung, 2008; Y F Liaw et al., 2008; Zoulim & Perrillo, 2008).

Tenofovir (TDF) is an oral anti-viral drug and has been approved for the treatment of CHB in 2008 (Ayoub & Keeffe, 2008; A S Lok & McMahon, 2009). It belongs to the same family of nucleotide analogs as ADV (Ayoub & Keeffe, 2008; Keeffe et al., 2008; A S Lok & McMahon, 2009; Zoulim & Perrillo, 2008). It has been shown to be more potent than ADV particularly in early suppression of HBV (Ayoub & Keeffe, 2008; Keeffe et al., 2008; Lai & Yuen, 2008; Leung, 2008; Marcellin et al., 2008). In a phase III clinical trial in HBeAg positive patients, TDF resulted in a significantly higher percentage of patients with undetectable HBV DNA levels compared with ADV (76% vs. 13%) after 48 weeks (Ayoub & Keeffe, 2008; Y F Liaw et al., 2008; Marcellin et al., 2008). No resistance mutations associated with TDF were found at week 48 and 72 (Ayoub & Keeffe, 2008; Keeffe et al., 2008; Lai & Yuen, 2008; Leung, 2008). The incidence of adverse events was similar in TDF and ADV (Ayoub & Keeffe, 2008; Keeffe et al., 2008). The incidence of ALT flares (>2 times baseline values) was higher in patients receiving TDF than those with ADV (11% vs. 4%) (Keeffe et al., 2008). Studies are still ongoing for long-term efficacy and safety.

### 2.2.3 Screening for HCC

As defined in the published guideline (Bruix, Sherman, & Practice Guidelines Committee, 2005), "screening refers to an application of diagnostic tests in patients at risk for HCC, but in whom there is no prior reason to suspect that HCC is present". It states clearly that screening is to detect the presence of HCC among the asymptomatic hepatitis B carriers. The ultimate goal of screening for HCC is to reduce morbidity and mortality (Bruix et al., 2005; Ying, 2009; Yuen & Lai, 2003). That means to detect early preclinical and early HCC that can be cured (resection).

Screening for disease should fulfill certain criteria to be medically and economically acceptable. Wilson's criteria are widely used to judge whether a disease should be screened for and they are shown as follows (Wilson & Jungner, 1968):-

i. The condition sought should be an important health problem;
ii. There should be an accepted treatment for patients with the recognized disease;
iii. Facilities for diagnosis and treatment should be available;
iv. There should be a latent or early symptomatic stage;
v. There should be a suitable test or examination;
vi. The test should be acceptable to the population;
vii. The natural history of the condition should be adequately understood;
viii. There should be an agreed policy on whom to treat as patients;
ix. The cost of case-finding (including diagnosis and treatment of patients diagnosed) should be economically balanced in relation to possible expenditure on medical care as a whole;
x. Case-finding should be a continuing process and not a once and for all project.

Although there are several published guidelines for HCC screening, there is no consensus regarding screening for HCC (Bruix et al., 2005; Keeffe et al., 2008; Y F Liaw et al., 2008; A S Lok & McMahon, 2009; Omata et al., 2010). A recent AASLD practice guideline has been published and recommended that HBV carriers at high risk should be screened with ultrasound (US) every 6-12 months and alpha-fetoprotein (AFP) alone if US is not available (A S Lok & McMahon, 2009). Ultrasound and AFP are currently two commonly used screening tests for HCC (A S Lok & McMahon, 2009). High risk group is defined as Asian men aged >40 years old, Asian women aged >50 years old, those with cirrhosis or family history of severe liver disease, with persistent or intermittent ALT elevation and/or high HBV DNA level >2000 IU/mL (A S Lok & McMahon, 2009). On the other hand, the latest Asia-Pacific consensus suggested that only male HBV carriers aged 40 or above with cirrhosis or family history of serious liver disease should be screened with US and AFP every 3-6 months (Y F Liaw et al., 2008). In general, HCC screening should be considered for patients with cirrhosis. However, it remains unclear whether screening for HCC in an asymptomatic population has beneficial outcomes, what is the best screening strategy and whether screening is cost-effective.

### 2.2.4 Health services for CHB in Hong Kong

The Hong Kong Government provides healthcare service to patients with HBV infection, but resources are limited and management has to be prioritized according to the severity of the illness. For patients found to be CHB carriers, the frequency of monitoring and types of laboratory tests differed by the severity of their diseases.

In Hong Kong, lamivudine (LVD), adefovir (ADV) and entecavir (ETV) are the standard antiviral drugs used for the treatment of CHB (Fung et al., 2008). Interferons are of doubtful use for Chinese patients (Fung et al., 2008). Telbivudine (LdT) is seldom used because of its cost and high resistance rate (Fung et al., 2008; Zoulim & Perrillo, 2008). The long-term effect of tenofovir (TDF) is unknown (Keeffe et al., 2008; Lai & Yuen, 2008; Y F Liaw et al., 2008).

Anti-viral drugs are expensive and the government provides subsidy for patients with cirrhosis and HCC only in public service. Most CHB patients with impaired liver function (ILF) need to pay for their full drug cost and HBV DNA assay. The costs of anti-viral treatment range from HKD 1,000 to HKD 3,000 per month depending on the drug choice (Yeo B, 2008). Patients' willingness to pay may influence treatment options which also affects the duration of treatment, effectiveness, drug resistance and side effects. Many patients cannot afford or are not willing to pay for treatment even though it is recommended by physicians. There is no policy on hepatitis B screening (Hong Kong (China). Dept. of Health., 1998), which is not routinely provided by the public service.

Free printed information on hepatitis is available from the Department of Health to educate the public about the prevention of spread of the disease, indication for treatment and treatment options (Department of Health). Primary care doctors or specialists can easily distribute these printed information to their patients during the consultation but this not often done because time is limited and the evaluation of disease pathology and its complication take top priority.

a. Management of Asymptomatic Hepatitis B (AHB) carriers

Most infected individuals are asymptomatic and CHB is usually diagnosed incidentally during blood donation, health assessment or when they develop liver complications such as cirrhosis or HCC. Asymptomatic hepatitis B (AHB) carriers may be followed-up yearly at General Outpatient Clinic (GOPC) or private primary care doctors with liver function test (LFT) and alpha fetoprotein (AFP) but many are not. According to a local study in a primary care setting, most of HBV carriers did not attend GOPC for following up of their disease (Kung, Lam, & Li, 2004). Furthermore, there were large variations in follow-up period and test intervals (Kung et al., 2004). It ranges from 1 to 14 months for follow-up, 2 to 36 for blood tests, and 6 to 60 months for ultrasound (Kung et al., 2004). One month follow-up may be given to those who were very anxious about their condition (Kung et al., 2004). Since they are asymptomatic population, they do not need to take anti-viral treatment unless liver-related complications developed (European Association For the study of the liver, 2008; Keeffe et al., 2008; Y F Liaw et al., 2008; A S Lok & McMahon, 2009). Both HCC screening and HBV DNA assay are not available for AHB carriers. AHB carriers are at risk of developing cirrhosis or HCC but screening is rarely done for these patients (Yuen et al., 2005).

b. Management of patients with Impaired Liver Function (ILF)

Patients with ILF usually have close monitoring and follow-up at Specialist Outpatient Clinics (SOPC) with LFT and AFP tests regularly. The frequency of follow-up contact may vary. It is determined by a combination of variables: results of LFT, degree of viral replication, and need of anti-viral drug. Patients with ILF who receive drug treatment often need to pay for their drug costs and HBV DNA assay. Screening for HCC is not available for patients with ILF.

c. Management of patients with cirrhosis or HCC

Patients with cirrhosis or HCC have close monitoring and follow-up at Specialist Outpatient Clinics (SOPC) with LFT and AFP tests regularly. Patients may receive anti-viral drug free of charge. Screening for HCC and HBV DNA assay are available for patients with cirrhosis.

Clinical guidelines have been established to provide guidance to healthcare providers and physicians for diagnosis and management of CHB infection to reduce the development of complications (Keeffe et al., 2008; Y F Liaw et al., 2008; A S Lok & McMahon, 2009). However, the following issues remain unresolved. Firstly, not the majority of infected individuals are identified. Secondly, many CHB patients do not receive adequate management and follow-up, in particular, for those who initially do not consider anti-viral drug treatment. Despite numerous studies on the epidemiology, natural history and management of CHB, little has been done on the gap in healthcare services and patients' willingness to pay for their CHB treatment. Understanding patients' perceived needs can help to make service more patient-centered and improve the quality of life to CHB patients.

### 2.2.5 HRQOL and service utilization

Studies have shown a significant inverse relationship between HRQOL and service utilization in Western population (Dominick & Ahern, 2004; Ethgen & Kahler, 2002; Nelson & McHorney, 1998; Parkerson & Gutman, 2000; Singh & Nelson, 2005). Nelson et al found that physical functioning and mental health were important indicators of both outpatient visits and hospitalization for patients with chronic disease after controlling for confounding variables (Nelson 1998). Another study by Mulunpalo et al showed that a significant linear relationship between HRQOL and outpatient physician visits for working-age population in Finland (Mulunpalo 1997). Furthermore, Dominick et al pointed out that HRQOL can be valuable tools for predicting future health care for older patients with osteoarthritis (Dominick 2004). Poorer general health was correlated with increased likelihood of analgesic or anti-inflammatory use (Dominick 2004). Poor mental health was associated with increased likelihood of analgesic or anti-inflammatory use (Dominick 2004).

There were several studies on the association between HRQOL and service utilization for Asian population (T. Chen & Li, 2009; C. L. K. Lam & Fong, 2002; Matsumura, 2000). A study by Matsumura in Japan found that subjects with Short Form-36 (SF-36) physical component summary (PCS) score below 40 were more likely to use outpatient services and to be hospitalized than those who had scores greater than 50 (Matsumura 2000). Subjects with both SF-36 physical and mental component summary scores below 40 were more likely to have taken sick leave than those who had scores greater than 50 (Matsumura, 2000). A large study in Hong Kong showed that a linear relationship between HRQOL and service utilization in the local Chinese population (C. L. K. Lam & Fong, 2002). Five out of eight SF-36 scores were independent determinants of consultation rates (C. L. K. Lam & Fong, 2002). Role limitation due to physical problem and bodily pain were associated with hospitalization (C. L. K. Lam & Fong, 2002).

A recent study assessing the effect of HRQOL on service utilization was conducted in 737 primary care patients in Mainland China (Chen 20009). Lower HRQOL scores were correlated with higher service utilization rates (Chen 20009). Three out of eight SF-36 scales were associated with both inpatient and outpatient consultation (Chen 20009).

Numerous studies reported on the relationship between HRQOL and service utilization for Western and Asian populations (T. Chen & Li, 2009; Dominick & Ahern, 2004; Ethgen & Kahler, 2002; C. L. K. Lam & Fong, 2002; Matsumura, 2000; Nelson & McHorney, 1998; Parkerson & Gutman, 2000; Singh & Nelson, 2005), but no data were available for CHB patients. More studies are needed to explore the effect of HRQOL on service utilization in patients with CHB.

### 2.3 Health-related Quality of Life (HRQOL) as a health outcome measure for Chronic Hepatitis B (CHB) patients

The goal of healthcare is to maintain, restore and improve health of patients. Traditionally, clinicians have focused primarily on 'hard' clinical outcomes, for instance, patient's mortality and morbidity (Eisen, Locke, & Provenzale, 1999). Clinicians are more likely to judge the effectiveness or efficacy of a therapy in terms of survival rate, biochemical parameters such as liver function, viral markers, and symptoms (Eisen et al., 1999). Traditional clinical outcomes (i.e. morbidity and mortality) are important but they do not adequately reflect patients' perceived health, feelings and the impact of illness on life. Health-related quality of life (HRQOL) can provide additional information on the effectiveness and quality of care.

Chronic hepatitis B (CHB) is a chronic debilitating condition that can lead to progressive impairment of physical and mental health as the disease progresses. Improvements in medical and surgical therapies in liver diseases have led to more people living with CHB. HRQOL should be considered an important outcome measures for assessing the impact of CHB and the effectiveness of treatment. The expansion from traditional clinical outcomes to include HRQOL outcomes will enable us to measure modern health care more sensitively (Younossi, 2001). HRQOL is more sensitive in capturing the effect of illness and interventions for those with uncomplicated disease (Bondini et al., 2007; Levy et al., 2008; Nokhodian, Ataei, Kassaian, Adibi, & Farajzadegan, 2009; S C Ong et al., 2008; Tan, Cheah, Teo, & Yang, 2008; Yi, 2006). Furthermore, HRQOL provides additional information for the prioritization of needs among patients with similar clinical severity defined by traditional clinical outcomes. The effect of an intervention on HRQOL has become a very important topic for both consumers and providers of health services (R. C. Martin, Eid, Scoggins, & McMasters, 2007; Poon et al., 2001; Yi, 2006).

The applications of HRQOL measures can be categorized as evaluative, discriminative and predictive (Preedy, Watson, & Lam, 2010; Yacavone, Locke, Provenzale, & Eisen, 2001). Evaluative measures are the most widely used in different populations or patients groups (Preedy et al., 2010). It is used to assess the impact of an illness, effectiveness or side effect of treatment, and quality of healthcare delivery (Preedy et al., 2010; Yacavone et al., 2001). Discriminative measures can be used to differentiate between groups in terms of HRQOL (Preedy et al., 2010; Yacavone et al., 2001). Predictive measures are used to identify people who are at risk or predict service needs for different populations or patient groups (Preedy et al., 2010). HRQOL measures can apply in economic evaluation in relation to treatment (Kanwal et al., 2005; Sun, Qin, Li, & Jiang, 2007; Takeda, Jones, Shepherd, Davidson, & Price, 2007; Veenstra, Spackman, Bisceglie, Kowdley, & Gish, 2008; Yuan, Iloeje, Li, Hay, & Yao, 2008).

The World Health Organization (WHO) states that 'health is a state of complete physical, mental and social well-being' (WHO, 1947). Well-being is the subjective perception of an individual's state of living, which has a similar concept as quality of life. It is noted that health is only one of many determinants of a person's quality of life, others include social environment, economy, religion etc. In the context of health services, the focus is on health-related quality of life (HRQOL) in an attempt to quantify the net consequence of a disease and its treatment on the patient's perception of his/her ability to live a useful and fulfilling life (Schipper, Clinch, & Olweny, 1996).

In the last few decades, there has been an increasing interest in the evaluation of HRQOL in patient groups, including those with chronic liver disease (Foster, Goldin, & Thomas, 1998; J. J. Gutteling, de Man, Busschbach, & Darlington, 2007; Younossi, 2001). The number of articles in gastroenterology on quality of life (QOL) or HRQOL has increased significantly in recent decades (Foster et al., 1998; L. M. Martin et al., 2006; L. M. Martin, Sheridan, & Younossi, 2002; L. M. Martin & Younossi, 2005; Younossi et al., 2001; Younossi, Kiwi, Boparai, Price, & Guyatt, 2000). HRQOL has become standard outcome measure in patients with chronic liver diseases in western countries especially in patients with chronic hepatitis C (CHC) (Chong et al., 2003; Foster, 1999; Foster et al., 1998; Kwan et al., 2008; Spiegel et al., 2005). It should also become an important outcome measure in CHB patients.

### 2.3.1 Impact of CHB on HRQOL

Although numerous studies have shown significant lower health-related quality of life (HRQOL) scores in patients with chronic liver diseases (CLD), there is relatively little attention on the impact of HRQOL in patients with hepatitis B virus (HBV) because most data come from western populations where CHB is uncommon (J. J. Gutteling et al., 2007; L. M. Martin et al., 2002). In general, studies showed a significant decline in HRQOL in patients with hepatitis C virus (HCV) (Foster et al., 1998; Heitkemper, Jarrett, Kurashige, & Carithers, 2001; Koff, 1999; Kwan et al., 2008; Miller, Hiller, & Shaw, 2001; Spiegel et al., 2005; Strauss & Dias Teixeira, 2006). Only a few papers explored the effect of CHB on HRQOL (Bondini et al., 2007; Levy et al., 2008; Nokhodian et al., 2009; S C Ong et al., 2008; Tan et al., 2008). The first paper on HRQOL of CHB was published by Foster et al in 1998, which evaluated the impact of chronic hepatitis C (CHC) and CHB by a generic measure of HRQOL, the Medical Outcomes Study Short Form-36 (SF-36) Health Survey (Foster et al., 1998). Patients with CHB had significant lower HRQOL scores in mental health and general health perception aspects, but their physical related HRQOL scores were comparable to the healthy control (Foster et al., 1998). The results indicated patients with CHB infection did not have significant lower scores in physical functions but the results were limited by a very small sample of CHB patients (Foster et al., 1998).

Studies with a larger sample size and patients with different stages of CHB are needed in order to provide more precise measures of HRQOL. One study found that CHB patients had similar HRQOL scores to the healthy control group, as measured by both generic (Short Form-36 Health Survey, SF-36) and disease-specific (Chronic Liver Disease Questionnaire, CLDQ) questionnaires (Bondini et al., 2007). CHB patients had lower HRQOL scores in only two (fatigue and worry) out of six CLDQ scales and two (physical functioning and vitality) out of eight SF-36 scales compared to the norm (Bondini et al., 2007). However, health preference values (utility) of CHB patients were lower than the population norm (Bondini et al., 2007).

Recently, two large studies showed that CHB infection had a negative impact on HRQOL (Levy et al., 2008; S C Ong et al., 2008). Asymptomatic hepatitis B (AHB) carriers, CHB patients with impaired liver function (ILF), and compensated cirrhosis (CC) patients had a small to moderate but significant effect on HRQOL, and decompensated cirrhosis (DC) and hepatocellular carcinoma (HCC) patients had the lowest HRQOL scores (S C Ong et al., 2008). Ong et al demonstrated that HRQOL measured by the generic HRQOL measures, the SF-36 Health Survey and EQ-5D, in Chinese AHB carriers was comparable to healthy controls, although those with ILF and CC patients showed a significant reduction in general health and mental health dimensions (S C Ong et al., 2008). Patients with more advanced stages of CHB (DC and HCC) had the lowest HRQOL scores in all dimensions (S C Ong et al., 2008). The results indicated deterioration in physical health while the disease progresses (S C Ong et al., 2008).

Another study by Tan et al showed that hepatitis B carriers in Singapore had good physical and mental health measured by both generic (SF-36 Health Survey) and disease-specific (Hepatitis Quality of Life Questionnaire) HRQOL measures (Tan et al., 2008). There was no significant difference in HRQOL between the 108 hepatitis B carriers in the study and general population, except in social functioning (Tan et al., 2008).

A recent study assessing HRQOL in patients with CHB infection was conducted using a disease-specific HRQOL measure (Chronic Liver Disease Questionnaire) in Iran (Nokhodian et al., 2009). A sample of 61 patients with CHB infection and 60 age and sex-matched healthy control were recruited in this study (Nokhodian et al., 2009). Patients had lower (worse) scores in three out of six CLDQ scales, including fatigue, abdominal and systemic symptoms, as compared to controls (Nokhodian et al., 2009). Surprisingly, CHB patients had a higher score on the worry scale, i.e. less worry, than the control groups (Nokhodian et al., 2009).

Findings from a multi-country study on health preference values found that health states related to CHB infection had significant reduction in HRQOL (Levy et al., 2008). Health preference is a composite HRQOL value that ranges from 0 (death) to 1 (perfect health), with higher scores implying better HRQOL (Brazier, Roberts, & Deverill, 2002). Patients with ILF and CC had a moderate impact on HRQOL with health preference values ranging from 0.68 to 0.80 (Levy et al., 2008). On the other hand, patients with DC or HCC had a stronger impact with health preference values ranging from 0.35 to 0.41 (Levy et al., 2008). Variation in health preference values was found between countries with lower health preference values found in Hong Kong and Mainland China than countries (Levy et al., 2008).

These studies provided some evidence on the negative HRQOL impact of CHB but they are limited by small sample size, inconsistent results and a lack of differentiation between CHB patient types (Bondini et al., 2007; Foster et al., 1998; S C Ong et al., 2008; Tan et al., 2008). Although studies have reported that HCC or cirrhosis patients had poorer overall HRQOL scores compared with the general population (Chong et al., 2003; A. A. Dan et al., 2008; S C Ong et al., 2008), it is still unclear whether patients with asymptomatic, CHB infection with or without ILF have poorer HRQOL than the general population, and whether any significant difference in HRQOL was found among different CHB groups.

An analytic investigation on factors affecting HRQOL enables better targeting of management. Previous studies suggested that biochemical markers, socio-demographic and psychosocial factors did affect HRQOL in patients with CLD but it has not been fully examined in Chinese CHB patients (Afendy et al., 2009; Bianchi et al., 2003; J J Gutteling et al., 2006; Hauser, Schnur, Steder-Neukamm, Muthny, & Grandt, 2004; Hussain et al., 2001; Marchesini et al., 2001; Sobhonslidsuk et al., 2006; Sumskiene, Sumskas, Petrauskas, & Kupcinskas, 2006; Younossi et al., 2001; Younossi et al., 2000). Disease severity, as measured by Child-Pugh scores or stage of CHB illness (asymptomatic, impaired liver function, cirrhosis and HCC), was one of the commonest factors that had a negative relationship with HRQOL (Bianchi et al., 2003; J J Gutteling et al., 2006; Marchesini et al., 2001; Sobhonslidsuk et al., 2006; Sumskiene et al., 2006; Younossi et al., 2001; Younossi et al., 2000). However, some studies did not find any significant effect between HRQOL and disease severity (Hauser, Holtmann, & Grandt, 2004; Hauser, Zimmer, Schiedermaier, & Grandt, 2004). One large cross-sectional study in Singapore found that disease severity was an important determinant of HRQOL of Chinese patients with CHB, controlling for demographic characteristics (S C Ong et al., 2008). Unfortunately, this study did not include some important clinical and co-morbidity variables in regression model, for instance, duration of illness and chronic co-morbidity (S C Ong et al., 2008).

One study examining the impact of liver cirrhosis found that the presence of cirrhosis was associated with lower HRQOL scores (Bondini et al., 2007). But Dan et al did not find any significant relationship between presence of cirrhosis and HRQOL (A. A. Dan et al., 2008). These two studies only included a small number of patients with CHB infection (Bondini et al., 2007; A. A. Dan et al., 2008). More studies are needed to confirm the relationship between the severity of liver disease and HRQOL in patients with CHB infection.

Liver biomarkers, such as alanine transaminase (ALT), was not found to have any significant association with HRQOL (Bondini et al., 2007; Hussain et al., 2001; Miller et al., 2001), though it is an important clinical markers to assess the severity of liver and determine indication for treatment (Fung et al., 2008; Keeffe et al., 2008; Y F Liaw et al., 2008; A S Lok & McMahon, 2009; McMahon, 2006). However, Kondo et al found an association between HRQOL and serum albumin (Kondo et al., 2007), which is a marker of severity of liver disease.

Physical symptoms, for instance, joint pain, muscle cramps, itching and abdominal pain, were also correlated with HRQOL (J. J. Gutteling et al., 2007; Marchesini et al., 2001; Younossi, 2001). Fatigue was also a concern for patients with chronic liver disease (J. J. Gutteling et al., 2007; J J Gutteling et al., 2006).

Anti-viral treatment may improve patients' HRQOL (Bernstein, Kleinman, Barker, Revicki, & Green, 2002; S. C. Chang, Ko, Wu, Peng, & Yang, 2008; Kang, Hwang, Lee, Chang, & Lee, 2005; McHutchison et al., 2001; Perrillo et al., 2004; Ware, Bayliss, Mannocchia, & Davis, 1999), but side effects can be a problem (Fung et al., 2008; Keeffe et al., 2008; Y F Liaw et al., 2008; A S Lok & McMahon, 2009). Foster et al showed that patients with HCV receiving anti-viral treatment of 6-12 months had decreased HRQOL because of side effects (Foster, 1999). Other studies demonstrated a sustained response to treatment was associated with improved HRQOL in patients with HCV infection (Bernstein et al., 2002; S. C. Chang et al., 2008; Kang et al., 2005; McHutchison et al., 2001; Perrillo et al., 2004; Ware et al., 1999). Studies are needed to confirm the effect of anti-viral treatment on HRQOL.

Socio-demographic factors also play an important role in HRQOL, including age, gender, education levels, marital status and socio-economic status (J. J. Gutteling et al., 2007; L. M. Martin et al., 2002). Previous studies found a significant effect of age and gender on HRQOL in patients with chronic liver disease, including patients with CHC and CHB (J. J. Gutteling et al., 2007; L. M. Martin et al., 2002). Older age was associated with lower HRQOL in patients with chronic liver disease (Afendy et al., 2009; J J Gutteling et al., 2006; Kondo et al., 2007; Sobhonslidsuk et al., 2006; Younossi et al., 2001), but insignificant or positive effect on physical or mental HRQOL (Bianchi et al., 2003; Bondini et al., 2007; A. A. Dan et al., 2008; Hauser, Holtmann, et al., 2004; Hauser, Zimmer, et al., 2004; Hussain et al., 2001; Sumskiene et al., 2006). Consistently, females were more likely to have poorer HRQOL than males (Afendy et al., 2009; Bianchi et al., 2003; A. A. Dan et al., 2008; J J Gutteling et al., 2006; Hussain et al., 2001; Sobhonslidsuk et al., 2006). This pattern is found on the general population as well as patients with CLD (C. L. Lam, Lauder, Lam, & Gandek, 1999; E. T. Lam, Lam, Lo, & Grandek, 2008). Very few data have demonstrated the effect of other socio-demographic factors (Hauser, Holtmann, et al., 2004; Hussain et al., 2001; Sobhonslidsuk et al., 2006), such as education level, marital status and social class/ socio-economic status. Studies showed that level of education was positively correlated with HRQOL (Hussain et al., 2001; Sobhonslidsuk et al., 2006). Data from Hussain et al found there was weak correlation between level of education and physical HRQOL (Hussain et al., 2001). On the other hand, another study proved that patients with lower education level had significant lower mental HRQOL scores (Sobhonslidsuk et al., 2006).

Chronic co-morbidity also affected HRQOL in patients with chronic liver disease (Hauser, Holtmann, et al., 2004; Hauser, Zimmer, et al., 2004; Hussain et al., 2001). Hauser et al examined 94 patients with CHC attending a liver clinic and showed that psychiatric co-morbidities was one of important determinant of mental component summary (MCS) score of SF-36 (Hauser, Zimmer, et al., 2004). The number of active co-morbidities was associated with the SF-36 physical component summary (PCS) score (Hauser, Zimmer, et al., 2004).

### 2.3.2 HRQOL measures applicable to CHB

Health-related quality of life (HRQOL) can be measured by generic and disease specific measures (M.S. Bayliss, 1999; Brown, 1999; Eisen et al., 1999; J. J. Gutteling et al., 2007; Yacavone et al., 2001; Younossi, 2001; Younossi & Guyatt, 1998). Generic HRQOL measures can be applied to different patient populations (M.S. Bayliss, 1999; Eisen et al., 1999; J. J. Gutteling et al., 2007; Yacavone et al., 2001; Younossi, 2001; Younossi & Guyatt, 1998). The advantage of using this instrument is that it can compare with other types of diseases or healthy control population (M.S. Bayliss, 1999; Eisen et al., 1999; J. J. Gutteling et al., 2007; Yacavone et al., 2001; Younossi, 2001; Younossi & Guyatt, 1998). Therefore, it is widely used in health services and comparative studies. However, generic measures may not detect small but important clinical changes specific to a particular patient group. The Medical Outcomes Study Short Form-36 (SF-36) is the most commonly used (J. J. Gutteling et al., 2007; Yacavone et al., 2001; Younossi, 2001; Younossi & Guyatt, 1998). It showed in a study by Foster et al. that CHB patients had significant lower HRQOL scores in mental health and general health perception aspects, but their physical related HRQOL scores were comparable to the healthy control (Foster et al., 1998). Previous studies on the use of SF-36 on CHB patients have demonstrated that patients with less severe disease had lower HRQOL scores in general health compared to those with general population or healthy controls (Bondini et al., 2007; Foster et al., 1998; S C Ong et al., 2008; Tan et al., 2008). Once they developed complications, lower HRQOL scores was found in both physical and mental health (S C Ong et al., 2008). The effectiveness of anti-viral treatment was detected by the SF-36 in a longitudinal study on 150 Chinese CHB patients at different stages of illness receiving LVD treatment (Yi, 2006).

A disease-specific measure theoretically can detect small but clinically important changes on HRQOL that are unique to the particular condition although it does not allow for comparison with the general population or other disease groups (M.S. Bayliss, 1999; Eisen et al., 1999; Younossi, 2001; J. J. Gutteling et al., 2007; Yacavone et al., 2001). Several HRQOL measures specific for chronic liver disease patients, such as the Chronic Liver Disease Questionnaire (CLDQ) (Younossi, Guyatt, Kiwi, Boparai, & King, 1999), the Hepatitis Quality of Life Questionnaire (HQLQ) (M. S. Bayliss et al., 1998), the Liver Disease Quality of Life Questionnaire (LDQOL) (Gralnek et al., 2000), the Liver Disease Symptom Index (LDSI 1.0 and 2.0) (Unal et al., 2001; van der Plas et al., 2004), the Hepatitis B Quality of Life (HBQOL) (Spiegel et al., 2007) and Chronic Liver Disease-Specific Quality of Life (CLD-QOL) (Lee et al., 2007) are available. Each instrument has its advantages and disadvantages. Table 1 presents the characteristics of these disease-specific HRQOL measures.

| | HQLQ | CLDQ | LDQOL | HBQOL | CLD-QOL |
|---|---|---|---|---|---|
| Author | Bayliss et al | Younossi et al | Granlnek et al | Spiegel et al | Lee et al |
| Year | 1998 | 1999 | 2000 | 2007 | 2007 |
| Country | USA | USA | USA | USA | Korea |
| # of items | 69 | 29 | 111 | 31 | 27 |
| # of scales | 13 | 6 | 20 | 6 | 5 |
| Total score | No | Yes | Yes | Yes | No |
| Scales | 8 scales from SF-36 | Fatigue | 8 scales from SF-36 | Psychological well-being | Specific symptoms |
| | Positive well-being | Activity | Symptoms of LD | Anticipation anxiety | Social function |
| | Sleep somnolence | Emotional function | Effects of LD | Vitality | Emotional status |
| | Health distress | Abdominal | Concentration | Stigmatization | General |
| | Limitations | Systemic | Memory | Vulnerability | Uncertain |
| | Health distress | Worry | Quality of social | Transmission | |
| | | | Health distress | | |
| | | | Sleep | | |
| | | | Loneliness | | |
| | | | Hopelessness | | |
| | | | Stigma of LD | | |
| | | | Sexual | | |

Table 1. Characteristics of Disease-specific HRQOL Measures

The Chronic Liver Disease Questionnaire (CLDQ) is the first disease-specific HRQOL measure for evaluating patients with chronic liver disease (CLD) developed by Younossi et al (Younossi et al., 1999). The CLDQ has 29 items generated by patients with chronic liver disease, hepatologists, and a review of literature (Younossi et al., 1999). The CLDQ has six scales measuring fatigue, activity, emotional function, abdominal symptoms, systemic symptoms and worry (Younossi et al., 1999), which captures the important problems associated with CHB infection and its complications. It is scored with six domain and one summary scores (Younossi et al., 1999). This short measure can be completed in less than 15 minutes, a criterion for assuring a good response rate (Cella & Tulsky, 1990; McColl,

Christiansen, & Konig-Zahn, 1997). Patients with different types and stages of liver disease were included in the development and validation process supporting its broad application in hepatology research (Younossi et al., 1999). It has been shown to have adequate internal reliability, validity and sensitivity (Younossi et al., 1999). The CLDQ has been shown to be suitable for cross-cultural adaptation to different cultures (Ferrer et al., 2006; Hauser, Schnur, et al., 2004; Rucci et al., 2005; Sobhonslidsuk, Silpakit, Kongsakon, Satitpornkul, & Sripetch, 2004; Wu, Deng, Ji, & Yan, 2003) including Italian, German, Chinese (Mainland) and Thai. Recently, it has also been translated into Portuguese and Bengali (Mucci, Citero Vde, Gonzalez, De Marco, & Nogueira-Martins, 2010; Ray, Dutta, Basu, & De, 2010). However, the responsiveness of the CLDQ has not been investigated widely. Further research is needed to demonstrate its ability to detect change over time or with intervention.

The other liver disease specific HRQOL measures are less widely used because they are either much longer or have relatively few data supporting their validity or sensitivity. The HQLQ developed by Bayliss has 69 items combining the generic SF-36 scales with three additional generic scales (positive well-being, sleep and health distress) and two hepatitis C specific scales (health distress and limitations because of hepatitis C ) and was intended for patients with chronic hepatitis C (CHC) infection (M. S. Bayliss et al., 1998). It has been shown to be sensitive in patients with CHC but data on patients with CHB infection are few (M. S. Bayliss et al., 1998). The instrument was recently translated and validated in patients with CHB in Singapore (S. C. Ong, Lim, & Li, 2009, 2010). The main disadvantage of the HQLQ is many liver disease specific symptoms, such as abdominal pain, are not addressed despite its length (M. S. Bayliss et al., 1998). Furthermore, significant ceiling effects of three scales were observed (M. S. Bayliss et al., 1998), and the instrument's responsiveness remains unknown (S. C. Ong et al., 2009, 2010).

The Liver Disease Quality of Life instrument (LDQOL) was developed by Gralnek et al consisting of generic and disease-specific scales with a total of 101 items (Gralnek et al., 2000). It is not very widely used because its length limits its acceptability. It is applicable mainly to patients with advanced liver disease or waiting for liver transplantation (Casanovas et al., 2003; Dias Teixeira, de Fatima Gomes de Sa Ribeiro, & Strauss, 2005). In other words, it was not designed for patients with less severe liver disease. The LDQOL has been translated and adapted into Spanish and Catalan in transplant patients as well as Brazilian Portuguese in patients with chronic liver disease (Casanovas et al., 2003; Dias Teixeira et al., 2005). Pilot testing has supported the reliability and validity of the LDQOL but it has not been tested in longitudinal studies (Dias Teixeira et al., 2005; Gralnek et al., 2000). Recently, a short form (36 items) of the liver disease quality of life instrument (SF-LDQOL) was validated on patients with advanced liver disease (Kanwal et al., 2008). However, its validity may not be generalizable to patients with asymptomatic hepatitis B or an early stage of liver disease (Kanwal et al., 2008).

The Liver Disease Symptom Index (LDSI) is a short instrument that consists of 18 items that measure nine disease-specific symptoms and the hindrance that patients experience from these symptoms (Unal et al., 2001; van der Plas et al., 2004). It has been validated on 374 patients but the data on its validity and other psychometric properties on CHB patients are limited (Unal et al., 2001).

The Hepatitis B Quality of Life instrument (HBQOL) is the first HRQOL measures designed for specifically hepatitis B patients without cirrhosis (Spiegel et al., 2007). It is a 31 items questionnaire including items assessing psychological well-being, anticipation anxiety, vitality, disease stigma, vulnerability, and transmissibility (Spiegel et al., 2007). It has shown to be valid and reliable in English-speaking patients in the United States (Spiegel et al., 2007). The validity and applicability of this instrument on CHB patients with complications and other cultures are not known.

The Chronic Liver Disease-Quality of Life questionnaire (CLD-QOL) was designed to measure HRQOL of Asian patients with chronic liver disease, the first of its kind (Lee et al., 2007). There are 27 items which are organized into the domains of specific symptoms, social function, emotional status, general symptoms and uncertain future (Lee et al., 2007). Lee et al found a significant difference in HRQOL scores between patients with mild stage of cirrhosis and moderate to severe stage of cirrhosis, supporting construct validity of CLD-QOL (Lee et al., 2007). Further evaluation on its psychometric properties on patients without cirrhosis is needed before the instrument can be applied more widely.

### 2.3.3 Preference-based measure (utility) of HRQOL

Cost-effectiveness analysis (CEA) is an area of increasing interest among researchers, physicians and policy makers (Sun et al., 2007). CEA is a method of summarizing the health benefits and resources used by health programmes, therefore policy makers can select among them (Russell, Gold, Siegel, Daniels, & Weinstein, 1996; Weinstein, 1990; Weinstein, Siegel, Gold, Kamlet, & Russell, 1996). It summarizes all programme costs and benefits (effectiveness), and uses economic theory to aid choice between competing health programmes when resources are scarce (Russell et al., 1996; Weinstein, 1990; Weinstein et al., 1996). CEA can express health benefits in more generic terms, such as quality adjusted life years (QALYs) gained (Weinstein, 1990). It provides a common unit to allow comparisons between different disease groups or intervention programmes (Weinstein, Torrance, & McGuire, 2009). This method is particularly useful in the analysis of preventive health programmes, such as anti-viral treatment in CHB patients (Kanwal et al., 2005; Sullivan et al., 2007; Sun et al., 2007; Yuan et al., 2008).

Most HRQOL measures give a profile of domain scores that are not designed for economic evaluation. Treatment evaluation by profile scores may give inconsistent results and lead to a piecemeal understanding of the impact of an intervention because of variations in the effect on different domains. For example, one scale indicates a beneficial effect whereas other scales may give negative results. Therefore, there is a need for methods to combine multidimensional information in more systematic ways. Research has shown that multi-dimensional HRQOL states can be converted to a composite preference value expressed on a numerical scale ranging from 0 (death) to 1 (perfect health) (Brazier et al., 2002), based on preference valuation by subjects from the general population (Guide to the methods of technology appraisal). It is possible to have negative preference for states that are worse than being dead (Preedy et al., 2010).

An important application of preference based measures is a measure of effectiveness in health economic evaluation (Preedy et al., 2010). Quality adjusted life year (QALY) is increasingly used as a measure of health outcomes in the past 20 years (Neumann, Greenberg, Olchanski, Stone, & Rosen, 2005). QALYs give a single index combining morbidity and mortality and is easy to calculate if the preference of health status is known

(Weinstein et al., 2009). It provides a common metric to compare with different treatment options with the other, to compare treatment side-effects versus benefit, or to compare intervention programs with another one (Preedy et al., 2010; Weinstein et al., 2009). QALYs have been applied to different diseases or intervention programs, for instance, treatment of coronary heart disease and screening for breast cancer (Chan, Nallamothu, Gurm, Hayward, & Vijan, 2007; Wong, Kuntz, Cowling, Lam, & Leung, 2007). Information on the preference values of different CHB states can be combined with life years gain in the evaluation of the cost-effectiveness of different anti-viral treatment strategies for CHB (Kanwal et al., 2005; Sullivan et al., 2007; Veenstra et al., 2008; Yuan et al., 2008).

Three most commonly used preference based measures of health are the Short Form-6D (SF-6D), the Health Utilities Index (HUI) and the EuroQol EQ-5D (Brazier et al., 2002; Brooks, 1996; Feeny, Furlong, Boyle, & Torrance, 1995). They are most useful for the evaluation of the cost-effectiveness of anti-viral treatment for CHB. Table 2 summarizes the domains of the commonly used generic HRQOL measures including the SF-6D, HUI and EQ-5D. They may give different results and interpretations because of different dimensions and methods of preference valuation. Preference values are also population specific that scoring algorithms derived from America or Europe may not apply to the Chinese. The SF-6D is the only measure that has been translated for and validated in the Chinese population in Hong Kong (C. L. K. Lam, Brazier, & McGhee, 2008).

| | SF-6D | HUI | EQ-5D |
|---|---|---|---|
| HRQOL | Utility | Utility | Utility |
| Author | Brazier et al | Feeney et al | EuroQol Group |
| Year | 2002 | 1995 | 1990 |
| Country | UK | USA | |
| # of items | 10 | 31 | 5 |
| # of scales | 6 | 8 | 5 |
| Total score | Yes | Yes | Yes |
| Scales | Physical functioning | Vision | Mobility |
| | Role limitations | Hearing | Self-care |
| | Social functioning | Speech | Usual activity |
| | Pain | Ambulation | Pain/discomfort |
| | Mental Health | Dexterity | Anxiety/depression |
| | Vitality | Emotion | |
| | | Cognition | |
| | | Pain | |

Table 2. The Comparison of Content Domains among Different HRQOL Measures

Several studies have assessed health preference in chronic liver diseases, but the majority of them were on chronic hepatitis C (CHC) (Chong et al., 2003; McLernon, Dillon, & Donnan, 2008; Thein, Krahn, Kaldor, & Dore, 2005). Only two large studies evaluating health preference of CHB values were found in the literature (Levy et al., 2008; S C Ong et al., 2008). The first one was a multi-center study to elicit utilities for six hypothetical states from infected and uninfected individuals by Levy et al (Levy et al., 2008). The results found that health preference values declined with disease progressing from 0.68 in uncomplicated CHB to 0.35 in decompensated cirrhosis (DC) (Levy et al., 2008). Patients with DC and hepatocellular carcinoma (HCC) had very low preference values (Levy et al., 2008), indicating a strong impact of CHB. The results of Levy's study had limitations because it rated preference values on disease-specific health states (Levy et al., 2008), which is in contrary from NICE's recommendation that health preference should be measured by generic measures based on valuations by the general public (Guide to the methods of technology appraisal). The other study was conducted in Singapore by Ong et al, which found significantly lower health preference values measured by EQ-5D in patients with DC and HCC compared with asymptomatic hepatitis B (AHB) carriers (S C Ong et al., 2008). A small study on 140 patients with chronic liver diseases, with 36% having CHB found that patients with CHB had better health preference values than patients with other liver diseases (A. A. Dan et al., 2008).

More studies on health preference values associated with each stage of CHB from AHB, to CHB with ILF, cirrhosis and HCC, using locally validated preference-based measures, are needed to provide more accurate estimates of the change in preference value with disease progression. Such information is useful for the evaluation the cost-effectiveness of anti-viral treatments.

## 3. Conclusion

Hepatitis B is a significant health problem in Southern China and Hong Kong. Chronic hepatitis B (CHB) is a chronic disease that puts significant demand on health services. Regular monitoring is needed for progression of disease and development of complications. Anti-viral treatments may be needed for the eradication of the virus and other interventions are required when complications develop. Understanding the impact of illness on quality of life can make health care more responsive to patients' needs. Studies have shown significant lower health-related quality of life (HRQOL) scores in CHB patients especially in the presence of complications. Data on HRQOL in patients with CHB are limited. Generic and disease specific measures can complement each other in the evaluation of the impact of CHB on HRQOL. The Chronic Liver Disease Questionnaire (CLDQ) is a liver disease-specific HRQOL measure applicable to patients with chronic liver disease at different stages of illness. It has the best face validity for adaptation to be used in Chinese patients with CHB in Hong Kong. There are lots of potential applications of HRQOL data of CHB patients. It can inform policy and practice to make health service more patient-centered. HRQOL may also be used as an outcome measure of effectiveness of treatment and quality of care. HRQOL can be converted into a preference value for the calculation of quality adjusted life year (QALYs) in cost-effectiveness analysis of medical intervention.

## 4. References

Afendy, A., et al. (2009). Predictors of health-related quality of life in patients with chronic liver disease. *Aliment Pharmacol Ther, 30*(5), 469-476.

Ayoub, W. S., & Keeffe, E. B. (2008). Review article: current antiviral therapy of chronic hepatitis B. *Aliment Pharmacol Ther.*

Bayliss, M. S. (1999). Methods in outcomes research in hepatology: definitions and domains of quality of life. *Hepatology, 29 (Supp 1)*, 3S-6S.

Bayliss, M. S., et al. (1998). A questionnaire to assess the generic and disease-specific health outcomes of patients with chronic hepatitis C. *Qual Life Res, 7*(1), 39-55.

Bernstein, D., et al. (2002). Relationship of health-related quality of life to treatment adherence and sustained response in chronic hepatitis C patients. *Hepatology, 35*(3), 704-708.

Bianchi, G., et al. (2003). Reduced quality of life of patients with hepatocellular carcinoma. *Dig Liver Dis, 35*(1), 46-54.

Bondini, S., et al. (2007). Health-related quality of life in patients with chronic hepatitis B. *Liver Int, 27*, 1119-1125.

Brazier, J. E., et al. (2002). The estimation of a preference-based measure of health from the SF-36. *J Health Econ, 21*, 271-292.

Brooks, R. (1996). EuroQol: the current state of play. *Health Policy, 37*(1), 53-72.

Brown, R. S. (1999). Strategies and pitfalls in quality of life research. *Hepatology, 29 (Suppl 1)*, 9S-12S.

Bruix, J., et al. (2005). Management of hepatocellular carcinoma. *Hepatology, 42*(5), 1208-1236.

Casanovas, T., et al. (2003). Validation of the Spanish version of the Liver Disease Quality of Life questionnaire in transplant patients. *Transplant Proc, 35*(5), 1803-1805.

Cella, D. F., & Tulsky, D. S. (1990). Measuring quality of life today: methodological aspects. *Oncology (Williston Park), 4*(5), 29-38; discussion 69.

Chan, H. L., et al. (2007). Treatment of hepatitis B e antigen positive chronic hepatitis with telbivudine or adefovir: a randomized trial. *Ann Intern Med, 147*(11), 745-754.

Chan, P. S., et al. (2007). Incremental benefit and cost-effectiveness of high-dose statin therapy in high-risk patients with coronary artery disease. *Circulation, 115*(18), 2398-2409.

Chang, S. C., et al. (2008). Factors associated with quality of life in chronic hepatitis C patients who received interferon plus ribavirin therapy. *J Formos Med Assoc, 107*(6), 454-462.

Chang, T. T., et al. (2006). A comparison of entecavir and lamivudine for HBeAg-positive chronic hepatitis B. *N Engl J Med, 354*(10), 1001-1010.

Chen, C. J., et al. (2000). Epidemiology of hepatitis B virus infection in the Asia-Pacific region. *J Gastroenterol Hepatol, 15*(Suppl), E3-E6.

Chen, T., & Li, L. (2009). Influence of health-related quality of life on health service utilization in addition to socio-demographic and morbidity variables among primary care patients in China. *Int J Public Health, 54*(5), 325-332.

Chong, C. A., et al. (2003). Health-state utilities and quality of life in hepatitis C patients. *Am J Gastroenterol, 98*(3), 630-638.

Cooksley, W. G., et al. (2003). Peginterferon alpha-2a (40 kDa): an advance in the treatment of hepatitis B e antigen-positive chronic hepatitis B. *J Viral Hepat, 10*(4), 298-305.

Custer, B., et al. (2004). Global epidemiology of hepatitis B virus. *J Clin Gastroenterol, 38*(10 Suppl), S158-168.

Dan, A. A., et al. (2008). Impact of chronic liver disease and cirrhosis on health utilities using SF-6D and the health utility index. *Liver Transpl, 14*, 321-326.

Dan, Y., et al. (2008). The economics of treating chronic hepatitis B in Asia. *Hepatology International, 2*(3), 284-295.

Department of Health, H. K. S. A. R. Viral Hepatitis Preventive Service. 2010, from http://www.info.gov.hk/hepatitis/big5/index.htm

Department of Health HKSAR. (1998). *Viral hepatitis & liver cancer and unintentional injuries in children*. Hong Kong (China).

Dias Teixeira, M. C., et al. (2005). A new insight into the differences among non-cirrhotic and cirrhotic patients using the liver disease quality of life instrument (LDQOL). *Ann Hepatol, 4*(4), 264-271.

Dienstag, J. L., et al. (1999). Lamivudine as initial treatment for chronic hepatitis B in the United States. *N Engl J Med, 341*(17), 1256-1263.

Dominick, K. L., & Ahern, F. M. (2004). Health-related quality of life and health service use among older adults with osteoarthritis. *Arthritis Rheum, 51*(3), 326-331.

Eisen, G. M., et al. (1999). Health-related quality of life: a primer for gastroenterologists. *Am J Gastroenterol, 94*(8), 2017-2021.

Ethgen, O., & Kahler, K. (2002). The effect of health related quality of life on reported use of health care resources in patients with osteoarthritis and rheumatoid arthritis: a longitudinal analysis. *J Rheumatol, 29*(6), 1147-1155.

European Association For the study of the liver. (2008). EASL Clinical practice guidelines: management of chronic hepatitis B. *Journal of hepatology, 50*, 227-242.

Fattovich, G., et al. (2008). Natural history of chronic hepatitis B: special emphasis on disease progression and prognostic factors. *J Hepatol, 48*(2), 335-352.

Feeny, D., et al. (1995). Multi-attribute health status classification systems. Health Utilities Index. *Pharmacoeconomics, 7*(6), 490-502.

Ferrer, M., et al. (2006). Validity of the Spanish version of the Chronic Liver Disease Questionnaire (CLDQ) as a standard outcome for quality of life assessment. *Liver Transpl, 12*(1), 95-104.

Foster, G. R. (1999). Hepatitis C virus infection: quality of life and side effects of treatment. *J Hepatol, 31*(Suppl 1), 250-254.

Foster, G. R., et al. (1998). Chronic hepatitis C virus infection causes a significant reduction in quality of life in the absence of cirrhosis. *Hepatology, 27*, 209-212.

Fung, J., et al. (2007). Adefovir dipivoxil monotherapy and combination therapy with lamivudine for the treatment of chronic hepatitis B in an Asian population. *Antivir Ther, 12*(1), 41-46.

Fung, J., et al. (2008). New paradigms for the treatment of chronic hepatitis B. *J Gastroenterol Hepatol.*

Gralnek, I. M., et al. (2000). Development and evaluation of the Liver Disease Quality of Life instrument in persons with advanced, chronic liver disease--the LDQOL 1.0. *Am J Gastroenterol, 95*(12), 3552-3565.

Guide to the methods of technology appraisal. from http://www.nice.org.uk/niceMedia/pdf/TAP_Methods.pdf

Gust, I. D. (1996). Epidemiology of hepatitis B infection in the Western Pacific and South East Asia. *Gut, 38 Suppl 2*, S18-23.

Gutteling, J. J., et al. (2007). Overview of research on health-related quality of life in patients with chronic liver disease. *Neth J Med, 65*(7), 227-234.

Gutteling, J. J., et al. (2006). Determinants of quality of life in chronic liver patients. *Aliment Pharmacol Ther, 23*, 1629-1635.

Hadziyannis, S. J., et al. (2005). Long-term therapy with adefovir dipivoxil for HBeAg-negative chronic hepatitis B. *N Engl J Med, 352*(26), 2673-2681.

Hadziyannis, S. J., et al. (2006). Long-term therapy with adefovir dipivoxil for HBeAg-negative chronic hepatitis B for up to 5 years. *Gastroenterology, 131*(6), 1743-1751.

Hadziyannis, S. J., et al. (2003). Adefovir dipivoxil for the treatment of hepatitis B e antigen-negative chronic hepatitis B. *N Engl J Med, 348*(9), 800-807.

Hauser, W., et al. (2004). Determinants of health-related quality of life in patients with chronic liver diseases. *Clin Gastroenterol Hepatol, 2*(2), 157-163.

Hauser, W., et al. (2004). Validation of the German version of the Chronic Liver Disease Questionnaire. *Eur J Gastroenterol Hepatol, 16*(6), 599-606.

Hauser, W., et al. (2004). Biopsychosocial predictors of health-related quality of life in patients with chronic hepatitis C. *Psychosom Med, 66*(6), 954-958.

Heitkemper, M., et al. (2001). Chronic hepatitis C. Implications for health-related quality of life. *Gastroenterol Nurs, 24*(4), 169-175; quiz 176-167.

Hong Kong (China). Dept. of Health. (1998). *Viral Hepatitis & Liver Cancer and Unintentional Injuries in Children*. Hong Kong: Dept. of Health.

Hong Kong Cancer Registry. (2006). *Fast Stats for Liver Cancer 2006.* Retrieved from http://www3.ha.org.hk/cancereg/data/liver.pdf.

Hong Kong Cancer Registry, H. A. (2008). Hong Kong Cancer Stat 2006.

Hussain, K. B., et al. (2001). Comorbid illness is an important determinant of health-related quality of life in patients with chronic hepatitis C. *Am J Gastroenterol, 96*, 2737-2744.

Jacobson, I. M. (2006). Therapeutic options for chronic hepatitis B: considerations and controversies. *Am J Gastroenterol, 101 Suppl 1*, S13-18.

Kang, S. C., et al. (2005). Health-related quality of life and impact of antiviral treatment in Chinese patients with chronic hepatitis C in Taiwan. *World J Gastroenterol, 11*, 7494-7498.

Kanwal, F., et al. (2005). Treatment alternatives for chronic hepatitis B virus infection: a cost-effectiveness analysis. *Ann Intern Med, 142*(10), 821-831.

Kanwal, F., et al. (2008). Prospective validation of the short form liver disease quality of life instrument. *Aliment Pharmacol Ther, 28*(9), 1088-1101.

Keeffe, E. B., et al. (2008). A Treatment Algorithm for the Management of Chronic Hepatitis B Virus Infection in the United States: 2008 Update. *Clinical Gastroenterology and Hepatology*.

Koff, R. S. (1999). Impaired health-related quality of life in chronic hepatitis C: the how, but not the why. *Hepatology, 29*(1), 277-279.

Kondo, Y., et al. (2007). Health-related quality of life of chronic liver disease patients with and without hepatocellular carcinoma. *J Gastroenterol Hepatol, 22*, 197-203.

Kung, K., et al. (2004). Screening in chronic hepatitis B carriers - A retrospective study in a primary care clinic. *H.K. Pract, 26*, 221-227.

Kwan, J. W., et al. (2008). The impact of chronic hepatitis C and co-morbid illnesses on health-related quality of life. *Qual Life Res, 17*(5), 715-724.

Lai, C. L., et al. (1998). A one-year trial of lamivudine for chronic hepatitis B. Asia Hepatitis Lamivudine Study Group. *N Engl J Med, 339*(2), 61-68.

Lai, C. L., et al. (2005). A 1-year trial of telbivudine, lamivudine, and the combination in patients with hepatitis B e antigen-positive chronic hepatitis B. *Gastroenterology, 129*(2), 528-536.

Lai, C. L., et al. (2003). Viral hepatitis B. *Lancet, 362*, 2089-2094.

Lai, C. L., et al. (2002). Entecavir is superior to lamivudine in reducing hepatitis B virus DNA in patients with chronic hepatitis B infection. *Gastroenterology, 123*(6), 1831-1838.

Lai, C. L., et al. (2006). Entecavir versus lamivudine for patients with HBeAg-negative chronic hepatitis B. *N Engl J Med, 354*(10), 1011-1020.

Lai, C. L., & Yuen, M. F. (2008). Chronic hepatitis B--new goals, new treatment. *N Engl J Med, 359*(23), 2488-2491.

Lam, C. L., et al. (1999). Population based norming of the Chinese (HK) version of the SF-36 Health Survey. *HK Pract, 21*, 460-470.

Lam, C. L. K., et al. (2008). Valuation of the SF-6D health states is feasible, acceptable, reliable, and valid in a Chinese population. *Value Health, 11*, 295-303.

Lam, C. L. K., & Fong, D. Y. T. (2002). The effect of health-related quality of life (HRQOL) on health service utilisation of a Chinese population. *Soc Sci Med, 55*(9), 1635-1646.

Lam, E. T., et al. (2008). Psychometrics and population norm of the Chinese (HK) SF-36 Health Survey version 2. *HK Pract, 30*, 185-198.

Lampertico, P., et al. (2005). Adefovir rapidly suppresses hepatitis B in HBeAg-negative patients developing genotypic resistance to lamivudine. *Hepatology, 42*(6), 1414-1419.

Lampertico, P., et al. (2007). Low resistance to adefovir combined with lamivudine: a 3-year study of 145 lamivudine-resistant hepatitis B patients. *Gastroenterology, 133*(5), 1445-1451.

Lavanchy, D. (2004). Hepatitis B virus epidemiology, disease burden, treatment, and current and emerging prevention and control measures. *J Viral Hepat, 11*(2), 97-107.

Lavanchy, D. (2005). Worldwide epidemiology of HBV infection, disease burden, and vaccine prevention. *J Clin Virol, 34 Suppl 1*, S1-3.

Lee, E. H., et al. (2007). Development and psychometric evaluation of a chronic liver disease-specific quality of life questionnaire. *J Gastroenterol Hepatol, 23*, 231-238.

Leung, N. (2008). Recent data on treatment of chronic hepatitis B with nucleos(t)ide analogues. *Hepatol Int, 2*(2), 163-178.

Levy, A. R., et al. (2008). The impact of chronic hepatitis B on quality of life: a multinational study of utilities from infected and uninfected persons. *Value Health, 11*, 527-538.

Liaw, Y. F., et al. (2009). 2-Year GLOBE trial results: telbivudine Is superior to lamivudine in patients with chronic hepatitis B. *Gastroenterology, 136*(2), 486-495.

Liaw, Y. F., et al. (2008). Asian-Pacific consensus statement on the management of chronic hepatitis B: a 2008 update. *Hepatology International, 2*(3), 263-283.

Liaw, Y. F., et al. (2004). Lamivudine for patients with chronic hepatitis B and advanced liver disease. *N Engl J Med, 351*(15), 1521-1531.

Lok, A. S., & McMahon, B. J. (2009). Chronic hepatitis B: update 2009. *Hepatology, 50*(3), 661-662.

Lok, A. S., et al. (1992). A controlled trial of interferon with or without prednisone priming for chronic hepatitis B. *Gastroenterology, 102*(6), 2091-2097.

Maddrey, W. C. (2000). Hepatitis B: an important public health issue. *J Med Virol, 61*(3), 362-366.

Manolakopoulos, S., et al. (2008). Long-term therapy with adefovir dipivoxil in hepatitis B e antigen-negative patients developing resistance to lamivudine. *Aliment Pharmacol Ther, 27*(3), 266-273.

Marcellin, P., et al. (2005). Treatment of chronic hepatitis B. *Rev Prat, 55*(6), 624-632.

Marcellin, P., et al. (2003). Adefovir dipivoxil for the treatment of hepatitis B e antigen-positive chronic hepatitis B. *N Engl J Med, 348*(9), 808-816.

Marcellin, P., et al. (2008). Tenofovir disoproxil fumarate versus adefovir dipivoxil for chronic hepatitis B. *N Engl J Med, 359*(23), 2442-2455.

Marchesini, G., et al. (2001). Italian Study Group for Quality of Life in Cirrhosis: Factors associated with poor health-related quality of life of patients with cirrhosis. *Gastroenterology, 120*, 170-178.

Martin, L. M., et al. (2006). Measurement of health-related quality of life in patients with chronic liver disease. *Liver Transpl, 12*(1), 22-23.

Martin, L. M., et al. (2002). The impact of liver disease on health-related quality of life: a review of the literature. *Curr Gastroenterol Rep, 4*(1), 79-83.

Martin, L. M., & Younossi, Z. M. (2005). Health-related quality of life (HRQL) in chronic liver disease. *Dig Liver Dis, 37*(11), 819-820.

Martin, R. C., et al. (2007). Health-related quality of life: return to baseline after major and minor liver resection. *Surgery, 142*, 676-684.

Matsumura, S. (2000). Perceived health status as a predictor of utilization of health-care resources and the number of sick-leave days in Japan. *Quality of Life Research, 9*(9), 1063.

Maynard, J. E. (1990). Hepatitis B: global importance and need for control. *Vaccine, 8 Suppl*, S18-20; discussion S21-13.

McColl, E., et al. (1997). Making the right choice of outcome measure *Cross Cultural Health Outcome Assessment: A User's Guide* (pp. 12-26): ERGHO, European Research Group on Health Outcomes.

McHutchison, J. G., et al. (2001). The effects of interferon alpha-2b in combination with ribavirin on health related quality of life and work productivity. *J Hepatol, 34*(1), 140-147.

McLernon, D. J., et al. (2008). Health-state utilities in liver disease: a systematic review. *Med Decis Making, 28*(4), 582-592.

McMahon, B. J. (2006). Selecting appropriate management strategies for chronic hepatitis B: who to treat. *Am J Gastroenterol, 101 Suppl 1*, S7-12.

McMahon, B. J. (2008). Natural history of chronic hepatitis B - clinical implications. *Medscape J Med, 10*(4), 91.

Merican, I., et al. (2000). Chronic hepatitis B virus infection in Asian countries. *J Gastroenterol Hepatol, 15*(12), 1356-1361.

Miller, E. R., et al. (2001). Quality of life in HCV-infection: lack of association with ALT levels. *Aust N Z J Public Health, 25*(4), 355-361.

Mucci, S., et al. (2010). [Cross-cultural adaptation of the Chronic Liver Disease Questionnaire (CLDQ) to the Brazilian population]. *Cad Saude Publica, 26*(1), 199-205.

Nelson, E. C., & McHorney, C. A. (1998). A longitudinal study of hospitalization rates for patients with chronic disease: results from the Medical Outcomes Study. *Health Serv Res, 32*(6), 759-774.

Neumann, P. J., et al. (2005). Growth and quality of the cost-utility literature, 1976-2001. *Value Health, 8*, 3-9.

Nguyen, M. H., & Keeffe, E. B. (2009). Chronic hepatitis B: early viral suppression and long-term outcomes of therapy with oral nucleos(t)ides. *J Viral Hepat, 16*(3), 149-155.

Nokhodian, Z., et al. (2009). Assessment of quality of life in hepatitis B patients in Iran. *Indian J Gastroenterol, 28*(3), 116-117.

Omata, M., et al. (2010). Asian Pacific Association for the Study of the Liver consensus recommendations on hepatocellular carcinoma. *Hepatol Int, 4*(2), 439-474.

Ong, S. C., et al. (2009). Cultural adaptation and validation of a questionnaire for use in hepatitis B patients. *J Viral Hepat, 16*(4), 272-278.

Ong, S. C., et al. (2010). Reliability and validity of a Chinese version's health-related quality of life questionnaire for hepatitis B patients. *Value Health, 13*(2), 324-327.

Ong, S. C., et al. (2008). Health-related quality of life in chronic hepatitis B patients. *Hepatology, 47*, 1108-1117.

Parkerson, G. R., Jr., & Gutman, R. A. (2000). Health-related quality of life predictors of survival and hospital utilization. *Health Care Financ Rev, 21*(3), 171-184.

Perrillo, R., et al. (2004). Comparison of quality of life, work productivity and medical resource utilization of peginterferon alpha 2a vs the combination of interferon alpha 2b plus ribavirin as initial treatment in patients with chronic hepatitis C. *J Viral Hepat, 11*(2), 157-165.

Perz, J. F., et al. (2006). The contributions of hepatitis B virus and hepatitis C virus infections to cirrhosis and primary liver cancer worldwide. *J Hepatol, 45*(4), 529-538.

Peters, M. G., et al. (2004). Adefovir dipivoxil alone or in combination with lamivudine in patients with lamivudine-resistant chronic hepatitis B. *Gastroenterology, 126*(1), 91-101.

Poon, R. T., et al. (2001). A prospective longitudinal study of quality of life after resection of hepatocellular carcinoma. *Arch Surg, 136*, 693-699.

Preedy, V. R., et al. (2010). Subjective Quality of Life Measures - General Principles and Concepts *Handbook of Disease Burdens and Quality of Life Measures* (pp. 381-399): Springer New York.

Rapti, I., et al. (2007). Adding-on versus switching-to adefovir therapy in lamivudine-resistant HBeAg-negative chronic hepatitis B. *Hepatology, 45*(2), 307-313.

Ray, I., et al. (2010). Quality of life assessment of patients with chronic liver disease in eastern India using a Bengali translation chronic liver disease questionnaire. *Indian J Gastroenterol.*

Rucci, P., et al. (2005). Validity and reliability of the Italian version of the Chronic Liver Disease Questionnaire (CLDQ-I) for the assessment of health-related quality of life. *Dig Liver Dis, 37*(11), 850-860.

Russell, L. B., et al. (1996). The role of cost-effectiveness analysis in health and medicine. Panel on Cost-Effectiveness in Health and Medicine. *Jama, 276*(14), 1172-1177.

Schipper, H., et al. (1996). Quality of life and pharmacoeconomics in clinical trials *Quality of life studies. Definition and conceptual issues.* (2nd ed., pp. 11-24). Philadelphia: Lippincott-Raven.

Singh, J. A., & Nelson, D. B. (2005). Health-related quality of life predicts future health care utilization and mortality in veterans with self-reported physician-diagnosed arthritis: the veterans arthritis quality of life study. *Semin Arthritis Rheum, 34*(5), 755-765.

Sobhonslidsuk, A., et al. (2004). Chronic liver disease questionnaire: translation and validation in Thais. *World J Gastroenterol, 10*(13), 1954-1957.

Sobhonslidsuk, A., et al. (2006). Factors influencing health-related quality of life in chronic liver disease. *World J Gastroenterol, 12*, 7786-7791.

Spiegel, B. M., et al. (2007). Development and validation of a disease-targeted quality of life instrument in chronic hepatitis B: the hepatitis B quality of life instrument, version 1.0. *Hepatology, 46*(1), 113-121.

Spiegel, B. M., et al. (2005). Impact of hepatitis C on health related quality of life: a systematic review and quantitative assessment. *Hepatology, 41*(4), 790-800.

Strauss, E., & Dias Teixeira, M. C. (2006). Quality of life in hepatitis C. *Liver Int, 26*(7), 755-765.

Sullivan, S. D., et al. (2007). Cost-effectiveness of peginterferon alpha-2a compared to lamivudine treatment in patients with hepatitis B e antigen positive chronic hepatitis B in Taiwan. *J Gastroenterol Hepatol, 22*(9), 1494-1499.

Sumskiene, J., et al. (2006). Disease-specific health-related quality of life and its determinants in liver cirrhosis patients in Lithuania. *World J Gastroenterol, 12*(48), 7792-7797.

Sun, X., et al. (2007). Comparative cost-effectiveness of antiviral therapies in patients with chronic hepatitis B: a systematic review of economic evidence. *J Gastroenterol Hepatol, 22*(9), 1369-1377.

Takeda, A., et al. (2007). A systematic review and economic evaluation of adefovir dipivoxil and pegylated interferon-alpha-2a for the treatment of chronic hepatitis B. *J Viral Hepat, 14*(2), 75-88.

Tan, N. C., et al. (2008). Patients with chronic hepatitis B infection: what is their quality of life? *Singapore Med J, 49*(9), 682-687.

Thein, H. H., et al. (2005). Estimation of utilities for chronic hepatitis C from SF-36 scores. *Am J Gastroenterol, 100*(3), 643-651.

Unal, G., et al. (2001). A psychometric comparison of health-related quality of life measures in chronic liver disease. *J Clin Epidemiol, 54*, 587-596.

van der Plas, S. M., et al. (2004). The Liver Disease Symptom Index 2.0; validation of a disease-specific questionnaire. *Qual Life Res, 13*, 1469-1481.

van der Poorten, D., et al. (2007). Combination adefovir-lamivudine prevents emergence of adefovir resistance in lamivudine-resistant hepatitis B. *J Gastroenterol Hepatol, 22*(9), 1500-1505.

Veenstra, D. L., et al. (2008). Evaluating anti-viral drug selection and treatment duration in HBeAg-negative chronic hepatitis B: a cost-effectiveness analysis. *Aliment Pharmacol Ther.*

Ware, J. E. J., et al. (1999). Health-related quality of life in chronic hepatitis C: impact of disease and treatment response. The Interventional Therapy Group. *Hepatology, 30,* 550-555.

Weinstein, M. C. (1990). Principles of cost-effective resource allocation in health care organizations. *International Journal of Technology Assessment in Health Care, 6,* 93-103.

Weinstein, M. C., et al. (1996). Recommendations of the Panel on Cost-effectiveness in Health and Medicine. *Jama, 276*(15), 1253-1258.

Weinstein, M. C., et al. (2009). QALYs: the basic. *Value Health, 12 (Suppl 1),* S5-S9.

WHO. (1947). Constitution of the World Health Organization. Geneva: WHO.

Wilson, J. M. G., & Jungner, G. (1968). *Principles and Practice of Screening for Disease.* Geneva: WHO.

Wong, I. O., et al. (2007). Cost effectiveness of mammography screening for Chinese women. *Cancer, 110*(4), 885-895.

Wright, T. L. (2006). Introduction to chronic hepatitis B infection. *Am J Gastroenterol, 101 Suppl 1,* S1-6.

Wu, C. H., et al. (2003). Preliminary Use of the CLDQ in Chronic Hepatitis B Patients. *Chin J Clin Psychol, 11*(1), 60-62.

Yacavone, R. F., et al. (2001). Quality of life measurement in gastroenterology: what is available? *Am J Gastroenterol, 96*(2), 285-297.

Yeo B. (2008). Monthly Index of Medical Specialties (MIMS). from http://www.mims.com/

Yi, L. X. (2006). Effect of lamivudine treatment on the quality of life of chronic hepatitis B. *J Cent South Univ (Med Sci), 31,* 396-399.

Ying, A. C. H. (2009). Guidelines on Cancer Prevention, Early Detection & Screening - Liver Cancer. from http://www.hkacs.org.hk/content/anti_cancer_society.php?page=234

Younossi, Z. M. (2001). Chronic liver disease and health-related quality of life. *Gastroenterology, 120*(1), 305-307.

Younossi, Z. M., et al. (2001). Health-related quality of life in chronic liver disease: the impact of type and severity of disease. *J Gastroenterol, 96,* 2199-2205.

Younossi, Z. M., & Guyatt, G. (1998). Quality-of-life assessments and chronic liver disease. *Am J Gastroenterol, 93*(7), 1037-1041.

Younossi, Z. M., et al. (1999). Development of a disease specific questionnaire to measure health related quality of life in patients with chronic liver disease. *Gut, 45*(2), 295-300.

Younossi, Z. M., et al. (2000). Cholestatic liver diseases and health-related quality of life. *Am J Gastroenterol, 95,* 497-502.

Yuan, Y., et al. (2008). Economic implications of entecavir treatment in suppressing viral replication in chronic hepatitis B (CHB) patients in China from a perspective of the Chinese Social Security program. *Value Health, 11 Suppl 1,* S11-22.

Yuen, M. F. (2007). Revisiting the natural history of chronic hepatitis B: impact of new concepts on clinical management. *J Gastroenterol Hepatol, 22*(7), 973-976.

Yuen, M. F., & Lai, C. L. (2001). Treatment of chronic hepatitis B. *Lancet Infect Dis, 1*(4), 232-241.

Yuen, M. F., & Lai, C. L. (2003). Screening for hepatocellular carcinoma: survival benefit and cost-effectiveness. *Ann Oncol, 14*(10), 1463-1467.

Yuen, M. F., et al. (2007). Long-term lamivudine therapy reduces the risk of long-term complications of chronic hepatitis B infection even in patients without advanced disease. *Antivir Ther, 12*(8), 1295-1303.

Yuen, M. F., et al. (2005). Prognostic determinants for chronic hepatitis B in Asians: therapeutic implications. *Gut, 54,* 1610-1614.

Zoulim, F., & Perrillo, R. (2008). Hepatitis B: reflections on the current approach to antiviral therapy. *J Hepatol, 48 Suppl 1,* S2-19.